Clinical and Epidemiological Aspects of Antimicrobial Resistance

Clinical and Epidemiological Aspects of Antimicrobial Resistance

Editor: Steven Blair

AMERICAN
MEDICAL PUBLISHERS
www.americanmedicalpublishers.com

AMERICAN
MEDICAL PUBLISHERS
www.americanmedicalpublishers.com

Cataloging-in-Publication Data

Clinical and epidemiological aspects of antimicrobial resistance / edited by Steven Blair.
p. cm.
Includes bibliographical references and index.
ISBN 978-1-63927-883-1
1. Drug resistance in microorganisms. 2. Anti-infective agents. 3. Epidemiology.
4. Emerging infectious diseases--Epidemiology. 5. Communicable diseases--Epidemiology.
6. Emerging infectious diseases--Treatment. 7. Communicable diseases--Treatment. 8. Cli I. Blair, Steven.
QR177 .C55 2023
616.904 1--dc23

American Medical Publishers,
41 Flatbush Avenue,
1st Floor, New York,
NY 11217, USA

ISBN 978-1-63927-883-1 (Hardback)

Contents

Preface

Antimicrobial resistance (AMR) occurs when microbes develop mechanisms to protect themselves from the effects of antimicrobials. It appears in bacteria as a result of protein upregulation, which enables a subpopulation of resistant bacteria to multiply through the process of natural selection. A few of the major causes of AMR are lack of sanitation, accessibility to clean water and hygiene, and a lack of access to quality and reasonably priced vaccines, medications and diagnostics. A few other factors which can result in AMR are lack of legislative enforcement, overuse and misuse of antimicrobials, inadequate disease and infection prevention in health-care facilities, as well as a lack of knowledge and awareness. Treatment of bacterial infections has become more challenging due to rising AMR and multiple resistances. It can be prevented by limiting the duration of antibiotic treatment and usage of antibiotics. This book elucidates the concepts and innovative models around prospective developments with respect to antimicrobial resistance. It contains a detailed explanation of the various clinical and epidemiological aspects of antimicrobial resistance. This book is appropriate for students seeking detailed information in this area of study as well as for experts.

This book unites the global concepts and researches in an organized manner for a comprehensive understanding of the subject. It is a ripe text for all researchers, students, scientists or anyone else who is interested in acquiring a better knowledge of this dynamic field.

I extend my sincere thanks to the contributors for such eloquent research chapters. Finally, I thank my family for being a source of support and help.

Editor

1

Prevalence of Extended-Spectrum Cephalosporin-Resistant *Escherichia coli* in a Farrowing Farm: ST1121 Clone Harboring IncHI2 Plasmid Contributes to the Dissemination of *bla*CMY-2

Hui Deng[1,2†], Hong-Bin Si[3†], Shu-Yi Zeng[1,2], Jian Sun[1,2], Liang-Xing Fang[1,2], Run-Shi Yang[1,2], Ya-Hong Liu[1,2,4] and Xiao-Ping Liao[1,2]*

[1] National Risk Assessment Laboratory for Antimicrobial Resistance of Animal Original Bacteria, South China Agricultural University, Guangzhou, China, [2] College of Veterinary Medicine, South China Agricultural University, Guangzhou, China, [3] College of Animal Science and Technology, Guangxi University, Nanning, China, [4] Jiangsu Co-Innovation Centre for Prevention and Control of Important Animal Infectious Diseases and Zoonoses, Yangzhou, China

***Correspondence:**
Xiao-Ping Liao
xpliao@scau.edu.cn

† These authors have contributed equally to this work.

During a regular monitoring of antimicrobial resistance in a farrowing farm in Southern China, 117 *Escherichia coli* isolates were obtained from sows and piglets. Compared with the isolates from piglets, the isolates from sows exhibited higher resistance rates to the tested cephalosporins. Correspondingly, the total detection rate of the $bla_{\text{CMY-2}}/bla_{\text{CTX-M}}$ genes in the sow isolates (34.2%) was also significantly higher than that of the piglet isolates (13.6%; $p < 0.05$). The $bla_{\text{CMY-2}}$ gene had a relatively high prevalence (11.1%) in the *E. coli* isolates. MLST and PFGE analysis revealed the clonal spread of ST1121 *E. coli* in most (7/13) of the $bla_{\text{CMY-2}}$-positive isolates. An indistinguishable IncHI2 plasmid harboring $bla_{\text{CMY-2}}$ was also identified in each of the seven ST1121 *E. coli* isolates. Complete sequence analysis of this IncHI2 plasmid (pEC5207) revealed that pEC5207 may have originated through recombination of an IncHI2 plasmid with a $bla_{\text{CMY-2}}$-carrying IncA/C plasmid like pCFSAN007427_01. In addition to $bla_{\text{CMY-2}}$, pEC5207 also carried other resistance determinants for aminoglycosides (*aacA7*), sulfonamides (*sul1*), as well as heavy metals ions, such as Cu and Ag. The susceptibility testing showed that the pEC5207 can mediate both antibiotic and heavy metal resistance. This highlights the role of pEC5207 in co-selection of $bla_{\text{CMY-2}}$-positive isolates under the selective pressure of heavy metals, cephalosporins, and other antimicrobials. In conclusion, clonal spread of an ST1121 type *E. coli* strain harboring an IncHI2 plasmid contributed to the dissemination of $bla_{\text{CMY-2}}$ in a farrowing farm in Southern China. We also have determined the first complete sequence analysis of a $bla_{\text{CMY-2}}$-carrying IncHI2 plasmid.

Keywords: *Escherichia coli*, clonal spread, $bla_{\text{CMY-2}}$, IncHI2 plasmid, farrowing farm

INTRODUCTION

Antimicrobial agents are often used as feed and water additives in food animals to treat or prevent disease and to promote general overall health (McEwen and Fedorka-Cray, 2002; Cabello et al., 2013). However, antimicrobial resistance driven by the intensive use of antimicrobial agents in animal husbandry is increasing worldwide (Witte, 1998). In the swine industry, antimicrobial resistance patterns can be traced to particular farms associated with certain management practices (Rasschaert et al., 2012; Brooks et al., 2014). In farrowing farms, antimicrobial resistance in piglets has been shown to be a reflection of antimicrobial use in sows (Mathew et al., 2005; Callens et al., 2015), because sows are an important reservoir of antimicrobial resistant bacteria for their offspring (Callens et al., 2012; Crombe et al., 2013). Additionally, piglet transfer from farrowing to finishing farms increases the likelihood of the transmission of resistant bacteria, thus increasing the risk of antimicrobial resistance transfer between swine farms (Sandvang et al., 2000; van Duijkeren et al., 2008). Therefore, surveillance for antimicrobial resistance in the farrowing farm is important for controlling the dissemination of antimicrobial resistance.

Escherichia coli is an important cause of intestinal and extraintestinal diseases in animals and humans worldwide, and β-lactams are widely used in veterinary medicine to treat colibacillosis. However, the use of extended-spectrum cephalosporins (ESCs) in animals has contributed to β-lactam resistance in *E. coli* (Greko et al., 2009). Resistance to ESCs in *E. coli* has been associated with the extended-spectrum β-lactamases (ESBLs) and plasmid-mediated Ambler class C cephamycinases (pAmpC β-lactamases; Seiffert et al., 2013). ESBLs are the major contributors to ESC resistance in *E. coli* and confer resistance to cephalosporins with an oxyimino side chain (cefotaxime, ceftriaxone, and ceftazidime; Bradford, 2001).

Unlike ESBLs, pAmpC β-lactamases exhibit activity against cephamycins, such as cefoxitin and cannot be inactivated by β-lactamase inhibitor clavulanate (Bradford, 2001; Jacoby, 2009). Among them, CMY-2, the most common pAmpC β-lactamase, has been documented worldwide in bacteria of human and animal origin (Li et al., 2007; Jacoby, 2009). The bla_{CMY-2} gene which likely originated from the chromosomal AmpC locus of *Citrobacter freundii* has been horizontally transmitted through plasmids in *E. coli* from different sources (Martin et al., 2012). Various plasmid types are associated with bla_{CMY-2}, including IncA/C, IncF, IncI1, IncL/M, IncP, IncK, and IncHI2. Of these, IncA/C and IncI1 plasmid are the most common carriers of bla_{CMY-2} (Verdet et al., 2009; Folster et al., 2011; Martin et al., 2012; Bortolaia et al., 2014; Guo et al., 2014).

The bla_{CMY-2} gene is prevalent in ESC-resistant *E. coli* of livestock (Li et al., 2007; Seiffert et al., 2013). In swine, the detection rate of bla_{CMY-2} in *E. coli* is quite different, ranging from 0 to up to 80% (Seiffert et al., 2013). Although the detection methods of CMY-2 vary between reports, this may still reflect the different prevalence of bla_{CMY-2} worldwide. In mainland China, the bla_{CMY-2} gene was detected for the first time in *E. coli* of swine origin in Tian et al. (2012), Zheng et al. (2012), and subsequently occured in swine *E. coli* isolates carrying plasmid-mediated quinolone resistance (PMQR) genes (Liu et al., 2013a). Recently, a surveillance study identified bla_{CMY-2} mainly in *E. coli* of pig origin, highlighting the role of CMY-2 in the ESC resistance of swine *E. coli* (Guo et al., 2014). In the present study, we make an investigation on the prevalence of drug resistance and ESBL/pAmpC genes in *E. coli* isolates from a swine farm in Southern China. The bla_{CMY-2}-positive isolates were further analyzed to characterize the transmission mechanisms of the bla_{CMY-2} gene.

MATERIALS AND METHODS

Bacterial Isolates and Antimicrobial Susceptibility Testing

In August 2011, a regular monitoring of antimicrobial resistance was conducted in a farrowing farm in Southern China. This farm had been in operation about 8 years and consisted of 2,300 sows with production of about 40,000 piglets for market annually. Rectal swab samples were randomly taken from one pig in every batch pen. The rectal swabs were taken by inserting the sterile swab about 2 cm into the rectum, rotated gently and then immersed in sterile PBS. After collection, the swabs were immediately brought to the laboratory in cool conditions. A total of 137 swab samples were collected from sows (1–5 years-old) and piglets (1–60 days-old). The collected samples were plated on MacConkey agar and then incubated at 37°C for 24 h. One suspected colony with typical *E. coli* morphology was selected from each sample and was identified with API 20E system (BioMerieux, France). Minimal inhibitory concentrations (MICs) of ampicillin (AMP), ceftazidime (CAZ), cefoxitin (FOX), cefotaxime (CTX), ceftiofur (CEF), amikacin (AMK), kanamycin (KAN), florfenicol (FFC), doxycycline (DOX), enrofloxacin (ENR), and trimethoprim-sulfamethoxazole (SXT) were determined by the agar dilution method in accordance with the standard provided by the Clinical and Laboratory Standards Institute (2013a,b). *E. coli* ATCC 25922 was used as the quality control strain.

Detection of ESBL/pAmpC Genes

Extended-spectrum β-lactamase genes (bla_{TEM}, bla_{SHV}, $bla_{CTX-M-1G}$, $bla_{CTX-M-9G}$, $bla_{CTX-M-2G}$, and $bla_{CTX-M-25G}$) among the *E. coli* isolates were analyzed by PCR amplification using previously published primers and protocols (Liu et al., 2013a). Purified PCR products were sequenced and compared using the β-lactamase classification system[1] to confirm the subtypes. Detection of pAmpC genes was performed by a multiplex PCR as previously described (Perez-Perez and Hanson, 2002). For amplification of the entire bla_{CMY-2} gene, PCR-positive isolates were re-amplified and sequenced with specific primers (Perez-Perez and Hanson, 2002).

Molecular Typing

All bla_{CMY-2}-positive isolates were classified according to *XbaI*-pulsed-field gel electrophoresis (PFGE) type (Tenover et al.,

[1] http://www.lahey.org/studies/webt.asp

1995). Comparison of PFGE patterns was performed by BioNumerics®v6.6 (Applied Maths, Ghent, Belgium) with a cut-off at 90% of the similarity values to indicate identical PFGE types. Multilocus sequence typing (MLST) was performed by using the primers and protocol specified at the *E. coli* MLST web site[2].

Transferability of bla_{CMY-2}

Conjugation experiments were performed as previously described (Chen et al., 2007a), using *E. coli* C600 (streptomycin-resistant; MIC >2000 μg/ml) as a recipient. Putative transconjugants were selected on MacConkey agar plates with streptomycin (2000 μg/ml) and cefoxitin (32 μg/ml), examined for the presence of bla_{CMY-2} by PCR assay, and finally confirmed by ERIC-PCR (Versalovic et al., 1991). All transconjugants were tested for antimicrobial susceptibility as described above.

The susceptibility of transconjugant EC5207-35T to heavy metals (Cu, Ag) was tested by microdilution in an aerobic atmosphere, as previously described, with some modifications (Mourao et al., 2015). Briefly, the transconjugant was incubated in Mueller–Hinton broth with serial dilutions of $CuSO_4$ (0.25, 0.5, 1, 2, 4, 8, 12, 16, 20, 24, 32, and 36 mM, adjusted to pH 7.2) and $AgNO_3$ (0.0125, 0.025, 0.06, 0.08, 0.125, 0.16, 0.25, 0.32, 0.5, 1.0, 1.5, and 3 mM, adjusted to pH 7.4). *E. coli* C600 was used as the reference strain.

Plasmid Analysis

Plasmids of the transconjugants were typed with PCR-based replicon typing (PBRT; Carattoli et al., 2005). The size of bla_{CMY-2}-carrying plasmid in the transconjugants was determined using S1 nuclease-digested (TaKaRa Biotechnology, Dalian, China) genomic DNA followed by PFGE and Southern blot hybridization with a bla_{CMY-2}-specific probe (Barton et al., 1995). Plasmid DNA from the transconjugants was extracted using the QIAGEN Plasmid Midi Kit, and was further analyzed by restriction fragment length polymorphism (RFLP) using *XbaI* (TaKaRa Biotechnology, Dalian, China).

Complete Sequence of bla_{CMY-2}-carrying IncHI2 Plasmid pEC5207

In order to further characterize the bla_{CMY-2}-carrying IncHI2 plasmids of the ST1121 clone in this study, the plasmid pEC5207 from transconjugant EC5207-35T was sequenced using SMRT sequencing approach and assembled by HGAP2.2.0 method (Chin et al., 2013). Open reading frames (ORFs) prediction and annotation were performed with the RAST tools (Aziz et al., 2008). Sequence comparison and map generation were performed using BLAST[3] and Easyfig version 2.1 (Sullivan et al., 2011).

[2]http://mlst.ucc.ie/mlst/dbs/Ecoli
[3]http://blast.ncbi.nlm.nih.gov

Statistical Methods

Statistical significance for the comparison of prevalence data was determined by the χ^2 test. Differences were considered statistically significant at $p < 0.05$.

Nucleotide Sequence Accession Number

The complete DNA sequence of plasmid pEC5207 was assigned GenBank accession number KT347600.

RESULTS

Antimicrobial Susceptibility

Rectal swab samples were randomly taken from one pig in every batch pen and 117 *E. coli* samples were isolated from 137 sow and piglet rectal swabs. The incidence for each group was approximately 85% (**Table 1**). Antimicrobial susceptibility tests showed that part of the isolates were resistant to CEF (30.8%), CTX (27.4%), FOX (14.5%), and CAZ (11.1%). Except for CAZ, cephalosporin resistance rates for sow isolates were significantly higher than those for isolates from piglets ($p < 0.05$). However, the resistance rate to CAZ for isolates from sows was still three times of that for piglet isolates (**Table 2**). In addition to cephalosporins, different levels of resistance to other classes of antimicrobials, including SXT (100%), DOX (98.3%), FFC (96.6%), AMP (94.0%), KAN (83.8%), ENR (64.1%) and AMK (29.9%), were also observed in the tested isolates (**Table 2**). The vast majority of the isolates (95.7%) exhibited a multidrug resistance (MDR) phenotype, and were resistant to four or more tested antimicrobial agents.

Detection of ESBL/pAmpC Genes

Among the 117 *E. coli* isolates, CTX-M-type ESBL genes were detected in 18 isolates (15.4%). The most common bla_{CTX-M}-type were $bla_{CTX-M-122}$ ($n = 8$), followed by $bla_{CTX-M-65}$ ($n = 5$), $bla_{CTX-M-55}$ ($n = 3$) and $bla_{CTX-M-64}$ ($n = 2$). TEM- and SHV-type ESBL genes were not detected in any of the isolates. Compared with the diverse bla_{CTX-M} genes detected in this study, bla_{CMY-2} was the only identified pAmpC gene, and was found in 13 isolates (11.1%). All the bla_{CMY-2}-positive isolates were resistant to FOX with MICs ranging from 64 to 256 μg/ml, and also exhibited multi-resistance to AMP, CTX, CEF, KAN, FFC, DOX, ENR, and SXT (**Figure 1**).

The co-existence of ESBL and pAmpC genes was not observed in any of the isolates. The total detection rate of

TABLE 1 | Information on the samples and *Escherichia coli* isolates in this study.

Sample source	No. of samples	No. (%) of *E. coli* isolates
Sow	84	73 (86.9)
Piglet	53	44 (83.0)
Total	137	117 (85.4)

TABLE 2 | Susceptibility of 117 *E. coli* isolates to 11 antimicrobial agents.

Antimicrobial agent[a]	MIC range (μg/ml)	MIC_{50} (μg/ml)	MIC_{90} (μg/ml)	Resistant (%)		
				Sow ($n = 73$)	Piglet ($n = 44$)	Total ($n = 117$)
CAZ	0.06–64	0.25	16	15.1	4.5	11.1
FOX	2–256	4	64	20.5	4.5*	14.5
CEF	<0.125–>256	1	128	38.4	18.2*	30.8
CTX	0.03–>256	0.125	32	35.6	13.6*	27.4
AMP	4–>512	>512	>512	94.5	93.2	94.0
AMK	1–>256	2	>256	17.8	50.0*	29.9
KAN	1–>512	>512	>512	78.1	93.2	83.8
FFC	4–512	256	512	95.9	97.7	96.6
DOX	4–256	64	128	97.3	100	98.3
ENR	0.016–128	4	32	60.3	70.5	64.1
SXT	2/38–>16/304	>16/304	>16/304	100	100	100

[a]*CAZ, ceftazidime; FOX, cefoxitin; CEF, ceftiofur; CTX, cefotaxime; AMP, ampicillin; AMK, amikacin; KAN, kanamycin; FFC, florfenicol; DOX, doxycycline; ENR, enrofloxacin; SXT, trimethoprim-sulfamethoxazole.*

$^*p < 0.05$ for resistance rate of isolates from piglets vs. sows.

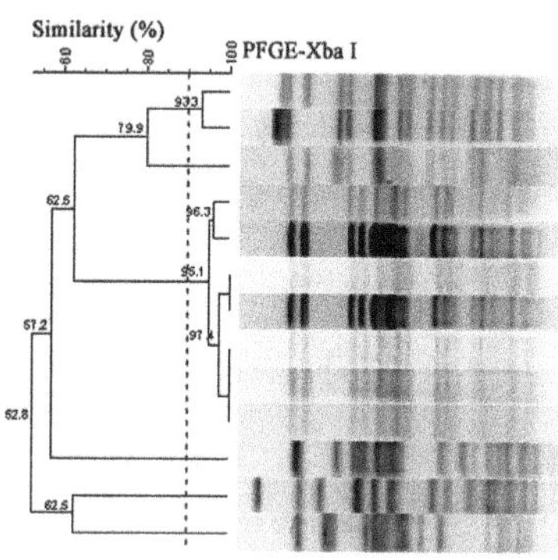

Isolate	Source	Resistance profile	Phylogroup	MLST	Plasmid characteristics	
					Size (kb)	PBRT
EC6413	Sow	AMP,FOX,CEF,CTX,CAZ,FFC,KAN,DOX,ENR,SXT	A	ST641	—	—
EC4103	Sow	AMP,FOX,CEF,CTX,CAZ,FFC,KAN,DOX,ENR,SXT	A	ST641	—	—
EC5106	Sow	AMP,FOX,CEF,CTX,FFC,KAN,DOX,ENR,SXT	B	ST641	—	—
EC3602	Sow	AMP,FOX,CEF,CTX,CAZ,FFC,KAN,DOX,ENR,SXT	C	ST1121	~290	HI2
EC5207	Sow	AMP,FOX,CEF,CTX,CAZ,FFC,KAN,DOX,ENR,SXT	C	ST1121	~290	HI2
EC6419	Sow	AMP,FOX,CEF,CTX,CAZ,FFC,KAN,DOX,ENR,SXT	C	ST1121	~290	HI2
EC5320	Sow	AMP,FOX,CEF,CTX,CAZ,FFC,KAN,DOX,ENR,SXT	C	ST1121	~290	HI2
EC5423	Sow	AMP,FOX,CEF,CTX,CAZ,FFC,KAN,DOX,ENR,SXT	C	ST1121	~290	HI2
EC1125	Piglet	AMP,FOX,CEF,CTX,CAZ,FFC,KAN,DOX,ENR,SXT	C	ST1121	~290	HI2
EC5417	Sow	AMP,FOX,CEF,CTX,CAZ,FFC,KAN,DOX,ENR,SXT	C	ST1121	~290	HI2
EC4105	Sow	AMP,FOX,CEF,CTX,FFC,KAN,DOX,ENR,SXT	D	ST4234	—	—
EC5422	Sow	AMP,FOX,CEF,CTX,CAZ,FFC,KAN,DOX,ENR,SXT	E	ST164	~290	HI2,FII
EC6208	Piglet	AMP,FOX,CEF,CTX,CAZ,FFC,KAN,DOX,ENR,SXT	F	ST2603	—	—

FIGURE 1 | Clonal relationship and plasmid characteristics of the 13 bla_{CMY-2}-positive *Escherichia coli* isolates. -, not detected. AMP, CAZ, FOX, CEF, CTX, KAN, FFC, DOX, ENR, and SXT are represented as in **Table 2**.

the bla_{CMY-2}/bla_{CTX-M} genes in the sow isolates (34.2%) was significantly higher than that in the piglet isolates (13.6%; $p < 0.05$). The distribution of ESBL/pAmpC genes among the isolates are listed in **Table 3**.

TABLE 3 | Distribution of ESBL/pAmpC genes among *E. coli* isolates.

Gene type	No. isolates (%)		Total ($n = 117$)
	Sow ($n = 73$)	Piglet ($n = 44$)	
ESBL	14 (19.2)	4 (9.1)	18 (15.4)
$bla_{CTX-M-55}$	3 (4.1)		3 (2.6)
$bla_{CTX-M-64}$	1 (1.4)	1 (2.3)	2 (1.7)
$bla_{CTX-M-65}$	4 (5.5)	1 (2.3)	5 (4.3)
$bla_{CTX-M-122}$	6 (8.2)	2 (4.5)	8 (6.8)
pAmpC			
bla_{CMY-2}	11 (15.1)	2 (4.5)	13 (11.1)
Total	25 (34.2)	6 (13.6)*	31 (26.5)

$^*p < 0.05$ for gene detection rate of isolates from piglets vs. sows.

Molecular Typing

We used cluster analysis of the bla_{CMY-2}-positive isolates to generate dendrograms from PFGE profiles (**Figure 1**). Six phylogenetic groups (designated A–F) each with more than 90% similarity were represented in these 13 isolates. Group C contained seven isolates, Group A two, and the other four groups one each.

Multilocus sequence typing analysis of the 13 bla_{CMY-2}-positive isolates identified five different STs including a novel one (ST4234). The most prevalent STs were ST1121 ($n = 7$) and ST641 ($n = 3$). The remaining isolates were each of a single ST type (**Figure 1**). Interestingly, the seven ST1121 isolates from six sows and one piglet were all contained in Group C. The three ST641 isolates from sows were divided between two groups (**Figure 1**).

Conjugation Assays and Plasmid Analysis

Eight bla_{CMY-2}-positive transconjugants were successfully obtained from the seven ST1121 and one ST164 *E. coli* isolates. S1 nuclease-PFGE analysis identified a single plasmid in each of the seven transconjugants from ST1121 isolates. Two plasmids were identified in the transconjugant EC5422-25T derived from the ST164 isolate EC5422 (Supplementary Figure S1). Subsequently, Southern blot hybridization identified the bla_{CMY-2} gene located on a ~290 kb plasmid in each of the transconjugants (Supplementary Figure S1). Replicon typing revealed the presence of the IncHI2 replicon in each of the eight transconjugants, but one of them (EC5422-25T) carried two replicons (IncHI2 and IncFII; **Figure 1**).

The IncHI2 plasmids of the ST1121 isolates shared indistinguishable RFLP profiles that were generated using *XbaI* digestion (data not shown). All of the transconjugants were resistant to FOX, CEF,CTX, AMP, KAN, and AMK. In addition, transfer of resistance to FFC, DOX, and SXT was also observed in the transconjugant EC5422-25T.

The metal susceptibility testing showed that the MICs of $CuSO_4$ and $AgNO_3$ for transconjugant EC5207-35T were higher than that of *E. coli* C600 (MIC_{CuSO4} = 12 vs. 8 mM; MIC_{AgNO3} = 1 vs. 0.0125 mM).

Complete Sequence of Plasmid pEC5207

We determined the DNA sequence of the plasmid derived from the bla_{CMY-2}-positive transconjugants that were obtained from the seven ST1121 isolates. This plasmid pEC5207 is 272,865 bp in length with a GC content of 46.16% and harbors 253 predicted ORFs. The plasmid backbone is organized similarly to that of pSH111_227 (GenBank JN983042) from *Salmonella* sp. and encodes typical IncHI2 plasmid replication, partition, maintenance and transfer functions (**Figure 2**). The replication region of pEC5207 included a *repHI2* gene. The *parA* and *parB* genes were involved in the plasmid partition. Two *tra* transfer regions and a *hipAB* toxin-antitoxin gene cluster were associated with the transfer and maintenance function of pEC5207. Interestingly, pEC5207 also contained a large number of genes encoding resistance to heavy metals including tellurium (*terABCDEFWXYZ*), silver (*silABCEPRS*) and copper (*copABCE*; **Figure 2**).

The bla_{CMY-2} gene in pEC5207 is contained within a 48,888 bp variable region (**Figure 2**). The variable portion is located in a region between *umuD* and *dcm* in pEC5207, where is the *hp161* locus in pSH111_227. The variable region showed high homology (>99%) with two parts of the bla_{CMY-2}-carrying IncA/C plasmid pCFSAN007427_01 (GenBank CP009413) from *Salmonella* and contained an IS*26* and a truncated Tn*As1* at the ends. In addition to bla_{CMY-2}, a new class I integron harboring aminoglycoside resistance gene *aacA7* and sulfonamide resistance gene *sulI* was also found in this variable region.

DISCUSSION

Antimicrobial susceptibility testing showed different resistance levels to cephalosporins and other classes of antimicrobials in *E. coli* isolates from a farrowing farm in Southern China. The antimicrobial usage records for this farm showed that doxycycline and the first generation cephalosporin cefradine were frequently added to drinking water or compound feeds as prophylactics. Other antimicrobials such as ceftiofur, enrofloxacin, florfenicol, and sulfamethoxazole were also commonly used for treatment during production. This background may be favorable for developing resistance to cephalosporins and other antimicrobials in this farm. The ESC-resistant *E. coli* usually carry additional genes conferring resistance to other veterinary antimicrobial agents like quinolone, aminoglycoside and florfenicol. In our previous study, the ESBL and pAmpC genes were detected in 67.5% of the PMQR-positive *E. coli*, indicating a strong association between ESC and quinolone resistance (Liu et al., 2013a). The 16S rRNA methylase genes, especially *rmtB*, and the florfenicol resistance gene *floR* are also commonly identified in ESBLs and pAmpC-producing *E. coli* isolates (Kang et al., 2009; Wu et al., 2009; Yu et al., 2010; Deng et al., 2011; Liu et al., 2013b; Guo et al., 2014). The use of different antimicrobial agents may increase the potential risk for selection of multidrug resistant isloates, and contribute to the MDR phenotypes of *E. coli* isolates in this farm.

Compared with the isolates from piglets, the isolates from sows showed significantly higher resistance rates to FOX, CEF and CTX, as well as a relatively higher resistance rate to CAZ. This coincided with the higher occurrence of the bla_{CMY-2} and bla_{CTX-M} genes in the isolates from sows than in the isolates from piglets. Previous studies have shown that cephalosporin treatment can result in the selection of ESBL and AmpC producing *E. coli* in animals and aggravate the problem of cephalosporin resistance (Tragesser et al., 2006; Cavaco et al., 2008; Kanwar et al., 2013; Barton, 2014). The longer antibiotic exposure times of the sows may promote the persistence of ESBL/AmpC-producing *E. coli* in the gastrointestinal tract, thus resulting in the serious cephalosporin resistance and relatively high prevalence of ESBL/AmpC genes observed in sow isolates.

In this study the prevalence of the bla_{CMY-2} gene (11.1%) was lower than that of the bla_{CTX-M} genes (15.4%). However, this level was much higher than those in our previous study (2.9%; Fang et al., 2015) and others' (1.0–3.0%) in China (Liu et al., 2007; Guo et al., 2014; Rao et al., 2014). Previous studies have shown that cefoxitin/ceftiofur-resistant isolates from *E. coli* and *Salmonella* had a high degree of association with the production of CMY enzymes (Barton, 2014). Therefore, the use of ceftiofur in this farm probably contributed to the selection of bla_{CMY-2}-producing *E. coli* isolates. MLST typing revealed a major ST type, ST1121, in seven of the thirteen bla_{CMY-2}-positive isolates. Since they shared a high similarity (>95%) in PFGE profiles, this suggested a clonal spread of these ST1121 isolates. Furthermore, plasmid analysis of the transconjugants from the seven ST1121 isolates revealed an indistinguishable IncHI2 plasmid harboring bla_{CMY-2} in these isolates. Thus, the clonal spread of ST1121 isolates harboring IncHI2 plasmid may play an important role in the dissemination of bla_{CMY-2} in this farm. Notably, among the 13 bla_{CMY-2}-positive isolates, one of the ST1121 isolates and the ST2603 isolate were isolated from piglets for market, which would indicate that the bla_{CMY-2}-positive isolates may have been introduced into other swine farms by piglet trading and therefore would accelerate the spread of bla_{CMY-2}. Further surveillance is necessary to determine

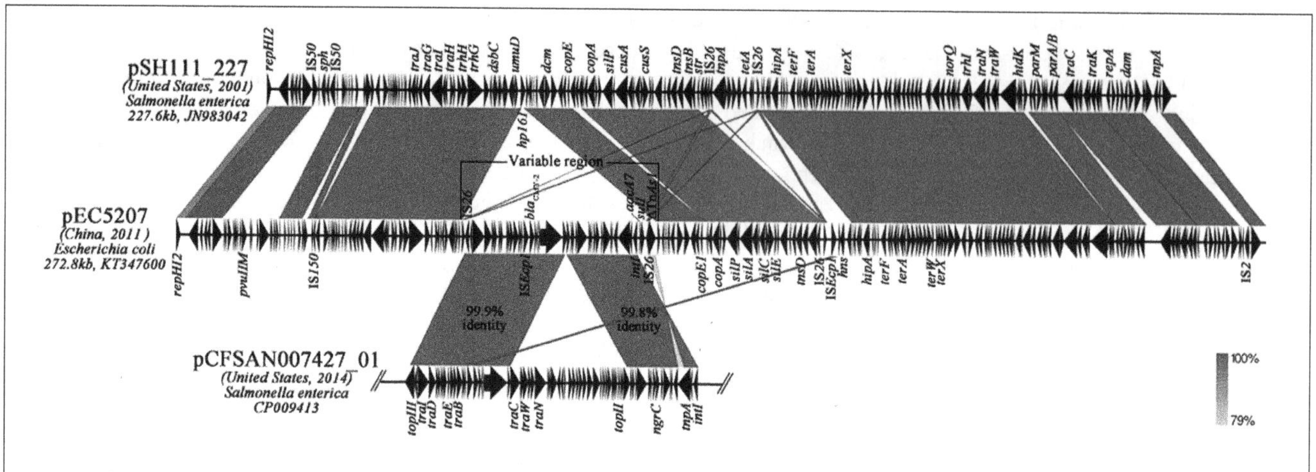

FIGURE 2 | Linear comparison of IncHI2 plasmids pEC5207, pSH111_227 and $bla_{\text{CMY-2}}$-carrying IncA/C plasmid pCFSAN007427_01. The arrows represent the positions and transcriptional direction of the ORFs. Regions of homology are shaded in gray.

the prevalence of $bla_{\text{CMY-2}}$-positive isolates in these swine farms.

Since its first identification on plasmid from *Klebsiella pneumoniae* (Bauernfeind et al., 1990), the $bla_{\text{CMY-2}}$ gene has been associated with various plasmid types. In our previous surveillance study, the $bla_{\text{CMY-2}}$ gene was identified on IncA/C, IncHI2, and IncX plasmids (Fang et al., 2015). In the present study, $bla_{\text{CMY-2}}$-carrying IncHI2 plasmids were not only detected in the clonal ST1121 isolates but also in a ST164 isolate. Additionally, the strong association of $bla_{\text{CMY-2}}$ with IncHI2 plasmid was also observed in *Salmonella* (Shi, 2015). This highlighted the role of the IncHI2 plasmid in the transfer of $bla_{\text{CMY-2}}$. Besides $bla_{\text{CMY-2}}$, IncHI2 plasmid is also associated with another pAmpC gene $bla_{\text{CMY-8}}$ (Chen et al., 2007b). In addition, IncHI2 plasmids have been implicated in the spread of $bla_{\text{CTX-M}}$ genes and are also frequently linked with the other antimicrobial resistance genes such as bla_{SHV}, bla_{IMP}, bla_{VIM}, *armA*, *qnrA1*, *qnrS1*, and *qnrB2* (Garcia Fernandez et al., 2007; Veldman et al., 2010; Coelho et al., 2012). Together, our data indicate that the IncHI2 plasmid played a significant role in the dissemination of antimicrobial resistance. However, to the best of our knowledge, there was no complete sequence analysis of a $bla_{\text{CMY-2}}$-carrying IncHI2 plasmid to date. Therefore, in order to further characterize the $bla_{\text{CMY-2}}$-carrying IncHI2 plasmids of ST1121 isolates, plasmid pEC5207 was sequenced in our study.

This plasmid possesses a typical IncHI2 plasmid backbone organized similarly to that of pSH111_227. A portion of *hp161* in pSH111_227 was replaced with a $bla_{\text{CMY-2}}$-harboring variable region in pEC5207. A sequence comparison revealed that this variable region might originate from IncA/C plasmid pCFSAN007427_01, and is flanked with IS*26* and a truncated Tn*As1*. Considering the potential for genetic rearrangements by insertion sequence and transposon (Hallet and Sherratt, 1997; Bennett, 2004), we speculate that IS*26* and Tn*As1* transposition into the *hp161* locus of a pSH111_227-like IncHI2 plasmid was followed by recombination with a pCFSAN007427_01-like $bla_{\text{CMY-2}}$-carrying IncA/C plasmid. This could set the stage for the integration of $bla_{\text{CMY-2}}$ into the IncHI2 plasmid.

Apart from the $bla_{\text{CMY-2}}$ gene, pEC5207 also carried other resistance determinants for aminoglycosides (*aacA7*), sulfonamides (*sul1*), as well as heavy metals ions, such as Cu and Ag. And the result of susceptibility tests also confirm the functionality of pEC5207 in the transfer of copper and silver resistance. Copper is often present as trace element feed additives for animal production in China (Wang et al., 2013). Silver is used as disinfectants in water or surfaces in the animal production setting (Mourao et al., 2015). Under the selective pressure of heavy metals, cephalosporins, and other antimicrobials, plasmid pEC5207 could play a critical role in the persistence of host bacteria in the intestine of pigs, thereby increasing the risk for co-selection of isolates carrying $bla_{\text{CMY-2}}$ gene. This may further explain the high prevalence of $bla_{\text{CMY-2}}$ in this farm.

CONCLUSION

The present study revealed a relatively high prevalence of $bla_{\text{CMY-2}}$ in a farrowing farm in Southern China. The clonal spread of ST1121 type *E. coli* harboring an IncHI2 plasmid mediated the dissemination of $bla_{\text{CMY-2}}$ in this farm. Nucleotide sequence analysis and comparisons indicated that the $bla_{\text{CMY-2}}$-carrying IncHI2 plasmid pEC5207 may have been generated by recombination with an IncA/C plasmid. pEC5207 may play an important role in the persistence of host bacteria under the selective pressure of heavy metal and antimicrobials. Although limited to a farrowing farm, our study indicates that there is a serious risk of dissemination of the $bla_{\text{CMY-2}}$ gene by clonal spread and piglet training. Broad and longitudinal studies to determine the prevalence of $bla_{\text{CMY-2}}$-positive *E. coli* in swine farms are required in the future.

ACKNOWLEDGMENTS

This work was supported by the Program for Changjiang Scholars and Innovative Research Team at University of Ministry of Education of China (Grant No. IRT13063), the Special Fund for Agro-scientific Research in the Public Interest (Grant No. 201203040), the National Natural Science Foundation (Grant No.31272609), and the Science and Technology Program of Guangzhou, China(Grant No. 2011J2200054).

REFERENCES

Aziz, R. K., Bartels, D., Best, A. A., Dejongh, M., Disz, T., Edwards, R. A., et al. (2008). The RAST Server: rapid annotations using subsystems technology. *BMC Genomics* 9:75. doi: 10.1186/1471-2164-9-75

Barton, B. M., Harding, G. P., and Zuccarelli, A. J. (1995). A general method for detecting and sizing large plasmids. *Anal. Biochem.* 226, 235–240. doi: 10.1006/abio.1995.1220

Barton, M. D. (2014). Impact of antibiotic use in the swine industry. *Curr. Opin. Microbiol.* 19, 9–15. doi: 10.1016/j.mib.2014.05.017

Bauernfeind, A., Schweighart, S., Dornbusch, K., and Giamarellou, H. (1990). "A transferable cephamycinase in *Klebsiella pneumoniae*, abstr. A190," in *Program and Abstracts of the 30th Interscience Conference on Antimicrobial Agents and Chemotherapy*. Washington, DC: American Society for Microbiology.

Bennett, P. M. (2004). Genome plasticity: insertion sequence elements, transposons and integrons, and DNA rearrangement. *Methods Mol. Biol.* 266, 71–113.

Bortolaia, V., Hansen, K. H., Nielsen, C. A., Fritsche, T. R., and Guardabassi, L. (2014). High diversity of plasmids harbouring blaCMY-2 among clinical *Escherichia coli* isolates from humans and companion animals in the upper Midwestern USA. *J. Antimicrob. Chemother.* 69, 1492–1496. doi: 10.1093/jac/dku011

Bradford, P. A. (2001). Extended-spectrum β-lactamases in the 21st century: characterization, epidemiology, and detection of this important resistance threat. *Clin. Microbiol. Rev.* 14, 933–951. doi: 10.1128/CMR.14.4.933-951.2001

Brooks, J. P., Adeli, A., and Mclaughlin, M. R. (2014). Microbial ecology, bacterial pathogens, and antibiotic resistant genes in swine manure wastewater as influenced by three swine management systems. *Water Res.* 57, 96–103. doi: 10.1016/j.watres.2014.03.017

Cabello, F. C., Godfrey, H. P., Tomova, A., Ivanova, L., Dolz, H., Millanao, A., et al. (2013). Antimicrobial use in aquaculture re-examined: its relevance to antimicrobial resistance and to animal and human health. *Environ. Microbiol.* 15, 1917–1942. doi: 10.1111/1462-2920.12134

Callens, B., Faes, C., Maes, D., Catry, B., Boyen, F., Francoys, D., et al. (2015). Presence of antimicrobial resistance and antimicrobial use in sows are risk factors for antimicrobial resistance in their offspring. *Microb. Drug Resist.* 21, 50–58. doi: 10.1089/mdr.2014.0037

Callens, B., Maes, D., Boyen, F., Haesebrouck, F., and Dewulf, J. (2012). "Antimicrobial resistance profile in faecal *Escherichia coli* of sows and their offspring in the farrowing unit and their interaction," in *Proceeding of the 13th International Symposium on Veterinary Epidemiology and Economics (ISVEE XIII)*, Wageningen: Wageningen Academic Publishers.

Carattoli, A., Bertini, A., Villa, L., Falbo, V., Hopkins, K. L., and Threlfall, E. J. (2005). Identification of plasmids by PCR-based replicon typing. *J. Microbiol. Methods* 63, 219–228. doi: 10.1016/j.mimet.2005.03.018

Cavaco, L. M., Abatih, E., Aarestrup, F. M., and Guardabassi, L. (2008). Selection and persistence of CTX-M-producing *Escherichia coli* in the intestinal flora of pigs treated with amoxicillin, ceftiofur, or cefquinome. *Antimicrob. Agents Chemother.* 52, 3612–3616. doi: 10.1128/AAC.00354-08

Chen, L., Chen, Z. L., Liu, J. H., Zeng, Z. L., Ma, J. Y., and Jiang, H. X. (2007a). Emergence of RmtB methylase-producing *Escherichia coli* and *Enterobacter cloacae* isolates from pigs in China. *J. Antimicrob. Chemother.* 59, 880–885. doi: 10.1093/jac/dkm065

Chen, Y. T., Lauderdale, T. L., Liao, T. L., Shiau, Y. R., Shu, H. Y., Wu, K. M., et al. (2007b). Sequencing and comparative genomic analysis of pK29, a 269-kilobase conjugative plasmid encoding CMY-8 and CTX-M-3 beta-lactamases in *Klebsiella pneumoniae*. *Antimicrob. Agents Chemother.* 51, 3004–3007. doi: 10.1128/AAC.00167-07

Chin, C. S., Alexander, D. H., Marks, P., Klammer, A. A., Drake, J., Heiner, C., et al. (2013). Nonhybrid, finished microbial genome assemblies from long-read SMRT sequencing data. *Nat. Methods* 10, 563–569. doi: 10.1038/nmeth.2474

Clinical and Laboratory Standards Institute (2013a). *Performance Standards for Antimicrobial Susceptibility Testing; 23rd Informational Supplement M100–S23.* Wayne, PA: Clinical and Laboratory Standards Institute.

Clinical and Laboratory Standards Institute (2013b). *Performance Standards for Antimicrobial Disk and Dilution Susceptibility Tests for Bacteria Isolated From Animals; Approved Standard-Fourth Edition. CLSI document VET01-A4.* Wayne, PA: Clinical and Laboratory Standards Institute.

Coelho, A., Piedra-Carrasco, N., Bartolome, R., Quintero-Zarate, J. N., Larrosa, N., Cornejo-Sanchez, T., et al. (2012). Role of IncHI2 plasmids harbouring blaVIM-1, blaCTX-M-9, aac(6')-Ib and qnrA genes in the spread of multiresistant *Enterobacter cloacae* and *Klebsiella pneumoniae* strains in different units at Hospital Vall d'Hebron. Barcelona, Spain. *Int. J. Antimicrob. Agents* 39, 514–517. doi: 10.1016/j.ijantimicag.2012.01.006

Crombe, F., Argudin, M. A., Vanderhaeghen, W., Hermans, K., Haesebrouck, F., and Butaye, P. (2013). Transmission dynamics of methicillin-resistant staphylococcus aureus in pigs. *Front. Microbiol.* 4:57. doi: 10.3389/fmicb.2013.00057

Deng, Y., He, L., Chen, S., Zheng, H., Zeng, Z., Liu, Y., et al. (2011). F33:A-:B- and F2:A-:B- plasmids mediate dissemination of rmtB-blaCTX-M-9 group genes and rmtB-qepA in *Enterobacteriaceae* isolates from pets in China. *Antimicrob. Agents Chemother.* 55, 4926–4929. doi: 10.1128/AAC.00133-11

Fang, L. X., Sun, J., Li, L., Deng, H., Huang, T., Yang, Q. E., et al. (2015). Dissemination of the chromosomally encoded CMY-2 cephalosporinase gene in *Escherichia coli* isolated from animals. *Int. J. Antimicrob. Agents* 46, 209–213. doi: 10.1016/j.ijantimicag.2015.04.003

Folster, J. P., Pecic, G., Mccullough, A., Rickert, R., and Whichard, J. M. (2011). Characterization of blaCMY-encoding plasmids among *Salmonella* isolated in the United States in 2007. *Foodborne Pathog. Dis.* 8, 1289–1294. doi: 10.1089/fpd.2011.0944

Garcia Fernandez, A., Cloeckaert, A., Bertini, A., Praud, K., Doublet, B., Weill, F. X., et al. (2007). Comparative analysis of IncHI2 plasmids carrying blaCTX-M-2 or blaCTX-M-9 from *Escherichia coli* and *Salmonella enterica* strains isolated from poultry and humans. *Antimicrob. Agents Chemother.* 51, 4177–4180. doi: 10.1128/AAC.00603-07

Greko, C., Badiola, J. I., Catry, B., Moreno, M. A., Pyörälä, S., Ruzauskas, M., et al. (2009). Reflection paper on the use of third and fourth generation cephalosporins in food producing animals in the European Union: development of resistance and impact on human and animal health. *J. Vet. Pharmacol. Ther.* 32, 515–533. doi: 10.1111/j.1365-2885.2009.01075.x

Guo, Y. F., Zhang, W. H., Ren, S. Q., Yang, L., Lu, D. H., Zeng, Z. L., et al. (2014). IncA/C plasmid-mediated spread of CMY-2 in multidrug-resistant *Escherichia coli* from food animals in China. *PLoS ONE* 9:e96738. doi: 10.1371/journal.pone.0096738

Hallet, B., and Sherratt, D. J. (1997). Transposition and site-specific recombination: adapting DNA cut-and-paste mechanisms to a variety of genetic rearrangements. *FEMS Microbiol. Rev.* 21, 157–178. doi: 10.1111/j.1574-6976.1997.tb00349.x

Jacoby, G. A. (2009). AmpC β-lactamases. *Clin. Microbiol. Rev.* 22, 161–182. doi: 10.1128/CMR.00036-08

Kang, H. Y., Kim, J., Seol, S. Y., Lee, Y. C., Lee, J. C., and Cho, D. T. (2009). Characterization of conjugative plasmids carrying antibiotic resistance genes encoding 16S rRNA methylase, extended-spectrum beta-lactamase, and/or plasmid-mediated AmpC beta-lactamase. *J. Microbiol.* 47, 68–75. doi: 10.1007/s12275-008-0158-3

Kanwar, N., Scott, H. M., Norby, B., Loneragan, G. H., Vinasco, J., Mcgowan, M., et al. (2013). Effects of ceftiofur and chlortetracycline treatment strategies on antimicrobial susceptibility and on tet(A), tet(B), and blaCMY-2 resistance genes among *E. coli* isolated from the feces of feedlot cattle. *PLoS ONE* 8:e80575. doi: 10.1371/journal.pone.0080575

Li, X. Z., Mehrotra, M., Ghimire, S., and Adewoye, L. (2007). Beta-Lactam resistance and beta-lactamases in bacteria of animal origin. *Vet. Microbiol.* 121, 197–214. doi: 10.1016/j.vetmic.2007.01.015

Liu, B. T., Liao, X. P., Yue, L., Chen, X. Y., Li, L., Yang, S. S., et al. (2013a). Prevalence of beta-lactamase and 16S rRNA methylase genes among clinical *Escherichia coli* isolates carrying plasmid-mediated quinolone resistance genes from animals. *Microb. Drug Resist.* 19, 237–245. doi: 10.1089/mdr.2012.0179

Liu, B. T., Yang, Q. E., Li, L., Sun, J., Liao, X. P., Fang, L. X., et al. (2013b). Dissemination and Characterization of Plasmids Carrying oqxAB-blaCTX-M Genes in *Escherichia coli* Isolates from Food-Producing Animals. *PLoS ONE* 8:e73947. doi: 10.1371/journal.pone.0073947

Liu, J. H., Wei, S. Y., Ma, J. Y., Zeng, Z. L., Lu, D. H., Yang, G. X., et al. (2007). Detection and characterisation of CTX-M and CMY-2 β-lactamases among *Escherichia coli* isolates from farm animals in Guangdong Province of China. *Int. J. Antimicrob. Agents* 29, 576–581. doi: 10.1016/j.ijantimicag.2006.12.015

Martin, L. C., Weir, E. K., Poppe, C., Reid-Smith, R. J., and Boerlin, P. (2012). Characterization of blaCMY-2 plasmids in *Salmonella* and *Escherichia coli* isolates from food animals in Canada. *Appl. Environ. Microbiol.* 78, 1285–1287. doi: 10.1128/AEM.06498-11

Mathew, A. G., Garner, K. N., Ebner, P. D., Saxton, A. M., Clift, R. E., and Liamthong, S. (2005). Effects of antibiotic use in sows on resistance of E. coli and *Salmonella enterica* Typhimurium in their offspring. *Foodborne Pathog. Dis.* 2, 212–220. doi: 10.1089/fpd.2005.2.212

McEwen, S. A., and Fedorka-Cray, P. J. (2002). Antimicrobial use and resistance in animals. *Clin. Infect. Dis.* 34 (Suppl. 3), S93–S106. doi: 10.1086/340246

Mourao, J., Novais, C., Machado, J., Peixe, L., and Antunes, P. (2015). Metal tolerance in emerging clinically relevant multidrug-resistant *Salmonella enterica* serotype 4,[5],12:i:- clones circulating in Europe. *Int. J. Antimicrob. Agents* 45, 610–616. doi: 10.1016/j.ijantimicag.2015.01.013

Perez-Perez, F. J., and Hanson, N. D. (2002). Detection of plasmid-mediated AmpC β-lactamase genes in clinical isolates by using multiplex PCR. *J. Clin. Microbiol.* 40, 2153–2162. doi: 10.1128/JCM.40.6.2153-2162.2002

Rao, L., Lv, L., Zeng, Z., Chen, S., He, D., Chen, X., et al. (2014). Increasing prevalence of extended-spectrum cephalosporin-resistant *Escherichia coli* in food animals and the diversity of CTX-M genotypes during 2003-2012. *Vet. Microbiol.* 172, 534–541. doi: 10.1016/j.vetmic.2014.06.013

Rasschaert, G., Michiels, J., Arijs, D., Wildemauwe, C., De Smet, S., and Heyndrickx, M. (2012). Effect of farm type on within-herd *Salmonella* prevalence, serovar distribution, and antimicrobial resistance. *J. Food Prot.* 75, 859–866. doi: 10.4315/0362-028X.JFP-11-469

Sandvang, D., Jensen, L. B., Baggesen, D. L., and Baloda, S. B. (2000). Persistence of a *Salmonella enterica* serotype typhimurium clone in Danish pig production units and farmhouse environment studied by pulsed field gel electrophoresis (PFGE). *FEMS Microbiol. Lett.* 187, 21–25. doi: 10.1111/j.1574-6968.2000.tb09130.x

Seiffert, S. N., Hilty, M., Perreten, V., and Endimiani, A. (2013). Extended-spectrum cephalosporin-resistant Gram-negative organisms in livestock: an emerging problem for human health? *Drug Resist. Updat.* 16, 22–45. doi: 10.1016/j.drup.2012.12.001

Shi, C. (2015). "Screening and characterization of antibiotic-resistant plasmids in *Salmonella*," in *Proceeding of the 2015 Annual Meeting July 25–28, 2015* (Portland: International Association for Food Protection).

Sullivan, M. J., Petty, N. K., and Beatson, S. A. (2011). Easyfig: a genome comparison visualizer. *Bioinformatics* 27, 1009–1010. doi: 10.1093/bioinformatics/btr039

Tenover, F. C., Arbeit, R. D., Goering, R. V., Mickelsen, P. A., Murray, B. E., Persing, D. H., et al. (1995). Interpreting chromosomal DNA restriction patterns produced by pulsed-field gel electrophoresis: criteria for bacterial strain typing. *J. Clin. Microbiol.* 33, 2233–2239.

Tian, G. B., Wang, H. N., Zhang, A. Y., Zhang, Y., Fan, W. Q., Xu, C. W., et al. (2012). Detection of clinically important beta-lactamases in commensal *Escherichia coli* of human and swine origin in western China. *J. Med. Microbiol.* 61, 233–238. doi: 10.1099/jmm.0.036806-0

Tragesser, L. A., Wittum, T. E., Funk, J. A., Winokur, P. L., and Rajala-Schultz, P. J. (2006). Association between ceftiofur use and isolation of *Escherichia coli* with reduced susceptibility to ceftriaxone from fecal samples of dairy cows. *Am. J. Vet. Res.* 67, 1696–1700. doi: 10.2460/ajvr.67.10.1696

van Duijkeren, E., Ikawaty, R., Broekhuizen-Stins, M. J., Jansen, M. D., Spalburg, E. C., De Neeling, A. J., et al. (2008). Transmission of methicillin-resistant *Staphylococcus aureus* strains between different kinds of pig farms. *Vet. Microbiol.* 126, 383–389. doi: 10.1016/j.vetmic.2007.07.021

Veldman, K., Dierikx, C., Van Essen-Zandbergen, A., Van Pelt, W., and Mevius, D. (2010). Characterization of multidrug-resistant, qnrB2-positive and extended-spectrum-β-lactamase-producing *Salmonella* Concord and *Salmonella* Senftenberg isolates. *J. Antimicrob. Chemother.* 65, 872–875. doi: 10.1093/jac/dkq049

Verdet, C., Gautier, V., Chachaty, E., Ronco, E., Hidri, N., Decre, D., et al. (2009). Genetic context of plasmid-carried blaCMY-2-like genes in *Enterobacteriaceae*. *Antimicrob. Agents Chemother.* 53, 4002–4006. doi: 10.1128/AAC.00753-08

Versalovic, J., Koeuth, T., and Lupski, J. R. (1991). Distribution of repetitive DNA sequences in eubacteria and application to fingerprinting of bacterial genomes. *Nucleic Acids Res.* 19, 6823–6831. doi: 10.1093/nar/19.24.6823

Wang, H., Dong, Y., Yang, Y., Toor, G. S., and Zhang, X. (2013). Changes in heavy metal contents in animal feeds and manures in an intensive animal production region of China. *J. Environ. Sci. (China)* 25, 2435–2442. doi: 10.1016/S1001-0742(13)60473-8

Witte, W. (1998). Medical consequences of antibiotic use in agriculture. *Science* 279, 996–997. doi: 10.1126/science.279.5353.996

Wu, Q., Zhang, Y., Han, L., Sun, J., and Ni, Y. (2009). Plasmid-mediated 16S rRNA methylases in aminoglycoside-resistant *Enterobacteriaceae* isolates in Shanghai. China. *Antimicrob. Agents Chemother.* 53, 271–272. doi: 10.1128/AAC.00748-08

Yu, F. Y., Yao, D., Pan, J. Y., Chen, C., Qin, Z. Q., Parsons, C., et al. (2010). High prevalence of plasmid-mediated 16S rRNA methylase gene rmtB among *Escherichia coli* clinical isolates from a Chinese teaching hospital. *BMC Infect. Dis.* 10:184. doi: 10.1186/1471-2334-10-184

Zheng, H., Zeng, Z., Chen, S., Liu, Y., Yao, Q., Deng, Y., et al. (2012). Prevalence and characterisation of CTX-M beta-lactamases amongst *Escherichia coli* isolates from healthy food animals in China. *Int. J. Antimicrob. Agents* 39, 305–310. doi: 10.1016/j.ijantimicag.2011.12.001

2

Draft Genomic Analysis of an Avian Multidrug Resistant *Morganella morganii* Isolate Carrying *qnrD1*

***Daniela Jones-Dias*[1,2]*, Lurdes Clemente*[3]*, Inês B. Moura*[1,2]*, Daniel A. Sampaio*[4]*, Teresa Albuquerque*[3]*, Luís Vieira*[4]*, Vera Manageiro*[1,2]** and Manuela Caniça*[1]**

[1] National Reference Laboratory of Antibiotic Resistances and Healthcare Associated Infections, Department of Infectious Diseases, National Institute of Health Doutor Ricardo Jorge, Lisbon, Portugal, [2] Centre for the Studies of Animal Science, Institute of Agrarian and Agri-Food Sciences and Technologies, Oporto University, Oporto, Portugal, [3] Microbiology and Mycology Laboratory, Instituto Nacional de Investigação Agrária e Veterinária, Lisbon, Portugal, [4] Innovation and Technology Unit, Human Genetics Department, National Institute of Health Doutor Ricardo Jorge, Lisbon, Portugal

***Correspondence:**
Vera Manageiro
vera.manageiro@insa.min-saude.pt

Morganella morganii is a commensal bacterium and opportunistic pathogen often present in the gut of humans and animals. We report the 4.3 Mbp draft genome sequence of a *M. morganii* isolated in association with an *Escherichia coli* from broilers in Portugal that showed macroscopic lesions consistent with colisepticemia. The analysis of the genome matched the multidrug resistance phenotype and enabled the identification of several clinically important and potentially mobile acquired antibiotic resistance genes, including the plasmid-mediated quinolone resistance determinant *qnrD1*. Mobile genetic elements, prophages, and pathogenicity factors were also detected, improving our understanding toward this human and animal opportunistic pathogen.

Keywords: *qnrD1*, plasmid, multidrug resistance, *Morganella morganii*, WGS

INTRODUCTION

The Gram negative *Morganella morganii* belongs to the tribe *Proteeae* of the family *Enterobacteriaceae* (O'Hara et al., 2000). This species, along with other elements of *Proteus* and *Providencia* genera can be found in the normal flora of humans, reptiles and in the wider environment (O'Hara et al., 2000; Lee and Liu, 2006; Dipineto et al., 2014). However, *M. morganii* isolates also constitute clinically relevant opportunistic pathogens, which can cause a variety of infections. Nosocomial outbreaks have been reported, suggesting that infections caused by *M. morganii* can lead to major clinical problems, such as wounds, urinary tract infections and septicemia (Nicolle, 2001; Tsanaktsidis et al., 2003; Falagas et al., 2006; Lee and Liu, 2006; Lin et al., 2015).

This bacterium has also been associated with infections in animals and with human animal bite wound infections, which suggests that *M. morganii* may also cause zoonotic infectious diseases (Ono et al., 2001; Choi et al., 2002; Abrahamian and Goldstein, 2011; Zhao et al., 2012; Di Ianni et al., 2015).

Several factors can affect the progression and severity of an infection. The presence of pathogenicity determinants is essential to the success of *M. morganii* in any environment, particularly in food animal farms, where the pressure caused by antibiotic treatments and the lack of prophylactic measures to avoid the spread of infectious diseases are usually noteworthy (Chen et al., 2012; Lin et al., 2015). It is globally accepted that horizontal gene transfer plays an important role in the dissemination of antibiotic resistance genes and pathogenicity factors (Huddleston, 2014). Considering that *M. morganii* may share the habitat with other clinically relevant pathogens, the investigation of any multidrug resistant isolate recovered from poultry is an important assignment.

Resistance to quinolones and fluoroquinolones has been increasingly reported among human and veterinary isolates, very likely as a consequence of the great usage of those antibiotics (Tamang et al., 2011). The *qnrD* gene, now denominated *qnrD1* due to the report of a second variant of the gene (Abgottspon et al., 2014), is a relatively uncommon antibiotic resistance gene, which has been described in members of the *Proteeae* family from different origins (Mazzariol et al., 2012; Zhang et al., 2013; Nasri Yaiche et al., 2014). This plasmid-mediated quinolone resistance (PMQR) determinant encodes a protein that protects DNA gyrases and topoisomerases from quinolone inhibition (Cavaco et al., 2009; Jacoby et al., 2014). Carriage of PMQR-encoding genes frequently confers modest increases to the minimum inhibitory concentrations (MIC) of fluoroquinolones (Poirel et al., 2012). Current studies have identified the environment, particularly animals and aquatic habitats, as a reservoir of PMQR genes (Poirel et al., 2012).

The aim of this study was to investigate the molecular background sustaining the multidrug resistance and pathogenicity of a *M. morganii* isolate. In this study, we report the antibiotic susceptibility and the draft genome sequence of a *qnrD1*-harboring avian isolate. The data gathered from bioinformatics analysis may improve our understanding toward this opportunistic pathogen.

MATERIALS AND METHODS

Bacterial Isolation, Antibiotic Susceptibility, and Molecular Characterization

Morganella morganii INSRALV892a was recovered in association with *E. coli* INSRALV892b in 2012 from a 13-days old broiler, recovered from a poultry industrial unit in Portugal. Samples consisted of organs (macerates of liver and spleen) collected during post-mortem examination that were submitted for bacteriological analysis. During post-mortem examination, the birds showed macroscopic lesions consistent with colisepticemia: aerosaculitis, acute enteritis, perihepatitis, and fibrinous peritonitis. Suspected *Enterobacteriaceae* colonies obtained in MacConkey agar plates were isolated in non selective media and identification was performed using API 20E strips (BioMérieux, Marcy-l'Étoile).

Minimum inhibitory concentrations were determined for both isolates by agar dilution method to ten antibiotics: ampicillin, cefotaxime, ceftazidime, meropenem, ciprofloxacin, gentamicin, chloramphenicol, trimethoprim, colistin, and tigecycline. To assess non-susceptibility, interpretation of results was performed according to the clinical breakpoints of the European Committee on Antimicrobial Susceptibility Testing (EUCAST)[1].

Plasmid-mediated quinolone resistance [QnrA, QnrB, QnrC, QnrD, QnrS, QepA, OqxAB, and Aac(6′)-Ib-cr]-, β-lactamase (TEM, SHV, OXA-G1, and CTX-M)-, and integrase (class 1, 2, and 3)-encoding genes were identified by PCR and confirmed by sequencing using DNA of both isolates, as previously described (Clemente et al., 2013).

The transference ability of specific antibiotic resistance genes from *M. morganii* INSRALV892a and *E. coli* INSRALV892b was assessed by broth mating out assays using *E. coli* J53 $NaN3^R$ as recipient strain, as described elsewhere (Jones-Dias et al., 2016). Resistant *E. coli* J53 transconjugants were then selected on MacConkey agar plates containing amoxicillin (100 mg/l) or ciprofloxacin (0.06 mg/l) together with sodium azide (200 mg/l), according with the antibiotic susceptibility profile of the donor isolates. To confirm the acquisition of the antibiotic resistance genes, we detected and identified the determinants in the transconjugants, following the methodology described above in this section.

Genome Sequencing and Analysis

Genomic DNA of *M. morganii* INSRALV892a was extracted using DNeasy Blood and Tissue Kit (Qiagen, Aarhus), and DNA quantification was performed by Qubit Fluorometric Quantitation (Thermo Fisher Scientific, Carlsbad, CA, USA), according to the manufacturer's instructions. Libraries were prepared from 1 ng of genomic DNA using the Nextera XT DNA Sample Preparation Kit (Illumina, San Diego, CA, USA), also following manufacturer's instructions. Whole Genome Sequencing (WGS) was performed using 150 bp paired-end reads on a MiSeq (Illumina, San Diego, CA, USA).

Sequence reads were then trimmed and filtered according to quality criteria. Briefly, reads were assembled *de novo* using CLC genomics workbench version 8.5 (Qiagen, Aarhus), which is based on Smith and Waterman algorithm. The raw FASTQ reads were first processed by quality score trimming (quality score limit = 0.05), removing all reads containing more than two ambiguous nucleotides or shorter than 50 bp. Trimmed reads were then *de novo* assembled with automatic bubble, word size and paired distance detection, using mapping mode "map reads back to contigs" (including scaffolding, and minimum contig length of 400 nucleotides). The NCBI prokaryotic genome automatic annotation pipeline (PGAAP) was used for annotation[2]. All *de novo* contigs were BLAST searched against the GenBank's non-redundant nucleotide collection (nr/nt). PathogenFinder 1.1, ResFinder 2.1, and PlasmidFinder 1.3 were used to estimate the number and type of pathogenicity determinants, antibiotic resistance genes and plasmids, respectively, within the genome (Zankari et al., 2012; Cosentino et al., 2013; Carattoli et al., 2014). PHAST search web

[1] http://www.eucast.org

[2] http://www.ncbi.nlm.nih.gov/genome/annotation_prok/

tool was used to identify and annotate any prophage sequence present in the draft genome (Zhou et al., 2011). ISsaga semi-automatic annotation system was also applied to detect the presence of insertion sequences (IS) (Varani et al., 2011).

Contigs containing antibiotic resistance genes were searched for identity through blastn[3] against the nr/nt NCBI database, and further mapped against the closest bacterial plasmids or genomes using CLC Genomics Workbench version 8.5.

Nucleotide Sequence GenBank Accession Numbers

This Whole Genome Shotgun project has been deposited at DDBJ/EMBL/GenBank under the accession LGYC00000000. The version described in this paper is the LGYC01000000[4].

RESULTS AND DISCUSSION

Morganella morganii INSRALV892a was found to be non-susceptible to ampicillin (>64 mg/L), cefotaxime (>4 mg/L), ceftazidime (2 mg/L), ciprofloxacin (>8 mg/L), chloramphenicol (16 mg/L), gentamicin (>32 mg/L), trimethoprim (>32 mg/L), colistin (>16 mg/L), and tigecycline (0.5 mg/L). However, it is important to highlight that *M. morganii* is intrinsically resistant to colistin, while tigecycline has also been shown to have poor activity against this species[5]. Among the antibiotics tested, the isolate was susceptible only to meropenem (0.125 mg/L). The *E. coli* INSRALV892b was also characterized with regard to antibiotic susceptibility and found to be non-susceptible to ampicillin (>64 mg/L), cefotaxime (>4 mg/L), ceftazidime (2 mg/L) and trimethoprim (>32 mg/L), and susceptible to meropenem (≤0.03 mg/L), ciprofloxacin (0.125 mg/L), chloramphenicol (≤8 mg/L), gentamicin (≤0.5 mg/L), colistin (≤1 mg/L), and tigecycline (0.5 mg/L). The molecular characterization of the isolates showed the presence of *qnrD1* and a class 2 integron in *M. morganii* INSRALV892a, and $bla_{\mathrm{CTX-M-1}}$ gene flanked by an IS*Ecp1* and *orf477*, as well as a class 1 integron in *E. coli* INSRALV892b. Conjugation experiments only revealed the transference of $bla_{\mathrm{CTX-M-1}}$ from *E. coli* INSRALV892b to isogenic *E. coli* J53 strain.

The WGS assembly of *M. morganii* INSRALV892a yielded 74 contigs (each >200 bp long and >100-fold coverage), which together comprised 4,267,817 bp, showing a GC content of 50.6%. The largest contig was 523,676 bp long and the N50 statistic, which stands for the minimum contig length of at least 50% of the contigs, was 342,352 bp. The average length of the obtained contigs was 34,190 bp. Among the obtained data, six contigs, ranging from 802 to 8,575 in length and showing a minimum coverage of 117.7-fold, matched plasmid sequences of different species. Overall, the genome sequence comprised 4,116 putative genes, among which 3,950 consisted of protein encoding sequences.

In silico analysis of the antibiotic resistance genes (90% identity and 40% minimum length) revealed the presence of loci for acquired resistance to aminoglycosides [*aadA1y*, *aph(3′)-Ic*, and *strA-strB*], β-lactam ($bla_{\mathrm{OXA-1}}$), fluoroquinolones (*qnrD1*, *aac(6′)-Ib-cr*), phenicols (*catA2 and catB3*), rifampicin (Δ*arr*), sulphonamides (*sul2*), trimethoprim (*dfrA1*), tetracycline (*tetY*), and streptothricin (*sat2*). Non-susceptibility to third generation cephalosporins such as cefotaxime and ceftazidime was not associated to any extended-spectrum β-lactamase, suggesting the involvement of inducible or stably derepressed *M. morganii* chromosomal *ampC* gene, the $bla_{DHA-type}$ gene (Harris and Ferguson, 2012).

The *dfrA1*, *catB2*, *sat2*, and *aadA1y* genes were enclosed in an In*2-17* class 2 integron that has already been described, for instance, in *Proteus vulgaris* isolates from China (HQ386830) (**Figure 1A**). Genes encoding resistance to tetracycline (*tetY*) and streptomycin (*strA-strB*) were detected in association with each other, and with proteins linked to DNA transfer processes, such as IS*Aba14* and an incomplete Tn*5393* (**Figure 1B**). The sulphonamide resistance gene *sul2* was flanked upstream by a *glmM*-containing region and ISCR2, while the downstream region consisted of a chromosomal region typical of *M. morganii* (**Figure 1C**); the *glmM* gene (formerly called *ureC*) encodes a phosphoglucosamine mutase that is considered a housekeeping gene essential for the cell wall synthesis (Tavares et al., 2003). The aminoglycoside resistance gene *aph(3′)-Ic* was associated to an IS*26* IR and a unknown *orf* (**Figure 1D**), and the genes Δ*arr*, *catB3*, $bla_{\mathrm{OXA-1}}$, and *aac(6′)-Ib*-cr were enclosed together, as gene cassettes of an integron variable region that has been previously found, for instance, in *S. enterica* from livestock (**Figure 1E**). However, in the latter, the array was flanked up and downstream by truncated inverted repeats of IS*26* while no conserved integron regions were found. The genetic regions where antibiotic resistance genes were incorporated were highly similar to other plasmid-borne structures, previously described in different Gram-negative bacteria, suggesting acquisition of resistance determinants through horizontal gene transfer (**Figure 1**).

The *qnrD1* gene was enclosed in an 8,449 bp length contig (LGYC01000051: mean coverage of 183.9-fold and a total read count of 13,382), matching a Col3M plasmid. Indeed, the *qnrD1* gene is frequently located on small non-conjugative plasmids harbored by *Proteeae*, which was corroborated by our conjugation assay (Zhang et al., 2013). Furthermore, the *qnrD1* gene has been located in plasmids showing similarities with a specific *Providencia vermicola* plasmid, suggesting that these small non-conjugative plasmids might be the product of recombination between an unknown *qnrD*-bearing region and a native plasmid from *Proteeae*.

This contig accommodated a 2,683 bp sequence showing 99% identity with previously described *qnrD1*-harboring plasmids, such as pGHS09-09a (HQ834473) and pCGS49 (JQ776507), reported in France and China, respectively. The three *qnrD1*-encoding sequences shared a *rep* gene (also reported as *orf4*) and two additional *orfs* (**Figure 1F**) (Guillard et al., 2012; Zhang et al., 2013). Six single nucleotide variants (SNVs) were detected between *qnrD1*-INSRALV892a and the pGHS09-09a plasmid,

[3]http://blast.ncbi.nlm.nih.gov/Blast.cgi

[4]http://www.ncbi.nlm.nih.gov/nuccore/LGYC00000000.1

[5]http://www.eucast.org

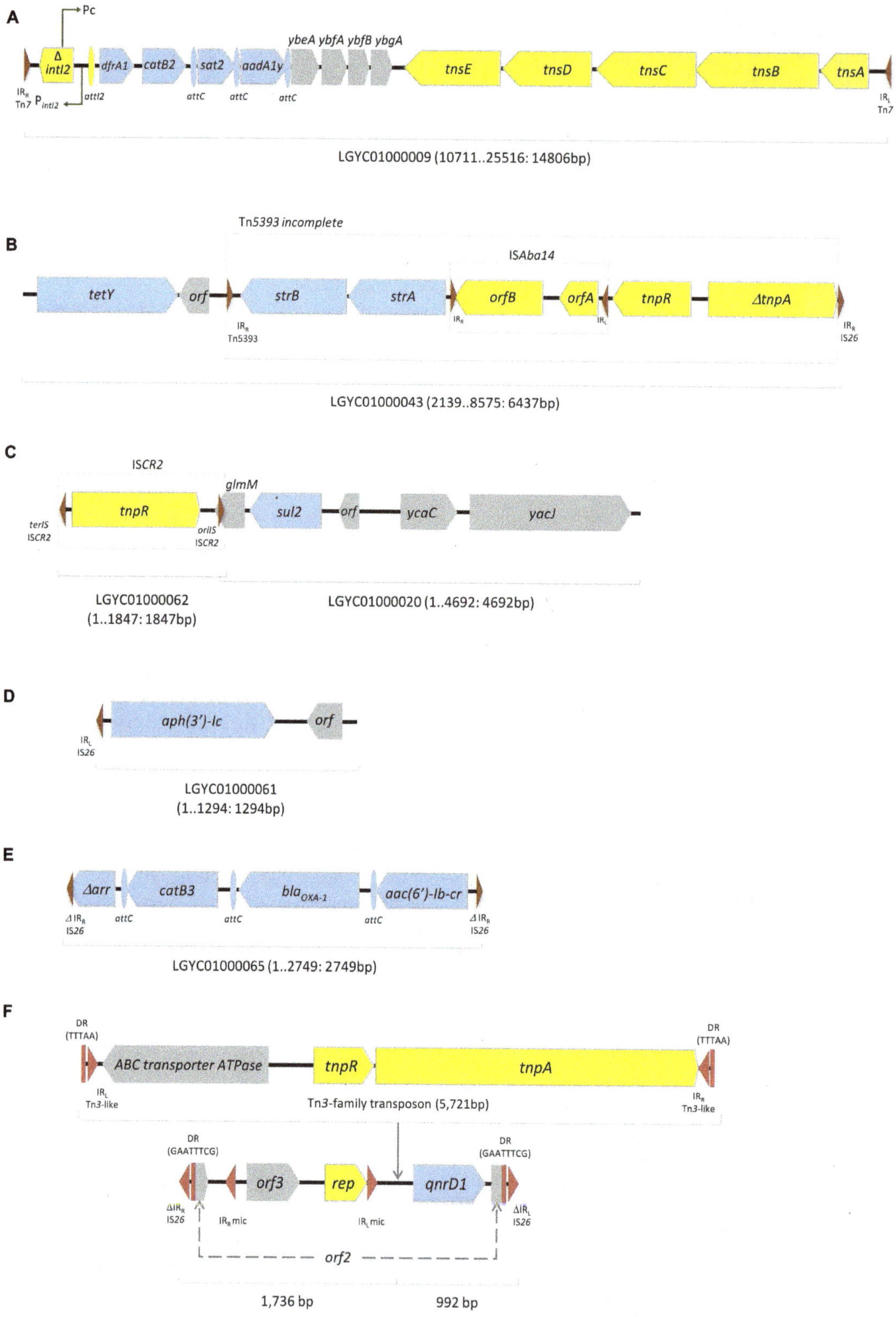

FIGURE 1 | Examples of contigs containing antibiotic resistance genes in *Morganella morganii* INSRALV892a. (A) *In2-17* class 2 integron encoding *dfrA1*, *catB2*, *sat2*, and *aadA1y*; **(B)** *tetY* and *strA-strB* associated to transposable elements; **(C)** *sul2* flanked upstream by IS*CR2*; **(D)** *aph(3')-Ic* associated to an IS*26* IR; **(E)** Δ*arr*, *catB3*, *bla*$_{OXA-1}$, and *aac(6')-Ib-cr* are bracketed by truncated IS*26* IR. **(F)** *qnrD1*-containing region. Blue, antibiotic resistance genes; Yellow, mobile genetic elements; Gray, other genes. Right and left inverted repeats (IR_R and IR_L) and direct repeats (DR) are indicated as red triangles and squares, respectively; mic, mobile insertion cassette.

two within the *rep* gene. Only one SNP was found with relation to pCGS49 in a non-coding region. The *qnrD1* gene was located within a mobile insertion cassette (mic) element bracketed by two inverted repeats, as previously described (Guillard et al., 2014) (**Figure 1F**).

Comparative bioinformatics analyses revealed the disruption of *orf2* caused by the insertion of IS*26* left and right inverted repeats flanking a region containing *orf3* and *rep*, within a mic, followed by *qnrD1*. In fact, this shows that is possible that LGYC01000051 contig could be either a Col3M plasmid missing an IS*26*-flanked region or a *qnrD1*-containing region that has become incorporated into a larger plasmid.

In addition, this region (**Figure 1F**) included three additional open reading frames: besides an ABC transporter-encoding gene perfectly matching a protein from *Aeromonas hydrophila*, this region harbored Tn*3*-like resolvases- and transposase-encoding genes, displaying *E. coli* plasmid pH226B (KX129784) as its best blast hit.

Mobile genetic elements are crucial tools for the acquisition of genetic diversity (Huddleston, 2014). Thus, we decided to search for and characterize the elements detected in the *M. morganii*'s genome. We identified 10 prophage regions, among which six were incomplete and four were intact, comprising 381 prophage-related genes. Intact prophage regions presented between 24.2 and 41.7 Kb and harbored 13–56 coding DNA sequences. The intact phages showing highest scores were assigned to Enterobacteria phage SfV, which is associated with O-antigen modification and serotype conversion in *Shigella flexneri*, and Enterobacteria phage mEp235 that consists of an unclassified Lambda-like virus (Sun et al., 2013). The bioinformatics detection of IS resulted in the identification of seven transposable elements: IS*3*, Tn*3*, IS*L3*, IS*256*, IS*6*, IS*91*, and IS*As1*. Besides the already mentioned Col3M no other typable plasmids were detected within the *M. morganii* genome, according with the PlasmidFinder tool.

Based on the probability scores assigned by PathogenFinder web-server (Cosentino et al., 2013), the isolate has a probability of acting as a human pathogen of 68.9%, which is in line with the opportunistic nature of this species. *M. morganii*'s genome matched 22 pathogenic families and 5 non-pathogenic families. Pathogenic factors showed diversity of functions and hosts, and included, for instance, transposase *insA* from IS*91* of *Salmonella enterica*, transposition protein *tnsE* of the Tn7 transposon of *S. flexneri*, and transcriptional regulator LysR family protein from *S. enterica*.

Multidrug resistant *M. morganii* isolates are rare and normally associated with non invasive nosocomial opportunistic infections in humans (Nicolle, 2001; Falagas et al., 2006). The detection of an avian *M. morganii* isolate harboring multiple and mobile antibiotic resistance genes and pathogenicity factors raises concerns regarding the dissemination of infection in birds and potential risk of zoonotic transmission. Several factors may affect the susceptibility of poultry to bacterial diseases, namely environmental stressors and previous antibiotic treatments, which are crucial to the development of infections involving different *Enterobacteriaceae* (Burkholder et al., 2008). The detection of an avian *M. morganii* isolate harboring multiple and mobile antibiotic resistance genes and pathogenicity factors raises concerns regarding the dissemination of infection in birds and potential risk of zoonotic transmission.

M. morganii is a well characterized opportunistic pathogen (Lee and Liu, 2006). However, its detection in poultry flocks, co-habiting the same hosts as other clinically important pathogens, makes it susceptible to the acquisition and donation of pathogenicity factors by horizontal gene transfer (Huddleston, 2014). To the best of our knowledge this report represents the first genome analysis of an isolate from animal origin carrying *qnrD1*. This genome sequence represents a valuable resource for studies on the epidemiology of zoonotic *M. morganii* isolates, and its features may be used as markers for the study of antibiotic resistance.

AUTHOR CONTRIBUTIONS

DJ-D designed the study, performed molecular experiments, analyzed the data and wrote the manuscript. LC performed the microbiological experiments and reviewed the manuscript. IM analyzed the data and reviewed the manuscript. TA, acquired laboratory data. DS and LV performed genome sequencing experiments. VM designed the study, analyzed the data and reviewed the manuscript. MC designed the study, reviewed and edited the manuscript. All authors read and approved the final manuscript.

FUNDING

DJ-D has received research funding from Fundação para a Ciência e a Tecnologia (FCT, grant number SFRH/BD/80001/2011). VM was supported by FCT fellowship (grant SFRH/BPD/77486/2011), financed by the European Social Funds (COMPETE-FEDER) and national funds of the Portuguese Ministry of Education and Science (POPH-QREN). We thank the support of FCT grant number PEst-OE/AGR/UI0211/2011-2014 and UID/MULTI/00211/2013.

REFERENCES

Abgottspon, H., Zurfluh, K., Nüesch-Inderbinen, M., Hächler, H., and Stephan, R. (2014). Quinolone resistance mechanisms in *Salmonella enterica* serovars Hadar, Kentucky, Virchow, Schwarzengrund, and 4,5,12:i:-, isolated from humans in Switzerland, and identification of a novel *qnrD* variant, *qnrD2*, in S. Hadar. *Antimicrob. Agents Chemother.* 58, 3560–3563. doi: 10.1128/AAC.02404-14

Abrahamian, F. M., and Goldstein, E. J. C. (2011). Microbiology of animal bite wound infections. *Clin. Microbiol. Rev.* 24, 231–246. doi: 10.1128/CMR.00041-10

Burkholder, K. M., Thompson, K. L., Einstein, M. E., Applegate, T. J., and Patterson, J. A. (2008). Influence of stressors on normal intestinal microbiota, intestinal morphology, and susceptibility to *Salmonella enteritidis* colonization in broilers. *Poult. Sci.* 87, 1734–1741. doi: 10.3382/ps.2008-00107

Carattoli, A., Zankari, E., Garcia-Fernandez, A., Voldby Larsen, M., Lund, O., Villa, L., et al. (2014). PlasmidFinder and pMLST: in silico detection and typing of plasmids. *Antimicrob. Agents Chemother.* 58, 3895–3903. doi: 10.1128/AAC.02412-14

Cavaco, L. M., Hasman, H., Xia, S., and Aarestrup, F. M. (2009). qnrD, a novel gene conferring transferable quinolone resistance in *Salmonella enterica* serovar Kentucky and Bovismorbificans strains of human origin. *Antimicrob. Agents Chemother.* 53, 603–608. doi: 10.1128/AAC.00997-08

Chen, Y. T., Peng, H. L., Shia, W. C., Hsu, F. R., Ken, C. F., Tsao, Y. M., et al. (2012). Whole-genome sequencing and identification of *Morganella morganii* KT pathogenicity-related genes. *BMC Genomics* 13(Suppl. 7):S4. doi: 10.1186/1471-2164-13-S7-S4

Choi, J. H., Yoo, H. S., Park, J. Y., Kim, Y. K., Kim, E., and Kim, D. Y. (2002). Morganelliasis pneumonia in a captive jaguar. *J. Wildl. Dis.* 38, 199–201. doi: 10.7589/0090-3558-38.1.199

Clemente, L., Manageiro, V., Ferreira, E., Jones-Dias, D., Correia, I., Themudo, P., et al. (2013). Occurrence of extended-spectrum β-lactamases among isolates of *Salmonella enterica* subsp. *enterica* from food-producing animals and food products, in Portugal. *Int. J. Food Microbiol.* 167, 221–228. doi: 10.1016/j.ijfoodmicro.2013.08.009

Cosentino, S., Voldby Larsen, M., Møller Aarestrup, F., and Lund, O. (2013). PathogenFinder: distinguishing friend from foe using bacterial whole genome sequence data. *PLoS ONE* 8:e77302. doi: 10.1371/journal.pone.0077302

Di Ianni, F., Dodi, P. L., Cabassi, C. S., Pelizzone, I., Sala, A., Cavirani, S., et al. (2015). Conjunctival flora of clinically normal and diseased turtles and tortoises. *BMC Vet. Res.* 10:91. doi: 10.1186/s12917-015-0405-x

Dipineto, L., Russo, T. P., Calabria, M., De Rosa, L., Capasso, M., Menna, L. F., et al. (2014). Oral flora of *Python regius* kept as pets. *Lett. Appl. Microbiol.* 58, 462–465. doi: 10.1111/lam.12214

Falagas, M. E., Kavvadia, P. K., Mantadakis, E., Kofteridis, D. P., Bliziotis, I. A., Saloustros, E., et al. (2006). *Morganella morganii* infections in a general tertiary hospital. *Infection* 34, 315–321. doi: 10.1007/s15010-006-6682-3

Guillard, T., Cambau, E., Neuwirth, C., Nenninger, T., Mbadi, A., Brasme, L., et al. (2012). Description of a 2,683-base-pair plasmid containing *qnrD* in two *Providencia rettgeri* isolates. *Antimicrob. Agents Chemother.* 56, 565–568. doi: 10.1128/AAC.00081-11

Guillard, T., Grillon, A., de Champs, C., Cartier, C., Madoux, J., Berçot, B., et al. (2014). Mobile insertion cassette elements found in small non-transmissible plasmids in *Proteeae* may explain *qnrD* mobilization. *PLoS ONE* 9:e87801. doi: 10.1371/journal.pone.0087801

Harris, P. N. A., and Ferguson, J. K. (2012). Antibiotic therapy for inducible AmpC β-lactamase-producing Gram-negative bacilli: what are the alternatives to carbapenems, quinolones and aminoglycosides? *Int. J. Antimicrob. Agents* 40, 297–305. doi: 10.1016/j.ijantimicag.2012.06.004

Huddleston, J. R. (2014). Horizontal gene transfer in the human gastrointestinal tract: potential spread of antibiotic resistance genes. *Infect. Drug Resist.* 7, 167–176. doi: 10.2147/IDR.S48820

Jacoby, G., Strahilevitz, J., and Hooper, D. (2014). Plasmid-mediated quinolone resistance. *Microbiol. Spectr.* 2:PLAS-0006-2013. doi: 10.1128/microbiolspec.PLAS-0006-2013

Jones-Dias, D., Manageiro, V., and Caniça, M. (2016). Influence of agricultural practice on mobile *bla* genes: IncI1-bearing CTX-M, SHV, CMY and TEM in *Escherichia coli* from intensive farming soils. *Environ. Microbiol.* 18, 260–272. doi: 10.1111/1462-2920.13021

Lee, I., and Liu, J. (2006). Clinical characteristics and risk factors for mortality in *Morganella morganii* bacteremia. *J. Microbiol. Immunol. Infect.* 39, 328–334.

Lin, T. Y., Chan, M. C., Yang, Y. S., Lee, Y., Yeh, K. M., Lin, J. C., et al. (2015). Clinical manifestations and prognostic factors of *Morganella morganii* bacteremia. *Eur. J. Clin.Microbiol. Infect. Dis.* 34, 231–236. doi: 10.1007/s10096-014-2222-8

Mazzariol, A., Kocsis, B., Koncan, R., Kocsis, E., Lanzafame, P., and Cornaglia, G. (2012). Description and plasmid characterization of *qnrD* determinants in *Proteus mirabilis* and *Morganella morganii*. *Clin. Microbiol. Infect.* 18, E46–E48. doi: 10.1111/j.1469-0691.2011.03728.x

Nasri Yaiche, M., Denden Rafraf, I., Guo, Q., Mastouri, M., Aouni, M., and Wang, M. (2014). Type II and type IV topoisomerase mutations in clinical isolates of *Morganella morganii* harbouring the *qnrD* gene. *Ann. Clin. Microbiol. Antimicrob.* 13:34. doi: 10.1186/s12941-014-0034-4

Nicolle, L. E. (2001). Urinary tract pathogens in complicated infection and in elderly individuals. *J. Infect. Dis.* 183(Suppl. 1), S5–S8. doi: 10.1086/318844

O'Hara, C. M., Brenner, F. W., and Miller, J. M. (2000). Classification, identification, and clinical significance of *Proteus*, *Providencia*, and *Morganella*. *Clin. Microbiol. Rev.* 13:534–546. doi: 10.1128/CMR.13.4.534-546.2000

Ono, M., Namimatsu, T., Ohsumi, T., Mori, M., Okada, M., and Tamura, K. (2001). Immunohistopathologic demonstration of pleuropneumonia associated with *Morganella morganii* in a piglet. *Vet. Pathol.* 38, 336–339. doi: 10.1354/vp.38-3-336

Poirel, L., Cattoir, V., and Nordmann, P. (2012). Plasmid-mediated quinolone resistance; interactions between human, animal, and environmental ecologies. *Front. Microbiol.* 3:24. doi: 10.3389/fmicb.2012.00024

Sun, Q., Lan, R., Wang, Y., Wang, J., Wang, Y., Li, P., et al. (2013). Isolation and genomic characterization of SfI, a serotype-converting bacteriophage of *Shigella flexneri*. *BMC Microbiol.* 17:39. doi: 10.1186/1471-2180-13-39

Tamang, M. D., Nam, H. M., Kim, A., Lee, H. S., Kim, T. S., Kim, M. J., et al. (2011). Prevalence and mechanisms of quinolone resistance among selected nontyphoid *Salmonella* isolated from food animals and humans in Korea. *Foodborne Pathog. Dis.* 8, 1199–1206. doi: 10.1089/fpd.2011.0899

Tavares, I. M., Leitão, J. H., and Sá-Correia, I. (2003). Chromosomal organization and transcription analysis of genes in the vicinity of *Pseudomonas aeruginosa glmM* gene encoding phosphoglucosamine mutase. *Biochem. Biophys. Res. Commun.* 302, 363–371. doi: 10.1016/S0006-291X(03)00169-4

Tsanaktsidis, G., Agarwal, S. A., Maloof, A. J., Chandra, J., and Mitchell, P. (2003). Postoperative *Morganella morganii* endophthalmitis associated with subclinical urinary tract infection. *J. Cataract Refract. Surg.* 29, 1011–1013. doi: 10.1016/S0886-3350(02)01847-3

Varani, A. M., Siguier, P., Gourbeyre, E., Charneau, V., and Chandler, M. (2011). ISsaga is an ensemble of web-based methods for high throughput identification and semi-automatic annotation of insertion sequences in prokaryotic genomes. *Genome Biol.* 12:R30. doi: 10.1186/gb-2011-12-3-r30

Zankari, E., Hasman, H., Cosentino, S., Vestergaard, M., Rasmussen, S., Lund, O., et al. (2012). Identification of acquired antimicrobial resistance genes. *J. Antimicrob. Chemother.* 67, 2640–2644. doi: 10.1093/jac/dks261

Zhang, S., Sun, J., Liao, X.-P., Hu, Q.-J., Liu, B.-T., Fang, L.-X., et al. (2013). Prevalence and plasmid characterization of the qnrD determinant in *Enterobacteriaceae* isolated from animals, retail meat products, and humans. *Microb. Drug Resist.* 19, 331–335. doi: 10.1089/mdr.2012.0146

Zhao, C., Tang, N., Wu, Y., Zhang, Y., Wu, Z., Li, W., et al. (2012). First reported fatal *Morganella morganii* infections in chickens. *Vet. Microbiol.* 156, 452–455. doi: 10.1016/j.vetmic.2011.11.021

Zhou, Y., Liang, Y., Lynch, K. H., Dennis, J. J., and Wishart, D. S. (2011). PHAST: a fast phage search tool. *Nucleic Acids Res.* 39, W347–W352. doi: 10.1093/nar/gkr485

3

Regulation of the Two-Component Regulator CpxR on Aminoglycosides and β-lactams Resistance in *Salmonella enterica* serovar Typhimurium

Hui Huang [1†], ***Yawei Sun*** [1,2†], ***Li Yuan*** [1†], ***Yushan Pan*** [1], ***Yanlin Gao*** [3], ***Caihui Ma*** [1] **and** ***Gongzheng Hu*** [1*]

[1] *College of Veterinary Medicine, Henan Agricultural University, Zhengzhou, China,* [2] *College of Animal Science and Technology, Henan Institute of Science and Technology, Xinxiang, China,* [3] *Animal Husbandry Bureau of Henan Province, Zhengzhou, China*

***Correspondence:**
Gongzheng Hu
yaolilab@126.com

[†] *These authors have contributed equally to this work.*

The two-component signal transduction system CpxAR is especially widespread in Gram-negative bacteria. It has been reported that CpxAR contributes to the multidrug resistance (MDR) in *Escherichia coli*. CpxR is a response regulator in the two-component CpxAR system. The aim of this study was to explore the role of *cpxR* in the MDR of *S. enterica* serovar Typhimurium. The minimal inhibitory concentrations (MICs) of various antibiotics commonly used in veterinary medicine for strains JS (a multidrug-susceptible standard strain of *S. enterica* serovar Typhimurium), JS△*cpxR*, JS△*cpxR*/p*cpxR*, JS△*cpxR*/p*cpxR**, JS△*cpxR*△*acrB*, JS△*cpxR*△*acrB*/p*cpxR*, JS△*cpxR*△*acrB*/p*cpxR**, 9 *S. enterica* serovar Typhimurium isolates (SH1–9), and SH1–9△*cpxR* were determined by the 2-fold broth microdilution method. The relative mRNA expression levels of *ompF*, *ompC*, *ompW*, *ompD*, *tolC*, *acrB*, *acrD*, *acrF*, *mdtA*, *marA*, and *soxS* in strains JS, JS△*cpxR*, and JS△*cpxR*/p*cpxR* were detected by real-time PCR. The results showed 2- to 4-fold decreases in the MICs of amikacin (AMK), gentamycin (GEN), apramycin (APR), neomycin (NEO), ceftriaxone (CRO), ceftiofur (CEF), and cefquinome (CEQ) for strain JS△*cpxR*, as compared to those for the parental strain JS. Likewise, SH1–9△*cpxR* were found to have 2- to 8-fold reduction in resistance to the above antibiotics, except for NEO, as compared to their parental strains SH1–9. Furthermore, 2- to 4-fold further decreases in the MICs of AMK, GEN, APR, and CEF for strain JS△*cpxR*△*acrB* were observed, as compared to those for strain JS△*acrB*. In addition, CpxR overproduction in strain JS△*cpxR* led to significant decreases in the mRNA expression levels of *ompF*, *ompC*, *ompW*, *ompD, tolC*, *acrB*, *marA*, and *soxS*, and significant increases in those of *stm3031* and *stm1530*. Notably, after all strains were induced simultaneously by GEN to the 15th passage at subinhibitory concentrations, strain JS△*cpxR*/p*cpxR* showed significant increases in mRNA expression levels of the efflux pump *acrD* and *mdtA* genes, as compared to strain JS△*cpxR*. Our results indicate that the two-component regulator CpxR contributes to resistance of *S. enterica* serovar Typhimurium to aminoglycosides and β-lactams by influencing the expression level of the MDR-related genes.

Keywords: *S. enterica* serovar Typhimurium, CpxR, aminoglycosides, β-lactams, resistance, AcrD

INTRODUCTION

Salmonella enterica serovar Typhimurium is a food-borne pathogen that causes gastroenteritis in humans (Scherer and Miller, 2001) and fowl typhoid in poultry (Barrow et al., 2004). The prevalence of multidrug-resistant (MDR) *S. enterica* species in many parts of the world has become a significant public health concern. Drug resistance in many cases is attributable to synergy between reduced drug intake (mainly due to low outer membrane permeability) (Pagès et al., 2008; Li and Nikaido, 2009) and active drug export (via efflux pumps) (Zgurskaya and Nikaido, 2000; Pagès et al., 2010). Resistance nodulation-cell division (RND)-family efflux systems (including AcrAB, AcrAD, AcrEF, MdtEF, and MdtABC) are especially effective in generating resistance in Gram negative bacteria (Nikaido, 1996) and often have a wide substrate specificity (Nikaido and Pagès, 2012). In *Escherichia coli*, all five RND-family drug exporters confer resistance to β-lactam antibiotics (Nishino et al., 2003), and *acrD* is also known to participate in the efflux of aminoglycosides (Rosenberg et al., 2000; Nishino and Yamaguchi, 2001a; Aires and Nikaido, 2005; Nishino et al., 2007). Some outer membrane proteins, especially OmpF, OmpC, and OmpW, have been shown to contribute to antibiotic resistance in *E. coli* and *Salmonella* typhimurium (Nikaido, 2003). In addition, OmpD, STM3031, and STM1530 are associated with ceftriaxone (CRO) resistance in *S. enterica* serovar Typhimurium (Hu et al., 2011), and OmpW participates in resistance to neomycin (NEO) and ampicillin (AMP) in *E. coli* (Wu et al., 2012).

Two-component signal transduction systems (TCSs) are key in the sensory response of bacteria (Parkinson and Kofoid, 1992). Studies have elucidated that the TCSs EvgA and BaeR contribute to MDR by modulating production of the multidrug transporter in *E. coli* (Nishino and Yamaguchi, 2001b; Baranova and Nikaido, 2002; Nishino and Yamaguchi, 2002). The Cpx envelope stress response is controlled by a TCS consisting of the membrane localized sensor kinase CpxA and the regulator CpxR. CpxR mediates the output response as a transcriptional regulator through phosphorylation of its receiver domain with an aspartate (D51) moiety (Stephenson and Hoch, 2002; MacRitchie et al., 2008). Phosphorylated CpxR (CpxR-P), which functions as a transcription factor, activates and, in a small number of cases, represses transcription of target genes by binding to the promoter of target genes at the consensus sequence 5′-GTAAAN$_5$GTAAA-3′ (De Wulf et al., 2002; Price and Raivio, 2009). In addition, the response regulator CpxR is also activated by some signals without the involvement of CpxA. For example, some cytoplasmic or growth signals, as well as excess carbon (glucose or pyruvate) in growth medium both activate CpxR independently of CpxA (Cuny et al., 2007; Wolfe et al., 2008).

In recent years, the CpxAR two-component system conferring resistance to antibacterial agent has received special attention. In *E. coli*, CpxR overproduction was found to confer resistance to β-lactams in an *acrB*-free background (Hirakawa et al., 2003a). CpxR-P also confers resistance to fosfomycin by directly repressing the expression of two genes, *glpT* and *uhpT*, in the enterohemorrhagic *E. coli* (EHEC) strain O157:H7 (Kurabayashi et al., 2014). Moreover, the CpxAR pathway contributes to *E. coli* resistance to antimicrobial peptides, such as ApoEdpl-W, polymyxin B, and melittin (Audrain et al., 2013) and protamine (Weatherspoon-Griffin et al., 2014). In *Klebsiella pneumoniae*, CpxR was able to directly bind to the promoter regions of *ompC*^{KP}and *kpnEF*, which contribute to the *K. Pneumoniae* MDR phenotype (Srinivasan et al., 2012; Srinivasan and Rajamohan, 2013). In *S. enterica* serovar Typhimurium, studies about the effect of *cpxR* on the resistance are still very limited, only few reports showed CpxAR confers resistance to CRO (Hu et al., 2011) and the antimicrobial peptides protamine, magainin, and melittin (Weatherspoon-Griffin et al., 2011). However, whether CpxAR plays a role in resistance of *S. enterica* serovar Typhimurium especially clinical isolates to aminoglycosides and β-lactams and the molecular mechanisms underlying resistance to aminoglycosides and β-lactams remain unknown. In this study, we systematically investigated the role of *cpxR* in aminoglycoside and β-lactam resistance in both susceptible strains and clinical isolates of *S. enterica* serovar Typhimurium, and also explored the molecular mechanisms of CpxAR that confer resistance to aminoglycosides and β-lactams.

MATERIALS AND METHODS

Bacterial Strains, Plasmids, and Bacteriophage

The bacterial strains, plasmids, and bacteriophage used in this study are listed in **Table 1**. *Salmonella enterica* serovar Typhimurium strain CVCC541, a clinical susceptible strain isolated from chicken in Changchun City, China, was supplied by the China Institute of Veterinary Drug Control (Beijing, China) and designated as JS in this report. Strains JS△*cpxR* and JS△*acrB* were generated from JS using the one-step inactivation of chromosomal genes method. Strain JS△*acrB*△*cpxR* was constructed by the phage P22-mediated transduction method using strain JS△*cpxR* as the donor and JS△*acrB* as the recipient. In this study, nine *S. enterica* serovar Typhimurium isolates were isolated from chickens collected from nine different regions of Henan province in China and named SH1–9.

Construction of the Expression Plasmids pBAD-CpxR and pBAD-CpxR*

The complete open reading frame of *cpxR* was amplified by PCR with primers *Xho*lI-*cpxR*-F/*Hind*III-*cpxR*-R (**Table 2**) from the genomic DNA of strain JS. The mutation sequence *cpxR**, which encodes a CpxR variant with an alanine residue at position 51 in place of aspartate, was engineered by overlapping PCR (Urban et al., 1997; Huang et al., 1999). The mutation site was generated through the design of primers Fm and Rm (**Table 2**). Three PCR reactions were performed to obtain the mutation sequence *cpxR**. Primers *Xho*lI-*cpxR*-F/Rm were used for amplification of the anterior segment of *cpxR*, primers Fm/*Hind*III-*cpxR*-R were used for amplification of the second part of *cpxR*, and the primers *Xho*lI-*cpxR*-F/*Hind*III-*cpxR*-R were used for splicing by overlap extension PCR. Finally, the expression plasmids pBAD-CpxR and pBAD-CpxR* were generated by inserting the target fragment to the multiple cloning site of vector pBAD. The expression level of

TABLE 1 | Bacterial strains, plasmids, and phage used in this study.

Strain, plasmid, or phage	Relevant characteristics	References or source
STRAINS		
JS	*S. enterica* Serovar Typhimurium CVCC541	Supplied by China Institute of Veterinary Drug Control
JSΔ*cpxR*	Derivative of JS that lacks *cpxR*	Huang et al., 2015
JSΔ*acrB*	Derivative of JS that lacks *acrB*	Huang et al., 2016
JSΔ*acrB*Δ*cpxR*	Derivative of JS that lacks both *cpxR* and *acrB*, Δ*cpxR::kan*	Huang et al., 2016
SH(1–9)	Clinical isolates from chicken in Henan province in China	This study
SH(1–9) Δ*cpxR*	Derivative of SH(1–9) that lack *cpxR*, Δ*cpxR::kan*	This study
PLASMIDS		
pKD4	Gene knowout help vector: $rep_{R6K\gamma}$ Ap^R FRT Km^R FRT	From *E. coli* Genetic Stock Center in Yale University
pKD46	Gene knowout help vector: rep^{ts}_{pSC101} Ap^R P_{araBAD} γ β exo	
pBAD	Expression vector: $rep_{pBR322}Ap^R$ araC P_{BAD}	Invitrogen Corporation
pBAD-CpxR	cpxR gene cloned to pBAD; Ap^R	This study
pBAD-CpxR*	Mutation sequence CpxR* cloned to pBAD; Ap^R	This study
PHAGE		
P22HT105/int	Transduction medium of *Salmonella*	Supplied by Microbial Genomics Research Center of Harbin Medical University

target proteins were determined according to the concentration of the inducer L-arabinose (Guzman et al., 1995).

Construction of *cpxR*-Deficient Mutants of *S. enterica* Serovar Typhimurium Isolates

The generation of strain JSΔ*cpxR::kan* was described in our previous study (Huang et al., 2015). The deletions were then transferred to nine *S. enterica* serovar Typhimurium isolates (SH1–9) by P22HT105/int transductions as previously described (Davis et al., 1980; Mann and Slauch, 1997). Nine *cpxR*-deficient mutants were designated as SH1–9Δ*cpxR* in this study.

Antibiotic Susceptibility Testing

The minimal inhibitory concentrations (MICs) of selected antibiotics for all strains were determined by the 2-fold broth microdilution method according to the CLSI guidelines (Clinical and Laboratory Standards Institute, 2008, 2012). The antibiotics used for susceptibility determination were gentamycin (GEN), amikacin (AMK), apramycin (APR), NEO, CRO, ceftiofur (CEF), CEQ. *E. coli* ATCC 25922 was used for quality control in all susceptibility tests. All tests were performed independently at least three times.

GEN Induction Testing

A single colony of each tested strain (JS, JSΔ*cpxR*, and JSΔ*cpxR*/p*cpxR*) was cultured in Luria-Bertani (LB) medium containing a 50% MIC of GEN at 37°C for 18 h. After growth overnight at 37°C, the cultures was diluted 1:100 in LB medium and cultured at 37°C for 18 h, and simultaneously the inducer GEN was added at subinhibitory concentrations. GEN induction testing of the strains was performed for 15 generations in this way.

Expression Levels of MDR-Related Genes

Total RNA was isolated from bacterial cultures using the MiniBEST Universal RNA Extraction Kit (TaKaRa Bio, Inc. Shiga, Japan) according to the manufacturer's instructions. OD260/OD280 values of total RNA were detected using a trace nucleic acid protein analyzer spectrophotometer (NanoDrop; Thermo Fisher Scientific, Waltham, MA, USA). Bulk cDNA samples were synthesized from total RNA using the PrimeScript™RT reagent Kit with gDNA Eraser (TaKaRa Bio, Inc.). The synthesized cDNA was confirmed by PCR and stored at -20°C until used. Real-time PCR was performed using the LightCycler®480 System (Roche Diagnostics, Indianapolis, IN, USA) with specific primer pairs (**Table 2**), cDNA template, and TaKaRa SYBR Premix Ex Taq II (TaKaRa Bio, Inc.). The 16S rRNA gene was chosen as a housekeeping gene. To precisely test the relative expression level of the genes of interest, standard curves of the amplification of all detected genes were individually established. CT values tested came within the linearity range for PCR amplification. Each sample was independently run at least twice. The $2^{-\Delta(\Delta CT)}$ method was used to calculate altered folds of the gene tested in the mutants, as compared to that in JS. Three independent experiments were performed under the same conditions.

Statistical Analysis

Statistical analysis was performed using SPSS version 17.0 software (IBM-SPSS, Inc., Chicago, IL, USA). Data were compared using the Student's *t*-test. A probability (p) value of > 0.05 was considered statistically significant.

RESULTS

Deletion of *cpxR* Increases Susceptibility of JS to aminoglycosides and β-lactams

To examine whether the response regulator CpxR contributes to the drug resistance of *S. enterica* serovar Typhimurium, a *cpxR* deletion mutant, JSΔ*cpxR*, was generated from strain JS, and the complementary strain JSΔ*cpxR*/p*cpxR* was prepared through the introduction of the expression plasmid pBAD-CpxR into

TABLE 2 | Sequences of primers used in this study.

Function	Primer	Sequence (5′ → 3′)	References or source
Amplification of *cpxR* gene	*XhoI*-*cpxR*-F *HindIII*-*cpxR*-R	CGCTCGAGATGAATAAAATCCTGTTAGT GCAAGCTTTCATGAAGCGGAAACCATCA	This study
Preparation of *cpxR**	*XhoI*-*cpxR*-F Rm	CGCTCGAGATGAATAAAATCCTGTTAGT ACTTTTGCTTGCCGTCATGATGCCGAAG	This study
	Fm *Hind* III-*cpxR*-R	CTTCGGCATCATGACGGCAAGCAAAAGT GCAAGCTTTCATGAAGCGGAAACCATCA	This study
REAL-TIME RELATIVE QUANTITATIVE PCR			
ompF	*ompF*-F *ompF*-R	CCTGGCAGCGGTGATCC AAATTTCTGCTGCGTTTGCG	Tatavarthy and Cannons, 2010
ompC	*ompC*-F *ompC*-R	TCGCAGCCTGCTGAACCAGAAC ACGGGTTGCGTTATAGGTCTGAG	Hu et al., 2011
ompD	*ompD*-F *ompD*-R	GCAACCGTACTGAAAGCCAGGG GCCAAAGAAGTCAGTGTTACGGT	Hu et al., 2011
ompW	*ompW*-F *ompW*-R	CAGCAGCAAAGTGCGTCCTTATGT AGACAGAGGCGCCAATTAACCAGT	Hu et al., 2011
stm3031	*stm3031*-F *stm3031*-R	TGCAAGCAGGGAGTAATAACGGGT TCACTTGGATACGCCCAGTCCCAT	Hu et al., 2011
stm1530	*stm1530*-F *stm1530*-R	CGTCTCGGTTTTGCTGGTTTGG GCCGTCATTTTTACCCTGATACTGC	Hu et al., 2011
acrB	*acrB*-F *acrB*-R	CGTGAGCGTTGAGAAGTCCT GGCGTCAGTTGGTATTTGGT	Li et al., 2009
acrD	*acrD*-F *acrD*-R	TCCGGCCAAATTGAATAGTT TCGGAACCGTCCTGATTAAC	Eaves et al., 2004
acrF	*acrF*-F *acrF*-R	TATCTGGCTGGATGCGAATCTGCT ACTTTGCCGAACTCTTCCGGATCT	Eaves et al., 2004
mdtA	*mdtA*-F *mdtA*-R	GAATGCGCGTCGTGATCTG TCCAGTTCCTGACGGGAAAC	Nishino et al., 2007
marA	*marA*-F *marA*-R	ATACATCCGCAGCCGTAAAA GTGATTCGCCATGCATATTG	Li et al., 2009
soxS	*soxS*-F *soxS*-R	TACGGTAACGCATCAAACA ACAGGCGGTGACGGTAAT	Li et al., 2009
16SrRNA	16SrRNA-F 16SrRNA-R	TTAGATACCCTGGTAGTCCACGC TTGCGGGACTTAACCCAAC	Li et al., 2009

The underlined bases are restriction sites.

JS△*cpxR*. The MICs of a number of antibiotics for strain JS and JS△*cpxR* were then determined. As shown in **Table 3**, strain JS△*cpxR* showed 2–4-fold decreases in the MICs of GEN, AMK, APR, NEO, CRO, CEF, and CEQ, as compared to the parental strain JS. The MICs of the above antibiotics increased by 4-fold for the complementary strain JS△*cpxR*/p*cpxR*, as compared to those for JS△*cpxR*. These results clearly suggest that *cpxR* plays an important role in conferring resistance of *S. enterica* serovar Typhimurium to aminoglycosides and β-lactams. In addition, JS△*cpxR*/p*cpxR** exhibited the same susceptibility as JS△*cpxR* to the tested antibiotics except for CEQ, which demonstrates that the susceptibility changes of *S. enterica* serovar Typhimurium to the tested antibiotics was mediated by CpxR-P.

Effects of Deletion of *acrB* on *cpxR*-Mediated Multidrug Resistance

In susceptible *S. enterica* serovar Typhimurium, the AcrAB efflux pump is constitutively expressed and plays a predominant role in intrinsic and acquired resistance (Mazzariol et al., 2000; Nishino et al., 2006). It has wild substrate spectrum and can capture substrates from the periplasm or the outer leaflet of the cytoplasmic membrane (Yu et al., 2003). Therefore, AcrAB may mask partial function of some efflux pumps located in the cytoplasmic membrane (Hirakawa et al., 2003a,b; Eaves et al., 2004; Nishino et al., 2007). To clarify the role of CpxR in resistance conferred by other efflux pumps, an *acrB* deletion mutant (JS△*acrB*) and a double deletion mutant (JS△*acrB*△*cpxR*) were generated from strain JS. The *cpxR* complementary strain JS△*acrB*△*cpxR*/p*cpxR* was prepared as described above. The MICs of various antibiotics for strains JS△*acrB*, JS△*acrB*△*cpxR*, and JS△*acrB*△*cpxR*/p*cpxR* were then determined. As shown in **Table 3**, strain JS△*acrB*△*cpxR* showed 2–4-fold decreases in the MICs of GEN, AMK, APR, NEO, and CEF, as compared to strain JS△*acrB*, while the complementary strain JS△*acrB*△*cpxR*/p*cpxR* exhibited 2–8-fold increases in the MICs of GEN, AMK, APR, NEO, CRO, CEF, and CEQ, as compared to strain JS△*acrB*△*cpxR*.

TABLE 3 | Susceptibility of *S. enterica* serovar Typhimurium to several antibiotics.

Strain	MICs (μg/mL)								
	AMK	GEN	APR	NEO	CRO	CEF	CEQ	ENR	CIP
JS	0.5	0.25	2	0.4	0.02	0.32	0.08	0.032	0.016
JSΔ*cpxR*	0.125	0.0625	1	0.1	0.01	0.08	0.04	0.032	0.016
JSΔ*cpxR*/p*cpxR*	0.5	0.25	4	0.4	0.04	0.32	0.16	0.032	0.016
JSΔ*cpxR*/p*cpxR**	0.125	0.0625	1	0.1	0.01	0.08	0.16	0.032	0.016
JSΔ*acrB*	0.25	0.25	2	0.2	0.01	0.0025	0.02	0.001	0.001
JSΔ*acrB*Δ*cpxR*	0.0625	0.0625	0.5	6.4▲	0.01	0.00125	0.02	0.001	0.001
JSΔ*acrB*Δ*cpxR*/p*cpxR*	0.5	0.25	2	25.6▲	0.02	0.005	0.08	0.001	0.001
JSΔ*acrB*Δ*cpxR*/p*cpxR*▲	0.0625	0.0625	0.5	6.4▲	0.01	0.00125	0.04	0.001	0.001

AMK, Amikacin; GEN, Gentamycin; APR, Apramycin; NEO, Neomycin; CRO, Ceftriaxone; CEF, Ceftiofur; CEQ, Cefquinome; ENR, Enrofloxacin; CIP, Ciprofloxacin.
▲High NEO resistance is present in strains because of the replacement of cpxR gene by kanamycin-resistant gene (ΔcpxR::kan).

TABLE 4 | Susceptibilities of *S. enterica* serovar Typhimurium isolates to antibiotics after *cpxR* were deleted.

Strains	MICs (μg/mL)						
	AMK	GEN	APR	NEO	CRO	CEF	CEQ
SH1	1.25	1	2	0.8	0.5	4	1
SH1Δ*cpxR*	0.625	0.125	0.5	12.8▲	0.5	2	1
SH2	5	32	4	0.4	0.5	4	0.5
SH2Δ*cpxR*	1.25	16	2	6.4▲	0.25	2	0.25
SH3	2	0.2	4	0.4	0.1	0.8	0.05
SH3Δ*cpxR*	0.5	0.1	1	6.4▲	0.05	0.4	0.05
SH4	1	0.4	2	0.4	0.05	0.8	0.1
SH4Δ*cpxR*	0.5	0.1	1	6.4▲	0.05	0.4	0.05
SH5	1	0.4	4	0.4	0.05	0.8	0.1
SH5Δ*cpxR*	0.5	0.2	2	3.2▲	0.05	0.4	0.05
SH6	0.4	0.2	8	0.8	0.1	0.2	0.1
SH6Δ*cpxR*	0.1	0.05	2	12.8▲	0.05	0.2	0.1
SH7	1.6	12.8	1024	1.6	0.1	1.6	0.2
SH7Δ*cpxR*	0.4	3.2	256	12.8▲	0.05	0.8	0.1
SH8	0.4	0.2	4	0.8	0.2	0.4	0.1
SH8Δ*cpxR*	0.2	0.1	2	12.8▲	0.05	0.1	0.05
SH9	0.8	0.4	4	0.8	0.1	0.8	0.05
SH9Δ*cpxR*	0.1	0.05	1	12.8▲	0.05	0.4	0.025

AMK, Amikacin; GEN, Gentamycin; APR, Apramycin; NEO, Neomycin; CRO, Ceftriaxone; CEF, Ceftiofur; CEQ, Cefquinome.
▲High NEO resistance is present in strains because of the replacement of cpxR gene by the kanamycin-resistant gene (ΔcpxR::kan).

These results revealed that CpxR can modulate resistance of *S. enterica* serovar Typhimurium to aminoglycosides and β-lactams in both *acrB* and Δ*acrB* backgrounds.

Role of *cpxR* in drug Resistance of *S. enterica* Serovar Typhimurium Isolates

To determinate the role of *cpxR* in regulating drug resistance of *S. enterica* serovar Typhimurium isolates, nine *cpxR*-deficient mutants (SH1–9Δ*cpxR*) derived from nine *S. enterica* serovar Typhimurium isolates (SH1–9) were constructed. The MICs for SH1–9 and SH1–9Δ*cpxR* to the above antibiotics were then determined. As shown in **Table 4**, among the nine *cpxR* deletion strains, all showed 2–4-fold decreases in the MICs of GEN, AMK, APR, and CEF, six revealed 2–4-fold decreases in the MIC of CRO, and six revealed 2–4-fold decreases in the MIC of CEQ, compared with their parental strains. These results indicate that *cpxR* also plays an important role in resistance of *S. enterica* serovar Typhimurium isolates to aminoglycosides and β-lactams.

Effects of *cpxR* on the expression Levels of a Series of MDR-Related Genes

In *E. coli*, it has been confirmed that *cpxR* can modulate the expression of the outer membrane proteins OmpF and OmpC (Batchelor et al., 2005), and the transporter MdtABC (Hirakawa et al., 2005). In *S. enterica* serovar Typhimurium, the expression of OmpD, STM3031, and STM1530 plays important roles in *cpxR*-mediated CRO resistance (Hu et al., 2011). In order to determine whether the drug resistance mediated by *cpxR* is due to altered expression levels of MDR-related genes, we detected the relative mRNA expression of a series of MDR-related genes. As shown in **Figure 1**, JS△*cpxR* showed no significant differences in the mRNA expression levels of all tested genes, as compared to strain JS, while the mRNA expression levels of *ompF*, *ompC*, *ompW*, *ompD*, *acrB*, *tolC*, *marA*, and *soxS* genes in strain JS△*cpxR*/p*cpxR* were significantly decreased ($p < 0.01$ or $p < 0.05$) relative to strain JS△*cpxR* (**Figures 1A,C,D**) and the mRNA levels of *stm3031* and *stm1530* in strain JS△*cpxR*/p*cpxR* were significantly increased ($p < 0.01$ or $p < 0.05$) relative to strain JS△*cpxR* (**Figure 1B**). There were no significant differences in mRNA expression levels of *acrD* and *mdtA* among strains JS, JS△*cpxR*, and JS△*cpxR*/p*cpxR* (**Figure 1C**). The expression levels of AcrF in these three strains were all very low and almost undetectable (data not shown). However, after all strains were induced by GEN at subinhibitory concentrations to the 15th passage simultaneously, strain JS△*cpxR*/p*cpxR* showed significant ($p < 0.01$) increases in the mRNA expression levels of *mdtA* and *acrD*, as compared to JS△*cpxR* (**Figure 1E**). These results suggest that the overexpression of *cpxR* can downregulate the expression levels of OmpF, OmpC, OmpW, OmpD, AcrB, TolC, MarA, and SoxS and upregulate those of STM3031 and STM1530 in susceptible *S. enterica* serovar Typhimurium strains,

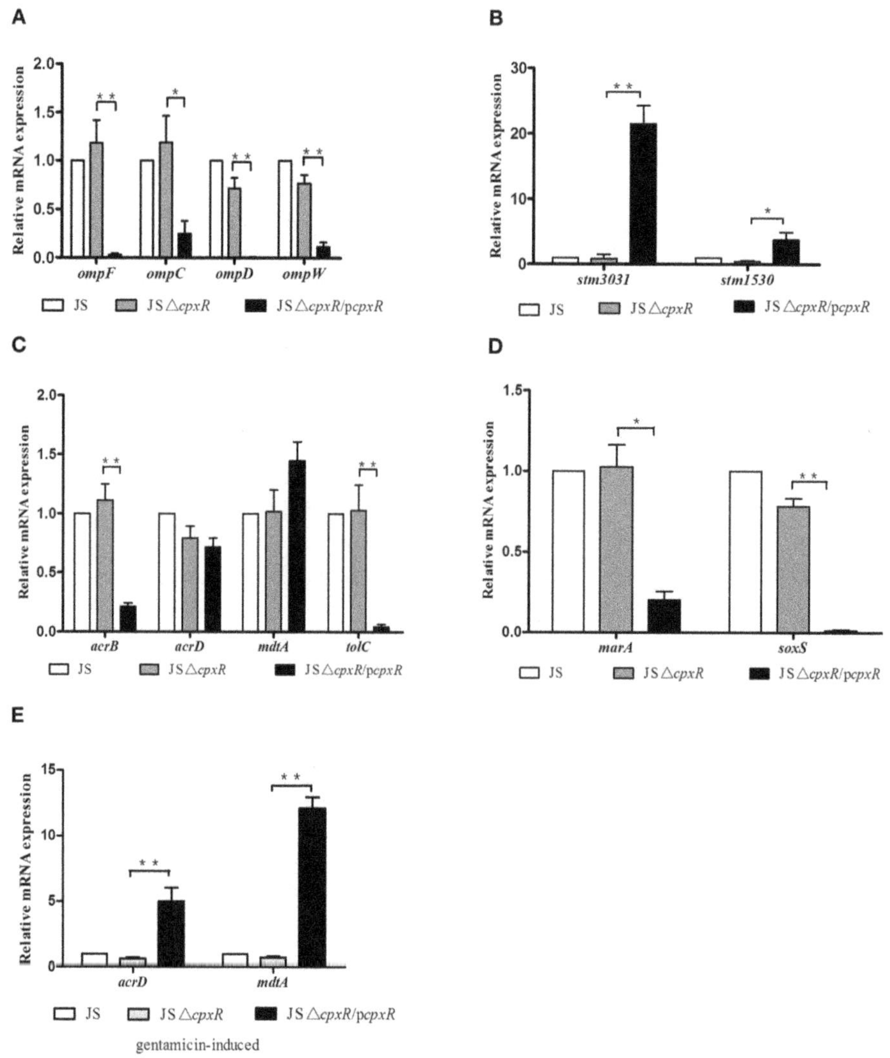

FIGURE 1 | Relative mRNA expression levels (n-fold) determined by real-time PCR. The expression level of each mRNA in strain JS represents 1-fold. The expression of the 16S rRNA gene was used as an internal control. Each bar represents the average value of three independent experiments. **(A)** Relative mRNA expression levels of the outer membrane proteins genes *ompF*, *ompC*, *ompD*, and *ompW*; **(B)** Relative mRNA expression levels of the outer membrane protein genes *stm3031* and *stm1530*; **(C)** Relative mRNA expression levels of the efflux pumps genes *acrB*, *acrD*, *mdtA*, and *tolC*; **(D)** Relative mRNA expression levels of the transcription factor genes *marA* and *soxS*. **(E)** Relative mRNA expression levels of the efflux pump genes *acrD* and *mdtA* in all tested strains induced by GEN to the 15th passage at subinhibitory concentrations. $^*p < 0.05$, $^{**}p < 0.01$.

and it also upregulated the expression levels of the efflux pumps AcrD and MdtA under the pressure of GEN.

DISCUSSION

In this study, we analyzed the effect of CpxR on the drug resistance of a susceptible strain and nine clinical isolates of *S. enterica* serovar Typhimurium and found 2- to 4-fold decreases in resistance to aminoglycosides and β-lactams by deletion of *cpxR* (**Tables 3, 4**). These results are similar to those of previous studies reporting that the overexpression of *cpxR* in *E. coli* caused 2-fold increases in resistance to β-lactams (Hirakawa et al., 2003a), but different from the findings that the *cpxA-cpxR* deleted mutant R200(Δ*cpxAR*) showed more remarkable decreases (>2048-fold) than strain JSΔ*cpxR* in the MIC of CRO, as compared to their parental strain (Hu et al., 2011). Obviously, R200, generated by a multistep resistance selection method, is a CRO-resistant strain. Therefore, we concluded that the influence of *cpxR* on the drug resistance of resistant strains is greater than that of susceptible strains.

It is known that OmpF and OmpC are the most abundant outer membrane proteins of *S. enterica* serovar Typhimurium. Many antimicrobial agents have been found to alter the expression of these proteins. Moreover, it has been confirmed that decreased level of OmpD, and increased levels of STM3031 and STM1530 are associated with *S. enterica* serovar Typhimurium CRO resistance (Hu et al., 2009, 2011). In this study, we found significant reductions in the levels of OmpF, OmpC, OmpD, and OmpW, and significant increases in levels of STM3031 and STM1530 when *cpxR* was reverted to strain JSΔ*cpxR*. Thus, the altered levels of the above-mentioned outer membrane proteins influenced by CpxR may be closely associated with the CpxR-mediated resistance of *S. enterica* serovar Typhimurium to β-lactams.

In Gram-negative bacteria, transporters belonging to the RND family are particularly effective in generating resistance, and MDR often results from the overexpression of multidrug efflux transporters (Grkovic et al., 2002). In this study, before the strains were induced with GEN, CpxR overexpression led to significant reductions in levels of AcrB, TolC, MarA, and SoxS. MarA and SoxS are global regulatory factors (Wall et al., 2009). Once overexpressed, MarA further activates AcrAB/TolC efflux and alters the expression of some membrane proteins (Sulavik et al., 1997). To our knowledge, the influence of CpxR on the mRNA levels of *marA* and *soxS* genes has not been demonstrated. Our results can give two suggestions. One is that the decrease in AcrAB–TolC, mediated by the complementation of *cpxR*, is associated with the decrease of the regulatory factors MarA and SoxS. The other is the expression levels of AcrB and TolC do not play a decisive role in CpxR-mediated resistance of *S. enterica* serovar Typhimurium to aminoglycoside and β-lactams. Our finding that CpxR can influence the susceptibility of *S. enterica* serovar Typhimurium to aminoglycosides and β-lactams in both *acrB* and Δ*acrB* backgrounds also supports the second suggestion. Nevertheless, more studies should be carried out to elucidate the reciprocal relationship among CpxR, outer membrane protein genes, efflux genes, and regulative genes.

In this study, the up-regulatory effect of CpxR on the expression levels of AcrD and MdtA were observed in the GEN-induced strains. Aminoglycoside uptake in Gram-negative bacteria includes three consecutive steps. The first step is an electrostatic interaction between aminoglycosides and the bacteria cell envelope through displacement of Mg^{2+} and Ca^{2+} ions that link adjacent lipopolysaccharide molecules, which damages the bacteria outer membrane and enhances its permeability. The second step is energy-dependent phase I of uptake, which leads to a small quantity of antibiotic molecules transversing the cytoplasmic membrane. The third step is energy-dependent phase II of uptake, in which misfolded proteins are produced due to the binding of incoming antibiotics to the ribosome. Some of these proteins are incorporated in the cytoplasmic membrane leading to the loss of membrane integrity. Therefore, additional quantities of aminoglycosides are transported across the damaged cytoplasmic membrane (Taber et al., 1987). Thus, CpxR may be activated by GEN in the inducing experiment *in vitro*. It has been reported that the promoter regions of *acrD* and *mdtABC* harbor binding sites for the response regulator BaeR (Nishino et al., 2007). CpxR also can bind to the *cpxR* box located in the promoter region of target genes. In common, the consensus *cpxR* box includes a tandem repeated GTAAA sequence that is separated by a 5-bp space (Batchelor et al., 2005). The DNA binding feature of CpxR encouraged us to analyze the promoter region of *acrD* and *mdtA* in the chromosome of *S. enterica* serovar Typhimurium LT2 (accession number: AE006468) for the presence of putative CpxR binding sites. Interestingly, our analysis revealed the presence of two similar sequences located 173 bp (site 1: GTAAA-gaacg-GCAAA) and 106 bp (site2: GTAAA-agcgc-ATGAT) upstream of the *acrD* translational start site, respectively. Among them, site 1 was also found 328 bp upstream of the *kpnEF* translational start site. Furthermore, it has been confirmed that purified CpxR from a strain of *K. Pneumoniae* can directly bind to site 1 (Srinivasan and Rajamohan, 2013). Because CpxR of *K. Pneumoniae* exhibits the highest level of homology to CpxR of *S. enterica* serovar Typhimurium (96%), CpxR of *S. enterica* serovar Typhimurium may directly bind to the promoter region of *acrD*. As we know, AcrD participates in the efflux of aminoglycosides, thus our analysis indicates that CpxR contributes to AcrD-mediated resistance of *S. enterica* serovar Typhimurium to GEN, which belongs to aminoglycosides.

Moreover, in this study, there were no significant differences in the mRNA expression levels of all tested genes in strain JSΔ*cpxR*, as compared to strain JS. It has been demonstrated that histidine kinase (HK) also possess response regulator phosphatase activity, which may ensure that the response regulator remains inactive in the absence of activating signals (Raivio and Silhavy, 1997). Therefore, we think that the response regulator CpxR is always in a pre-stimulated resting state and does not modulate mRNA levels at physiological levels. Biochemical data suggest that CpxR can become phosphorylated by the low-molecular-weight phospho-donor acetyl phosphate and, further, that this form (CpxR-P) has a greater affinity for binding to the promoters of target genes (Pogliano et al., 1997). Similarly, it has been demonstrated that, in the absence of CpxA, CpxR can transcriptionally activate downstream target genes, suggesting that CpxR-P is responsible for transcriptional activation of target genes (Danese et al., 1995; De Wulf and Lin, 2000; Batchelor et al., 2005). In this scenario, we conclude that CpxR overproduction in JS△*cpxR* encourages the emergence of CpxR-P, which acts as a modulator of gene expression.

In summary, we have reported the first systematical and extensive study about the role of CpxR in aminoglycoside and β-lactams resistance in both susceptible strains and clinical isolates of *S. enterica* serovar Typhimurium. Our results not only clearly confirmed that CpxR contributes to resistance of *S. enterica* serovar Typhimurium to aminoglycoside and β-lactams but also indicated that the effect of CpxR on the expression levels of MDR-related genes is closely associated with CpxR-mediated resistance of *S. enterica* serovar Typhimurium to aminoglycoside and β-lactams. This is the first time that the effect of CpxR on the expression levels of *marA* and *soxS* genes have been investigated in *S. enterica* serovar Typhimurium. Further studies are obviously required to investigate the reciprocal relationship among CpxR, MDR-related outer membrane protein genes, efflux pump genes and regulative genes including *marA* and *soxS*.

AUTHOR CONTRIBUTIONS

HH, YS, and GH conceived of the study, and participated in its design and coordination. YG, CM isolated the *S. enterica* Serovar Typhimurium isolates. HH carried out the antibiotics susceptibility testing and molecular biology studies, including gene deletion, construction of expression vector and RT-PCR. HH and YP performed the statistical analysis. HH drafted the manuscript. YS, LY, and GH revised the manuscript.

ACKNOWLEDGMENTS

We thank Professor Chenzhang Wang for assistance with the real-time PCR.

REFERENCES

Aires, J. R., and Nikaido, H. (2005). Aminoglycosides are captured from both periplasm and cytoplasm by the AcrD multidrug efflux transporter of *Escherichia coli*. *J. Bacteriol.* 187, 1923–1929. doi: 10.1128/JB.187.6.1923-1929.2005

Audrain, B., Ferrières, L., Zairi, A., Soubigou, G., Dobson, C., Coppée, J. Y., et al. (2013). Induction of the Cpx envelope stress pathway contributes to *Escherichia coli* tolerance to antimicrobial peptides. *Appl. Environ. Microbiol.* 79, 7770–7779. doi: 10.1128/AEM.02593-13

Baranova, N., and Nikaido, H. (2002). The baeSR two-component regulatory system activates transcription of the yegMNOB (mdtABCD) transporter gene cluster in *Escherichia coli* and increases its resistance to novobiocin and deoxycholate. *J. Bacteriol.* 184, 4168–4176. doi: 10.1128/JB.184.15.4168-4176.2002

Barrow, P. A., Bumstead, N., Marston, K., Lovell, M. A., and Wigley, P. (2004). Faecal shedding and intestinal colonization of *Salmonella enterica* in in-bred chicked: the effect of host genetic background. *Epidemiol. Infect.* 132, 117–126. doi: 10.1017/S0950268803001274

Batchelor, E., Walthers, D., Kenney, L. J., and Goulian, M. (2005). The *Escherichia coli* CpxA-CpxR envelope stress response system regulates expression of the porins OmpF and OmpC. *J. Bacteriol.* 187, 5723–5731. doi: 10.1128/JB.187.16.5723-5731.2005

Clinical and Laboratory Standards Institute (2008). *Performance Standards for Antimicrobial Disk and Dilution Susceptibility Tests for Bacteria Isolated from Animals; Approved Standard, 3rd Edn.* Wayne, PA: CLSI. (Informational Supplement, M31–A3).

Clinical and Laboratory Standards Institute (2012). *Performance Standards for Antimicrobial Susceptibility Testing; Twenty-second Informational Supplement.* Wayne, PA: CLSI (Twenty-Two Informational Supplement M100–S22).

Cuny, C., Lesbats, M., and Dukan, S. (2007). Induction of a global stress response during the first step of *Escherichia coli* plate growth. *Appl. Environ. Microbiol.* 73, 885–889. doi: 10.1128/AEM.01874-06

Danese, P. N., Snyder, W. B., Cosma, C. L., Davis, L. J., and Silhavy, T. J. (1995). The Cpx two-component signal transduction pathway of *Escherichia coli* regulates transcription of the gene specifying the stress-inducible periplasmic protease, DegP. *Genes Dev.* 9, 387–398. doi: 10.1101/gad.9.4.387

Davis, R. W., Bolstein, D., and Rorh, J. R. (1980). *Advanced Bacterial Genetics.* Cold Spring Harbor, NY: Cold Spring Harbor Laboratory Press.

De Wulf, P., and Lin, E. C. (2000). Cpx two-component signal transduction in *Escherichia coli*: excessive CpxR-P Levels underlie CpxA* phenotypes. *J. Bacteriol.* 182, 1423–1426. doi: 10.1128/JB.182.5.1423-1426.2000

De Wulf, P., McGuire, A. M., Liu, X., and Lin, E. C. (2002). Genome-wide profiling of promoter recognition by the two-component response regulator CpxR-P in *Escherichia coli*. *J. Biol. Chem.* 277, 26652–26661. doi: 10.1074/jbc.M203487200

Eaves, D. J., Ricci, V., and Piddock, L. J. (2004). Expression of *acrB*, *acrF*, *acrD*, *marA*, and *soxS* in *Salmonella enterica* Serovar Typhimurium: role in multiple antibiotic resistance. *Antimicrob. Agents Chemother.* 48, 1145–1150. doi: 10.1128/AAC.48.4.1145-1150.2004

Grkovic, S., Brown, M. H., and Skurray, R. A. (2002). Regulation of bacterial drug export systems. *Microbiol. Mol. Biol. Rev.* 66, 671–701. doi: 10.1128/MMBR.66.4.671-701.2002

Guzman, L. M., Belin, D., Carson, M. J., and Beckwith, J. (1995). Tight regulation, modulation, and high-level expression by vectors containing the arabinose pBAD promoter. *J. Bacteriol.* 177, 4121–4130.

Hirakawa, H., Inazumi, Y., Masaki, T., Hirata, T., and Yamaguchi, A. (2005). Indole induces the expression of multidrug exporter genes in *Escherichia coli*. *Mol. Microbiol.* 55, 1113–1126. doi: 10.1111/j.1365-2958.2004.04449.x

Hirakawa, H., Nishino, K., Hirata, T., and Yamaguchi, A. (2003b). Comprehensive studies of drug resistance mediated by overexpression of response regulators of two-component signal transduction systems in *Escherichia coli*. *J. Bacteriol.* 185, 1851–1856. doi: 10.1128/JB.185.6.1851-1856.2003

Hirakawa, H., Nishino, K., Yamada, J., Hirata, T., and Yamaguchi, A. (2003a). β-Lactam resistance modulated by the overexpression of response regulators of two-component signal transduction systems in *Escherichia coli*. *J. Antimicrob. Chemother.* 52, 576–582. doi: 10.1093/jac/dkg406

Hu, W. S., Chen, H. W., Zhang, R. Y., Huang, C. Y., and Shen, C. F. (2011). The expression levels of outer membrane proteins STM1530 and OmpD, which are influenced by the CpxAR and BaeSR two-component systems, play important roles in the ceftriaxone resistance of *Salmonella enterica* Serovar Typhimurium. *Antimicrob. Agents Chemother.* 55, 3829–3837. doi: 10.1128/AAC.00216-11

Hu, W. S., Lin, J. F., Lin, Y. H., and Chang, H. Y. (2009). Outer membrane protein STM3031 (Ail/OmpX-like) plays a key role in the ceftriaxone resistance of *Salmonella enterica* serovar Typhimurium. *Antimicrob. Agents Chemother.* 53, 3248–3255. doi: 10.1128/AAC.00079-09

Huang, H., Liu, B. G., Sun, Y. W., Ma, C. H., Cheng, L. P., Yuan, L., et al. (2016). Construction of *cpxR* and *acrB* double gene deletion strain of *Salmonella enterica* Serovar Typhimurium and analysis of its susceptibility to antibacterial agents. *Acta Vet. Zootech. Sin.* 47, 595–602. doi: 10. 11843/j. issn. 0366-6964. 2016.03.00

Huang, H., Tian, Y. K., Sun, Y. W., Cheng, L. P., Yuan, L., Liu, J. H., et al. (2015). Construction of *cpxR* gene deleted *Salmonella* typhimurium and analysis of its susceptibility to antibiotics. *Chin. J. Prev. Vet. Med.* 37, 756–760. doi: 10. 3969/j.issn.1008-0589.2015.10.06

Huang, P. T., Yu, W. Y., and Chen, T. M. (1999). *PCR Lab Manual* (Translate). Beijing: Science Press.

Kurabayashi, K., Hirakawa, Y., Tanimoto, K., Tomita, H., and Hirakawa, H. (2014). Role of the CpxAR two-component signal transduction system in control of fosfomycin resistance and carbon substrate uptake. *J. Bacteriol.* 196, 248–256. doi: 10.1128/JB.01151-13

Li, L., Wang, Y. P., Wu, Y. N., Wu, C. M., and Shen, J. Z. (2009). Association of marR, soxR and acrR mutations with multiple antibiotic resistance in ciprofloxacin-selected *Salmonella* mutants. *Food Saf. Qual. Detect. Technol.* 1, 1–9.

Li, X. Z., and Nikaido, H. (2009). Efflux-mediated drug resistance in bacteria: an update. *Drugs* 69, 1555–1623. doi: 10.2165/11317030-000000000-00000

MacRitchie, D. M., Buelow, D. R., Price, N. L., and Raivio, T. L. (2008). Two-component signaling and gram negative envelope stress response systems. *Adv. Exp. Med. Biol.* 631, 80–110. doi: 10.1007/978-0-387-78885-2_6

Mann, B. A., and Slauch, J. M. (1997). Transduction of low-copy number plasmids by bacteriophage P22. *Genetics* 146, 447–456.

Mazzariol, A., Cornaglia, G., and Nikaido, H. (2000). Contributions of the AmpC β-lactamase and the AcrAB multidrug efflux system in intrinsic resistance of *Escherichia coli* K-12 to β-lactams. *Antimicrob. Agents Chemother.* 44, 1387–1390. doi: 10.1128/AAC.44.5.1387-1390.2000

Nikaido, H. (1996). Multidrug efflux pumps of gram-negative bacteria. *J. Bacteriol.* 178, 5853–5859.

Nikaido, H. (2003). Molecular basis of bacterial outer membrane permeability revisited. *Microbiol. Mol. Biol. Rev.* 67, 593–656. doi: 10.1128/MMBR.67.4.593-656.2003

Nikaido, H., and Pagès, J. M. (2012). Broad-specificity efflux pumps and their role in multidrug resistance of Gram-negative bacteria. *FEMS Microbiol. Rev.* 36, 340–363. doi: 10.1111/j.1574-6976.2011.00290.x

Nishino, K., Latifi, T., and Groisman, E. A. (2006). Virulence and drug resistance roles of multidrug efflux systems of *Salmonella enterica* serovar Typhimurium. *Mol Microbiol.* 1, 126–141. doi: 10.1111/j.1365-2958.2005.04940.x

Nishino, K., Nikaido, E., and Yamaguchi, A. (2007). Regulation of multidrug efflux systems involved in multidrug and metal resistance of *Salmonella enterica* serovar Typhimurium. *J. Bacteriol.* 189, 9066–9075. doi: 10.1128/JB.01045-07

Nishino, K., Yamada, J., Hirakawa, H., Hirata, T., and Yamaguchi, A. (2003). Roles of TolC-dependent multidrug transporters of *Escherichia coli* in resistance to β-Lactams[J]. *Antimicrob. Agents Chemother.* 47, 3030–3033. doi: 10.1128/AAC.47.9.3030-3033.2003

Nishino, K., and Yamaguchi, A. (2001a). Analysis of the complete library of putative drug transporter genes in *Escherichia coli*. *J. Bacteriol.* 183, 5803–5812. doi: 10.1128/JB.183.20.5803-5812.2001

Nishino, K., and Yamaguchi, A. (2001b). Overexpression of the response regulator evgA of the two-component signal transduction system modulates multidrug resistance conferred by multidrug resistance transporters. *J. Bacteriol.* 183, 1455–1458. doi: 10.1128/JB.183.4.1455-1458.2001

Nishino, K., and Yamaguchi, A. (2002). EvgA of the two-component signal transduction system modulates production of the yhiUV multidrug transporter in *Escherichia coli*. *J. Bacteriol.* 184, 2319–2323. doi: 10.1128/JB.184.8.2319-2323.2002

Pagès, J. M., Alibert-Franco, S., Mahamoud, A., Bolla, J. M., Davin-Regli, A., Chevalier, J., et al. (2010). Efflux pumps of gram-negative bacteria, a new target for new molecules. *Curr. Top. Med. Chem.* 8, 1848–1857. doi: 10.2174/156802610793176620

Pagès, J. M., James, C. E., and Winterhalter, M. (2008). The porin and the permeating antibiotic: a selective diffusion barrier in Gram-megative bacteria. *Nat. Rev. Microbiol.* 6, 893–903. doi: 10.1038/nrmicro1994

Parkinson, J. S., and Kofoid, E. C. (1992). Communication modules in bacterial signaling proteins. *Annu. Rev. Genet.* 26, 71–112. doi: 10.1146/annurev.ge.26.120192.000443

Pogliano, J., Lynch, A. S., Belin, D., Lin, E. C. C., and Beckwith, J. (1997). Regulation of *Escherichia coli* cell envelope proteins involved in protein folding and degradation by the Cpx two-component system. *Genes Dev.* 11, 1169–1182. doi: 10.1101/gad.11.9.1169

Price, N. L., and Raivio, T. L. (2009). Characterization of the Cpx regulon in *Escherichia coli* strain MC4100. *J. Bacteriol.* 191, 1798–1815. doi: 10.1128/JB.00798-08

Raivio, T. L., and Silhavy, T. J. (1997). Transduction of envelope stress in *Escherichia coli* by the Cpx two-component system. *J. Bacteriol.* 179, 7724–7733.

Rosenberg, E. Y., Ma, D., and Nikaido, H. (2000). AcrD of *Escherichia coli* is an aminoglycoside efflux pump. *J. Bacteriol.* 182, 1754–1756. doi: 10.1128/JB.182.6.1754-1756.2000

Scherer, C. A., and Miller, S. I. (2001). "Molecular pathogenesis of Salmonella," in *Principles of Bacterial Pathogenesis*, ed E. A. Groisman (New York, NY: Academic Press, Inc.), 266–333.

Srinivasan, V. B., and Rajamohan, G. (2013). KpnEF, a new member of the *Klebsiella pneumoniae* cell envelope stress response regulon, is an SMR-Type efflux pump involved in broad-spectrum antimicrobial resistance. *Antimicrob. Agents Chemother.* 57, 4449–4462. doi: 10.1128/AAC.02284-12

Srinivasan, V. B., Vaidyanathan, V., Mondal, A., and Rajamohan, G. (2012). Role of the two-component signal transduction system CpxAR in conferring cefepime and chloramphenicol resistance in *Klebsiella pneumoniae* NTUH-K2044. *PLoS ONE* 7:e33777. doi: 10.1371/journal.pone.0033777

Stephenson, K., and Hoch, J. A. (2002). Two-component and phosphorelay signal-transduction systems as therapeutic targets. *Curr. Opin. Pharmacol.* 2, 507–512. doi: 10.1016/S1471-4892(02)00194-7

Sulavik, M. C., Dazer, M., and Miller, P. F. (1997). The Salmonella typhimurium mar locus: molecular and genetic analyses and assessment of its role in virulence. *J. Bacteriol.* 179, 1857–1866.

Taber, H. W., Mueller, J. P., Miller, P. F., and Arrow, A. S. (1987). Bacterial uptake of aminoglycoside antibiotics. *Microbiol. Rev.* 51, 439–457.

Tatavarthy, A., and Cannons, A. (2010). Real-time PCR detection of *Salmonella* species using a novel target: the outer membrane porin F gene (*ompF*). *Lett. Appl. Microbiol.* 50, 645–652. doi: 10.1111/j.1472-765X.2010.02848.x

Urban, A., Neukirchen, S., and Jaeger, K. E. (1997). A rapid and efficient method for site-directed mutagenesis using one-step over-lap extension PCR. *Nucleic. Acids Res.* 25, 2227–2228. doi: 10.1093/nar/25.11.2227

Wall, M. E., Markowitz, D. A., Rosner, J. L., and Martin, R. G. (2009). Model of transcriptional activation by MarA in *Escherichia coli*. *PLoS Comput. Biol.* 5:e1000614. doi: 10.1371/journal.pcbi.1000614

Weatherspoon-Griffin, N., Yang, D., Kong, W., Hua, Z., and Shi, Y. (2014). The CpxA/CpxR two-component regulatory system up-regulates the multidrug resistance cascade to facilitate Escherichia coli resistance to a model antimicrobial peptide. *J. Biol. Chem.* 289, 32571–32582. doi: 10.1074/jbc.M114.565762

Weatherspoon-Griffin, N., Zhao, G., Kong, W., Kong, Y., Morigen, Andrews-Polymenis, H., et al. (2011). The CpxR/CpxA two-component system up-regulates two tat-dependent peptidoglycan amidases to confer bacterial resistance to antimicrobial peptide. *J. Biol. Chem.* 286, 5529–5539. doi: 10.1074/jbc.M110.200352

Wolfe, A. J., Parikhm, N., Lima, B. P., and Zemaitaitis, B. (2008). Signal integration by the two-component signal transduction response regulator CpxR. *J. Bacteriol.* 190, 2314–2322. doi: 10.1128/JB.01906-07

Wu, X. B., Zou, H. J., Tian, L. H., Pan, J. Y., and Zhao, F. K. (2012). Construction of *ompW* knock-out mutants of *Escherichia coli* to increase sensitivity to neomycinsulphate and ampicillin. *Acta Microbiol. Sin.* 52, 1021–1026. doi: 10.13343/j.cnki.wsxb.2012.08.012

Yu, E. W., McDermott, G., Zgurskaya, H. I., Nikaido, H., and Koshland, D. E. Jr. (2003). Structural basis of multiple drug-binding capacity of the AcrB multi drug efflux pump. *Science* 300, 976–980. doi: 10.1126/science.1083137

Zgurskaya, H. I., and Nikaido, H. (2000). Multidrug resistance mechanisms: drug efflux across two membranes. *Mol. Microbiol.* 37, 219–225. doi: 10.1046/j.1365-2958.2000.01926.x

4

The Risk of Some Veterinary Antimicrobial Agents on Public Health Associated with Antimicrobial Resistance and their Molecular Basis

Haihong Hao [1,2], Pascal Sander[3], Zahid Iqbal[1], Yulian Wang[2], Guyue Cheng[1] and Zonghui Yuan [1,2]*

[1] *China MOA Laboratory for Risk Assessment of Quality and Safety of Livestock and Poultry Products, Huazhong Agricultural University, Wuhan, China,* [2] *National Reference Laboratory of Veterinary Drug Residues (HZAU) and MOA Key Laboratory for the Detection of Veterinary Drug Residues in Foods, Huazhong Agricultural University, Wuhan, China,* [3] *Laboratory of Fougères, French Agency for Food, Environmental and Occupational Safety, Fougères Cedex, France*

***Correspondence:**
Zonghui Yuan
yuan5802@mail.hzau.edu.cn

The risk of antimicrobial agents used in food-producing animals on public health associated with antimicrobial resistance continues to be a current topic of discussion as related to animal and human public health. In the present review, resistance monitoring data, and risk assessment results of some important antimicrobial agents were cited to elucidate the possible association of antimicrobial use in food animals and antimicrobial resistance in humans. From the selected examples, it was apparent from reviewing the published scientific literature that the ban on use of some antimicrobial agents (e.g., avoparcin, fluoroquinolone, tetracyclines) did not change drug resistance patterns and did not mitigate the intended goal of minimizing antimicrobial resistance. The use of some antimicrobial agents (e.g., virginiamycin, macrolides, and cephalosporins) in food animals may have an impact on the antimicrobial resistance in humans, but it was largely depended on the pattern of drug usage in different geographical regions. The epidemiological characteristics of resistant bacteria were closely related to molecular mechanisms involved in the development, fitness, and transmission of antimicrobial resistance.

Keywords: antimicrobial agents, food-producing animal, antimicrobial resistance, public health, molecular basis

INTRODUCTION

Antimicrobial agents have been used in food animal production since the 1950s. Antimicrobial agents have contributed significantly to the prevention and treatment of infectious diseases in food animals and some of them have played a very important role in the promotion of animal growth and feed efficiency (Dibner and Richards, 2005; Niewold, 2007). Since many classes of antimicrobial agents used in food animals are also used in human medicine, there is the potential for selection, and spread of antimicrobial resistant bacteria in animals to humans through the food supply. Human health consequences have been raised concerning whether the use of antimicrobial agents in food animals may minimize the effectiveness of the same classes of medically important antimicrobial agents to treat antimicrobial resistant infectious diseases in humans (Salisbury et al., 2002). In this respect, the administration of low doses (5–40 mg/kg.feed) of antimicrobial growth-promoters in animal feed were banned by Europe (EU) in 2006 to protect public health, and this ban drew a great attention of other countries and international organizations (Marshall and Levy, 2011) since this low dose drug exposure over a long period of time could elicit selective pressure leading to the emergence of resistant bacteria.

For comprehensive surveillance monitoring of antimicrobial resistance in food-borne pathogens, many countries have established antimicrobial resistance monitoring systems, such as the National Antimicrobial Resistance Monitoring System (NARMS) in United States of America (USA) and Danish Integrated Antimicrobial Resistance Monitoring and Research Program (DANMAP). The Food and Agriculture Organization (FAO), World Health Organization (WHO), and World Organization for Animal Health (OIE) have organized expert workshops on the risk assessment and management of non-human antimicrobial usage and their resistance(FAO/OIE/WHO, 2003, 2004, 2006). WHO/FAO/OIE have jointly carried out systematic evaluation of veterinary antimicrobial resistance for the impact on public health (FAO/OIE/WHO, 2006). The European Medicines Agency (EMA), European Food Safety Authority (EFSA) and European Center for Disease Prevention and Control (ECDC) have also work together for the Joint Interagency Antimicrobial Consumption and Resistance Analysis (JIACRA) and have also published reports on antimicrobial use in food animals and antimicrobial resistance recently (ECDC/EFSA/EMA, 2015).

In the present review, results of risk assessments based on data from different antimicrobial resistance monitoring systems are reported to evaluate the stewardship programs of antimicrobial use in food animals. Resistance to some representative antimicrobial agents (e.g., cephalosporins, tetracyclines, fluoroquinolones, macrolides, glycopeptides, and streptogramins) in some selected pathogens (e.g., *Enterococci spp*, *Campylobacter spp*, *Salmonella spp*, and *Escherichia coli*) were taken as examples to describe the relationship between antimicrobial resistance and drug usage in food animals. The molecular mechanism involved in the development, fitness, and transmission of antimicrobial resistance was also integrated into the review to provide a comprehensive understanding of the antimicrobial resistance and to identify the need for risk management of antimicrobial drugs.

AVOPARCIN AND GLYCOPEPTIDE-RESISTANT ENTEROCOCCI

Avoparcin, a vancomycin analog, was effective against gram-positive bacteria by disturbing their cell wall synthesis. Avoparcin had been widely used as a feed additive in food animals during 1940s–1990s. As a member of glycopeptides, there was concern that the misuse of avoparcin may confer cross-resistance to glycopeptides and in particular vancomycin which is known as one of the important last-line antimicrobials in human medicine. In 1993, isolation and frequency of vancomycin-resistant *Enterococci* (VRE) from food-producing animals in Great British drew public health concern about the consequences of wide use of avoparcin as a growth promoter in animals. From 1995 to 2000, Denmark, United Kingdom, EU members, Japan and China gradually banned the use of avoparcin in food-producing animals.

It is important to keep in mind that the term of VRE includes several combinations of bacterial species (e.g., *Enterococcus faecium and Enterococcus faecalis*) and resistance genes (*vanA, B, C, D, E, G, L, M,* and *N*). The characteristics of *van A-N* genes are summarized in **Table 1**. The *vanA, B, D, E, G, L, M,* and *N* are acquired genetic determinants in *E. faecium* and/or *E. faecalis*, while *vanC* is intrinsic gene present in *E. gallinarum* and *E. casseliflavus*/*E. flavescens* (Cetinkaya et al., 2000; Boyd et al., 2008). Among those, *E. faecium* with *vanA* type vancomycin resistance is clinically most important because *vanA* is an acquired and transferable gene which is resistant to both vancomycin and teicoplanin (Nilsson, 2012). The *vanB* and *vanN* are transferable but is susceptible to teicoplanin (Nomura et al., 2012). The *vanM* is newly found in China and confirmed to have transferability and resistance to both vancomycin and teicoplanin (Xu et al., 2010; Chen et al., 2015).

Extensive use of avoparcin for animal growth promotion in most parts of Europe may be the reason for high prevalence of VRE in the intestinal microbiota of farm animals in Europe during the 1990s (Aarestrup, 1995; Klare et al., 1995). Once the use of avoparcin was prohibited, prevalence of VRE among farm animals decreased in some EU countries. According to DANMAP report, substantial reductions (from 80 to 0%) in the prevalence of VRE were observed between 1995 and 2013, after the ban on avoparcin as growth promoter in Denmark (DANMAP, 2013). Very few vancomycin resistant enterococci have been isolated from Danish livestock and produced meat during 2003–2013 (DANMAP, 2013).

However, it was noteworthy that ban on avoparcin did not effectively reduce incidence of vancomycin-resistant *E. faecium* in avian feces. A paper published in 2008 showed that vancomycin-resistant *E. faecium* was still highly prevalent in poultry in Europe (Werner et al., 2008). Even after 15 years of the EU ban on avoparcin, vancomycin-resistant *E. faecium* was still present in the food chain and could be detected in 47% of the broiler feces (Garcia-Migura et al., 2007; DANMAP, 2010). The proportion of broilers colonized with vancomycin-resistant *E. faecium* increased from less than 1% in 2000 to over 40% in 2005, even though Sweden had forbidden the use of avoparcin as growth promoter since 1986 (Nilsson et al., 2009). The high prevalence of vancomycin-resistant *E. faecium* in EU countries may be due to the transferability of *E. faecium* with the *vanA* gene (Nilsson et al., 2009). The *vanN* gene with transferability was also found in vancomycin-resistant *E. faecium* isolated from chicken meat (Nomura et al., 2012).

The most important concern is not only that VRE are present among farm animals but also their potential to transfer resistance genes to vancomycin susceptible enterococci and other Gram—positive bacteria that may be transmitted via food products to humans. Some earlier reports showed that hospital isolates of *E. faecium* generally clustered in subgroups which were different from those found in animals (Top et al., 2004; Willems et al., 2005). In contrast, some in *vivo* transfer studies indicated that *vanA* gene was located in transposon Tn1546 and may be

TABLE 1 | Characteristics of glycopetide-resistant genes in Enterococci.

Characteristics	*vanA*	*vanB*	*vanC*	*vanD*	*vanE*	*vanG*	*vanL*	*vanM*	*vanN*
Enterococcus species	***E. faecium; E. faecalis***	***E. faecium; E. faecalis***	***E. gallinarum, E. casseliflavus, E. flavescens***	***E. faecium***	***E. faecalis***	***E. faecalis***	***E. faecalis***	***E. faecium***	***E. faecium***
Vancomycin MIC (μg/mL)	64–1024	4–1024	2–32	16–64	16–32	16–32	8	>256	16
Teicoplanin MIC (μg/mL)	16–512	<1	<1	2–16	<0.5	<0.5	<0.5	96	0.5
Genetic determinant	acquired	acquired	intrinsic	acquired	acquired	acquired	acquired	acquired	acquired
transferable	Yes	Yes	No	No	No	No	No	Yes	Yes
New precursor of ligase	D-ala-D-lac	D-ala-D-lac	D-ala-D-ser	D-ala-D-lac	D-ala-D-ser	D-ala-D-ser	D-ala-D-ser	D-ala-D-lac	D-ala-D-ser
Expression	Inducible	Inducible	constitutive	constitutive	Constitutive or inducible	Constitutive or inducible	Constitutive or inducible	Inducible	constitutive

transferred between animal and human adapted enterococci (Jensen, 1998; Lester et al., 2006; Lester and Hammerum, 2010). The *vanM* gene was also located in transferable element and could transfer by conjugation (Xu et al., 2010). Similar strains of VRE have been isolated from both farm animal and human, indicating that some of those strains may adapt to farm animals and cause infectious diseases in humans (Freitas et al., 2011). However, the origin of Tn1546 element encoding *vanA* resistance in US hospitals was still unknown (Jensen, 1998; Lester et al., 2006; Lester and Hammerum, 2010). It was difficult to determine to what extent did the presence of VRE among farm animals actually affect public health (Nilsson, 2012).

Notably, a controversy was perceived in the geographical distribution of VRE among humans. In the United States, about 20,000 (or 40%) of *Enterococcus* healthcare-associated infections in 2013 were vancomycin resistant, including 77% of vancomycin resistant *E. faecium* (CDC, 2013). In Denmark, vancomycin resistance was detected in only 3.4% of *E.faecium* isolates from bloodstream infections in 2013 (DANMAP, 2013). In other Nordic countries, the level of vancomycin resistant *Enterococcus* was even lower than in Denmark in recent years (EARS-Net, 2012). Therefore, VRE was more common in US hospitals than that in European hospitals, although in the USA, avoparcin had never been approved for use in food animals (Gambarotto et al., 2000; Bonten et al., 2001). It was likely that the serious problem of VRE in US hospitals was not related to the use of avoparcin in food animals but to that of vancomycin use in human medicine, because therapeutic vancomycin treatment was much higher in the USA when compared with that in Europe (Acar et al., 2000).

VIRGINIAMYCIN AND STREPTOGRAMIN-RESISTANT *ENTEROCOCCI*

Virginiamycin is a streptogramin antimicrobial which could block the transpeptidation or translocation of protein synthesis in bacteria. It has been used for the prevention of *Clostridial enteritis* and enhancement of growth and feed efficiency in poultry, swine and cattle for more than 30 years in Japan, Canada, U.S.A, and other countries. However, EU prohibited its use in food-producing animals in 1999 because it was assumed to select for streptogramin-resistant *Enterococci* (SRE) and lead to treatment failure of patients in hospitals with pristinamycin and Synercid (Quinupristin-Dalfopristin) resistant *Enterococcus faecium* infections. Mechanisms conferring resistance to streptogramin in *E. faecium* was mediated via related acetyltransferases (VatD and VatE), erythromycin ribosomal methylase B (ErmB) and staphylococcal-type lactonase (VgbA) (Werner et al., 2002).

Some epidemiological investigations showed that streptogramin-resistant genes (*vat*) were detected in 25% of virginiamycin-resistant *E. faecium* isolated from pigs and chickens, and in 29% of isolates from farm workers in Denmark (Hammerum et al., 1998; Haroche et al., 2000). The NARMS report revealed that long-term use of virginiamycin for growth promotion was likely to result in the emergence of streptogramin-resistant *Enterococcus* which was present in 30–70% of poultry products purchased from supermarkets (NARMS, 2012).

Transferability of these *vat* genes was observed among *E. faecium* isolates from food-animals (Sørensen et al., 2001). The resistant strains may also spread indirectly to human beings from farms through the environment including raw manure or surface/ground water (Smith et al., 2003). Sørensen et al. (2001) found that streptogramin- resistant *E. faecium* from food animals was able to establish transient populations in the gut after experimental ingestion. Additionally, similar genetic patterns of *vanA* containing *Enterococci* isolates, from poultry and human, were reported in Spain (Robredo et al., 2000).

However, streptogramin-resistant *E. faecium* from poultry may be well-adapted to cloaca, but difficult to survive against the gastric barrier and colonization resistance in the gut (Smith et al., 2003). Despite the high rate of exposure in contaminated meat, prevalence of streptogramin resistant *E. faecium* remained low and therefore, bacteria with high resistance could rarely establish in human beings (McDonald et al., 2001). By using pulsed-field gel electrophoresis (PFGE) technique, Hershberger et al. (2005) found distinct gene cluster of streptogramin-resistant *E. faecium*, isolated from poultry and human beings. Additionally, numerous studies found the different genetic profiles of streptogramin- resistant *E. faecium*, isolated from food-animals (poultry and pork) and human beings, indicating that the bacterial strains might be highly host specific (Smith et al., 2003; Hershberger et al., 2005; Hammerum et al., 2010).

The US Food and Drug Administration and Center for Veterinary Medicine (FDA-CVM) reported that there was not enough data to show the transmission of SRE between animals and humans (FDV-CVM, 2004). A quantitative risk assessment performed by US FDA-CVM concluded that risk of SRE, caused by virginiamycin use in food animals, was about 1–14 heads per billion due to the treatment failure of VRE infections (FDV-CVM, 2004). A quantitative human health risk and benefits assessment for virginiamycin showed that human health benefits of virginiamycin withdrawal ranged from zero to less than one statistical life and withdrawal of the drug may cause more human illnesses than it would prevent (Cox and Popken, 2004; Cox, 2005). Phillips (2007) showed that human health risk from resistance among enterococci selected by virginiamycin was small (Phillips, 2007). Some scientists have disagreed with the conclusion that the ban of virginiamycin in EU could lead to an increased prevalence of streptogramin resistant enterococci (Hammerum et al., 2007). Although an investigation showed that the continued use of virginiamycin as growth promoter in poultry may increase the potential for streptogramin- resistant *E. faecium* infection in humans (Kieke et al., 2006).

FLUOROQUINOLONE AND RESISTANCE IN *CAMPYLOBACTER*

Fluoroquinolones, a family of synthetic broad-spectrum antimicrobial agents, played an important role in the treatment of bacterial infection in both veterinary medicine and in human medicine. Fluoroquinolones can inhibit the DNA synthesis of bacteria by selectively inhibiting their DNA gyrase and/or topoisomerase (Suto et al., 1992). The fluoroquinolone resistance in Campylobacter was mediated by mutations in the drug target enzyme (e.g., Thr-86-Ile mutation in GyrA) and/or by overexpression of efflux pumps (e.g., CmeABC) (Griggs et al., 2005).

Both enrofloxacin and ciprofloxacin were the second generation of fluroquinolones. They had similar structural and antimicrobial activity. The enrofloxacin was approved to treat bacterial infections in poultry in the USA before 2005, while ciprofloxacin was used in human medicine to treat foodborne infections such as *Campylobacter*, *Salmonella*, *E.coli*, and *Shigella*. When enrofloxacin was administrated into some food producing animal, it could be metabolized to ciprofloxacin (Gratacós-Cubars'i et al., 2007). The close relationship between fluoroquinolone drug in veterinary medicine and it use in human medicine may raise the risk of fluoroquinolone resistance from animal to human.

There was evidence that the use of enrofloxacin in poultry production would induce fluoroquinolone resistance in *Campylobacter jejuni* and these fluoroquinolone resistant bacteria transferred to humans and contributed to the treatment failure of campylobacterosis in humans via poultry exposure (FDA, 2002; Nelson et al., 2007). Some in *vitro* and in *vivo* studies have demonstrated that FQ-resistant strains would rapidly emerge when *Campylobacter* was exposed to FQs (e.g., enrofloxacin). The frequencies of emergence may range between approximately 10^{-6}–10^{-8}/cell/generation in culture media, indicating that resistant bacteria would inevitably emerge when cell population was sufficiently larger than 10^6 (Yan et al., 2006; Han et al., 2008). FQ-susceptible *C. jejuni* in chicken could rapidly attain FQ-resistance within 24 h after the initiation of treatment with enrofloxacin (McDermott et al., 2002; Luo et al., 2003; van Boven et al., 2003; Farnell et al., 2005; Griggs et al., 2005). The FQ-resistant *Campylobacter* population could eventually colonize into intestinal tract of birds and may be transmitted to human via the contaminated poultry meat (Luangtongkum et al., 2009).

Due to above reasons, US FDA withdrew the use of enrofloxacin in poultry in 2005 (USFDA, 2005). After withdrawal of enrofloxacin from poultry, the rate of FQ-resistance in *C. jejuni* decreased in chicken during 2005–2007 (NARMS, 2010). Human clinicians also observed a reduction in domestically acquired *Campylobacter* infections with decreased susceptibility to fluoroquinolones, and it was thought to be a great achievement regarding public health (Nelson et al., 2007). However, during 2008–2011, the positive rate of ciprofloxacin-resistant *C. jejuni* from retail chicken was again increased (14.6–22.7%) in the USA (NARMS, 2012). These studies suggest that the policy on the ban of fluoroquinolone use in poultry did not reduce or eliminate reservoirs of FQ -resistant *C. jejuni* with subsequent reemergence and persist in poultry products in the USA.

The spread of FQ-resistant *C. jejuni* in USA might result from high mutation rate and enhanced fitness of the bacteria in chicken reservoirs (Luangtongkum et al., 2009). Previous studies have demonstrated that resistant *C. jejuni*, carrying Thr-86-Ile mutation in GyrA, could colonize chicken caecum in the absence of antimicrobial selection pressure (Luo et al., 2005; Nelson et al., 2007; Han et al., 2012; Zeitouni et al., 2012). The Thr-86-Ile mutation in GyrA can modulate DNA supercoiling homeostasis and result in better survivability of FQ-resistant *C. jejuni* in chicken host (Han et al., 2012). Due to the enhanced fitness, it will be difficult to reduce the prevalence of FQ-resistance in *C. jejuni*, even though farmers have not used these antimicrobials in poultry. Additionally, the NARMS human data showed that ciprofloxacin resistant *C. jejuni* in USA kept increasing from 16.7 in 1997 to 25.3% in 2012 (NARMS, 2012).

Contrary to the situation in USA, the ECDC/EFSA/EMA JIACARA reported data showed no associations between the consumption of fluoroquinolones in food-producing animals and the occurrence of resistance in *Campylobacter spp* from cases of human infection (ECDC/EFSA/EMA, 2015). Although the growth promoting agents of fluoroquinolone were withdrawn in European countries earlier in the Twenty first century, the incidence of FQ -resistant *C. jejuni* in broilers raised from 5.3 in

2001 to 26% in 2013 (DANMAP, 2013). The relationship between fluorquinolone use in food animals and antimicrobial resistance in humans may be different based on the geographic region, poultry production environment and fluoquinolone surveillance monitoring protocols.

MACROLIDES AND RESISTANCE IN *CAMPYLOBACTER*

Macrolides inhibit bacteria protein biosynthesis by preventing peptidyltransferase location and/or inhibiting ribosomal translation (Tenson et al., 2003; Liang and Han, 2013). Macrolides were the first choice for treatment infections caused by Gram-positive bacteria in animal and campylobacterosis in human. Macrolide resistance develops in *Campylobacter* by point mutation in target genes of 23S rRNA, ribosomal protein and by overexpression of efflux pumps (Hao et al., 2013).

In food-producing animals, macrolide drugs, such as tylosin and tilmicosin, have been used as growth promoters for decades in USA and Canada. However, two macrolide members, tylosin, and spiramycin were banned for their use as animal growth promoters in Finland and EU since 1995 because exposure of animals to these drugs was implicated as a possible cause of treatment failure in *Campylobacter* infections in humans.

From the ECDC/EFSA/EMA JIACARA report, positive associations were noted for total consumption of macrolides in food-producing animals in 2011 and 2012 and the occurrence of resistance in *C. jejuni* from cases of human infection (ECDC/EFSA/EMA, 2015). However, the data obtained from European antimicrobial resistance monitoring systems, like DANMAP, revealed that macrolide resistance in *C. jejuni* isolates from Danish broilers kept at a relatively low level (lower than 1%) and there was no significant temporal variation during 2000–2012 (DANMAP, 2013).

Contrary to the ECDC/EFSA/EMA JIACARA report, the USA risk assessment data showed that tylosin and tilmicosin in food animals did not result in a risk to public health in relationship to the development and dissemination of macrolide resistant *Campylobacter* (Hurd et al., 2004). The probability of treatment failure of drug resistant *Campylobacter* infections was only one person in 2.36, 14, and 53 billion per year due to consumption of beef, poultry, and pork, respectively (Hurd et al., 2004). In other words, the probability of therapy failure of human campylobacteriosis due to resistant bacteria in food animals exposed to tylosin or tilmicosin, was much less than the mortality due to automobile accidents (1/7,000), shootings (1/10,000), motorcycle and car accidents (1/500,000), aircraft accidents (1/1,000,000), lightning strikes (1/3,000,000) and shark attacks (1/100,000,000) in USA (Hurd et al., 2004). Therefore, the two veterinary macrolide drugs (tylosin and tilmicosin) may have negligible risk for human health (Casewell et al., 2003; Phillips et al., 2004a,b; Turnidge, 2004). Data obtained from NARMS also revealed that macrolide resistance in *C. jejuni* isolates from American chicken breast kept at a relatively low level (lower than 1%) and there was no significant temporal variation during 2000–2012 (NARMS, 2012; DANMAP, 2013).

The mutation frequency for macrolide resistance in *Campylobacter* was reported to be about 10^{-10}/cell/generation which is approximately 10,000-fold lower than that of FQ resistance (Yan et al., 2006; Lin et al., 2007). The mutants obtained by single-step selection tend to have low-to-intermediate levels of macrolide resistance (Erythromycin MIC = 8–64 μg/ml) (Kim et al., 2006; Lin et al., 2007; Caldwell et al., 2008). These mutants generally had fitness cost in the absence of macrolide drugs (Kim et al., 2006; Caldwell et al., 2008). Acquisition of mutations in 23S rRNA, which conferred a high level of resistance to erythromycin (MIC ≥ 512 μg/ml), appeared to require stepwise selection and/or prolonged exposure to macrolide drugs (Lin et al., 2007; Caldwell et al., 2008). In the absence of macrolide selection pressure, most of the 23S rRNA mutations could be stably maintained without competition (Gibreel et al., 2005; Caldwell et al., 2008), but due to their fitness burden, they could be rapidly outcompeted by the erythromycin susceptive *C. jejuni* in both *vitro* or *vivo* environment (Hao et al., 2009; Almofti et al., 2011a,b; Luangtongkum et al., 2011; Zeitouni et al., 2012).

Since *Campylobacter coli* is the most common *Campylobacter* species in pigs, we also discuss the topic of macrolide resistant *C. coli* in this review. The ban on tylosin as growth promoter had a remarkable effect on the level of erythromycin resistance in *C. coli* from pigs, as it decreased from 66 to 20% in Denmark between 1998 and 2005 (Hammerum et al., 2007). However, DANMAP data showed that during 2006–2010, the macrolide resistance in *C. coli* varied within the range of 10–20% without significant reduction (DANMAP, 2010). The macrolide resistance in *C. coli* isolates, although more prevalent than that in *C. jejuni* isolates, also did not increase over the past 10 years since the beginning of the monitoring in the U.S.A (NARMS, 2010). A previous study demonstrated that *C. coli* were not intrinsically more mutable than *C. jejuni*, because no elevated mutation frequency for erythromycin was observed in *C. coli* (Lin et al., 2007).

TETRACYCLINES AND RESISTANCE IN *SALMONELLA*

Tetracyclines are protein synthesis inhibitors. They bind to the 30S ribosomal subunit and prevent the binding of aminoacyl-tRNA to mRNA-ribosome complex (Bassetti et al., 2013). Bacteria could develop resistance to tetracycline by efflux pumps (TetA, B, C, D, E, F, G, H, I, J, K, L, P(A), P(B),V, Y, Z, 30, OtrB, TcrC), ribosomal protection (TetM, O, Q, S, T, U, W, OtrA,), and enzymatic inactivation of drugs (TetX) (Linkevicius et al., 2015). Moreover, the tetracycline resistance genes are often located in some transferable elements including plasmids and integrons (Szmolka et al., 2015).

Tetracyclines have widely been used in human and veterinary medicine since the first discovery of tetracycline in 1948. In food animal production, tetracyclines, like oxytetracycline, and chlorotetracycline, were broadly used for growth promotion and prophylaxis (Chopra and Roberts, 2001). The data from antimicrobial resistance monitoring programs showed that tetracycline resistance was commonly detected in foodborne pathogens (DANMAP, 2014; EFSA, 2015). EU countries have banned the use of tetracyclines for growth promotion since 2006.

However, withdrawal of tetracycline growth promoters did not alter the epidemiology of tetracycline resistance in EU counties. DANMAP reported that tetracycline resistant *Salmonella* Typhimurium isolated from pigs had increased from less than 30% in 2001 to 47% in 2013 (DANMAP, 2013). It was also stated that 29,797 kg (active compound) of tetracyclines were sold to the pig industry in Denmark during 2013 and total consumption of the drugs in pig industry was increased by 2-fold in 2013 as compared to that in 2001 (DANMAP, 2013). The increased therapeutic use of tetracyclines might be a primary reflection of the increased occurrence of drug resistance in *S.* Typhimurium and *E.coli* isolates from pigs (DANMAP, 2010). Using logistic regression analysis, the results from a previous study also showed that both the *S.*Typhimurium phage type ($p < 0.0001$) and the increase in tetracycline consumption ($p = 0.0007$) were significantly associated with the antimicrobial resistance (Emborg et al., 2007). The ECDC/EFSA/EMA JIACARA reported positive associations for total consumption of tetracyclines and the occurrence of resistance in *Salmonella spp* from cases of human infection in 2011 and 2012 (ECDC/EFSA/EMA, 2015). Additionally, tetracycline-resistant *S.* Typhimurium also became more prevalent in human cases and reported as domestically acquired sporadic (36%) and outbreak related (21%) (Emborg et al., 2007).

The high prevalence of tetracycline resistance in zoonotic pathogens could be explained by the transfer of already established or new resistant clones rather than the conversion of well-established susceptible clones into resistant ones by uptake of resistance genes (Szmolka et al., 2015). The serotype of *Salmonella* may also decide the prevalence of resistance to tetracylines. It is known that *Salmonella* Enteritidis and *S.* Typhimurium are two general serotypes of *Salmonella* associated with public health. However, the resistance to tetracycline in *S.* Enteritidis (5%) from human was much lower than that in *S.* Typhimurium (DANMAP, 2010). The drug resistance among *S.* Typhimurium isolates might be due to the transferrable ability of tetracycline resistance determinants (e.g., class 1 integron and *Salmonella* genomic island 1) and the possible fitness of these determinants in pig host (Anjum et al., 2011).

CEPHALOSPORINS AND RESISTANCE IN *SALMONELLA* AND *E. COLI*

The cephalosporins are a class of β-lactams which can disrupt the synthesis of the peptidoglycan layer forming the bacterial cell wall. Cephalosporins have great significance in the treatment of bacterial infection in human medicine. The third and fourth generation cephalosporins are the most common antimicrobial drugs used as human medicine worldwide. However, the third generation cephalosporins, such as ceftiofur, has also been extensively used in many different food animals and the fourth-generation cephalosporin, like cefquinome, was approved by the US Food, and Drug Administration (US FDA) in 2007 soon after its approval by the European Union.

Gram-negative bacteria may develop resistance to β-lactams by producing β-lactamase to inactivate the drugs. The major public health concern is that use of third and fourth generation of cephalosporins in food animals might result in resistance development in foodborne pathogens (e.g., *Salmonella* and *E. coli*). Some evidence, provided by Keep Antibiotic Working (KAW), Union of Concerned Scientists (UCS), the American Medical Association (AMA) and the Infectious Diseases Society of America (IDSA), showed that approval of cefquinome might induce the development of resistance in foodborne pathogens and enhance the transfer risk of resistance to human which may compromise public health. Recently the FDA ordered to prohibit extra label use of cephalosporin drugs in food-producing animals (FDA, 2015).

Interestingly, NARMS data showed that there was no considerably change of cephalosporins resistance in *E. coli* and *Salmonella* isolates from ground turkey, ground beef and pork chop during 2002–2012 (NARMS, 2012). Although there was a transient increase in cephalosporin resistance of *Salmonella* from ground turkey during years of 2007–2009, yet it decreased again in the year 2012. During 2002–2012, antimicrobial resistance was increased (10–35%) in *Salmonella* isolates from chicken breast and the resistance rate was considerably lower in *E. coli* isolates than that in *Salmonella* isolates. In the case of *E. coli* from chicken breast, ground turkey and pork chop, resistance was lower than 10% (except for 11.7% in chicken breast in 2009) and even less than 1% for the ground beef bacteria from 2002 to 2010 (NARMS, 2010).

Additionally, the NARMS human data showed that cephalosporins resistance in *Salmonella* and *E.coli*O157 kept at a very low level (less than 1%) during 2000–2012 (NARMS, 2012). From the ECDC/EFSA/EMA JIACARA report, no associations were observed between the consumption of 3rd—and 4th—generation cephalosporins in food-producing animals and the occurrence of resistance to this sub-class in selected bacteria from human (ECDC/EFSA/EMA, 2015).

Concern of resistant bacteria carrying extended-spectrum β-lactamases (ESBLs) has been raised after the use of third and fourth generation of cephalosporins. The ESBLs encoding genes (e.g., *bla*OXA, *bla*PSE, *bla*SHV, *bla*TEM, *bla*CTX-M), as well as the plamid-mediated AmpC β-lactamases (PMAβ, such as *bla*CMY and *bla*FOX), and carbepenemases (e.g., *bla*IMP, *bla*KPC, *bla*VIM) could be involved in the resistance to extended-spectrum β–lactams (Liebana et al., 2013; Rubin and Pitout, 2014; Bae et al., 2015). There were many reports about the transmission of ESBL carrying bacteria (Hasman et al., 2005; Collignon and Aarestrup, 2007), but the possible zoonotic spread of ESBL is still controversial. Some investigators found that there was similarity between ESBL genes and bacterial properties in isolates from human, livestock and companion animal populations, indicating that exchange of ESBL genes and ESBL bacterial between these reservoirs (Valentin et al., 2014; Dahms et al., 2015). A review paper by Ewers et al. (2012) showed that the European, American and Asian countries (e.g., Japan) shared a similar population of ESBL subtypes, but ESBL subtype (bla_{CTX-M}) from human was similar to that from pets but significantly different with that from food-producing animals (Ewers et al., 2012). Largely unknown environmental factors might impact the spread of resistant pathogens and increase the complexity of development and transfer of resistance enzymes. For example, wild animals like waterfowl, prey and rodents carry similar subtype of ESBL *E. coli* to humans, indicating that wildlife could be an environmental reservoir and melting pot for enzymatic resistance. The bacteria might re-infect humans through the omnipresent bird feces. Similar to humans traveling, the birds migration might also contribute to the worldwide spread of the resistant organism (Guenther et al., 2009, 2010, 2011; Dolejska et al., 2011).

CONCLUSIONS

The relationship between use of antimicrobial agents in food animals and antimicrobial resistance associated with human public health is a complex and controversial subject (**Table 2**). The risk of the use of some antimicrobial agents in food-producing animals with consequences on human public health is still problematic because there are so many factors to consider from an antimicrobial resistance perspective (**Table 2**). There is not enough of compelling evidence to assert that the prevalence

TABLE 2 | Summary of risk assessment of some veterinary antimicrobial drugs on human public health associated with antimicrobial resistance and their molecular basis.

Veterinary drug Use and ban	Associated Public health	Resistance monitoring data in animasl	Resistance monitoring data in humans	Risk assessment; Risk association	Molecular basis
Avoparcin, Used 1940s–1990s; Banned 1995–2000; Not approved in USA for use in animal.	Vancomycin-resistant *Enterococci* (VRE), and *E. faecium* (VREF)	In EU, high prevalence of VRE in 1990s and in poultry after 2000; In Denmark, VRE reduced from 1995 to 2013; few VRE in livestock during 2003–2013.	In U. S. A, 40% VRE infections in 2013; In EU, <5% VRE in 2013.	Positive risk; Still some controversy questions	vanA gene located in transferable transposon Tn1546
Virginiamycin, Used as GP for 30 years; Banned in 1999 in EU	*streptogramin-resistant Enterococci (SRE),* and *E.faecium* (SREF)	In Denmark, 25% SREF from pigs and chickens; In USA, 30–70% SREF from poultry products in 2012.	Very rare in human hospital.	FDA-CVM: risk is little weight	VatD, VatE; ErmB; VgbA; Hard resistance development
Veterinary fluoroquinolones, e.g., enrofloxacin Banned use on poultry in 2005 in USA	fluoroquinolones resistant *Campylobacter jejuni*	In USA, high prevalence of FQ-resistant *C. jejuni* in poultry before 2005, resistance reduced during 2005–2007, resistance increased during 2008–2011.	In USA, ciprofloxacin resistant *C. jejuni* kept increasing from 16.7% in 1997 to 25.3% in 2012.	FDA-CVM: Positive risk ECDC/EFSA/EMA JIACARA: no risk associations	Thr-86-Ile mutation in GyrA; high mutation rate and enhanced fitness in chicken
Veterinary Macrolides e.g., tylosin, tilmicosin. EU banned tylosin and spiramycin as GP since 1995	Macrolide resistant *Campylobacter spp*	Resistant *C.jejuni* kept low level (<1%) in USA and Denmark; Resistant *C. coli* in pig reduced during 1998 –2005 and kept at about 10% during 2006–2010 in Denmark; kept at a stable level in USA in the past decade.	Erythromycin resistant *C. jejuni* is rare in human	FDA-CVM: negative risk ECDC/EFSA/EMA JIACARA: positive risk associations	point mutation in target genes of 23S rRNA; low mutation frequency and fitness cost of resistance
Veterinary tetracyclines EU banned tetracyclines as growth promotor since 2006	Tetracycline resistance in *Salmonella* Typhimurium	In Denmark, resistant *S.*Typhimurium from pigs had increased from less than 30% in 2001 to 47% in 2013.	High prevalent of tetracycline-resistant *S.* Typhimurium in human	ECDC/EFSA/EMA JIACARA report: positive associations	*Tet* genes were normally located in some transferable elements
Veterinary Cephalosporins	Cephalosporins resistance in *E. coli* and *Salmonella*	In USA, no significant change of resistance from animal product during 2002–2012;	Resistance kept at a very low level (<1%) during 2000–2012 in USA.	ECDC/EFSA/EMA JIACARA report: no risk associations	Complex distribution of ESBLs in animal, human and environment.

GP was Growth promotor; ESBL was extended-spectrum β-lactamases; ECDC/EFSA/EMA JIACARA was European center for disease prevention and control/European food safety authority/European Medicines Agency. Joint Interagency Antimicrobial Consumption and Resistance Analysis report. Risk association means the association between consumption of veterinary antimicrobial drugs in food-producing animal and the occurrence of resistance bacterial from human infection. The FDA-CVM risk means the relationship between the use of antimicrobial agents in food-producing animal and human public health associated with antimicrobial resistance in special foodborne pathogens.

of some resistant bacteria in humans was due to antimicrobial agents used in food animals (NAMI, 2010; Horigan et al., 2016). The zoonotic spread of antimicrobial resistant bacteria or resistant genes is also questionable because resistant pathogens could be found in soil, water and environment and long-term occurrence of antimicrobial resistant genes in nature was even known before the antimicrobial era (Casewell et al., 2003; Aminov and Mackie, 2007; Kobayashi et al., 2007; Aminov, 2010). Therefore, it is not wise to oversimplify the opinion that the resistant bacteria from food producing animal is a major origin of human infection and neglect the highly complex environment scenario.

Furthermore, the ban on some antimicrobial usage has not altered or decreased the incidence of resistance in foodborne pathogens. This may be due to the enhanced fitness or high transferability of some resistant determinants. To control the increased animal disease, therapeutic levels of some antimicrobial drugs (e.g., fluroquinolones and tetracyclines) has been increased. This may also be a reason for the increased detection of resistance to some therapeutic drugs in food borne pathogens isolated from food animals after the ban of growth promoters (Koluman and Dikici, 2013).

On the concept of "one health one world," international governments need to cooperate to establish an international antimicrobial resistance surveillance monitoring program and monitor the antimicrobial resistance trends in human and animals for a long time. Both the benefit and risk outcomes should be considered into the risk assessment and management. To find wise strategy to control antimicrobial resistance, it is necessary to considerate the chemotherapeutic medicine, microbiology and agricultural environment and fully understand molecular basis involved in the emergence of antimicrobial resistance.

AUTHOR CONTRIBUTIONS

The Idea and designation: HH, and ZY; Data collection and analysis: HH, PS, and YW; The writing and modification of this manuscript: HH, ZI, PS, and GC.

FUNDING

This article is financially supported by grants from National Basic Research Program of China (2013CB127206), National Key Research and Development Program (2016YFD0501302), Fundamental Research Funds for the Central Universities (2662015PY035), Morning Program of Wuhan in China (2015070404010191), National Program for Risk Assessment of Quality and Safety of Livestock and Poultry Products (GJFP2016008), National Natural Science Foundation of China (31101856/31302143/31272614), National Key Technology R&D Program (2012BAK01B00).

REFERENCES

Aarestrup, F. M. (1995). Occurrence of glycopeptide resistance among Enterococcus faecium isolates from conventional and ecological poultry farms. *Microb. Drug Resist.* 1, 255–257. doi: 10.1089/mdr.1995.1.255

Acar, J., Casewell, M., Freeman, J., Friis, C., and Goossens, H. (2000). Avoparcin and virginiamycin as animal growth promoters: a plea for science in decision-making. *Clin. Microbiol. Infect.* 6, 477–482. doi: 10.1046/j.1469-0691.2000.00128.x

Almofti, Y. A., Dai, M., Sun, Y., Haihong, H., and Yuan, Z. (2011a). Impact of erythromycin resistance on the virulence properties and fitness of *Campylobacter jejuni*. *Microb. Pathog.* 50, 336–342. doi: 10.1016/j.micpath.2011.02.009

Almofti, Y. A., Dai, M., Sun, Y., Hao, H., Liu, Z., Cheng, G., et al. (2011b). The physiologic and phenotypic alterations due to macrolide exposure in *Campylobacter jejuni*. *Int. J. Food Microbiol.* 151, 52–61. doi: 10.1016/j.ijfoodmicro.2011.08.002

Aminov, R. I. (2010). A brief history of the antibiotic era: lessons learned and challenges for the future. *Front. Microbiol.* 1:134. doi: 10.3389/fmicb.2010.00134

Aminov, R. I., and Mackie, R. I. (2007). Evolution and ecology of antibiotic resistance genes. *FEMS Microbiol. Lett.* 271, 147–161. doi: 10.1111/j.1574-6968.2007.00757.x

Anjum, M. F., Choudhary, S., Morrison, V., Snow, L. C., Mafura, M., Slickers, P., et al. (2011). Identifying antimicrobial resistance genes of human clinical relevance within Salmonella isolated from food animals in Great Britain. *J. Antimicrob. Chemother.* 66, 550–559. doi: 10.1093/jac/dkq498

Bae, D., Cheng, C. M., and Khan, A. A. (2015). Characterization of extended-spectrum beta-lactamase (ESBL) producing non-typhoidal Salmonella (NTS) from imported food products. *Int. J. Food Microbiol.* 214, 12–17. doi: 10.1016/j.ijfoodmicro.2015.07.017

Bassetti, M., Merelli, M., Temperoni, C., and Astilean, A. (2013). New antibiotics for bad bugs: where are we? *Ann. Clin. Microbiol. Antimicrob.* 12:22. doi: 10.1186/1476-0711-12-22

Bonten, M. J., Willems, R., and Weinstein, R. A. (2001). Vancomycin-resistant enterococci: why are they here, and where do they come from? *Lancet Infect. Dis.* 1, 314–325. doi: 10.1016/S1473-3099(01)00145-1

Boyd, D. A., Willey, B. M., Fawcett, D., Gillani, N., and Mulvey, M. R. (2008). Molecular characterization of *Enterococcus faecalis* N06-0364 with low-level vancomycin resistance harboring a novel D-Ala-D-Ser gene cluster, vanL. *Antimicrob. Agents Chemother.* 52, 2667–2672. doi: 10.1128/AAC.01516-07

Caldwell, D. B., Wang, Y., and Lin, J. (2008). Development, stability, and molecular mechanisms of macrolide resistance in *Campylobacter jejuni*. *Antimicrob. Agents Chemother.* 52, 3947–3954. doi: 10.1128/AAC.00450-08

Casewell, M., Friis, C., Marco, E., McMullin, P., and Phillips, I. (2003). The European ban on growth-promoting antibiotics and emerging consequences for human and animal health. *J. Antimicrob. Chemother.* 52, 159–161. doi: 10.1093/jac/dkg313

CDC (2013). *Antibiotic Resistance Threats in United States*. Available online at: http://www.fda.gov/AnimalVeterinary/SafetyHealth/AntimicrobialResistance/NationalAntimicrobialResistanceMonitoringSystem/default.htm

Cetinkaya, Y., Falk, P., and Mayhall, C. G. (2000). Vancomycin-resistant enterococci. *Clin. Microbiol. Rev.* 13, 686–707. doi: 10.1128/CMR.13.4.686-707.2000

Chen, C., Sun, J., Guo, Y., Lin, D., Guo, Q., Hu, F., et al. (2015). High prevalence of vanM in vancomycin-resistant *Enterococcus faecium* isolates from Shanghai, China. *Antimicrob. Agents Chemother.* 59, 7795–7798. doi: 10.1128/AAC.01732-15

Chopra, I., and Roberts, M. (2001). Tetracycline antibiotics: mode of action, applications, molecular biology, and epidemiology of bacterial resistance. *Microbiol. Mol. Biol. Rev.* 65, 232–260. doi: 10.1128/MMBR.65.2.232-260.2001

Collignon, P., and Aarestrup, F. M. (2007). Extended-spectrum beta-lactamases, food, and cephalosporin use in food animals. *Clin. Infect. Dis.* 44, 1391–1392. doi: 10.1086/516612

Cox, L. A. Jr. (2005). Potential human health benefits of antibiotics used in food animals: a case study of virginiamycin. *Environ. Int.* 31, 549–563. doi: 10.1016/j.envint.2004.10.012

Cox, L. A. Jr. and Popken, D. A. (2004). Quantifying human health risks from virginiamycin used in chickens. *Risk Anal.* 24, 271–288. doi: 10.1111/j.0272-4332.2004.00428.x

Dahms, C., Hübner, N. O., Kossow, A., Mellmann, A., Dittmann, K., and Kramer, A. (2015). Occurrence of ESBL-producing *Escherichia coli* in livestock and farm workers in mecklenburg-western pomerania, Germany. *PLoS ONE* 10:e0143326. doi: 10.1371/journal.pone.0143326

DANMAP (2010). *DANMAP 2010 - Use of Antimicrobial Agents and Occurrence of Antimicrobial Resistance in Bacteria from Food Animals, Food and Humans in Denmark.* Available online at: http://www.danmap.org

DANMAP (2013). *DANMAP 2013 - Use of Antimicrobial Agents and Occurrence of Antimicrobial Resistance in Bacteria from Food Animals, Food and Humans in Denmark.* Available online at: http://www.danmap.org

DANMAP (2014). *DANMAP 2014 - Use of Antimicrobial Agents and Occurrence of Antimicrobial Resistance in Bacteria from Food Animals Food and Humans in Denmark.* DANMAP.

Dibner, J. J., and Richards, J. D. (2005). Antibiotic growth promoters in agriculture: history and mode of action. *Poult. Sci.* 84, 634–643. doi: 10.1093/ps/84.4.634

Dolejska, M., Frolkova, P., Florek, M., Jamborova, I., Purgertova, M., Kutilova, I., et al. (2011). CTX-M-15-producing *Escherichia coli* clone B2-O25b-ST131 and *Klebsiella* spp. isolates in municipal wastewater treatment plant effluents. *J. Antimicrob. Chemother.* 66, 2784–2790. doi: 10.1093/jac/dkr363

EARS-Net (2012). *European Antimicrobial Resistance Surveillance Network.* Available online at: http://ecdc.europa.eu/en/activities/surveillance/EARS-Net/Pages/index.aspx

ECDC/EFSA/EMA (2015). "ECDC/EFSA/EMA first joint report on the integrated analysis of the consumption of antimicrobial agents and occurrence of antimicrobial resistance," in *Bacteria from Humans and Food-Producing Animals. Joint Interagency Antimicrobial Consumption and Resistance Analysis (JIACRA) Report* (Stockholm; Parma; london: EFSA Journal), 4006.

EFSA (2015). EU Summary Report on antimicrobial resistance in zoonotic and indicator bacteria from humans, animals and food in 2013. *EFSA J.* 13:4036. doi: 10.2903/j.efsa.2015.4036

Emborg, H. D., Vigre, H., Jensen, V. F., Vieira, A. R., Baggesen, D. L., and Aarestrup, F. M. (2007). Tetracycline consumption and occurrence of tetracycline resistance in *Salmonella typhimurium* phage types from Danish pigs. *Microb. Drug Resist.* 13, 289–294. doi: 10.1089/mdr.2007.746

Ewers, C., Bethe, A., Semmler, T., Guenther, S., and Wieler, L. H. (2012). Extended-spectrum beta-lactamase-producing and AmpC-producing *Escherichia coli* from livestock and companion animals, and their putative impact on public health: a global perspective. *Clin. Microbiol. Infect.* 18, 646–655. doi: 10.1111/j.1469-0691.2012.03850.x

FAO/OIE/WHO (2003). *Joint FAO/OIE/WHO Expert Workshop on Non-Human Antimicrobial Usage and Antimicrobial Resistance: Scientific assessment Geneva.* FAO/OIE/WHO.

FAO/OIE/WHO (2004). Second *Joint FAO/OIE/WHO Expert Workshop on Non-Human Antimicrobial Usage and Antimicrobial Resistance: Management Options.* OSLO: FAO/OIE/WHO.

FAO/OIE/WHO (2006). *Report of a Joint FAO/OIE/WHO Expert Consultation on Antimicrobial Use in Aquaculture and Antimicrobial Resistance* Seoul: FAO/OIE/WHO.

Farnell, M. B., Donoghue, A. M., Cole, K., Reyes-Herrera, I., Blore, P. J., and Donoghue, D. J. (2005). Campylobacter susceptibility to ciprofloxacin and corresponding fluoroquinolone concentrations within the gastrointestinal tracts of chickens. *J. Appl. Microbiol.* 99, 1043–1050. doi: 10.1111/j.1365-2672.2005.02712.x

FDA (2002). *Final Decision of the Commissioner Docket No. 2000N21571 with Drawal of Approval of the New Animal Drug Application for Enrofloxacin in Poultry [EB/OL].* Available online at: http://www.fda.gov/AnimalVeterinary/SafetyHealth/RecallsWithdrawals/ucm042004.htm

FDA (2015). *Limiting Antimicrobial Resistance. FDA-CVM.*

FDV-CVM (2004). "Risk assessment of streptogramin resistance in enterococcus faecium attributable to the use of streptogramins in animals," in *Virginiamycin Risk Assessment* (F. C. f. V. Medicine), Available online at: http://www.fda.gov/OHRMS/DOCKETS/98fr/2004n-0479-ra00001.pdf

Freitas, A. R., Coque, T. M., Novais, C., Hammerum, A. M., Lester, C. H., Zervos, M. J., et al. (2011). Human and swine hosts share vancomycin-resistant *Enterococcus faecium* CC17 and CC5 and *Enterococcus faecalis* CC2 clonal clusters harboring Tn1546 on indistinguishable plasmids. *J. Clin. Microbiol.* 49, 925–931. doi: 10.1128/JCM.01750-10

Gambarotto, K., Ploy, M. C., Turlure, P., Grélaud, C., Martin, C., Bordessoule, D., et al. (2000). Prevalence of vancomycin-resistant enterococci in fecal samples from hospitalized patients and nonhospitalized controls in a cattle-rearing area of France. *J. Clin. Microbiol.* 38, 620–624.

Garcia-Migura, L., Liebana, E., Jensen, L. B., Barnes, S., and Pleydell, E. (2007). A longitudinal study to assess the persistence of vancomycin-resistant *Enterococcus faecium* (VREF) on an intensive broiler farm in the United Kingdom. *FEMS Microbiol. Lett.* 275, 319–325. doi: 10.1111/j.1574-6968.2007.00911.x

Gibreel, A., Kos, V. N., Keelan, M., Trieber, C. A., Levesque, S., Michaud, S., et al. (2005). Macrolide resistance in *Campylobacter jejuni* and *Campylobacter coli*: molecular mechanism and stability of the resistance phenotype. *Antimicrob. Agents Chemother.* 49, 2753–2759. doi: 10.1128/AAC.49.7.2753-2759.2005

Gratacós-Cubarsí, M., García-Regueiro, J. A., and Castellari, M. (2007). Assessment of enrofloxacin and ciprofloxacin accumulation in pig and calf hair by HPLC and fluorimetric detection. *Anal. Bioanal. Chem.* 387, 1991–1998. doi: 10.1007/s00216-006-1000-6

Griggs, D. J., Johnson, M. M., Frost, J. A., Humphrey, T., Jørgensen, F., and Piddock, L. J. (2005). Incidence and mechanism of ciprofloxacin resistance in *Campylobacter* spp. isolated from commercial poultry flocks in the United Kingdom before, during, and after fluoroquinolone treatment. *Antimicrob. Agents Chemother.* 49, 699–707. doi: 10.1128/AAC.49.2.699-707.2005

Guenther, S., Ewers, C., and Wieler, L. H. (2011). Extended-spectrum beta-lactamases producing *E. coli* in wildlife, yet another form of environmental pollution? *Front. Microbiol.* 2:246. doi: 10.3389/fmicb.2011.00246

Guenther, S., Grobbel, M., Beutlich, J., Guerra, B., Ulrich, R. G., Wieler, L. H., et al. (2010). Detection of pandemic B2-O25-ST131 *Escherichia coli* harbouring the CTX-M-9 extended-spectrum beta-lactamase type in a feral urban brown rat (*Rattus norvegicus*). *J. Antimicrob. Chemother.* 65, 582–584. doi: 10.1093/jac/dkp496

Guenther, S., Grobbel, M., Lübke-Becker, A., Goedecke, A., Friedrich, N. D., Wieler, L. H., et al. (2009). Antimicrobial resistance profiles of *Escherichia coli* from common European wild bird species. *Vet. Microbiol.* 144, 219–225. doi: 10.1016/j.vetmic.2009.12.016

Hammerum, A. M., Heuer, O. E., Lester, C. H., Agersø, Y., Seyfarth, A. M., Emborg, H. D., et al. (2007). Comment on: withdrawal of growth-promoting antibiotics in Europe and its effects in relation to human health. *Int. J. Antimicrob. Agents* 30, 466–468. doi: 10.1016/j.ijantimicag.2007.07.012

Hammerum, A. M., Jensen, L. B., and Aarestrup, F. M. (1998). Detection of the satA gene and transferability of virginiamycin resistance in *Enterococcus faecium* from food-animals. *FEMS Microbiol. Lett.* 168, 145–151. doi: 10.1111/j.1574-6968.1998.tb13267.x

Hammerum, A. M., Lester, C. H., and Heuer, O. E. (2010). Antimicrobial-resistant enterococci in animals and meat: a human health hazard? *Foodborne Pathog. Dis.* 7, 1137–1146. doi: 10.1089/fpd.2010.0552

Han, J., Sahin, O., Barton, Y. W., and Zhang, Q. (2008). Key role of Mfd in the development of fluoroquinolone resistance in *Campylobacter jejuni*. *PLoS Pathog.* 4:e1000083. doi: 10.1371/journal.ppat.1000083

Han, J., Wang, Y., Sahin, O., Shen, Z., Guo, B., Shen, J., et al. (2012). A fluoroquinolone resistance associated mutation in gyrA Affects DNA supercoiling in *Campylobacter jejuni*. *Front. Cell. Infect. Microbiol.* 2:21. doi: 10.3389/fcimb.2012.00021

Hao, H., Dai, M., Wang, Y., Peng, D., Liu, Z., and Yuan, Z. (2009). 23S rRNA mutation A2074C conferring high-level macrolide resistance and fitness cost in *Campylobacter jejuni*. *Microb. Drug Resist.* 15, 239–244. doi: 10.1089/mdr.2009.0008

Hao, H., Yuan, Z., Shen, Z., Han, J., Sahin, O., Liu, P., et al. (2013). Mutational and transcriptomic changes involved in the development of macrolide resistance in *Campylobacter jejuni*. *Antimicrob. Agents Chemother.* 57, 1369–1378. doi: 10.1128/AAC.01927-12

Haroche, J., Allignet, J., Aubert, S., Van Den Bogaard, A. E., and El Solh, N. (2000). satG, conferring resistance to streptogramin A, is widely distributed in *Enterococcus faecium* strains but not in staphylococci.

Antimicrob. Agents Chemother. 44, 190–191. doi: 10.1128/AAC.44.1.190-191.2000

Hasman, H., Mevius, D., Veldman, K., Olesen, I., and Aarestrup, F. M. (2005). beta-Lactamases among extended-spectrum beta-lactamase (ESBL)-resistant Salmonella from poultry, poultry products and human patients in The Netherlands. *J. Antimicrob. Chemother.* 56, 115–121. doi: 10.1093/jac/dki190

Hershberger, E., Oprea, S. F., Donabedian, S. M., Perri, M., Bozigar, P., Bartlett, P., et al. (2005). Epidemiology of antimicrobial resistance in enterococci of animal origin. *J. Antimicrob. Chemother.* 55, 127–130. doi: 10.1093/jac/dkh508

Horigan, V., Kosmider, R. D., Horton, R. A., Randall, L., and Simons, R. R. (2016). An assessment of evidence data gaps in the investigation of possible transmission routes of extended spectrum beta-lactamase producing *Escherichia coli* from livestock to humans in the UK. *Prev. Vet. Med.* 124, 1–8. doi: 10.1016/j.prevetmed.2015.12.020

Hurd, H. S., Doores, S., Hayes, D., Mathew, A., Maurer, J., Silley, P., et al. (2004). Public health consequences of macrolide use in food animals: a deterministic risk assessment. *J. Food Prot.* 67, 980–992.

Jensen, L. B. (1998). Differences in the occurrence of two base pair variants of Tn1546 from vancomycin-resistant enterococci from humans, pigs, and poultry. *Antimicrob. Agents Chemother.* 42, 2463–2464.

Kieke, A. L., Borchardt, M. A., Kieke, B. A., Spencer, S. K., Vandermause, M. F., Smith, K. E., et al. (2006). Use of streptogramin growth promoters in poultry and isolation of streptogramin-resistant *Enterococcus faecium* from humans. *J. Infect. Dis.* 194, 1200–1208. doi: 10.1086/508189

Kim, J. S., Carver, D. K., and Kathariou, S. (2006). Natural transformation-mediated transfer of erythromycin resistance in *Campylobacter coli* strains from turkeys and swine. *Appl. Environ. Microbiol.* 72, 1316–1321. doi: 10.1128/AEM.72.2.1316-1321.2006

Klare, I., Heier, H., Claus, H., Reissbrodt, R., and Witte, W. (1995). vanA-mediated high-level glycopeptide resistance in *Enterococcus faecium* from animal husbandry. *FEMS Microbiol. Lett.* 125, 165–171. doi: 10.1111/j.1574-6968.1995.tb07353.x

Kobayashi, T., Nonaka, L., Maruyama, F., and Suzuki, S. (2007). Molecular evidence for the ancient origin of the ribosomal protection protein that mediates tetracycline resistance in bacteria. *J. Mol. Evol.* 65, 228–235. doi: 10.1007/s00239-007-9006-z

Koluman, A., and Dikici, A. (2013). Antimicrobial resistance of emerging foodborne pathogens: status quo and global trends. *Crit. Rev. Microbiol.* 39, 57–69. doi: 10.3109/1040841X.2012.691458

Lester, C. H., Frimodt-Møller, N., Sørensen, T. L., Monnet, D. L., and Hammerum, A. M. (2006). *In vivo* transfer of the vanA resistance gene from an *Enterococcus faecium* isolate of animal origin to an *E. faecium* isolate of human origin in the intestines of human volunteers. *Antimicrob. Agents Chemother.* 50, 596–599. doi: 10.1128/AAC.50.2.596-599.2006

Lester, C. H., and Hammerum, A. M. (2010). Transfer of vanA from an *Enterococcus faecium* isolate of chicken origin to a CC17 *E. faecium* isolate in the intestine of cephalosporin-treated mice. *J. Antimicrob. Chemother.* 65, 1534–1536. doi: 10.1093/jac/dkq170

Liang, J. H., and Han, X. (2013). Structure-activity relationships and mechanism of action of macrolides derived from erythromycin as antibacterial agents. *Curr. Top. Med. Chem.* 13, 3131–3164. doi: 10.2174/15680266113136660223

Liebana, E., Carattoli, A., Coque, T. M., Hasman, H., Magiorakos, A. P., Mevius, D., et al. (2013). Public health risks of enterobacterial isolates producing extended-spectrum beta-lactamases or AmpC beta-lactamases in food and food-producing animals: an EU perspective of epidemiology, analytical methods, risk factors, and control options. *Clin. Infect. Dis.* 56, 1030–1037. doi: 10.1093/cid/cis1043

Lin, J., Yan, M., Sahin, O., Pereira, S., Chang, Y. J., and Zhang, Q. (2007). Effect of macrolide usage on emergence of erythromycin-resistant Campylobacter isolates in chickens. *Antimicrob. Agents Chemother.* 51, 1678–1686. doi: 10.1128/AAC.01411-06

Linkevicius, M., Sandegren, L., and Andersson, D. I. (2015). Potential of tetracycline resistance proteins to evolve tigecycline resistance. *Antimicrob. Agents Chemother.* 60, 789–796. doi: 10.1128/AAC.02465-15

Luangtongkum, T., Jeon, B., Han, J., Plummer, P., Logue, C. M., and Zhang, Q. (2009). Antibiotic resistance in Campylobacter: emergence, transmission and persistence. *Future Microbiol.* 4, 189–200. doi: 10.2217/17460913.4.2.189

Luangtongkum, T., Shen, Z., Seng, V. W., Sahin, O., Jeon, B., Liu, P., et al. (2011). Impaired fitness and transmission of macrolide-resistant *Campylobacter jejuni* in its natural host. *Antimicrob. Agents Chemother.* 56, 1300–1308. doi: 10.1128/AAC.05516-11

Luo, N., Pereira, S., Sahin, O., Lin, J., Huang, S., Michel, L., et al. (2005). Enhanced *in vivo* fitness of fluoroquinolone-resistant *Campylobacter jejuni* in the absence of antibiotic selection pressure. *Proc. Natl. Acad. Sci. U.S.A.* 102, 541–546. doi: 10.1073/pnas.0408966102

Luo, N., Sahin, O., Lin, J., Michel, L. O., and Zhang, Q. (2003). *In vivo* selection of Campylobacter isolates with high levels of fluoroquinolone resistance associated with gyrA mutations and the function of the CmeABC efflux pump. *Antimicrob. Agents Chemother.* 47, 390–394. doi: 10.1128/AAC.47.1.390-394.2003

Marshall, B. M., and Levy, S. B. (2011). Food animals and antimicrobials: impacts on human health. *Clin. Microbiol. Rev.* 24, 718–733. doi: 10.1128/CMR.00002-11

McDermott, P. F., Bodeis, S. M., English, L. L., White, D. G., Walker, R. D., Zhao, S., et al. (2002). Ciprofloxacin resistance in *Campylobacter jejuni* evolves rapidly in chickens treated with fluoroquinolones. *J. Infect. Dis.* 185, 837–840. doi: 10.1086/339195

McDonald, L. C., Rossiter, S., Mackinson, C., Wang, Y. Y., Johnson, S., Sullivan, M., et al. (2001). Quinupristin-dalfopristin-resistant *Enterococcus faecium* on chicken and in human stool specimens. *N. Engl. J. Med.* 345, 1155–1160. doi: 10.1056/NEJMoa010805

NAMI (2010). *Antibiotic Use in Livestock Production: Ensuring Meat Safety.* N. A. M. Institute. Available online at: http://www.MeatAMI.com: AMI Fact Sheet

NARMS (2010). *Retail Meat Report-National Antimicrobial Resistance Monitoring System.* Available online at: http://www.fda.gov/AnimalVeterinary/SafetyHealth/AntimicrobialResistance/NationalAntimicrobialResistanceMonitoringSystem/default.htm

NARMS (2012). *Retail Meat Report-National Antimicrobial Resistance Monitoring System.* Available online at: http://www.fda.gov/AnimalVeterinary/SafetyHealth/AntimicrobialResistance/NationalAntimicrobialResistanceMonitoringSystem/default.htm

Nelson, J. M., Chiller, T. M., Powers, J. H., and Angulo, F. J. (2007). Fluoroquinolone-resistant Campylobacter species and the withdrawal of fluoroquinolones from use in poultry: a public health success story. *Clin. Infect. Dis.* 44, 977–980. doi: 10.1086/512369

Niewold, T. A. (2007). The nonantibiotic anti-inflammatory effect of antimicrobial growth promoters, the real mode of action? A hypothesis. *Poult. Sci.* 86, 605–609. doi: 10.1093/ps/86.4.605

Nilsson, O. (2012). Vancomycin resistant enterococci in farm animals - occurrence and importance. *Infect. Ecol. Epidemiol.* 2:16959. doi: 10.3402/iee.v2i0.16959

Nilsson, O., Greko, C., Top, J., Franklin, A., and Bengtsson, B. (2009). Spread without known selective pressure of a vancomycin-resistant clone of *Enterococcus faecium* among broilers. *J. Antimicrob. Chemother.* 63, 868–872. doi: 10.1093/jac/dkp045

Nomura, T., Tanimoto, K., Shibayama, K., Arakawa, Y., Fujimoto, S., Ike, Y., et al. (2012). Identification of VanN-type vancomycin resistance in an *Enterococcus faecium* isolate from chicken meat in Japan. *Antimicrob. Agents Chemother.* 56, 6389–6392. doi: 10.1128/AAC.00747-12

Phillips, I. (2007). Withdrawal of growth-promoting antibiotics in Europe and its effects in relation to human health. *Int. J. Antimicrob. Agents* 30, 101–107. doi: 10.1016/j.ijantimicag.2007.02.018

Phillips, I., Casewell, M., Cox, T., De Groot, B., Friis, C., Jones, R., et al. (2004a). Antibiotic use in animals. *J. Antimicrob. Chemother.* 53, 885. doi: 10.1093/jac/dkh149

Phillips, I., Casewell, M., Cox, T., De Groot, B., Friis, C., Jones, R., et al. (2004b). Does the use of antibiotics in food animals pose a risk to human health? A critical review of published data. *J. Antimicrob. Chemother.* 53, 28–52. doi: 10.1093/jac/dkg483

Robredo, B., Singh, K. V., Torres, C., and Murray, B. E. (2000). Streptogramin resistance and shared pulsed-field gel electrophoresis patterns in vanA-containing *Enterococcus faecium* and *Enterococcus hirae* isolated from humans and animals in Spain. *Microb. Drug Resist.* 6, 305–311. doi: 10.1089/mdr.2000.6.305

Rubin, J. E., and Pitout, J. D. (2014). Extended-spectrum beta-lactamase, carbapenemase and AmpC producing Enterobacteriaceae in companion animals. *Vet. Microbiol.* 170, 10–18. doi: 10.1016/j.vetmic.2014.01.017

Salisbury, J. G., Nicholls, T. J., Lammerding, A. M., Turnidge, J., and Nunn, M. J. (2002). A risk analysis framework for the long-term management of antibiotic resistance in food-producing animals. *Int. J. Antimicrob. Agents* 20, 153–164. doi: 10.1016/S0924-8579(02)00169-3

Smith, D. L., Johnson, J. A., Harris, A. D., Furuno, J. P., Perencevich, E. N., and Morris, J. G., et al. (2003). Assessing risks for a pre-emergent pathogen: virginiamycin use and the emergence of streptogramin resistance in *Enterococcus faecium*. *Lancet Infect. Dis.* 3, 241–249. doi: 10.1016/S1473-3099(03)00581-4

Sørensen, T. L., Blom, M., Monnet, D. L., Frimodt-Møller, N., Poulsen, R. L., and Espersen, F. (2001). Transient intestinal carriage after ingestion of antibiotic-resistant *Enterococcus faecium* from chicken and pork. *N.Engl. J. Med.* 345, 1161–1166. doi: 10.1056/NEJMoa010692

Suto, M. J., Domagala, J. M., Roland, G. E., Mailloux, G. B., and Cohen, M. A. (1992). Fluoroquinolones: relationships between structural variations, mammalian cell cytotoxicity, and antimicrobial activity. *J. Med. Chem.* 35, 4745–4750. doi: 10.1021/jm00103a013

Szmolka, A., Lestar, B., Paszti, J., Fekete, P., and Nagy, B. (2015). Conjugative IncF and IncI1 plasmids with tet(A) and class 1 integron conferring multidrug resistance in F18(+) porcine enterotoxigenic *E. coli*. *Acta Vet. Hung.* 63, 425–443. doi: 10.1556/004.2015.040

Tenson, T., Lovmar, M., and Ehrenberg, M. (2003). The mechanism of action of macrolides, lincosamides and streptogramin B reveals the nascent peptide exit path in the ribosome. *J. Mol. Biol.* 330, 1005–1014. doi: 10.1016/S0022-2836(03)00662-4

Top, J., Schouls, L. M., Bonten, M. J., and Willems, R. J. (2004). Multiple-locus variable-number tandem repeat analysis, a novel typing scheme to study the genetic relatedness and epidemiology of *Enterococcus faecium* isolates. *J. Clin. Microbiol.* 42, 4503–4511. doi: 10.1128/JCM.42.10.4503-4511.2004

Turnidge, J. (2004). Antibiotic use in animals–prejudices, perceptions and realities. *J Antimicrob. Chemother.* 53, 26–27. doi: 10.1093/jac/dkg493

USFDA (2005). *Withdrawal of Approval of Bayer Corporation's New Animal Drug Application (NADA).* USFDA.Available online at: http://www.fda.gov/animalveterinary/safetyhealth/recallswithdrawals/ucm042004.htm

Valentin, L., Sharp, H., Hille, K., Seibt, U., Fischer, J., Pfeifer, Y., et al. (2014). Subgrouping of ESBL-producing Escherichia coli from animal and human sources: an approach to quantify the distribution of ESBL types between different reservoirs. *Int. J. Med. Microbiol.* 304, 805–816. doi: 10.1016/j.ijmm.2014.07.015

van Boven, M., Veldman, K. T., de Jong, M. C., and Mevius, D. J. (2003). Rapid selection of quinolone resistance in *Campylobacter jejuni* but not in *Escherichia coli* in individually housed broilers. *J. Antimicrob. Chemother.* 52, 719–723. doi: 10.1093/jac/dkg402

Werner, G., Coque, T. M., Hammerum, A. M., Hope, R., Hryniewicz, W., Johnson, A., et al. (2008). Emergence and spread of vancomycin resistance among enterococci in Europe. *Euro Surveill.* 13:19046.

Werner, G., Klare, I., and Witte, W. (2002). Molecular analysis of streptogramin resistance in enterococci. *Int. J. Med. Microbiol.* 292, 81–94. doi: 10.1078/1438-4221-00194

Willems, R. J., Top, J., van Santen, M., Robinson, D. A., Coque, T. M., Baquero, F., et al. (2005). Global spread of vancomycin-resistant Enterococcus faecium from distinct nosocomial genetic complex. *Emerg. Infect. Dis.* 11, 821–828. doi: 10.3201/1106.041204

Xu, X., Lin, D., Yan, G., Ye, X., Wu, S., Guo, Y., et al. (2010). vanM, a new glycopeptide resistance gene cluster found in *Enterococcus faecium*. *Antimicrob. Agents Chemother.* 54, 4643–4647. doi: 10.1128/AAC.01710-09

Yan, M., Sahin, O., Lin, J., and Zhang, Q. (2006). Role of the CmeABC efflux pump in the emergence of fluoroquinolone-resistant Campylobacter under selection pressure. *J. Antimicrob. Chemother.* 58, 1154–1159. doi: 10.1093/jac/dkl412

Zeitouni, S., Collin, O., Andraud, M., Ermel, G., and Kempf, I. (2012). Fitness of macrolide resistant *Campylobacter coli* and *Campylobacter jejuni*. *Microb. Drug Resist.* 18, 101–108. doi: 10.1089/mdr.2011.0188

5

Integration of PK/PD for Dose Optimization of Cefquinome Against *Staphylococcus aureus* Causing Septicemia in Cattle

Ijaz Ahmad[1], Haihong Hao[2], Lingli Huang[2,3], Pascal Sanders[4], Xu Wang[2], Dongmei Chen[1,3], Yanfei Tao[1,3], Shuyu Xie[2,3], Kuang Xiuhua[2], Juan Li[2], Wan Dan[2] and Zonghui Yuan[1,2,3]*

[1] National Reference Laboratory of Veterinary Drug Residues and MAO Key Laboratory for Drug Residues Detection, Huazhong Agriculture University, Wuhan, China, [2] MOA Laboratory for Risk Assessment of Safety and Quality of Livestock and Poultry Products, Huazhong Agriculture University, Wuhan, China, [3] Hubei Collaborative Innovation Centre for feed Safety and Animal Nutrition, Huazhong Agricultural University, Wuhan, China, [4] Laboratory of Fougères, French Agency for Food, Environmental and Occupational Safety, Maisons-Alfort, France

***Correspondence:**
Zonghui Yuan,
National Reference Laboratory of Veterinary Drug Residues and MAO Key Laboratory for the Detection of Veterinary Drug Residues, Huazhong Agricultural University, No. 1, Shizhishan Street, Hongshan District, Wuhan, Hubei 430070, China
yuan5802@mail.hzau.edu.cn

Cefquinome is a fourth generation cephalosporin with antimicrobial activity against gram negative and gram positive bacterial species, including *Staphylococcus aureus*. The aim of our study was to observe the *ex-vivo* activity of cefquinome against *Staphylococcus aureus* strains by using bovine serum from intravenously treated cattle. Cefquinome kinetics were measured by liquid chromatography and UV detection. *In vitro* post antibiotic effects (PAEs) and mutant prevention concentrations were determined with *S. aureus* strain ATCC 12598. Cefquinome exhibited time-dependent killing and produced *in vitro* PAEs increasing with concentration and time of exposure. A pharmacokinetic-pharmacodynamic model was established to simulate the efficacy of cefquinome for different dosage regimens. A dosage of 2 mg/kg every 12 h for 3 days was expected to reach a bactericidal activity against *S. aureus* in case of septicemia.

Keywords: cefquinome, *Staphylococcus aureus*, cattle, PK/PD, septicemia

Introduction

Staphylococcus aureus is a gram positive bacteria, responsible for many animal and human diseases. It can cause an extensive variety of infections from skin and soft tissue infections to septicemia. If it is not treated efficiently, the sepsis can produce inflammatory response, organ dysfunction syndrome, shock, and finally death (Fecteau et al., 2009; Fluit, 2012). During the first day of life septicemia commonly occurs in calves. Bacteremia was observed during the neonatal period in 20–30% of diarrheic calves. In bacteremia or septicemia, the bacteria isolated included *Escherichia coli*, *Salmonella* spp, *Campylobacter* spp, *Klebsiella* spp., and *Staphylococcus* spp (Raboisson et al., 2010). Consequently, *S. aureus* has a documented effect on mortality, with related rate of mortality at 20–40% (Uramatsu et al., 2010). Since, staphylococcal diseases are usually treated with antibiotics there is an associated risk to select antibiotic resistance (Normand et al., 2000). Without treatment, the mortality rate will be high (Gordon, 1998).

Rational Antibiotic therapy needs to ensure clinical efficacy and to reduce the risk of antibiotic resistance selection and amplification (Toutain et al., 2002; Ambrose et al., 2007; Jacobs, 2007; Tam et al., 2007). The beta-lactam antiobiotic is safer in the target animals as compared to other antibiotics (Dumka et al., 2013). The beta lactam antibiotic is time dependent and its bactericidal activity is lower as compared to other bactericidal antibiotics. Also, it has no or a minimal post antibiotic effect. Therefore to optimize the efficacy, the drug concentration should be maintained above the MIC for a longer time during the dosing interval at the site of infection (McKellar et al., 2004; Owens and Ambrose, 2007; Zonca et al., 2011; Papich, 2014). Cefquinome is the fourth generation cephalosporin, mainly used in veterinary medicine. This drug has been developed especially for use in veterinary medicine (Smiet et al., 2012; Papich, 2014), and is registered in many countries worldwide. Cefquinome has been used for the treatment of many diseases including acute mastitis, respiratory diseases, food rot in cattle, calf septicemia, metritis-mastitits-agalactia syndrome in sows, foal septicemia and respiratory diseases in horses (Uney et al., 2011; Liu et al., 2012; Dumka et al., 2013; Shan et al., 2014). The advantages of cefquinome include broad spectrum antibacterial activity, stability against β-lactamase, enhanced potency, and bioavailability and the ability to penetrate easily into gram negative bacteria (Dumka et al., 2013). Cefquinome pharmacokinetics (PK) have been studied in several animal species such as camels, horses, ducks, cows, wild boars, piglet, rabbits and cattle (Allan and Thomas, 2003; Ehinger et al., 2006; Li et al., 2008; Al-Taher, 2010; Hwang et al., 2011; Liguo et al., 2011; Liu et al., 2012; Shan et al., 2014).

In human medicine, international guidelines for management of severe sepsis underline the needs to base the choice of antibiotics on the knowledge of their pharmacokinetics and their pharmacodynamics (PK/PD) (Dellinger et al., 2008; Solomkin et al., 2010; Duszyńska et al., 2012). The use of PK/PD modeling has also become common in the veterinary literature. PK-PD principles are an important tool to be used by the regulatory authority when studying the application of an antimicrobial. It was also stated that the single most important factor responsible for the emergence of resistance is bacterial exposure to sub optimal concentration of an antibiotic (Papich, 2014). Therefore, some strategies have been established for dosage regimens to attain appropriate PK/PD targets in severe infection and to minimize selection of antibiotic resistance (Drusano, 2004; Olofsson and Cars, 2007; Duszyńska et al., 2012). Recently, one researcher investigated the pharmacokinetics and *ex-vivo* pharmacodynamics activity of cefquinome by using tissue cage fluid and serum obtained from pigs (Zhang et al., 2014). Efficacy of different dosage regimens was investigated in a *Staphylococcus aureus* infection in a thigh model of neutropenic mouse (Wang et al., 2014).

The objectives of the present study were to examine the PK and, establish *in vitro* PD parameters and *ex-vivo* PD characteristics of cefquinome in serum for integration in a PK-PD model for cefquinome for treatment of *Staphylococcus aureus* systemic infections in calves.

Materials and Methods

Animals

All the experimental procedure in this study were performed according to the guidelines of the committee on the use and care of the laboratory animals in Hubei province China. The study was approved by the Animal Care Center, Hubei Science and Technology Agency in China (SYXK 2013–0044). All the animals were monitored throughout the study for any adverse effect signs. The study was conducted in 6 healthy cattle calves of 6–10 months of age. Body weights (BW) was 185 ± 10 kg. They were housed in a 8 × 10 m cattle pen, and the pen was cleaned daily. The room temperature was 25 ± 2°C and a relative humidity of 45 65% was maintained in the animal house. All animals were allowed a 15 days acclimation period before the study began. The water and feed for the animals was available *ad libitum*. None of the animals had been treated with antibiotics before.

Drug Administration and Sample Collection

Each calf received cefquinome (Cefquinome sulfate 2.5%, Shanghai Tongren Pharmaceutical Company Ltd.) at a dosage of 1 mg/kg BW. The drug was administered intravenously to 6 cattle by jugular vein at the dose rate of 1 mg/kg. The blood samples (5 mL) were collected before and at 0.25, 0.5, 1, 2, 3, 4, 6, 8, 12, and 24 h after cefquinome administration from opposite jugular vein. Blood samples were collected into EDTA tubes and tubes without anticoagulant. Plasma and serum were obtained immediately by centrifugation at 3000 *g* for 20 min at 4°C and the supernatants (plasma or serum) were stored at −20°C until analysis.

Drug Analysis

Chemicals and Reagents

The cefquinome reference standard (95% purity) was kindly supplied by Dr. Ehrenstorfer (Augsburg, Germany). The reagents used were of analytical grade. Formic acid, methanol (MeOH), and acetonitrile (ACN) were provided by TEDIA (USA). Solid phase extraction (SPE) cartridges (Waters Oasis™ HLB, waters) were used in the analytical method. De-ionized water (Milli-Q Millipore Corp.) was used during the study.

Development of HPLC Method

Plasma samples were analyzed using a Waters 2695 series high performance liquid chromatography (HPLC) and a Waters 2587 UV detector set at a wavelength of 268 nm. The chromatographic separation was achieved with an analytical ZORBAX SB-$C_{18\ column}$ (250 × 4.6 mm i.d., 5 μm; Agilent Technology, USA) at 30 ± 5°C. The separation was on isocratic mode with mobile phase A containing 0.1% formic acid and B acetonitrile (90/10, v/v) at 0.9 ml/min flow rate. The injection volume was 50 μL.

After thawing at room temperature, aliquots of 250 μL cattle plasma were collected in 1.5 mL tubes. Then, 500 μL methanol was added, tubes were shaken for 20 s, and were centrifuged (8000 *g*) for 10 min at 4°C. After centrifugation, the supernatant was pipetted into a tube and 10 mL water was added. The mixture was then cleaned up on a HLB SPE cartridge (3 mL, Waters Corp., Milford, MA, USA), preconditioned with 3 mL methanol and 3 mL water. After transfer, the cartridge was washed with 3 mL water and 3 mL (10% methanol). The analytes were eluted with 3 mL acetonitrile. The samples were dried with a stream of nitrogen at 50°C. The residue remaining after evaporation with nitrogen was reconstituted with 500 μL of 15% acetonitrile.

After Vortex mixing for 20 s, the samples were filtered through 0.22 μm nylon Millipore chromatographic syringe filter into an autosampler vial.

For calibration, 250 μL blank plasma were spiked with 0.01–5 μL of a series of diluted cefquinome working standard solutions and analyzed as above. The cefquinome concentrations in the prepared standard samples were 0.01, 0.02, 0.04, 0.08, 0.16, 1, 2, and 5 μg/mL. Spiked quality control samples were prepared at the concentrations of 0.04, 0.08, and 0.16 μg/mL. Retention time for cefquinome in plasma was 13.40 min. The limit of detection (LOD) and limit of quantification (LOQ) were 0.01 and 0.04 μg/mL. Cefquinome quantification is linear within a range of 0.01–5 μg/mL ($r^2 > 0.999$). The recovery of cefquinome from plasma was 76.24 ± 2.55% (mean ± SD). The coefficient of variability (CV %) was all <15% for intra- and inter-day variation.

Pharmacokinetic Analysis

Pharmacokinetic analysis was performed using Win-Nonlin (version 5.2.1, Pharsight Corporation, Mountain View, CA, USA). The data obtained after plasma concentration determination were analyzed by compartmental methods. The compartmental analysis was evaluated based on Akaike Information Criteria estimates and coefficient of determination application for the best fit model (Liu et al., 2012). The data were analyzed by non-compartment modeling. To find the values of the area under the concentration-time curve (AUC) and area under the first moment curve (AUMC), we used the linear trapezoidal route. The apparent volume of distribution at steady state (VSS) and volume of distribution (VDarea) were calculated according the following equation.

$$VD_{area} = \frac{Dose}{AUC \times \beta}$$

$$VSS = \frac{Dose/AUC}{AUMC/AUC}$$

The pharmacokinetic parameters are presented as mean ± SD.

Pharmacodynamics

Bacterial Strain and Animals

Staphylococcus aureus Rosenbach (ATCC BAA-934), subsp. Aureus (ATCC-12598), and ATCC-29213 strains were purchased from the American Type Culture Collection (ATCC). *Staphylococcus aureus* subsp. Aureus Rosenbach (ATCC-12598) was isolated from septic arthritis (www.atcc.org). Thirty *S. aureus* strains isolated from healthy cattle in Huazhong Agriculture University Wuhan, China were also evaluated. The strains were stored at −80°C. Prior to each experiment, the bacteria were grown freshly on Chrom agar and MH agar and incubated at 37°C.

Determination of Minimal Inhibitory Concentration, Minimal Bactericidal Concentration, Mutant Prevention Concentration, and Post Antibiotic Effect

The minimal inhibitory concentration (MIC) of cefquinome against *S. aureus* strains were determined in both broth and serum by micro dilution method according to the CLSI (Clinical and Laboratory standards Institute, 2008), at concentrations between 8 and 0.015 μg/mL. Microplates were incubated at 37°C for 24 h. MIC was determined as the lowest cefquinome concentration where at the end of the incubation period for 24 h, growth of visible bacteria was inhibited. For the minimal bactericidal concentration (MBC) of cefquinome against *S. aureus* strains, 100 μL from each well were successively diluted in 0.85% sodium chloride solution by 1:10 steps and 10 μL were spread on MH agar plates for colony forming unit (cfu) counting and incubated at 37°C for 24 h. MBC was defined as the lowest drug concentration which resulted in a 99.9% reduction in the bacterial density. MBC is the result of five independent experiments. The mean was expressed as the final result.

The mutant prevention concentration (MPC) of cefquinome is determined by agar method. The inoculum of *Staphylococcus aureus* was concentrated to 10^{10} CFU/mL according (Balaje et al., 2013). Bacterial suspensions were inoculated on the agar plates containing serial dilutions of cefquinome and cultured for 96 h. MPC was the lowest drug concentration on agar plates without bacterial growth under anaerobic conditions. Drug range tested for MPC was 1 MIC, 2 MIC, 4 MIC, 8 MIC, 16 MIC, and 32 MIC.

Post-antibiotic effect (PAE) of cefquinome against *Staphylococcus aureus* is estimated with removal of drug methods. The strain of *S. aureus* was incubated with 1 MIC, 2 MIC, 4 MIC of drug. After one and two hours' incubation, the drug was eliminated by several times of centrifuge and wash with fresh medium. The colony forming units (CFU) per milliliter were determined at different time points. The recovery growth kinetic curves of bacteria were established in order to calculate the PAE.

In vitro and *Ex-vivo* Bacterial Killing Curves

After MIC and MBC determinations, different concentration of cefquinome were prepared in MHB ranging from 1/8 to 16 × MIC before bacterial inoculation (10^6 cfu/mL). Growth was checked with a control. The tubes containing bacteria and different concentration of cefquinome were incubated at 37°C and the viable counts of bacteria were determined at 2, 5, 8, and 24 h. At each time, 100 μL obtained were sampled, gradient diluted by saline and then colony forming units were counted. The limit of detection was 10 cfu/mL.

Serum samples obtained from calves that had received cefquinome intravenously were used. Controls were prepared from serum samples collected from the same calves before administration. A 10 μL volume of bacterial culture in stationary phase was added to 1 mL of serum to give a final suspension of approximately 10^6 cfu/mL. The tubes containing bacterial culture and serum were than incubated at 37°C, and viable counts were determined at 0, 2, 5, 8, and 24 h (Shan et al., 2014).

The time-kill curves obtained with serum were analyzed with a pharmacodynamic model described by the following equation

$$\frac{dB}{dt} = k_{net} \times \left(1 - \frac{B}{B_{max}}\right) \times B - \left(\frac{E_{max} + C^{\gamma}}{EC_{50}^{\gamma} + C^{\gamma}}\right) \times B$$

Where B, is the number of bacterial cell expressed as cfu/mL, k_{net} the net growth rate, B_{max} the maximum number of bacteria, E_{max}

the maximum killing rate, EC_{50}, the concentration to reach half of maximal killing rate and γ, the steepness.

The *ex-vivo* time kill curve was fitted with this model with the hypothesis of a decrease in cefquinome concentration according the incubation time using the proc lsqnonlin (Matlab).

Pharmacodynamic Analysis, PK-PD Integration and PK-PD Modeling Analysis

For cefquinome, the surrogate markers of antimicrobial activity, AUC_{24h}/MIC, C_{max}/MIC, and T>MIC, were determined by linking *in vitro* data and *in vivo* pharmacokinetic parameters for serum.

$$\frac{dB}{dt} = k_{net} \times \left(1 - \frac{B}{B_{max}}\right) \times B - k_{death} \times B - \left(\frac{E_{max} + C^{\gamma}}{EC_{50}^{\gamma} + C^{\gamma}}\right) \times B$$

The relationship between the *ex-vivo* AUC_{24h}/MIC ratio and thevariation between the initial bacterial count and the bacterial count after 24 h of incubation (cfu/mL) in serum content was established by using the inhibitory sigmoid E_{max} model (FS and Lees, 2001). This model is described by the following equation

$$E = E_{max} - \frac{(E_{max} - E_0) \cdot C^N}{C^N + EC_{50}^N}$$

where E is the effect of antibacterial agent measured as the change in $\log_{10}$ difference of bacterial count after 24 h incubation compared with the initial log cfu/mL in the serum sample; E_0 is the change in $\log_{10}$ difference in bacterial count of control sample between 0 and 24 h; E_{max} is the change in $\log_{10}$ difference in bacterial count between 0 and 24 h in the cefquinome containing samples; EC_{50} is the AUC_{24h}/MIC value producing 50% of the E_{max}; C is the AUC_{24h}/MIC ratio being examined; and N is the Hill coefficient that describes the steepness of the (AUC_{24h}/MIC) effect curve. These PD parameters were calculated using the GraphPad Prism software (version 5.01, USA).

The *ex-vivo* antibacterial effect of cefquinome after intravenous administration were quantified MIC from the sigmoid E_{max} equation by determining AUC_{24h}/MIC for four levels of effect: for bacteriostatic action (no change in bacterial count, that is $E = 0$), for 50% reduction in the bacterial count, for bactericidal action (a 99.9% reduction in bacterial count) and for bacterial elimination (a 99.99% reduction) (FS and Lees, 2001). The dose was calculated by the using the following formula.

$$Dose = \frac{(AUC_{24}/MIC) \cdot MIC \cdot CL}{fu \cdot F}$$

Cefquinome is time dependent drug and the PK/PD index responsible for the efficacy is T > *MIC*. To find *T > MIC*% we used the following formula

$$T \succ MIC = In\left(\frac{D}{Vd \cdot MIC}\right) \cdot \frac{T1/2\beta}{In2} \cdot \frac{100}{t}$$

Where $T > MIC$ (in percent) is the time interval during which the drug plasma concentration is above or equal to the minimal inhibitory concentration (MIC) values; D is the planned dose; $t_{1/2}$ the terminal elimination half-life; and t is the dose interval (Smiet et al., 2012).

To investigate the effect of different dosage regimens, the pharmacodynamic model describing bacterial growth rate in function of cefquinome concentration was combined with the pharmacokinetic model and simulations were performed with mlxplore software (version-1.1.0, Lixoft, Orsay, France).

Results

Pharmacokinetics of Cefquinome

No adverse reactions were observed after intravenous drug administration. The plasma concentration-time profiles are illustrated in (**Figure 1**). After intravenous administration, plasma concentration of cefquinome was best fitted with a two-compartment model (**Table 1**). The elimination half-life was 2.1 ± 0.45 h showing rapid elimination after intravenous administration. The area under the concentration time curve $AUC_{0-\infty}$ was 8.04 ± 0.34 µg.h/mL. The volume of distribution at steady state (Vss: 0.28 ± 0.02 L/kg) was low. The mean residence time up to last was 2.3 ± 0.3 h.

Pharmacodynamics

MIC, MBC, MPC, and PAE of Cefquinome against Staphylococcus *aureus* Strains

The MIC and MBC of cefquinome against *S. aureus* were for the three tested strains at 0.25 and 0.5 µg/mL in culture medium MHB and in serum (**Table 2**). MIC_{90} of 30 strains isolated from healthy cattle in our laboratory was 0.25 µg/mL. The mutant prevention concentration (MPC) of cefquinome against the 3 strains in MHB and serum were 2 µg/mL.

Post-antibiotic effect (PAE) of cefquinome for different concentrations (1x, 2x, 4x MIC) and time exposure (1, 2 h)

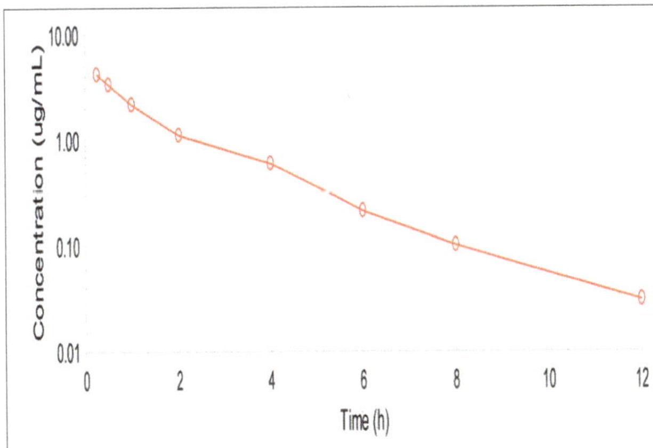

FIGURE 1 | Semi-logarithmic plot of mean serum concentration after intra venous administration of cefquinome (1 mg/kg) in cattle ($n = 6$). Two compartment method (Winonlin software) were used to observe the concentration-time curve.

is lower than 1 h and increases with time and concentration (**Table 3**).

In vitro and *Ex-vivo* Antimicrobial Activity

Time kill curves obtained against *S. aureus* ATCC-12598 for different concentrations of cefquinome expressed as multiple of MIC were reported (**Figure 2**). The curves were characteristics of time-dependent antibiotic activity. The net growth rate is lower for concentration below the MIC. Meanwhile the bactericidal activity increased with increasing concentration of the cefquinome up to 4 MIC. A further increase in concentration resulted in the same death rate.

Serum samples from six cattle that had been administered cefquinome intravenously collected at different time points were used to determine *ex-vivo* killing rate. The results show that at the highest concentration, the number of bacteria decreased slightly (**Figure 3**). A net killing rate is obtained with samples collected before 6 h and growth is observed for serum samples collected after 8 h. In the data set with serum, a phenomenon of decrease of bacteria number followed by a regrowth was observed on the time kill curves obtained with serum sampled at 8 and 12 h. After fitting, the net killing rate was $0.95\,h^{-1}$, the net growth rate was $k_{net} = 0.6915\,h^{-1}$, the maximum number of bacteria B_{max} was (10E9.25), the maximum killing rate was $E_{max} = 1.67\,h^{-1}$, $EC_{50} = 0.06\,\mu g/mL$, $\gamma = 0.70$ and cefquinome decrease rate = $0.15\,h^{-1}$.

PK/PD Integration

The mean values of the PK/PD indices C_{max}/MIC, AUC_{24}/MIC, C_{max}/MBC, AUC_{24}/MBC, and C_{max}/MPC, AUC_{24}/MPC of cefquinome against *staphylococcus aureus* are shown in (**Table 4**). The values determined for C_{max}/MIC and AUC_{24}/MIC were 16.72 and 32.16 h. The mean values for C_{max}/MPC and AUC_{24}/MPC were 2.09 and 4.02.

PK/PD Modeling

The association between AUC_{0-24}/MIC ratio and antibiotic efficacy was best described by using inhibitory sigmoid E_{max} model. The parameters obtained N, E_0, E_{max} and AUC_{0-24}/MIC values required for various degrees of antibacterial activity are shown in **Table 5**. The values of AUC_{0-24}/MIC ratios for bacteriostasis activity, bactericidal action and virtual eradication were 29.71, 51.97, and 67.51, respectively.

Estimation of Dose

The dose of cefquinome in cattle calves after a single intravenous administration, based on the observed AUC_{24h}/MIC values by modeling PK/PD data, MIC values and PAE values of our study and MIC_{90} required for bacteriostatic, bactericidal and bacterial eradication responses are 3.6, 6.4, and 8.3 mg/kg for bacteriostatic, bactericidal action and virtual eradication activity for 24 h dosage interval. The t > MIC for the above mentioned dose are 50, 57, and 60%.

TABLE 1 | Pharmacokinetics parameters after intravenous administration of Cefquinome in cattle at the dose (1 mg/kg) body weight.

PK parameters	Mean	SD
AUC (μg.h/mL)	8.04	0.34
K_{10} (l/h)	0.67	0.03
K_{12} (1/h)	0.39	0.09
K_{21} (1/h)	0.69	0.24
T ½α (h)	0.48	0.09
T 1/2 β (h)	2.10	0.45
V1 (L/kg)	0.18	0.00
CL (L/h.kg)	0.12	0.00
Vss (L/kg)	0.28	0.02
MRT (h)	2.30	0.30
AUMC (μg.h2/Ml)	18.56	2.19

AUC, Area under the concentration-time curve; K_{10}, First order elimination rate constant; K_{12}, First order transfer rate constant describing distribution between central and peripheral compartment; K_{21}, First order transfer rate constant describing distribution between peripheral and central compartment; T 1/2α, Half-life of distribution; T 1/2β, Half-life of elimination; CL, Systemic clearance; Vss, Volume of distribution at steady state; MRT, Mean residence time; AUMC, Area under the first moment-time curve.

TABLE 3 | Post antibiotic effect (PAE) after 1 and 2 h. (ATCC-12598).

Antibacterial concentration	PAE after 1 h (h)	PAE after 2 h (h)
1MIC	0.10	0.10
2MIC	0.20	0.20
4MIC	0.30	0.60

TABLE 2 | MIC, MBC and MPC (μg/ml) of Cefquinome against *staphylococcus aureus*.

Parameters	Matrix	Strain 1 (ATCC-29213)	Strain 2 (ATCC-BAA-934)	Strain 3 (ATCC-12598)	Mean ± SD
MIC	MHB	0.25	0.25	0.25	0.25 ± 00
	Serum	0.25	0.25	0.25	0.25 ± 00
MBC	MHB	0.5	0.5	0.5	0.50 ± 00
	Serum	0.5	0.5	0.5	0.50 ± 00
MBC/MIC	MHB	2	2	2	2 ± 00
	Serum	2	2	2	2 ± 00
MPC	MHB	4	2	2	2.66 ± 1.15
MPC/MIC	MHB	16	8	8	10.66 ± 4.61

MIC, Minimum inhibitory concentration; MBC, Minimum bactericidal concentration; MPC, Mutant prevention concentration.

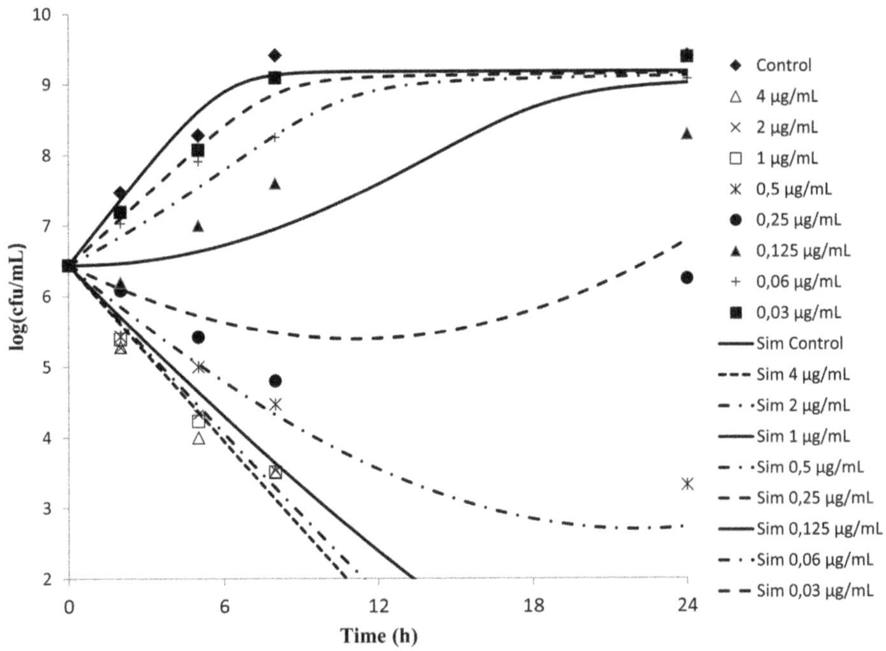

FIGURE 2 | *In vitro* antibacterial activity of cefquinome against *Staphylococcus aureus* in MH broth. The figures show that cefquinome exhibit time dependent activity when the concentration increases.

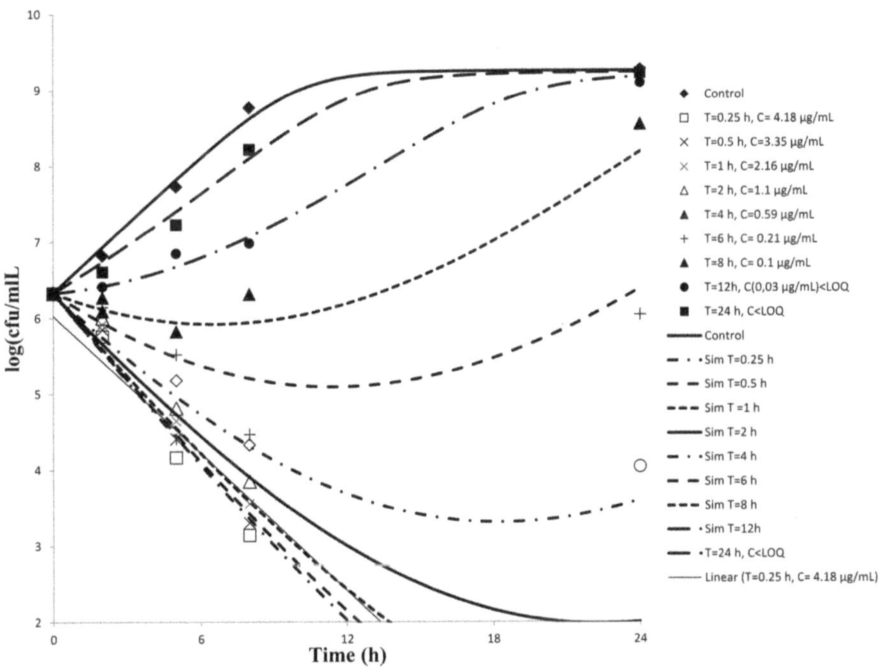

FIGURE 3 | *Ex-vivo* antibacterial activity of cefquinome in serum of cattle against *staphylococcus aureus* after intravenous administration (n = 6). The concentration of cefquinome in serum at different time interval shows its effect on *staphylococcus aureus.*

Using a PK/PD model with the PD parameters derived from *ex-vivo* analysis, actions of different doses (0.5, 1, 2.5, 5, 7.5 mg/kg) were simulated (**Figure 4**). According these figures, a dose of 1 mg/kg is not sufficient to reduce the bacterial load while a dose of 2 mg/kg lead to a net reduction of a factor of 10 after 12 h.

Different dosage regimen for 3 days of treatment (1 mg/kg every 12 h, 1 mg/kg every 24 h and 2 mg/kg every 24 h, 2 mg/kg

TABLE 4 | Integration of PK/PD data obtained after intra venous administration of Cefquinome (1 mg/kg) in cattle (n = 6).

Parameter	Unit	Mean
C_{MAX}	μg/ml	4.18
$AUC_{0-24\,h}$	μg.h/ml	8.04
MIC	μg/ml	0.25
MBC	μg/ml	0.50
MPC	μg/ml	2.00
C_{MAX}/MIC	–	16.72
$AUC_{0-24\,h}$/MIC	h	32.16
C_{MAX}/MBC	–	8.36
$AUC_{0-24\,h}$/MBC	H	16.08
C_{MAX}/MPC	–	2.09
$AUC_{0-24\,h}$/MPC	h	4.02

TABLE 5 | PK/PD Modeling of *ex-vivo* data after administration of Cefquinome in cattle (n = 6).

Parameters	Unit	Mean
E_0	Log_{10} CFU/ml	2.93
E_{MAX}	Log_{10} CFU/ml	−5.33
E_{MAX}-E_0	Log_{10} CFU/ml	8.26
Slope (N)	–	2.74
$AUC_{24\,h}$/MIC EC50	h	36.96
$AUC_{24\,h}$/MIC for bacteriostatic action	h	29.71
$AUC_{24\,h}$/MIC for bactericidal action (99.9% reduction)	h	51.97
$AUC_{24\,h}$/MIC for bacterial eradication (99.99% reduction)	h	67.51

E_0, difference in bacterial count in control sample (without drug) between 0 and 24 h; E_{max}, difference in bacterial count in sample incubated with Cefquinome between 0 and 24 h; AUC_{24h}/MIC EC_{50}:AUC_{24h}/MIC of drug producing 50% of maximal antibacterial effect; N, slope of the AUC_{24h}/MIC–response curve.

every 12 h, and 5 mg/kg every 24 h) (**Figure 5**) were simulated. A dosage regimen of 2 mg/kg every 12 h should be efficient to reach a bactericidal activity in serum (**Figure 5**).

Discussion

Pharmacokinetic properties of cefquinome have been studied previously in the serum of cattle after intravenous administration at 1 mg/kg (Shan et al., 2014). The reported terminal half life, clearance and Vss were respectively 2.4 ± 0.21 h, 0.11 ± 0.03 L/h.kg, 0.3 ± 0.5 L/kg and were very close to our values. The terminal elimination half-life of cefquinome is similar to values that were observed in piglet (Zhang et al., 2014), ducks (Liguo et al., 2011), rabbit (Hwang et al., 2011), and horses (Winther et al., 2011) in the range of (0.9–2.77 h) following IV administration. The volume of distribution at steady state was low which means that cefquinome was not as widely distributed as previously reported for piglet (Zhang et al., 2014), sheep (Uney et al., 2011), rabbits (Hwang et al., 2011), and horses (Winther et al., 2011) in the range (0.19–0.36 L/kg).

The MIC of cefquinome against *S. aureus* strains tested (0.25 μg/mL) were in the same range as those previously reported (Limbert et al., 1991; Wang et al., 2014). The MBC was determined to be two fold higher.

Cefquinome is considered to be a time-dependent agent and its activity is a function of the time remaining in excess of MIC. There was a regrowth observed in the inoculated bacteria on the *ex-vivo* time kill curves obtained for low concentration. A model with a decreasing of cefquinome concentration in serum was used to fit the data. This mathematical model is the simplest to describe a bacterial regrowth. As antimicrobial concentration in serum after 24 h of incubation was not measured, it was not supported by any data and must be considered as theoretical. A theoretical MIC value for the strain tested was calculated as 0.064 μg/mL. This value means a better susceptibility of *S. aureus* in serum than those observed after 24 h of culture in Mueller Hinton.

The PAE observed *in vitro* below 1 h is short in comparison of 2.9 h obtained *in vivo* in neutropenic mice thigh model of *staphylococcus aureus* (Wang et al., 2014). The *in vivo* PAE of cephalosporin were between 2 and 6 h in the former model. Then, PAE determined *in vitro* is a poor predictor of those observed *in vivo*. For our simulation, PAE will not be considered as our data are not enough to build a model to predict *in vivo* scenario.

The bactericidal action of a time dependent drug is relatively slow as compared to concentration dependent drugs (Levison, 2004), and little increase in bactericidal activity is seen when the concentration is increased more than maximal killing concentration, which is approximately equal to 4 times the MIC. These drugs have short or no PAE for gram negative bacilli and have short PAE for gram positive bacilli; the drug concentration above the MIC relative to dosing interval is important, consequently the dosing administration frequency is an important factor for the efficacy. Shorter dosing intervals will increase the duration of time at which the drug concentration is above the MIC of the causative agent (McKellar et al., 2004). For time dependent drugs, AUC/MIC is a poor predictor of efficacy while T > MIC is the best surrogate. To estimate this surrogate from PK and *in vitro* and *ex-vivo* data, it is necessary to estimate the maximum kill rate, EC_{50} and steepness from the time kill curve data using a differential model (Nielsen and Friberg, 2013). So use of mathematical model describing simultaneously the pharmacokinetics of a drug and the effect on bacterial growth is the best approach to investigate time dependent drugs.

The mutant selection window hypothesis was initially proposed using agar plate assays and then explored in several *in vitro* and *in vivo* models mainly for fluoroquinolones for which resistance appears by mutation. For time-dependent drugs such as cephalosporin, it was rarely reported and as far as we know, only one recent paper investigated *in vivo* the mutant selection window for cefquinome against *E. coli* in an *in vitro* model (Zhang et al., 2014). For *S. aureus*, the observed *in vitro* MPC (2 μg/mL) was 8 times higher than the MIC (0.25 μg/mL). Compared with the MIC definition, the mutant prevention concentration (MPC) is defined as the lowest drug concentration that prevents the growth of the least susceptible first-step

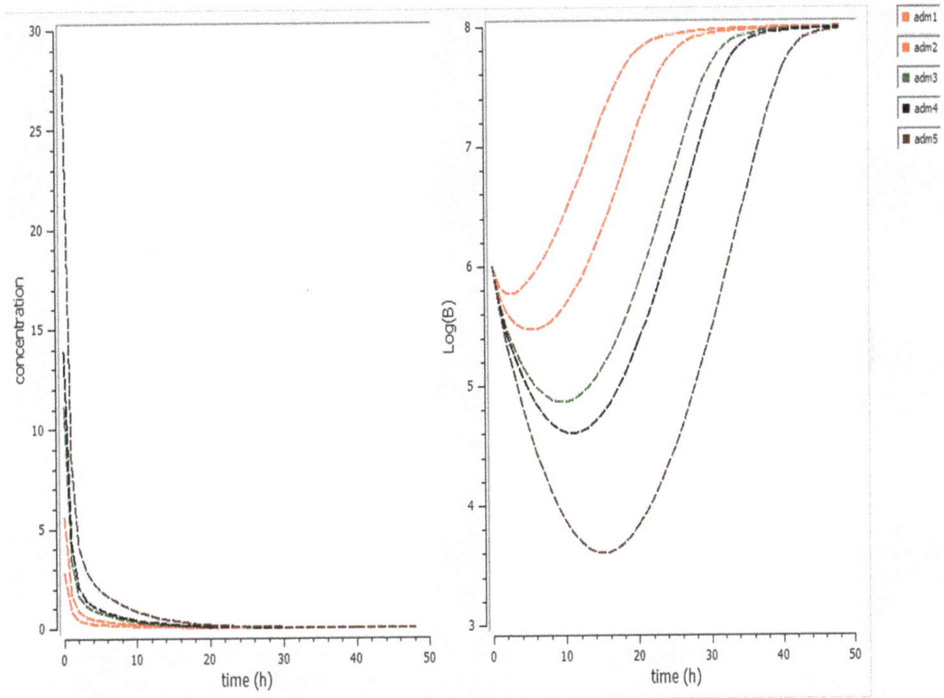

FIGURE 4 | Simulate the effect of different doses (0.5, 1, 2.5, 5, 7.5 mg/kg). The effect of different doses were observed on bacteria and its elimination.

resistant mutants. It has been proposed that the $AUC_{24\,h}$/MPC ratio could help as an indicator of drug exposure that stops the selection of drug-resistant mutants (Zhao and Drlica, 2001; Olofsson et al., 2006). Further investigations are needed to determine the mechanisms of resistance (induced or acquired) observed in our study. For this reason, mutant prevention concentration was not taken into account in our dosage regimen optimization.

PK/PD model helps as a bridge between *in vitro* and *in vivo* study and permits predicting the suitable dose for bacteriological bend and emergence. According our pharmacokinetic and pharmacodynamic parameters, single dose to reach bacteriostatic, bactericidal and eradication activity corresponding to 3.6, 6.4, and 8.3 mg/kg doses to maintain a concentration higher than the observed MIC (0.25 μg/mL) for a fraction of 50, 57, or 60% of a 24 h interval (**Figure 4**). For the treatment, we simulate different dosage regimen and show that a 3 day treatment of 2 mg/kg every 12 h should be efficient against *S. aureus* ATCC 12598 in cattle. These PK/PD interrelationships expect that cefquinome treatment is likely to be effective clinically against *S. aureus* strains with the same or lower MIC. Our model is based upon a single strain and with pharmacokinetic parameters derived from healthy animals. Rather it would be better to base our dose determination on the MIC_{90} values and to obtain more information about the population pharmacokinetics of cefquinome to take into account all the variability associate to animals and bacteria.

The therapeutic effect of an antimicrobial agent depends on several factors such as disease severity, animal immune response, pathogen load and strain virulence. The objective of the approach described here is to clear an organism of a pathogen, which was expected to be present in the central compartment during acute infection. Our model for *S. aureus* with a MIC of 0.25 μg/mL lead to $AUC_{24\,h}$/MIC for bacteriostasis and bactericidal action close 30 and 52 h which are higher than those (21 and 35 h, respectively) reported in piglet cage tissue fluid for a strain of *E. coli* with an MIC of 0.03 μg/mL (Zhang et al., 2014). The PK-PD surrogates have been widely used to provide dosages that aim to ensure clinical cures. These surrogates are less appropriate to prevent emergence of resistance strains and it has been suggested that the AUC/MPC ratio could serve as an indicator of drug exposure that prevents the selection of drug resistant mutant. However, this ratio should be a surrogate of the prevention of resistance selection at the target site. But, the same approaches must be applied to other body compartments such as the intestinal lumen where the microbiota can be exposed to selective concentration of the drug (Zhang et al., 2013).

Resistance to antimicrobials is a major threat for human health, the overuse and misuse is considered to be the main factor for increasing bacterial resistance in both humans and animals. The gut microbiota constitutes one of the key reservoirs of resistance genes between commensal bacterial ecosystems (Andremont, 2003; Phillips et al., 2004; Baquero et al., 2011; De Lastours et al., 2012; Vasseur et al., 2014). Antibiotic dosages presently used in humans and animals have not been developed to prevent the collateral choice on the gut microbiota and the selection and amplification of resistant strains (Fantin et al., 2009; De Lastours et al., 2012; Vasseur et al., 2014). An

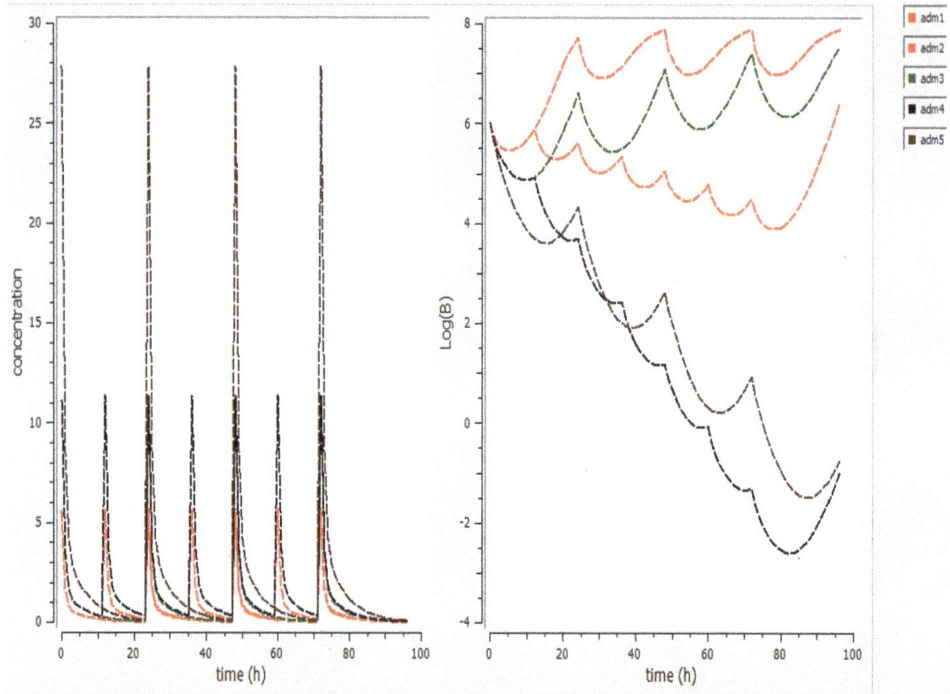

FIGURE 5 | Simulate different dosage regimen (1 mg/kg every 12 h, 1 mg/kg every 24 h, and 2 mg/kg every 24 h, 2 mg/kg every 12 h, and 5 mg/kg every 24 h). The different doses were simulated for different intervals of time to find the efficient dose and dose intervals

investigation of the interactions between microbial populations and antibiotics, as well as better understanding of the significant factors governing antimicrobial action and resistance range, might lead to the development of strategies combining maximum efficacy with minimum impact on the commensal bacterial ecosystems (Baquero et al., 2011; Cantón and Morosini, 2011; Martinez et al., 2012; Vasseur et al., 2014). For example, current studies confirmed that the degree of increasing of antimicrobial resistance in the gut microbiota was directly associated with the magnitude of the antibiotic dosage, irrespective of the route of administration (Nguyen et al., 2012; Zhang et al., 2013; Vasseur et al., 2014). Therefore there is an essential need to improve the antibiotic dose by taking this effect in the process of drug optimization.

Conclusion

The purpose of our study was to estimate a dosage regimen of cefquinome after intravenous administration that would be efficient for treatment of *S. aureus* septicemia in cattle. The dosage estimate was based on a pharmacokinetic analysis and some pharmacodynamic studies. As previously described we observed that cefquinome is a time dependent drug with a low *in vitro* PAE for *S. aureus*. Pharmacodynamic parameters were derived from the analysis of static time kill curves obtained *ex-vivo*. The dosage regimen was simulated using a mathematical model. For a time dependent drug, this approach for dose determination is better than the analysis of the relationship between AUC/MIC value and the number of viable bacteria after 24 h. A dosage regimen of 2 mg/kg every 12 h during 3 days should be efficient in the treatment of *S. aureus* septicemia.

Author Contributions

Design of the work: HH, LH, ZY. Analysis and interpretation of the work: PS, IA. Drafting the work or revising it critically for important intellectual content: DC, YT, SX, XW. Experimental procedure performed: IA. Paper writing: IA, JL, WD, KX.

Acknowledgments

This article is financially supported by National Natural Science Foundation of China (31101856/31302143), Grants from National Basic Research program of China (2013CB127200), National Key Technology R&D Program (2012BAK01B00), Fundamental Research Funds for the Central Universities (2662015PY035) and project supported by the morning program of Wuhan in China (2015070404010191).

References

Allan, M. J., and Thomas, E. (2003). Pharmacokinetics of cefquinome after parenteral administration of an aqueous solution in the horse. *J. Vet. Pharmacol. Ther.* 26, 82–307. doi: 10.1046/j.1365-2885.25.s1.1.x

Al-Taher, A. (2010). Pharmacokinetics of cefquinome in camels. *J. Anim. Vet. Adv.* 9, 848–852. doi: 10.3923/javaa.2010.848.852

Ambrose, P. G., Bhavnani, S. M., Rubino, C. M., Louie, A., Gumbo, T., Forrest, A., et al. (2007). Pharmacokinetics-Pharmacodynamics of antimicrobial therapy: it's not just for mice anymore. *Clin. Infect. Dis.* 44, 79–86. doi: 10.1086/510079

Andremont, A. (2003). Commensal flora may play key role in spreading antibiotic resistance. *ASM NEWS* 69, 601–607. Available online at: http://www.asm.org/ccLibraryFiles/FILENAME/0000000696/znw012030152p.pdf

Balaje, R. M., Sidhu, P. K., Kaur, G., and Rampal, S. (2013). Mutant prevention concentration and PK-PD relationships of enrofloxacin for Pasteurella multocida in buffalo calves. *Res. Vet. Sci.* 95, 1114–1124. doi: 10.1016/j.rvsc.2013.07.019

Baquero, F., Coque, T. M., and de la Cruz, F. (2011). Ecology and evolution as targets: the need for novel eco-evo drugs and strategies to fight antibiotic resistance?. *Antimicrob. Agents Chemother.* 55, 3649–3660. doi: 10.1128/AAC.00013-11

Cantón, R., and Morosini, M. I. (2011). Emergence and spread of antibiotic resistance following exposure to antibiotics. *FEMS Microbiol. Rev.* 35, 977–991. doi: 10.1111/j.1574-6976.2011.00295.x

CLSI. (2008). *Performance Standards for Antimicrobial Disk and Dilution Susceptibility Tests for Bacteria Isolated from Animals; Approved Standard*, 3rd Edn. Vol. 28, M31-A3, Wayne, PA.

De Lastours, V., Cambau, E., Guillard, T., Marcade, G., Chau, F., and Fantin, B. (2012). Diversity of individual dynamic patterns of emergence of resistance to quinolones in Escherichia coli from the fecal flora of healthy volunteers exposed to ciprofloxacin. *J. Infect. Dis.* 206, 1399–1406. doi: 10.1093/infdis/jis511

Dellinger, R., Levy, M., and Carlet, J. (2008). Surviving Sepsis Campaign: international guidelines for management of severe sepsis and septic shock 2008. *Crit. Care Med* 38, 296–327. doi: 10.1097/01.CCM.0000298158.12101.41

Drusano, G. L. (2004). Antimicrobial pharmacodynamics: critical interactions of 'bug and drug. *Nat. Rev. Microbiol.* 2, 289–300. doi: 10.1038/nrmicro862

Dumka, V. K., Dinakaran, V., Ranjan, B., and Rampal, S. (2013). Comparative pharmacokinetics of cefquinome following intravenous and intramuscular administration in goats. *Small Rumin. Res.* 113, 273–277. doi: 10.1016/j.smallrumres.2013.02.010

Duszyńska, W. (2012). Pharmacokinetic-pharmacodynamic modelling of antibiotic therapy in severe sepsis. *Anaesthesiol. Intensive Ther.* 44, 158–164. Available online at: http://czasopisma.viamedica.pl/ait/article/viewFile/19826/15538

Ehinger, A. M., Schmidt, H., and Kietzmann, M. (2006). Tissue distribution of cefquinome after intramammary and "systemic" administration in the isolated perfused bovine udder. *Vet. J.* 172, 147–153. doi: 10.1016/j.tvjl.2005.02.029

FS, A., and Lees, P. (2001). Pharmacokinetics and pharmacodynamics of danofloxacin in serum and tissue fluids of goats following intravenous and intramuscular administration. *Am. J. Vet. Res.* 62, 1979–1989. doi: 10.2460/ajvr.2001.62.1979

Fantin, B., Duval, X., Massias, L., Alavoine, L., Chau, F., Retout, S., et al. (2009). Ciprofloxacin dosage and emergence of resistance in human commensal bacteria. *J. Infect. Dis.* 200, 390–398. doi: 10.1086/600122

Fecteau, G., Smith, B. P., and George, L. W. (2009). Septicemia and meningitis in the newborn calf. *Vet. Clin. North Am. Food Anim. Pract.* 25, 195–208, vii–viii. doi: 10.1016/j.cvfa.2008.10.004

Fluit, A. C. (2012). Livestock-associated Staphylococcus aureus. *Clin. Microbiol. Infect.* 18, 735–744 doi: 10.1111/j.1469-0691.2012.03846.x,

Gordon, L. A. (1998). Staphylococcus aureus: a well-armed pathogen. *Clin. Infect. Dis.* 26, 1179–1181. doi: 10.1086/520289

Hwang, Y. H., Song, I. B., Lee, H. K., Kim, T. W., Kim, M. S., Lim, J. H., et al. (2011). Pharmacokinetics and bioavailability of cefquinome in rabbits following intravenous and intramuscular administration. *J. Vet. Pharmacol. Ther.* 34, 618–620. doi: 10.1111/j.1365-2885.2011.01289.x

Jacobs, M. R. (2007). Combating resistance: application of the emerging science of pharmacokinetics and pharmacodynamics. *Int. J. Antimicrob. Agents* 30(Suppl. 2), S122–S126. doi: 10.1016/j.ijantimicag.2007.07.036

Levison, M. E. (2004). Pharmacodynamics of antimicrobial drugs. *Infect. Clin. North Am.* 18, 451–465. doi: 10.1016/j.idc.2004.04.012

Li, X. B., Wu, W. X., Su, D., Wang, Z. J., Jiang, H. Y., and Shen, J. Z. (2008). Pharmacokinetics and bioavailability of cefquinome in healthy piglets. *J. Vet. Pharmacol. Ther.* 31, 523–527. doi: 10.1111/j.1365-2885.2008.00989.x

Liguo, Y., Jian, S., Rui, W., Lihua, S., Lixiang, Z., Xianyang, L., et al. (2011). Pharmacokinetics and bioavailability of cefquinome in healthy ducks. *Am. J. Vet. Res.* 72, 122–126. doi: 10.2460/ajvr.72.1.122

Limbert, M., Isert, D., Klesel, N., Markus, A., Seeger, K., Seibert, G., et al. (1991). Antibacterial activities *in vitro* and *in vivo* and pharmacokinetics of cefquinome (HR 111V), a new broad-spectrum cephalosporin. *Antimicrob. Agents Chemother.* 35, 14–19. doi: 10.1128/AAC.35.1.14

Liu, B., Zhang, C., Zhang, X., Yang, S., Yu, J., Sun, J., et al. (2012). Pharmacokinetics and bioavailability of cefquinome in crossbred wild boars. *J. Vet. Pharmacol. Ther.* 35, 611–614. doi: 10.1111/j.1365-2885.2011.01360.x

Martinez, M. N., Papich, M. G., and Drusano, G. L. (2012). Dosing regimen matters: the importance of early intervention and rapid attainment of the pharmacokinetic/pharmacodynamic target. *Antimicrob. Agents Chemother.* 56, 2795–2805. doi: 10.1128/AAC.05360-11

McKellar, Q. A., Sanchez Bruni, S. F., and Jones, D. G. (2004). Pharmacokinetic/pharmacodynamic relationships of antimicrobial drugs used in veterinary medicine. *J. Vet. Pharmacol. Ther.* 27, 503–514. doi: 10.1111/j.1365-2885.2004.00603.x

Nguyen, T. T., Chachaty, E., Huy, C., Cambier, C., de Gunzburg, J., Mentré, F., et al. (2012). Correlation between fecal concentrations of ciprofloxacin and fecal counts of resistant Enterobacteriaceae in piglets treated with ciprofloxacin: toward new means to control the spread of resistance? *Antimicrob. Agents Chemother.* 56, 4973–4975. doi: 10.1128/AAC.06402-11

Nielsen, E. I., and Friberg, L. E. (2013). Pharmacokinetic-pharmacodynamic modeling of antibacterial drugs. *Pharmacol. Rev.* 65, 1053–1090. doi: 10.1124/pr.111.005769

Normand, E. H., Gibson, N. R., Reid, S. W., Carmichael, S., and Taylor, D. J. (2000). Antimicrobial-resistance trends in bacterial isolates from companion-animal community practice in the UK. *Prev. Vet. Med.* 46, 267–278. doi: 10.1016/S0167-5877(00)00149-5

Olofsson, S. K., and Cars, O. (2007). Optimizing drug exposure to minimize selection of antibiotic resistance. *Clin. Infect. Dis.* 45, S129–136. doi: 10.1086/519256

Olofsson, S. K., Marcusson, L. L., Komp Lindgren, P., Hughes, D., and Cars, O. (2006). Selection of ciprofloxacin resistance in Escherichia coli in an *in vitro* kinetic model: relation between drug exposure and mutant prevention concentration. *J. Antimicrob. Chemother.* 57, 1116–1121. doi: 10.1093/jac/dkl135

Owens, R., and Ambrose, P. G. (2007). Antimicrobial stewardship and the role of pharmacokinetics-pharmacodynamics in the modern antibiotic era. *Diagn. Microb. Infect. Dis.* 57, 77S–83S. doi: 10.1016/j.diagmicrobio.2006.12.012

Papich, M. G. (2014). Pharmacokinetic-pharmacodynamic (PK-PD) modeling and the rational selection of dosage regimes for the prudent use of antimicrobial drugs. *Vet. Microbiol.* 171, 480–486. doi: 10.1016/j.vetmic.2013.12.021

Phillips, I., Casewell, M., Cox, T., De Groot, B., Friis, C., Jones, R., et al. (2004). Does the use of antibiotics in food animals pose a risk to human health? A critical review of published data. *J. Antimicrob. Chemother.* 53, 28–52. doi: 10.1093/jac/dkg483

Raboisson, D., Clément, J., Queney, N., Lebreton, P., and Schelcher, F. (2010). Detection of bacteriuria and bacteremia in newborn calves by a catalase-based urine test. *J. Vet. Intern. Med. Am. Coll. Vet. Intern. Med.* 24, 1532–1536. doi: 10.1111/j.1939-1676.2010.0602.x

Shan, Q., Yang, F., Wang, J., Ding, H., He, L., and Zeng, Z. (2014). Pharmacokinetic/pharmacodynamic relationship of cefquinome against *Pasteurella multocida* in a tissue-cage model in yellow cattle. *J. Vet. Pharmacol. Ther.* 37, 178–185. doi: 10.1111/jvp.12076

Smiet, E., Haritova, A., Heil, B. A., Fink-Gremmels, J., and Wijnberg, I. D. (2012). Comparing the pharmacokinetics of a fourth generation cephalosporin in three different age groups of New Forest ponies. *Equine Vet. J. Suppl.* 52–56. doi: 10.1111/j.2042-3306.2011.00501.x

Solomkin, J. S., Mazuski, J. E., Bradley, J. S., Rodvold, K. A., Goldstein, E. J. C., Baron, E. J., et al. (2010). Diagnosis and management of complicated intra-abdominal infection in adults and children: guidelines by the surgical infection society and the infectious diseases society of America. *Clin. Infect. Dis. Off. Publ. Infect. Dis. Soc. Am.* 50, 133–164. doi: 10.1086/649554

Tam, V. H., Louie, A., Deziel, M. R., Liu, W., and Drusano, G. L. (2007). The relationship between quinolone exposures and resistance amplification is characterized by an inverted U: a new paradigm for optimizing pharmacodynamics to counterselect resistance. *Antimicrob. Agents Chemother.* 51, 744–747. doi: 10.1128/AAC.00334-06

Toutain, P. L., Castillo, J. R. E., and Bousquet-Mélou (2002). The pharmacokinetic-pharmacodynamic approach to a rational dosage regimen for antibiotics. *Res. Vet. Sci.* 73, 105–114. doi: 10.1016/S0034-5288(02)00039-5

Uney, K., Altan, F., and Elmas, M. (2011). Development and validation of a high-performance liquid chromatography method for determination of cefquinome concentrations in sheep plasma and its application to pharmacokinetic studies. *Antimicrob. Agents Chemother.* 55, 854–859. doi: 10.1128/AAC.01126-10

Uramatsu, M., Matsumoto, T., Tateda, K., Shibuya, K., Miyazaki, S., Horino, T., et al. (2010). Involvement of endotoxin in the mortality of mice with gut-derived sepsis due to methicillin-resistant Staphylococcus aureus. *Microbiol. Immunol.* 54, 330–337. doi: 10.1111/j.1348-0421.2010.00217.x

Vasseur, M. V., Laurentie, M., Rolland, J.-G., Perrin-Guyomard, A., Henri, J., Ferran, A. A., et al. (2014). Low or high doeses of cefquinome targeting low or high bacterial inocula cure klebsiella pneumoniae lung infections but differentially impact the levels of antibiotic resistance in fecal flora. *Antimicrob. Agents Chemother.* 58, 1744–1748. doi: 10.1128/AAC.02135-13

Wang, J., Qi, S., Huanzhong, D., Chaoping, L., and Zhenling, Z. (2014). Pharmacodynamics of Cefquinome in a Neutropenic mouse Thigh model of Staphylococcus aureus infection. *Antimicrob. Agents Chemother.* 58, 3008–3012. doi: 10.1128/AAC.01666-13

Winther, L., Baptiste, K. E., and Friis, C. (2011). Antimicrobial disposition in pulmonary epithelial lining fluid of horses, part11. Cefquinome. *J. Vet. Pharmacol. Ther.* 34, 482–486. doi: 10.1111/j.1365-2885.2010.01248.x

Zhang, B. X., Lu, X. X., Gu, X. Y., Li, X. H., Gu, M. X., Zhang, N., et al. (2014). Pharmacokinetics and *ex-vivo* pharmacodynamice of sefquinome in porcine serrum and tissue cage fluids. *Vet. J.* 199, 399–405. doi: 10.1016/j.tvjl.2013.12.015

Zhang, L., Huang, Y., Zhou, Y., Buckley, T., and Wang, H. (2013). Antibiotic administration routes significantly influence the levels of antibiotic resistance in gut microbiota. *Antimicrob. Agents Chemother.* 57, 3659–3666. doi: 10.1128/AAC.00670-13

Zhao, X., and Drlica, K. (2001). Restricting the selection of antibioticresistant mutants: a general strategy derived from fluoroquinolone studies. *Clin. Infect. Dis.* 33, 147–156. doi: 10.1086/321841

Zonca, A., Gallo, M., Locatelli, C., Carli, S., Moroni, P., Villa, R., et al. (2011). Cefquinome sulfate behavior after intramammary administration in healthy and infected cows. *J. Dairy Sci.* 94, 3455–3461. doi: 10.3168/jds.2010-4109

6

Bacteriophages as Potential Treatment for Urinary Tract Infections

*Wilbert Sybesma[1], Reinhard Zbinden[2], Nino Chanishvili[3], Mzia Kutateladze[3], Archil Chkhotua[4], Aleksandre Ujmajuridze[4], Ulrich Mehnert[1] and Thomas M. Kessler[1]**

[1] Neuro-Urology, Spinal Cord Injury Center and Research, University of Zürich, Balgrist University Hospital, Zürich, Switzerland, [2] Institute of Medical Microbiology, University of Zürich, Zürich, Switzerland, [3] The Eliava Institute of Bacteriophage, Microbiology, and Virology, Tbilisi, Georgia, [4] Tsulukidze National Center of Urology, Tbilisi, Georgia

***Correspondence:**
Thomas M. Kessler
tkessler@gmx.ch

Background: Urinary tract infections (UTIs) are among the most prevalent microbial diseases and their financial burden on society is substantial. The continuing increase of antibiotic resistance worldwide is alarming so that well-tolerated, highly effective therapeutic alternatives are urgently needed.

Objective: To investigate the effect of bacteriophages on *Escherichia coli* and *Klebsiella pneumoniae* strains isolated from the urine of patients suffering from UTIs.

Material and methods: Forty-one *E. coli* and 9 *K. pneumoniae* strains, isolated from the urine of patients suffering from UTIs, were tested *in vitro* for their susceptibility toward bacteriophages. The bacteriophages originated from either commercially available bacteriophage cocktails registered in Georgia or from the bacteriophage collection of the George Eliava Institute of Bacteriophage, Microbiology and Virology. *In vitro* screening of bacterial strains was performed by use of the spot-test method. The experiments were implemented three times by different groups of scientists.

Results: The lytic activity of the commercial bacteriophage cocktails on the 41 *E. coli* strains varied between 66% (Pyo bacteriophage) and 93% (Enko bacteriophage). After bacteriophage adaptation of the Pyo bacteriophage cocktail, its lytic activity was increased from 66 to 93% and only one *E. coli* strain remained resistant. One bacteriophage of the Eliava collection could lyse all 9 *K. pneumoniae* strains.

Conclusions: Based on the high lytic activity and the potential of resistance optimization by direct adaption of bacteriophages as reported in this study, and in view of the continuing increase of antibiotic resistance worldwide, bacteriophage therapy is a promising treatment option for UTIs highly warranting randomized controlled trials.

Keywords: bacteriophages, antibiotics, urinary tract infection, bacteriophage adaptation, antibiotic resistance

---

Abbreviation: AM, ampicillin; AMC, amoxicillin/clavulanic acid; CIP, ciprofloxacin; CL, confluent lysis; CXM, cefuroxime; *E. coli, Escherichia coli;* ESBL, extended spectrum beta lactamase; EUCAST, European Committee on Antimicrobial Susceptibility Testing; F, female; I, intermediate; IP, individual clear or opaque plaques; *K. oxytoca, Klebsiella oxytoca; K. pneumonia, Klebsiella pneumoniae;* M, male; n, no (absent); ND, not done; NF, nitrofurantoin; NOR, norfloxacin; OL, overgrown lysis; *P. aeruginosa, Pseudomonas aeruginosa;* R, resistant; S, sensitive; SCL, semi-confluent lysis; SXT, sulfamethoxazole/trimethoprim or co-trimoxazole; tv, taches vierges; UTIs, urinary tract infections; y, yes (present).

INTRODUCTION

Urinary tract infections (UTIs) are among the most prevalent bacterial infections and their financial burden for the society is substantial. In the USA alone, UTIs are responsible for over 7 million physician visits annually (Foxman, 2002) and approximately 15% of all community-prescribed antibiotics are used for UTIs resulting in an annual cost in excess of 1 billion US dollars (Mazzulli, 2002). UTIs account for more than 100'000 hospital admissions annually in the USA (Foxman, 2002), most often for pyelonephritis. These infections are held responsible for at least 40% of all hospital-acquired infections, and the majority of cases are catheter-associated (Rüden et al., 1997). The wide and often uncritical use of antibiotics contributes to the global increase in resistant strains and the present state of microbial resistance is alarming (Carlet et al., 2011; Verbeken et al., 2014). Thus, there is an urgent need for effective, well-tolerated therapeutic alternatives.

After the discovery of bacteriophages by d'Hérelle in 1917, the use of bacteriophage therapy was proposed in the 1920s and has a long and colorful history. At present, bacteriophage therapy is a registered medicine in East European countries like Georgia, Armenia, Ukraine, and Russia, and well accepted by physicians and patients. Several researchers (Abedon et al., 2011; Chanishvili, 2012) have reviewed numerous examples of successfully applied bacteriophage therapy for a diverse area of medical specializations, including dermatology, surgery, wound treatment, intestinal infections, ophthalmology, gynecology and urology. In the Western world bacteriophages have been approved as food processing aid for the decontamination of food (e.g., ListShield^{TM}). However, the use of bacteriophages as treatment against selected bacterial infectious diseases has not yet been approved by regulatory authorities and a regulatory framework is still missing (Pirnay et al., 2011, 2015). Nevertheless, the interest from Western clinicians to collaborate with specialists in bacteriophage therapy is rising, as is illustrated by the growing number of scientific papers in peer reviewed journals, for instance regarding the identification of bacteriophages against the O104:H4 *E. coli* outbreak in Germany, (Merabishvili et al., 2012) and the treatment of *P. aeruginosa* and *Staphylococcus aureus* infections in burn wound patients (Merabishvili et al., 2013). In addition, a number of recent reviews have addressed the safety of bacteriophage therapy (Kutter et al., 2010; Pirnay et al., 2015).

Technically, bacteriophage therapy involves the application of bacteriophages that, upon encounter with specific pathogenic bacteria, can infect and kill the pathogenic bacteria. Bacteriophages can specifically dock on bacteria (host species), introduce their DNA, multiply by using the host cell machinery bacteria, and subsequently lyse the bacteria with release of virion progeny that can re-initiate the cycle. In this way, bacteriophages are unique among antibacterial agents in their ability to increase their numbers in the presence of specific bacterial targets.

Bacteriophages might be rather appropriate means to treat patients suffering from UTIs: compared to last generation of antibiotics, bacteriophages are relatively cheap and the treatment can be done under the control of medical personnel by using a catheter for intravesical instillation several times a day. In addition, bacteriophage therapy for UTI treatment will be applied locally and does not involve a systemic treatment. It is also likely that the absence of physical and metabolic barriers in this kind of treatment increases the potential efficacy and reduces the occurrence of potential adverse events. Thus, in view of the high prevalence of UTIs, the continuing increase of antibiotic resistance worldwide, and the renewed interest to apply bacteriophage therapy in the Western world, we investigated the effect of bacteriophages on *E. coli* and *K. pneumoniae* strains isolated from the urine of patients suffering from UTIs.

MATERIALS AND METHODS

Information on Bacterial Strains and Patients

Between February 2012 and January 2013, 41 *E. coli* and 9 *K. pneumoniae* strains were isolated from urinary cultures of 50 patients (22 women and 28 men) suffering from UTIs defined according to the European Association of Urology Guidelines on Neuro-Urology (Groen et al., 2016). Urine samples were collected by sterile catheterization at the Balgrist University Hospital Zürich and sent within 16 h to the microbiological laboratory of the University of Zürich, Switzerland. None of the patients received antibiotic treatment within 4 weeks before urinary culture. The mean age of the 50 patients was 55 ± 18 years. The causes of lower urinary tract dysfunction were spinal cord injury in 38 (76%), multiple sclerosis in 8 (16%) and spinal stenosis in 4 (4%) patients. Of the 50 patients, 34 (68%) relied on aseptic intermittent self-catheterization, 12 (24%) on an indwelling (transurethral $n = 4$, suprapubic $n = 8$) catheter and 4 (16%) voided spontaneously.

The urine samples were cultivated on sheep blood agar (COS, bioMérieux, Marcy l'Etoile, France), on sheep blood agar with colistin and nalidixic acid (CNA, bioMérieux) and on the chromogenic agar (Uriselect 4, Bio-Rad, Marnes - la Coquette, France). The isolated bacteria were identified according to standard procedures. The susceptibility testing was performed according to the EUCAST Version 3.1, 2013 (www.eucast.org). The strains were stored at −70°C in skimmed milk. Before shipping to Georgia, the isolated strains were sub-cultured and transferred to Amies transport agar (Copan, Brescia, Italy).

Bacteriophages

Four commercial bacteriophage preparations registered in Georgia, Pyo, Intesti, Ses, and Enko bacteriophages, along with 29 *E. coli* and 10 *K. pneumoniae* bacteriophages from the bacteriophage collection of the George Eliava Institute of Bacteriophage, Microbiology and Virology, were used in a bacterial cell lysis screening assay. In order to eliminate effects of batch to batch variations, the individual bacteriophage preparations used for the screening came from the same production batch. The bacteriophages composing the four commercial bacteriophage preparations were grown on a set of bacterial strains, and underwent titration by Appelmans method

(Appelmans, 1921) on each individual strain previously used for multiplication of the bacteriophages. In agreement with current regulation the average titer of the mixture is 10^{-4}–10^{-5} for at least 48 h (Appelmans method), which corresponds to titers of 10^7–10^9 pfu/mL.

The individual bacteriophages have been selected on basis of their capability to eliminate currently prevailing pathogenic microorganisms in Georgia, including *E. coli, P. aeruginosa, Staphylococcus* spp., *Shigella* spp., *Salmonella* spp., *Enterococcus* spp., and *Proteus* spp. More information of the composition and origin of the four bacteriophage preparations can be found in earlier work on Pyo and Intesti (Abedon et al., 2011) and Ses and Enko (Fitzgerald-Hughes et al., 2014).

The 29 *E. coli* bacteriophages were freshly prepared and originally isolated for their potential as antimicrobial agents for therapeutical applications from a broad range of different sources during the period 2000–2012, like sewage waters, agricultural farm isolates (Khurtsia et al., 2001) and clinical isolates (Ghudumidze et al., 2012).

The 10 *K. pneumoniae* bacteriophages (**Table 3**) were isolated between 2002 and 2012 from sewage samples (Karumidze et al., 2013) with the aim to treat patients suffering from UTIs and prostatitis using clinical *K. pneumoniae* strains or *K. oxytoca* strains as hosts. All bacteriophages used in this study were lytic bacteriophages, as was concluded on basis of a combination of analyses and observations, including plaque morphology and clarity of lytic zones on the lawn of bacterial agar, host range, time to infection, time of latent period, and concentration of progeny (Clokie and Kropinski, 2009).

Screening

Screening of bacterial strains for susceptibility to bacteriophages was performed by using a spot test method (Craigie and Yen, 1938) and then modified by different authors and adjusted for different species (Felix and Callow, 1943; Felix, 1956). Bacterial cultures were grown overnight (18–24 h at 37°C) to receive a concentration of 10^9 colony forming units (cfu) mL^{-1} and diluted 10 times up to a final concentration of 10^8 cfu mL^{-1}. 100 μL of the diluted culture was transferred into 2–3 mL of previously melted and cooled soft agar (0.7% Brain-Heart agar), vortexed for 30–60 s and poured on the top of solidified and previously dried Petri dishes containing 2% of Brain-Heart agar. After solidification of the top agar (30–60 min) at room temperature, 10 μL of bacteriophage suspension with a titer of

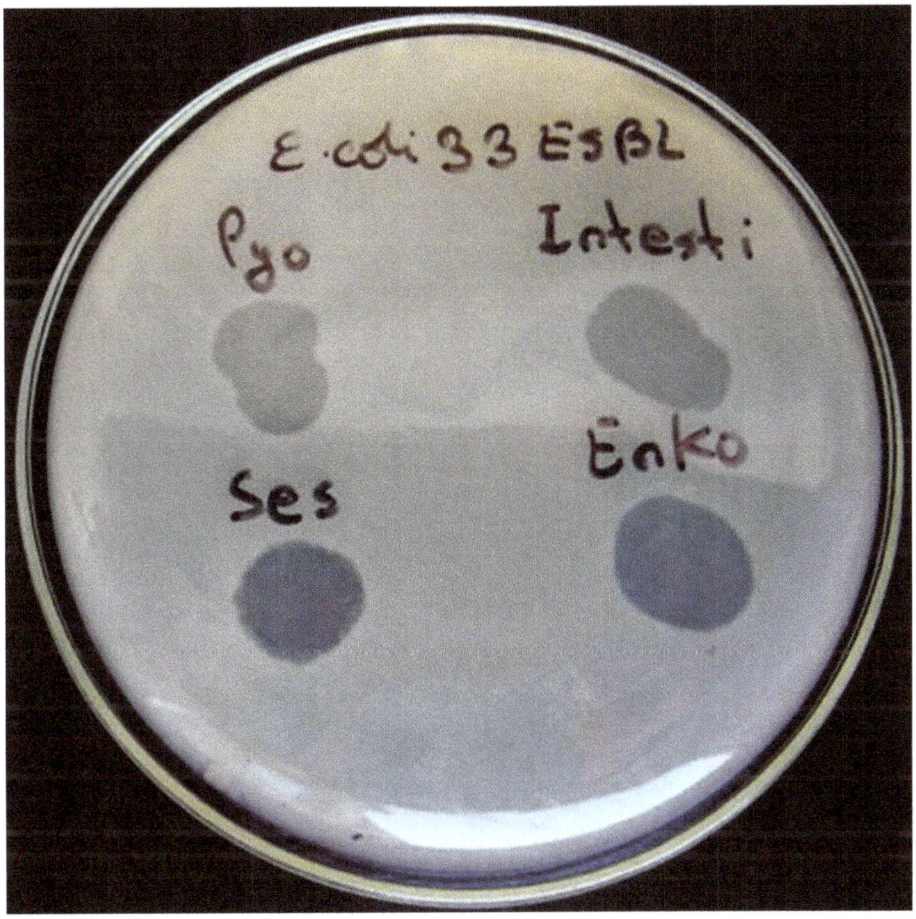

FIGURE 1 | Plaque morphology of *Escherichia coli* strain #33. The figure shows overgrown (partial) lysis (OL) in case of Pyo and Intesti bacteriophages and confluent (complete) lysis (CL) in case of Ses and Enko bacteriophages. All these results are positive.

10^7 plaques forming units (pfu) mL^{-1} was placed on top of the soft agar using an automatic pipette. The plates were let to dry for 20–30 min and then incubated overnight (18–24 h) at 37°C. Next, the results were visually evaluated.

Primary Outcome Measure

The primary outcome measure was the assessment of lytic activity of the bacteriophages on the bacteria, as could be identified by the plaque morphology in a double-layered plaque assay using *E. coli* or *K. pneumoniae* strains. A bacterial lawn inoculated with a range of bacteriophages gives different visual patterns, similar to a bacteriophage typing pattern and depending on the effect of the bacteriophage-host strain interaction. The clear zones usually differ by their intensity and structure (**Figures 1** and **2**). The positive reactions were classified as "CL" - confluent lysis, i.e., a full clear zone on the well-developed lawn of bacterial culture; "SCL" - semi-confluent lysis, i.e., a not fully cleared bacterial lawn; "OL" - overgrown lysis, i.e., single bacterial colonies that overgrew a complete clear zone; "IP" - individual clear or opaque plaques, which look like multiple small clear zones on the bacterial lawn within a drop contour, previously assigned by d'Hérelle as "tv" from "*taches vierges*" (Clokie and Kropinski, 2009; Chanishvili, 2012). The negative reactions were classified as "R" - resistant, i.e., no lysis.

Extension and Optimisation of the Bacteriophage Preparation Host-Range (Adaptation)

Expansion of the range of lytic activity of the Pyo bacteriophages cocktail was achieved by selection of mutant bacteriophages with extended host-range (h-mutants) and by increasing their titers in the bacteriophage preparation. For this purpose the bacteriophages were propagated in a suspension containing the bacterial cultures of choice with low or no susceptibility to these bacteriophages. The initial steps of adaptation technique are similar to Appelmans' method for titration in liquid media (Appelmans, 1921). The adapted bacteriophages were used for the repeated screening.

RESULTS

The antibiogram of the 41 *E. coli* and 9 *K. pneumoniae* strains shows the ESBL production capability of the strains and their sensitivity or resistance for each of seven tested

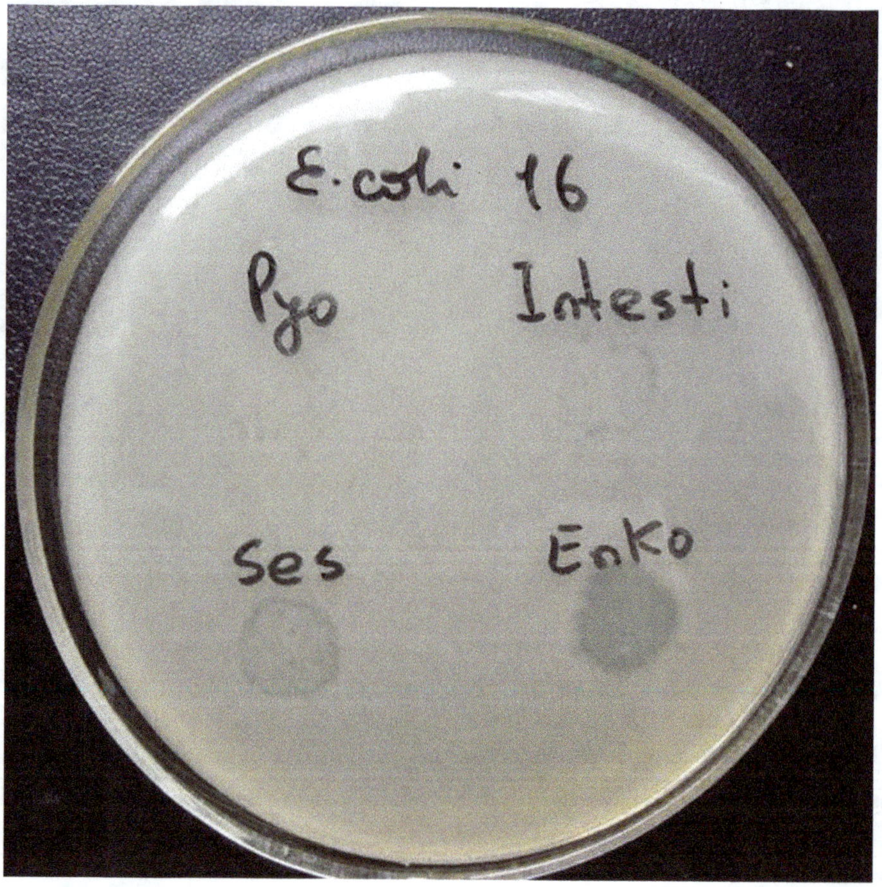

FIGURE 2 | Plaque morphology of *E. coli* strain #16. The figure shows individual plaques (IP) in case of Pyo and Intesti bacteriophages and two degrees of overgrown (partial) lysis (OL) in case of Ses and Enko bacteriophages. All these results are positive.

antibiotics, **Table 1**. In summary, the strain susceptibility varies between sensitive for all antibiotics to resistant for at least six of the seven tested antibiotics. The lytic (killing) activity of the commercial bacteriophage cocktails on the 41 *E. coli* strains varied between 66% (27 strains sensitive for Pyo bacteriophages) and 93% (38 strains sensitive for Enko bacteriophages), **Table 2**. From the 29 *E. coli* bacteriophages from the Eliava collection, the highest lytic activity came from the bacteriophages vB_*E. coli* _4t, vB_*E. coli* _4s, and vB_*E. coli* _Pic with 42, 39, and 24% coverage, respectively. Three of the *E. coli* strains (*E. coli* 5, *E. coli* 29, and *E. coli* 35 ESBL) showed complete resistance to all bacteriophage from any of the 4 commercial bacteriophage cocktails and 29 *E. coli* bacteriophages from the Eliava collection.

However, after adaptation of the Pyo bacteriophages the lytic activity could be increased from 27 to 38 sensitive strains (66 to 93%, **Table 2**), including two of the three previously mentioned resistance strains. In total, all but one *E. coli* strain could be lysed by one of the four commercial bacteriophage preparations and only strain *E. coli* 35 ESBL remained resistant, even after the adaptation of the Pyo bacteriophage preparation.

Regarding *K. pneumoniae* strains (**Table 3**), the best result was shown by bacteriophage v_B-KpS10 that could lyse all nine strains.

Bacteriophage and antibiotic susceptibility/resistance did not correlate. For example, *E. coli* strain #33 was resistant to all tested antibiotics except nitrofurantoin (NF; **Table 1**), while the same strain was susceptible to all tested bacteriophages (**Table 2**, **Figure 1**). On the contrary, *E. coli* strain #35 was resistant to all tested bacteriophages (**Table 2**), but showed susceptibility to two antibiotics, i.e., amoxicillin (AMC) and sulfamethoxazole (SXT; **Table 1**).

DISCUSSION

The *in vitro* lytic activity of bacteriophages has already been demonstrated in several studies (Chanishvili, 2012) but data

TABLE 1 | Antibiogram of 41 *Escherichia coli* and 9 *Klebsiella pneumoniae* strains isolated from the urine of patients suffering from UTIs.

	Antibiotic resistance profile							
	AM	**AMC**	**CXM**	**SXT**	**NOR**	**CIP**	**NF**	**ESBL**
***E. coli* strain number**								
3,9,10,13,17,19,21,22, 23,25,27,28,38,39,40	S	S	S	S	S	S	S	N
12	S	S	S	S	S	S	R	N
11,30	S	S	S	S	R	R	S	N
29,36	R	S	S	S	S	S	S	N
14,24	R	S	S	S	R	R	S	N
8	R	S	S	S	I	S	S	N
37	R	S	S	R	S	S	S	N
7,16,18,20	R	S	S	R	R	R	S	N
1,4	R	S	R	S	S	S	S	Y
5	R	S	R	S	S	S	S	N
2,31	R	S	R	S	R	R	S	Y
15	R	S	R	S	R	R	S	N
35	R	S	R	S	R	R	R	Y
41	R	S	R	R	R	R	S	Y
6	R	R	S	R	R	R	S	N
26	R	R	S	I	R	R	S	N
32	R	R	R	R	S	S	S	Y
33,34	R	R	R	R	R	R	S	Y
***K. pneumoniae* strain number**								
43	R	S	S	S	S	S	S	Y
46,50	R	S	S	S	S	S	S	N
42	R	S	S	S	S	S	ND	N
48	R	S	S	R	S	S	S	N
49	R	S	R	R	S	S	ND	Y
47	R	S	R	R	R	R	S	Y
44	R	S	R	R	I	I	R	N
45	R	R	R	R	R	R	ND	Y

*Strains were isolated from 22 different women and 28 different men with age between 25 and 80. Numbers 1–41 are E. coli strains with at least 18 different antibiotic resistance profiles. Numbers 42–50 are K. pneumoniae strains with at least seven different antibiotic resistance profiles. AM, ampicillin; AMC, amoxicillin/clavulanic acid; CXM, cefuroxime; SXT, sulfamethoxazole/trimethoprim or co-trimoxazole; NOR, norfloxacin; CIP, ciprofloxacin; NF, nitrofurantoin; ESBL, extended-spectrum-beta-lactamase; Y, yes (present); N, no (absent); R, resistant; S, sensitive; I, intermediate; ND, not done. Notwithstanding the occurrence of several identical antibiograms, all strains have different bacteriophage resistance/sensitivity profiles, except strains 14 and 24 (compare with **Tables 2** and **3**).*

TABLE 2 | Results of spot tests on 41 *E. coli* strains using commercial bacteriophage cocktails.

Strain number	Commercial bacteriophage cocktails				
	Pyo				
	Before adaptation	After adaptation	Intesti	Ses	Enko
39	CL	CL	CL	OL	OL
7	IP	IP	IP	OL	OL
20	IP	OL	IP	OL	OL
6,16	IP	SCL	IP	OL	OL
9	OL	CL	OL	OL	OL
1	OL	CL	OL	SCL	OL
23	OL	OL	CL	OL	OL
12,21,33	OL	OL	OL	CL	CL
31	OL	OL	OL	IP	SCL
4,8,14,24,26,30,34	OL	OL	OL	OL	OL
40	OL	OL	OL	SCL	OL
28	OL	OL	SCL	CL	CL
27,32	OL	OL	SCL	SCL	SCL
17	OL	OL	SCL	OL	OL
38	OL	SCL	CL	SCL	SCL
19	OL	SCL	OL	OL	OL
3	R	CL	OL	IP	OL
18,36,37	R	CL	OL	OL	OL
25	R	CL	R	R	OL
15	R	CL	R	SCL	OL
22	R	CL	R	SCL	SCL
2	R	CL	SCL	SCL	CL
5	R	IP	R	R	R
10	R	IP	SCL	SCL	SCL
11	R	R	R	OL	SCL
35	R	R	R	R	R
41	R	R	SCL	SCL	CL
29	R	SCL	R	R	R
13	SCL	SCL	SCL	CL	CL
Lytic activity	65.9%	92.7%	82.9%	90.2%	92.7%

CL, confluent lysis; SCL, semi-confluent lysis; OL, overgrown lysis; IP, individual plaques; R, resistant. Twenty-nine unique bacteriophage resistance/sensitivity profiles can be distinguished.

on the application of bacteriophages for treating UTIs are scarce (Perepanova et al., 1957; Arshba and Bagdoeva, 1965; Kolomeitsev et al., 1966; Danilova, 1996; Letkiewicz et al., 2010; Khawaldeh et al., 2011; Chanishvili, 2012). In the present study we showed for the first time the lytic activity of commercially existing bacteriophage cocktails on 41 *E. coli strains,* isolated from urinary cultures of patients suffering from UTIs. The applied spot test demonstrated the results of the bacteriophage–bacteria interactions: All reactions assigned as CL, SCL, OL, and IP were positive, which means that the bacteriophages lysed the bacteria, although with different degrees of effectiveness. In case of CL the bacteria could not develop bacteriophage resistance during the incubation period on the plate (18 h), indicating that this kind of bacteriophage–bacterium interaction can be considered as the most effective one. The other spot morphologies reflected less lytic activity, which could partially be caused by the different concentrations of specific bacteriophages in the commercial cocktails. Interestingly, our results show a similar order of lytic activity for the four commercial bacteriophages (before adaptation) as reported in an earlier bacteriophage sensitivity test on *E. coli* strains (Fitzgerald-Hughes et al., 2014). Furthermore, in the present study, we have shown that, as is common in the development of bacteriophages, the impact and activity of the bacteriophage cocktails can be increased in adaptation experiments, as illustrated by the change from IP into OL, or even CL (**Table 2**). The commercial bacteriophage preparations, after the adaptation experiments of the Pyo bacteriophage cocktail in successive series of adaptation, showed lytic activity on 40 of the 41 *E. coli* strains. *K. pneumoniae* bacteriophages from the Eliava collection could lyse all of the 9 *K. pneumoniae* strains tested. Besides adaptation, the efficacy of bacteriophage cocktails can also be increased by addition of new bacteriophages that show lytic activity toward the targeted clinical bacterial isolate.

TABLE 3 | Results of spot tests on 9 *K. pneumoniae* strains using laboratory bacteriophages from the Eliava collection.

	Bacteriophages									
Strain number	**vB_KlpR1**	**vB_KloxR2**	**vB_KlpR3**	**vB_KlpR4**	**vB_KlpR5**	**vB_KlpR6**	**vB_KlpR7**	**vB_KlpR8**	**v_BR KpM 9**	**v_BRKpS 10**
45,47	R	R	OL	OL	R	R	R	R	OL	OL
42	R	R	R	R	R	CL	R	CL	OL	OL
48	R	R	R	R	R	R	R	OL	R	SCL
50	R	R	R	R	R	R	R	R	OL	OL
43,44,46	R	R	R	R	R	R	R	R	R	OL
49	R	R	R	R	R	R	R	R	SCL	CL
Lytic activity	0%	0%	22%	22%	0%	11%	0%	22%	56%	100%

CL, confluent lysis; SCL, semi-confluent lysis; OL, overgrown lysis; IP, individual plaques; R, resistant. Six unique bacteriophage resistance/sensitivity profiles can be distinguished.

Since the mode of action of antimicrobial drugs like antibiotics differs considerably from bacteriophages, resistance mechanisms are consequently different, as can be concluded by comparing **Table 1** with **Tables 2** and **3**. Furthermore, these data also indicate that all but two bacterial strains with a similar antibiotic resistance profile have different bacteriophage resistance profiles, which indicates a broader (genetic) variability among the isolates than could have been expected on the basis of the antibiotic resistance profiles only. Although beyond the scope of this study, detailed genetic characterisation could indicate the effect of bacteriophages on specific serotypes or genotypes of *E. coli* and *K. pneumonia* and determine the spectrum of the (adapted) bacteriophage cocktails vs. the diversity of the strains. Full genome sequencing could further reveal which defense mechanisms by the bacteria and which counter-strategies by the bacteriophages may have been evolved (Samson et al., 2013).

The applied bacteriophage cocktails Pyo, Intesti, Ses, and Enko are allowed by the Georgian medicinal products legislation. In terms of safety, these bacteriophage preparations are already commercially available for more than 50 years and have been used millions of times without relevant incidence of adverse events. In addition, the bacteriophages in these cocktails are all lytic and do not have the ability to integrate and remain in the bacterial genome, contrarily to the temperate bacteriophages that after infection include their DNA into the host genome without making much harm to the host (see Materials and Methods). For a complete overview on quality and safety requirements for sustainable bacteriophage therapy products see (Pirnay et al., 2015).

Notwithstanding the potential of application of bacteriophage therapies in treating patients suffering from UTIs, and its broad acceptance in some East European countries, one major limitation today is the regulatory framework in the Western world (Verbeken et al., 2014; Pirnay et al., 2015), which requires a long and expensive road of assessments and randomized, placebo-controlled, double-blind trials. These studies should also investigate the best routes of administration, duration and dosage of treatment, adverse events, stability and definition of formulations and applicability for acute infections. Furthermore, and in order to accelerate potential regulatory approval for bacteriophage therapy, bacteriophages should not be considered in a similar way as chemical drugs, but, because of their typical mode of action, more like the components of the influenza vaccine, which is re-evaluated and changed yearly and does not require clinical trials for each revision (Pirnay et al., 2011). In addition, it may be appropriate to classify bacteriophages in different ways for different applications. For example as a drug for systemic applications, but as a medical device for more topical applications, as proposed for the treatment of UTIs (Pirnay et al., 2011). Recently, a set-up has been proposed where bacteriophage therapy is coordinated and standardized (in a first instance) by national bacteriophage therapy centers, which operate under the supervision of relevant public health authorities and in interaction with private stakeholders (Pirnay et al., 2015).

CONCLUSION

The results of this study have clearly shown the lytic activity of commercial bacteriophage cocktails on *E. coli* and *K. pneumonia* strains isolated from patients suffering from UTIs. In addition, the presented data has shown the potential of bacteriophage adaptation experiments with the aim to increase the lytic activity of the bacteriophage cocktails.

In times of increasing antibiotic resistance worldwide and in combination with the long history of safe use of bacteriophages in East European countries, our findings can be seen as a stimulus to invest in the set-up of randomized, placebo-controlled trials and investigate the efficacy of bacteriophage therapies in the Western world as a common alternative to strictly chemical-based treatment of bacterial infections.

In view of the high prevalence of UTIs, bacteriophages, as natural and self-amplifying antibacterial "drugs," might offer a non-systemic effective therapeutic option urgently warranting randomized controlled trials.

AUTHOR CONTRIBUTIONS

All authors had full access to all of the data in the study and take responsibility for the integrity of the data and the accuracy of data analysis. Study concept and design: WS, TMK. Acquisition, analysis, or interpretation of data: WS, RZ, MK, NC, AC, AU,

UM, TMK. Drafting of the manuscript: WS and TMK. Critical revision of the manuscript for important intellectual content: RZ, MK, NC, AC, AU, UM. Data analysis: WS, TMK. Obtained funding: UM, TMK. Study supervision: TMK. All authors read and approved the final version to be published.

ACKNOWLEDGMENTS

Marina Goderdzishvili, Nana Balarjishvili, Nino Ghudumidze, Darejan Zhgenti, Darejan Bolkvadze, Natia Skhirtladze, Natia Karumidze, and Khatuna Makalatia are acknowledged for technical assistance with the preparation of bacteriophages and related optimization protocols. Martina Marchesi is acknowledged for technical support in preparing all the strains for shipping. Harald Bruessow is acknowledged for providing valuable comments on the manuscript.

REFERENCES

Abedon, S. T., Kuhl, S. J., Blasdel, B. G., and Kutter, E. M. (2011). Phage treatment of human infections. *Bacteriophage* 1, 66–85. doi: 10.4161/bact.1.2.15845

Appelmans, R. (1921). Le dosage du bacteriophages. *C. R. Soc. Biol.* 85, 1098–1099.

Arshba, C., and Bagdoeva, K. (1965). Application of phage therapy against colibacterial infections of urinary tract. *Clin. Exp. Urol.* 3, 7–13.

Carlet, J., Collignon, P., Goldmann, D., Goossens, H., Gyssens, I. C., Harbarth, S., et al. (2011). Society's failure to protect a precious resource: antibiotics. *Lancet* 378, 369–371. doi: 10.1016/S0140-6736(11)60401-7

Chanishvili, A. (2012). *A Literature Review of the Practical Application of Bacteriophages*. New York City: Nova Science Publishers.

Clokie, M. R. J., and Kropinski, A. (2009). *Bacteriophages: Methods and Protocols*. New York City: Humana Press.

Craigie, J., and Yen, C. H. (1938). The demonstration of types of *B. typhosus* by means of preparation of type II Vi phage. *Can Public Health J.* 29, 448–463.

Danilova, T. M. (1996). Phage therapy of the inflammatory urogenital infections in women. *Proc. Dermatol. Venerol.* 5:75.

Felix, A. (1956). Phage typing of *Salmonella typhimurium*: its place in epidemiological and epizootiological investigations. *J. Gen. Microbiol.* 14, 208–222. doi: 10.1099/00221287-14-1-208

Felix, A., and Callow, B. R. (1943). Typing of paratyphoid *B. Bacilli* by Vi bacteriophage. *Br. Med. J.* 2, 127–130. doi: 10.1136/bmj.2.4308.127

Fitzgerald-Hughes, D., Bolkvadze, D., Balarjishvili, N., Leshkasheli, L., Ryan, M., Burke, L., et al. (2014). Susceptibility of extended-spectrum-beta-lactamase-producing *Escherichia coli* to commercially available and laboratory-isolated bacteriophages. *J. Antimicrob. Chemother.* 69, 1148–1150. doi: 10.1093/jac/dkt453

Foxman, B. (2002). Epidemiology of urinary tract infections: incidence, morbidity, and economic costs. *Am. J. Med.* 113(Suppl. 1A), 5S–13S. doi: 10.1016/S0002-9343(02)01054-9

Ghudumidze, N., Makalatia, K., Ediberidze, I., Kusradze, I., Karumidze, N., Merabishvili, M., et al. (2012). "Susceptibility of *Salmonella* and *E. coli* bacteriophages to environmental factors," in *Proceeding of the Conference: Bacteriophages and Probiotics - Alternatives to Antibiotics*, Tbilisi.

Groen, J., Pannek, J., Castro Diaz, D., Del Popolo, G., Gross, T., Hamid, R., et al. (2016). Summary of European association of urology (EAU) guidelines on neuro-urology. *Eur. Urol.* 69, 324–333. doi: 10.1016/j.eururo.2015.07.071

Karumidze, N., Kusradze, I., Rigvava, S., Goderdzishvili, M., Rajakumar, K., and Alavidze, Z. (2013). Isolation and characterisation of lytic bacteriophages of *Klebsiella pneumoniae* and *Klebsiella oxytoca*. *Curr. Microbiol.* 66, 251–258. doi: 10.1007/s00284-012-0264-7

Khawaldeh, A., Morales, S., Dillon, B., Alavidze, Z., Ginn, A. N., Thomas, L., et al. (2011). Bacteriophage therapy for refractory *Pseudomonas aeruginosa* urinary tract infection. *J. Med. Microbiol.* 60, 1697–1700. doi: 10.1099/jmm.0.029744-0

Khurtsia, N., Porchkhidze, K., Merabishvili, M., Tolordava, E., Burbutashvili, T., Giorkhelidze, T., et al. (2001). "Advances of clinical and theoretical Medicine and Biology," *Proceedings of the Conference Study of the Phage Susceptibility of the Strains Related to the Uro-Pathogenic E. coli and Enterococcus sp. Black-Sea Countries III International Conference*, Tskaltubo.

Kolomeitsev, N. B., Goroeinko, I. I., Shakmatov, V. K., and Brazhnik, P. K. (1966). "Treatment of urological infections with different antibiotics and specific coli-proteus bacteriophages," in *Strategy and Tactics of Antibiotic Therapy* (Krasnodar: Krasnodar Medical Institute), 172–174.

Kutter, E., De Vos, D., Gvasalia, G., Alavidze, Z., Gogokhia, L., Kuhl, S., et al. (2010). Phage therapy in clinical practice: treatment of human infections. *Curr. Pharm. Biotechnol.* 11, 69–86. doi: 10.2174/138920110790725401

Letkiewicz, S., Miedzybrodzki, R., Klak, M., Jonczyk, E., Weber-Dabrowska, B., and Gorski, A. (2010). The perspectives of the application of phage therapy in chronic bacterial prostatitis. *FEMS Immunol. Med. Microbiol.* 60, 99–112. doi: 10.1111/j.1574-695X.2010.00723.x

Mazzulli, T. (2002). Resistance trends in urinary tract pathogens and impact on management. *J. Urol.* 168, 1720–1722. doi: 10.1016/S0022-5347(05)64397-2

Merabishvili, M., De Vos, D., Verbeken, G., Kropinski, A. M., Vandenheuvel, D., Lavigne, R., et al. (2012). Selection and characterization of a candidate therapeutic bacteriophage that lyses the *Escherichia coli* O104:H4 strain from the 2011 outbreak in Germany. *PLoS ONE* 7:e52709. doi: 10.1371/journal.pone.0052709

Merabishvili, M., Vervaet, C., Pirnay, J. P., De Vos, D., Verbeken, G., Mast, J., et al. (2013). Stability of Staphylococcus aureus phage ISP after freeze-drying (lyophilization). *PLoS ONE* 8:e68797. doi: 10.1371/journal.pone.0068797

Perepanova, T. S., Debreeva, O. S., Koliatarova, G. A., Kondratieva, E. M., Aitskaia, I. M., Malysheva, V. T., et al. (1957). The efficacy of bacteriophages preparations in treatment of inflammatory urogenital diseases. *Urol. Nephrol.* 5, 14–17.

Pirnay, J. P., Blasdel, B. G., Bretaudeau, L., Buckling, A., Chanishvili, N., Clark, J. R., et al. (2015). Quality and safety requirements for sustainable phage therapy products. *Pharm. Res.* 32, 2173–2179. doi: 10.1007/s11095-014-1617-7

Pirnay, J. P., De Vos, D., Verbeken, G., Merabishvili, M., Chanishvili, N., Vaneechoutte, M., et al. (2011). The phage therapy paradigm: pret-a-porter or sur-mesure? *Pharm Res.* 28, 934–937. doi: 10.1007/s11095-010-0313-5

Rüden, H., Gastmeier, P., Daschner, F. D., and Schumacher, M. (1997). Nosocomial and community-acquired infections in Germany. Summary of the results of the first national prevalence study (NIDEP). *Infection* 25, 199–202.

Samson, J. E., Magadan, A. H., Sabri, M., and Moineau, S. (2013). Revenge of the phages: defeating bacterial defences. *Nat. Rev. Microbiol.* 11, 675–687. doi: 10.1038/nrmicro3096

7

Important Role of a Putative Lytic Transglycosylase Cj0843c in β-Lactam Resistance in *Campylobacter jejuni*

*Ximin Zeng, Barbara Gillespie and Jun Lin**

Department of Animal Science, The University of Tennessee, Knoxville, TN, USA

***Correspondence:**
Jun Lin
jlin6@utk.edu

Beta-lactam antibiotics are an important class of antibiotics for treating bacterial infections. Despite prevalent β-lactam resistance in *Campylobacter jejuni*, the leading bacterial cause of human diarrhea in developed countries, molecular mechanism of β-lactam resistance in *C. jejuni* is still largely unknown. In this study, *C. jejuni* 81–176 was used for random transposon mutagenesis. Screening of a 2,800-mutant library identified 22 mutants with increased susceptibility to ampicillin. Of these mutants, two mutants contains mutations in *Cj0843c* (a putative lytic transglycosylase gene) and in its upstream gene *Cj0844c*, respectively. Complementation experiment demonstrated that the Cj0843 contributes to β-lactam resistance. The *Cj0843c* insertional mutation was subsequently introduced to diverse *C. jejuni* clinical strains for MIC test, showing that Cj0843c contributes to both intrinsic and acquired β-lactam resistance of *C. jejuni*. Consistent with this finding, inactivation of Cj0843c also dramatically reduced β-lactamase activity. Genomic examination and PCR analysis showed *Cj0843c* is widely distributed in *C. jejuni*. High purity recombinant Cj0843c was produced for generation of specific antiserum. The Cj0843 was localized in the periplasm, as demonstrated by immunoblotting using specific antibodies. Turbidimetric assay further demonstrated the capability of the purified Cj0843c to hydrolyze cell walls. Inactivation of Cj0843c also significantly reduced *C. jejuni* colonization in the intestine. Together, this study identifies a mechanism of β-lactam resistance in *C. jejuni* and provides insights into the role of cell wall metabolism in regulating β-lactamase activity.

Keywords: beta-lactamase, peptidoglycan, random transposon mutagenesis, lytic transglycosylase

INTRODUCTION

Beta-lactam antibiotics, which inhibit biosynthesis of bacterial cell wall, are the most commercially available antibiotics in the market. For instance, in 2009, beta-lactam antibiotics account for more than half of the total antibiotic sales globally (Hamad, 2010). However, the efficacy of the β-lactam based therapy is severely threatened by a variety of β-lactam resistance mechanisms in bacteria, such as production of beta-lactamases (Korfmann and Wiedemann, 1988; Iaconis and Sanders, 1990; Jacoby, 2009), expression of the penicillin-binding proteins (PBPs) with reduced affinity for β-lactam antibiotics (Fuda et al., 2004), and extrusion of β-lactam using multi-drug efflux pumps (Nikaido, 1998; Vila and Martinez, 2008). Production of β-lactamase has been a major and threatening β-lactam resistance mechanism. Recently, increasing evidence demonstrate a direct link between cell wall metabolism and regulation of β-lactamase activity in Gram-negative bacteria, which provides insights into the development of innovative strategies to counteract β-lactam resistance in pathogenic bacteria (Zeng and Lin, 2013).

Campylobacter jejuni is the leading bacterial cause of human gastroenteritis in the developed countries (Humphrey et al., 2007). Clinical symptoms include fever and watery diarrhea in humans. In rare case, campylobacteriosis can cause severe sequelae such as Guillain–Barré syndrome, an acute flaccid paralysis that may lead to respiratory muscle compromise and death (Nachamkin et al., 1998; Hughes and Cornblath, 2005; Nyati and Nyati, 2013). The annual incidence of campylobacteriosis in the United States is approximately 1% (Poly and Guerry, 2008), resulting in 1.7 billion dollars cost in medical practice and productivity (Hoffmann et al., 2012). In parallel to its increased prevalence, *Campylobacter* is increasingly resistant to macrolides and fluoroquinolones, the two major clinical antibiotics (Luo et al., 2005; Caldwell et al., 2008; Koningstein et al., 2011). Recently, it has been proposed that an oral β-lactam, such as co-amoxiclav, may provide an alternative therapy for *Campylobacter* infection (Elviss et al., 2009; Griggs et al., 2009). However, β-lactam resistant *C. jejuni* strains have also been observed in epidemiological studies (Lachance et al., 1991; Griggs et al., 2009). Thus, understanding the mechanisms of β-lactam resistance in *C. jejuni* would help us develop effective therapeutic strategy that will allow the use of existing β-lactams against resistant *C. jejuni*. In *Campylobacter*, two beta-lactam resistance mechanisms have been characterized, which include the presence of CmeABC multi-drug efflux pump (Lin et al., 2002) and the production β-lactamase OXA-61 (Alfredson and Korolik, 2005; Griggs et al., 2009). Despite these progresses, the findings from recent studies strongly suggest the existence of novel β-lactamases and/or regulatory system in *C. jejuni* for β-lactam resistance (Griggs et al., 2009; Zeng et al., 2014).

In this study, using random mutagenesis, we identified a putative lytic transglycosylase (LT) Cj0843c that is required for intrinsic and acquired β-lactam resistance in *C. jejuni*. This finding was further validated by a series of molecular, biochemical and genomic examination. Consistent with this finding, inactivation of Cj0843c, which is highly conserved in *C. jejuni*, dramatically reduced β-lactamase activity. The role of Cj0843c in peptidoglycan metabolism was validated by a standard LT assay using purified Cj0843c. This study provides compelling evidence that Cj0843c, a putative LT, plays a critical role in regulating β-lactamase-mediated β-lactam resistance in *C. jejuni*.

MATERIALS AND METHODS

Bacterial Strains, Plasmids, and Culture Conditions

The major bacterial strains and plasmids used in this study are listed in **Table 1**. The *C. jejuni* strains were grown routinely in Müller-Hinton (MH) broth or agar at 42°C in tri-gas incubator (85% N_2, 10% CO_2, 5% O_2). *Escherichia coli* strains were grown routinely in Luria-Bertani (LB) broth with shaking (250 rpm) or on agar at 37°C overnight. When

TABLE 1 | Key bacterial plasmids and strains used in this study.

Plasmids or strains	Description	Source or reference
Plasmids		
pRY111	*Escherichia coli–Campylobacter* shuttle vector, kanamycin resistant	Yao et al., 1993
pCj843c	pRY111 derivative containing *Cj0843c, Cj0844c,* and *Cj0845c*	This study
pCj844c	pRY111 derivative containing *Cj0843c* and *Cj0844c*	This study
pET28b-Cj0843c	Expression vector for recombinant Cj0843c, Kan^r	Novagen
Strains		
Campylobacter jejuni		
JL241	NCTC 11168, human isolate	Parkhill et al., 2000
JL890	JL241 derivative with transposon inserted into *Cj0843c*, Kan^r	This study
JL990	JL890 derivative, complemented with pCj843c	This study
JL28	81–176, human isolate, for random transposon mutagenesis	Black et al., 1988
JL30	81–176 (JL28) derivative with transposon inserted into *cmeB* gene, Kan^r	Lin et al., 2002
JL916	JL28 derivative with EZ::TN <KAN-2> transposon inserted into *Cj0843c*, Kan^r	This study
JL926	JL916 derivative, complemented with pCj843c	This study
JL962	81–176 derivative, ampicillin resistant. The β-lactamase gene bla_{OXA-61} was introduced into chromosome via natural transformation using genomic DNA from ampicillin resistant *C. jejuni* 21190 (Zeng et al., 2014)	This study
JL963	JL962 derivative. The *Cj0843c::kan* mutation was introduced into chromosome via natural transformation using genomic DNA from JL916, Kan^r	This study
JL995	81–176 (JL28) derivative, Kan^r. The *pgp1::kan* mutation was introduced into JL28 chromosome via natural transformation using genomic DNA of the *pgp1* mutant (Frirdich et al., 2012)	This study
JL996	JL962 derivative. The *pgp1::kan* mutation was introduced into JL962 chromosome via natural transformation using genomic DNA of the *pgp1* mutant (Frirdich et al., 2012)	This study
E. coli		
DH5α	F- Φ80*lacZ*ΔM15 Δ(*lacZYA-argF*)U169 *recA1 endA1 hsdR17* (rk−, mk+) *phoA* supE44 thi-1 *gyrA96 relA1* λ-	Invitrogen
JL985	pET28b-Cj0843c in BL21(DE3)	This study

needed, culture media were supplemented with ampicillin (100 μg/ml), kanamycin (50 μg/ml), and chloramphenicol (Cm; 20 μg/ml).

Random Transposon Mutagenesis

We have successfully used *C. jejuni* 81–176 as a host strain for *in vivo* random transposon mutagenesis using EZ-Tn5 < KAN-2 > Tnp Transposome system (Epicentre; Lin et al., 2009; Hoang et al., 2011, 2012; Zeng et al., 2013b). In this study, the wild-type *C. jejuni* 81–176 (ampicillin Minimum inhibitory concentration (MIC) = 1 μg/ml) was subjected to *in vivo* random transposon mutagenesis; the procedure and screening strategy are detailed in previous publications (Lin et al., 2009; Hoang et al., 2011, 2012; Zeng et al., 2013b). The mutants with growth defects in MH broth containing kanamycin (50 μg/ml) and ampicillin (0.25 μg/mL) were identified. To determine transposon insertion site, genomic DNA extracted from the selected mutant was subjected to direct sequencing as described previously (Lin et al., 2009; Hoang et al., 2011; Zeng et al., 2013b).

Antimicrobial Susceptibility Test

The susceptibilities of *C. jejuni* strains to different antimicrobials (Fisher Bioreagents) were determined by a standard microtiter broth dilution method with an inoculum of 10^6 CFU/ml as described previously (Lin et al., 2002; Zeng et al., 2014). MIC for specific antimicrobial was defined by the lowest concentration of the antimicrobial showing complete inhibition of bacterial growth after 2 days of incubation at 42°C under microaerophilic condition.

Beta-lactamase Activity Assay

To measure β-lactamase activity in *C. jejuni* strains, standard assay was performed on cell lysates of different strains by following previous procedure (Griggs et al., 2009; Zeng et al., 2014) with minor modifications. Briefly, late-log phase bacterial cells were harvested from MH plates, washed with PBS, and adjusted to an optical density at 600 nm of approximately 1.2 in PBS. Bacterial suspensions were sonicated and centrifuged at 13,000 rpm for 5 min. The supernatant was subjected to protein concentration measurement using BCA Protein Assay kit (Pierce). One hundred microliter of supernatant containing 40 μg of protein was mixed with 0.8 ml of ice-chilled reaction buffer (0.1 M phosphate; 1 mM EDTA, pH 7.0). Then 100 μl of nitrocefin (500 μg/ml) was added to the above reaction mix followed by incubation at 37°C for 30 min. The activity was determined by spectrometric at 486 nm. The molar extinction coefficient of hydrolyzed nitrocefin at 486 nm is 20,500 M^{-1} cm^{-1}. The lysate from *C. jejuni* 81–176 was used as negative control. The β-lactamase activity was expressed as hydrolyzed nitrocefin (μM) per hr per mg of protein.

Complementation of *C. jejuni* 81–176 Transposon Mutants

The long fragment (containing the genes *Cj0843c*, *Cj0844c*, and *Cj0845c*) and the short fragment (containing the genes *Cj0844c* and *Cj0845c*) were PCR amplified from *C. jejuni* 81–176 using primer pairs of Cj0843c_F/Cj0843c_R and Cj0843c_F/Cj0844c_R (**Table 2**), respectively, with *Pfu*Ultra fusion II DNA polymerase (Stratagene). The resulting fragments were ligated into *Sma*I-digested shuttle vector pRY111 (Yao et al., 1993) and ligation mix was introduced into *E. coli* DH5α by heat shock transformation. The *E. coli* transformants containing the plasmid that bears the three-gene (named pCj843c) or the two-gene fragment (named pCj0844c) were identified and confirmed by sequencing. Both constructs were mobilized into *C. jejuni* 81–176 transposon mutants by triparental conjugation as described previously (Zeng et al., 2013a, 2014).

Natural Transformation

Natural transformation (biphasic method) was performed following standard procedure as described by Wang and Taylor (1990). Approximately 4 μg of *C. jejuni* genomic DNA was used for natural transformation. The insertional *Cj0843c* mutations in different strains were confirmed by PCR using primer pair Cj0843c_F1 and Cj0843c_R1 (**Table 2**).

Production of Recombinant Cj0843c and Generation of Polyclonal Antiserum

N-terminal histidine-tagged recombinant Cj0843c was produced in *E. coli* by using pET-28b(+) vector. Briefly, approximately 1568-bp fragment of *Cj0843c* was PCR amplified from *C. jejuni* NCTC 81–176 using primer pairs rCj0843c_F1(*Nde*I) and rCj0843c-pET28b_R(*Sal*I; **Table 2**). The amplified product and the vector pET-28b(+) were both digested with *Nde*I and *Sal*I and ligated with each other. Cloning, expression, and purification of rCj0843c were performed using the procedures described in our previous publication (Lin et al., 2005; Zeng et al., 2013a). The plasmid pET28b-Cj0843c in the *E. coli* BL21(DE3) clone (JL985) producing rCj0843c was sequenced to confirm the correct insertion. The fractions containing pure rCj0843c were pooled and dialyzed against 1 x PBS buffer (Fisher Bioreagents). The concentration of the purified rCj0843c was determined using BCA Protein Assay Kit (Pierce™). Approximately 4 mg of highly purified rCj0843c was used for the production of rabbit polyclonal antisera by Pacific Immunology Corp (Ramona, CA). Pre- and post-immune serum samples were analyzed by immunoblotting against pure rCj0843c to confirm the generation of specific Cj0843c antibody.

Enzymatic Activity of rCj0843c

The LT activity of rCj0843c was evaluated using turbidimetric assay as reported before with minor modification (Caldentey and Bamford, 1992). In brief, the isogenic *Cj0843c* mutant of *C. jejuni* 81–176 was harvested from three overnight-cultured MH agar plates and resuspended in 50 ml Tris-HCl buffer (50 mM, pH 7.5). Then 3 ml of chloroform was added in the suspension, which was kept at room temperature for 30 min with gently shaking. Subsequently, the chloroform-extracted cells (the crude cell walls) were pelleted by centrifugation at 13,000 rpm for 5 min, washed once with 50 mM Tris-HCl buffer (pH7.5), and resuspended in 50 ml of 50 mM Tris-HCl buffer (pH 7.5).

To perform turbidimetric assay, the crude cell walls were adjusted to final $OD_{450\ nm}$ of approximately 0.45 using 50 mM Tris-HCl buffer. Then the purified rCj0843c was added to 1 ml of such cell wall suspension with final concentration of 24 μg/ml; the cell wall suspension containing PBS instead of rCj0843c served as control. The decrease in turbidity at 450 nm was determined after 2.5 h of incubation at 37°C. The turbidimetric assay was performed with triplicate and the statistical analysis of a Student's t test was carried out using SAS (v9.4). A *P*-value less than 0.05 was considered significant.

Localization of the Cj0843c

To determine cellular localization of Cj0843c, the periplasmic and spheroplastic fractions were prepared using the PeriPreps™ Periplasting Kit (Epicentre) as detailed in our recent publication (Zeng et al., 2013a). Different cellular fractions were subsequently subjected to SDS-PAGE and immunoblotting analysis as described in our previous publications (Lin et al., 2002; Zeng et al., 2009, 2013a). Briefly, the protein samples were separated by SDS-PAGE with a 12% (wt/vol) polyacrylamide separating gel. After SDS-PAGE, proteins in the gels were then electrophoretically transferred to nitrocellulose membranes (Bio-Rad) at 60 V for 1 h at 4°C. The membranes were incubated with blocking buffer (5% Nestle skim milk powder in PBS) for 16 h at 4°C prior to incubation with primary antibodies (Rabbit anti-Cj0843c at 1:5000 dilution in the blocking buffer). To ensure the quality of periplasmic and spheroplastic fractions, antibodies directed against CmeR (cytoplasmic control, 1:2000 dilution) were also used as primary antibodies. After incubation at 25°C for 1 h, the blots were washed three times with PBS containing 0.05% Tween 20 and subsequently incubated with secondary antibodies (1:50,000 dilution of goat anti-rabbit IgG-HRP; Kirkegaard and Perry) at 25°C for 1 h. After washing, the blots were developed with the SuperSignal West Dura Chemiluminescent Substrate (Thermo Scientific). Prestained molecular weight markers (Bio-Rad) were coelectrophoresed and blotted to allow estimation of the sizes of the proteins.

Prevalence of Cj0843c in *C. jejuni*

Total 30 *C. jejuni* strains from different hosts and geographically diverse areas were grown microaerophilically to late exponential phase and harvested by centrifugation. The cell pellets were suspended in 100 μL of water and lysed by boiling for 5 min. After centrifugation, the supernatants were used as template in PCR assay with highly *Cj0843c*-specific primers Cj0843c_F1 and Cj0843c_R1 (**Table 2**). For bioinformatic analysis of *Cj0843c* prevalence among available genome sequences, total 103 *C. jejuni* genomes were extracted from Integrated Microbial Genomes[1] and the multi-sequence alignment was analyzed using Clustal Omega[2]. In addition, presence of *Cj0843c* homolog was also examined in the genomes of 49 *Campylobacter coli* and 298 *Helicobacter pylori* strains.

Chicken Colonization Experiment

Campylobacter jejuni 81-176 wild-type strain together with its isogenic *Cj0843c* mutant (JL916) and the complementation strain (JL926; **Table 2**) were used for colonization assay in a chicken model system as described in previous studies (Lin et al., 2002; Lin and Martinez, 2006; Hoang et al., 2011; Zeng et al., 2013a). The chicken study was approved by the Institutional Animal Care and Use Committee at The University of Tennessee (Protocol 1387 under oversight of the IACUC Chair Carla Sommardahl). Briefly, 1-day-old broiler chickens were obtained from a commercial hatchery (Hubbard Hatchery, Pikesville, TN, USA). The chickens were negative for *Campylobacter* as determined by culturing cloacal swabs prior to use in this study. Three groups of 4-days-old chickens (10 birds/group) were inoculated with different bacteria via oral gavage using a dose approximately 10^5 CFU of fresh late log-phase *C. jejuni* per bird. Notably, the motility of parent strain and its *Cj0843c* mutant was confirmed to be at a comparable level prior to challenge. The isogenic *Cj0843c* mutant displayed reduced growth in MH broth when compared to its parent strain. However, the fresh *C. jejuni* cultures with similar growth phase, reflected by the final $OD_{600\ nm}$ measurement, were used to challenge chickens; the bacteria in such cultures were assumed to be in the same

[1] https://img.jgi.doe.gov/cgi-bin/imgm_hmp/main.cgi

[2] http://www.ebi.ac.uk/Tools/msa/clustalo/

TABLE 2 | Major primers used in this study.

Primer	DNA Sequence (5′–3′)[a]	Product size (bp)	Target gene and function
Cj0843c_F	AACAAAATCCCAAGCTAAAGTCA	3,767	*Cj0843c, Cj0844c* and *Cj0845c* operon
Cj0843c _R	TTCTAGACAAGACAAGTAAAGATGATG		
Cj0844c_R	CAAGTGAATTTTCTTCCTTTTTGAG	2,028	With Cj0843c_F, to amplify *Cj0844c* and *Cj0845c*
Cj0843c_F1	GCTCAAACCTTTAAAAATCAAAGA	586	*Cj0843c* prevalence and validation of *Cj0843c* mutation
Cj0843c_R1	TTTGCCAAGCAAAAGGATCT		
rCj0843c_F1(NdeI)	GGAATTC<u>CATATG</u>CAATATAGTATAGAAAAACTCAAAAAGGAA	1,568	Recombinant Cj0843c
rCj0843c-pET28b_R(SalI)	GCGCAT<u>GTCGAC</u>CTAAGATTTGTTTAGATCATTTGCC		

[a] *Restriction sites are underlined in the primer sequence and the names are identified in parentheses.*

physiological state. For each group, 5 birds were euthanized and cecal samples were collected at 6 and 10 days post-inoculation. The cecal contents from each bird were weighed and diluted in MH broth. The diluted samples were plated onto MH agar plates with *Campylobacter* specific selective supplements (Oxoid, UK). The number of CFU per gram of cecal contents was calculated for each chicken and was used as an indicator of the colonization level. The detection limit of the plating methods was 10^2 CFU/g of cecal contents. A bird from which no *Campylobacter* colonies were detected was assigned a conservative value of 99 CFU/g of cecal contents for the purpose of calculating means and for statistical analysis. One-way analysis of variance (ANOVA) followed by a least-significant difference test was used to analyze the significant differences in colonization level (log transformed). A *P*-value less than 0.05 was considered significant.

RESULTS

Cj0843c, a Putative Lytic Transglycosylase, is Required for Ampicillin Resistance

The *C. jejuni* 81–176 strain was used as a host strain to generate a library consisting of 2,800 Tn5-insertional mutants. Individual mutant grown in microtiter plates was replicated into screening plates containing MH broth with sublethal concentration of ampicillin (0.25 μg/ml). A total of 22 mutants displayed increased susceptibility to ampicillin. The insertional sites of these mutants were mapped by direct sequencing. It's not surprising that most of them (20 mutants) contains transposon insertion in *cmeABC* locus which encodes CmeABC multidrug efflux pump system which was previously shown to be involved in ampicillin resistance (Lin et al., 2002, 2003). Specifically, transposon insertional mutations were identified in *cmeA* (two different sites with four mutants), *cmeB* (two different sites with four mutants), and *cmeC* (2 different sites with 12 mutants). Interestingly, the other two mutants have transposon insertion identified in two adjacent genes, the CJJ81176_0859 and CJJ81176_0860 (hereinafter, the corresponding universal locus names in *C. jejuni* NCTC 11168, *Cj0843c* and *Cj0844c*, were used). The Cj0843c was annotated as a putative secreted LT. Specifically, Cj0843c contains a highly conserved domain (COG0741, E-value is 3.53e-27) represented by MltE, an endo-specific LT from *E. coli* that catalyzes hydrolysis of glycan chains to generate short chains with 1,6-anhydro-MurNAc ends (Fibriansah et al., 2012). *Cj0844c* was annotated as putative integral membrane protein. Both mutants displayed fourfold MIC reduction for ampicillin when compared to that of wild type 81–176 (**Table 3**).

Genome analysis showed that the start codon of *Cj0843c* overlapped the stop codon of *Cj0844c* by 4 bp nucleotides. In addition, there is only 2 bp nucleotide gap between the start codon of *Cj0844c* and the stop codon of its upstream gene *Cj0845c*. Therefore, the *Cj0845c*, *Cj0844c*, and *Cj0843c* may form an operon. The transposon insertion into *Cj0844c* may cause polar effect, affecting the expression of downstream gene *Cj0843c*. To test this, two constructs with different length (pCj0843c and pCj0844c) was constructed for complementation (**Table 1**). The pCj0843c covers the whole three-gene operon while pCj0844c only contains two upstream genes *Cj0845c* and *Cj0844c*. As shown in **Table 3**, complementation with pCj0843c restored the MIC of both mutants to the level of wild type strain. However, complementation of the *Cj0844c* mutant with pCj0844c failed to restore MIC of ampicillin to wild-type level, indicating that the Cj0843c, not *Cj0844c*, is involved in ampicillin resistance in *C. jejuni* 81–176.

To examine the role of Cj0843c in ampicillin resistance in different strains, the *Cj0843c* transposon mutation was also introduced into *C. jejuni* NCTC 11168 via natural transformation. As shown in **Table 3**, the isogenic *Cj0843c* mutant of NCTC 11168 also displayed increased susceptibility to ampicillin (eightfold reduction) while the MIC of the complementation strain was the same as that of wild type strain.

Cj0843c is Involved in the Resistance to Various β-lactam Antibiotics in *Campylobacter*

We also examined if inactivation of Cj0843c affected susceptibilities of *C. jejuni* to different β-lactam antibiotics. As shown in **Table 4**, susceptibilities of *Cj0843c* mutant to various β-lactam antibiotics (penicillin G, ticarcillin, carbenicillin, and cloxacillin) significantly increased (fourfold) when compared to wild-type 81–176 strain. Complementation of the isogenic Cj0843c mutant with pCj0843c restored MIC of ampicillin to wild type level (**Table 4**). In terms of other types of antimicrobials, such as bile salts (cholic acid and deoxycholic acid), ciprofloxacin and ethidium bromide (**Table 4**), the susceptibilities of *Cj0843c* mutant did not change when compared to wild-type strain.

Cj0843c also Plays an Important Role in Acquired Ampicillin Resistance

Although *C. jejuni* 81–176 lacks beta-lactamase gene bla_{OXA-61} in the genome (Griggs et al., 2009), it could acquire high-level ampicillin resistance (Amp^r) due to the acquisition of active beta-lactamase bla_{OXA-61} from *C. jejuni* 21190 via natural transformation (Zeng et al., 2014). The MIC of ampicillin for the Amp^r derivative of 81–176 was 128 μg/mL, which is 128-fold higher than the MIC of wild-type 81–176 (**Figure 1**), as reflected by the dramatic change of the beta-lactamase activity (**Figure 1**). However, inactivation of *Cj0843c* in the Amp^r derivative of 81–176 dramatically reduced MIC (8 μg/mL) as well as the beta-lactamase activity in cell lysates (**Figure 1**). In contrast, although mutation in multidrug efflux pump gene *cmeB* (Lin et al., 2002) in the Amp^r derivative led to reduced MIC of ampicillin (16 μg/mL), the beta-lactamase activity was not changed (**Figure 1**). This finding clearly indicated that Cj0843c also plays an important role in β-lactamase-mediated ampicillin resistance by modulating the activity of β-lactamase Bla_{OXA-61} in *C. jejuni*.

TABLE 3 | Susceptibilities of two representative *C. jejuni* strains and their isogenic mutants to ampicillin.

Parent strain	MIC (μg/mL)						
	Wild type	*Cj0843c*⁻	*Cj0844c*⁻	*Cj0843c*⁻/pCj0843c	*Cj0844c*⁻/pCj0843c	*Cj0844c*⁻/pCj0844c	*CmeB*⁻
81–176	1	0.25	0.25	1	1	0.25	0.0625
NCTC 11168	16	2	ND[a]	16	ND	ND	4

[a] *ND, not determined.*

TABLE 4 | Cj0843 is only involved in *C. jejuni* resistance to various β-lactams.

Chemical	81–176 WT	*cj0843c::Tn5*	*cj0843c::Tn5*/pCj0843c
Penicillin G (μg/ml)	16	4	16
Ticarcillin (μg/ml)	256	64	256
Carbenicillin (μg/ml)	64	16	64
Cloxacillin (μg/ml)	512	128	512
Cholic acid (mg/ml)	12.5	12.5	N/D[a]
Ciprofloxacin (μg/ml)	0.25	0.25	N/D
Deoxycholic acid (mg/ml)	20	20	N/D
Ethidium bromide (μg/ml)	1	1	N/D

[a]*N/D, not determined.*

To determine the role of Pgp1, an identified gene involved cell wall metabolism in *C. jejuni* (Frirdich et al., 2012), in ampicillin resistance, the *pgp1::kan* mutation was introduced into the wild-type 81-176 and its Amp^r derivative in this study via natural transformation using genomic DNA of the *pgp1* mutant, creating isogenic *pgp1* mutant JL995 and JL996, respectively (**Table 1**). The MICs for JL995 and JL996 are 1 and 128 μg/mL, respectively, which are the same as those for their corresponding parent strains. Consistent with this finding, the beta-lactamase activity was not changed due to the inactivation of *pgp1*.

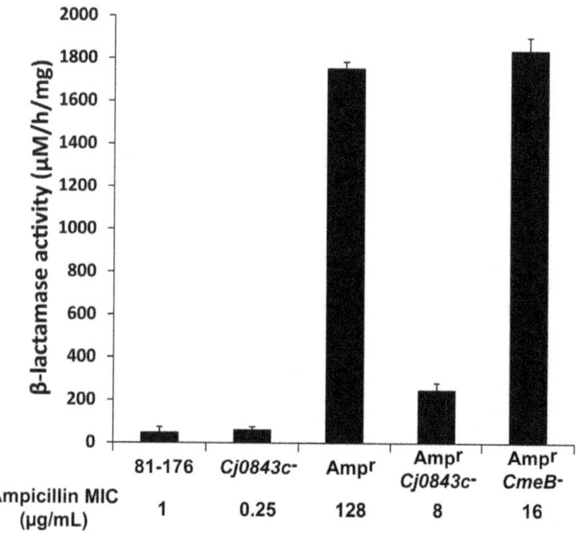

FIGURE 1 | Effect of *Cj0843c* mutation on intracellular β-lactamase activities and ampicillin resistance in *Campylobacter jejuni*. The ampicillin MIC values were listed below each corresponding strain. Amp^r, the 81–176 derivative with β-lactamase gene bla_{OXA-61} introduced into chromosome via natural transformation using genomic DNA from ampicillin resistant *C. jejuni* 21190 (Zeng et al., 2014). The procedure for nitrocefin-based β-lactamase activity assay was detailed in Materials and Methods. The activity was determined by spectrometric change at 486 nm. The molar extinction coefficient of hydrolyzed nitrocefin at 486 nm is 20,500 M^{-1} cm^{-1}. The β-lactamase activity was expressed as hydrolyzed nitrocefin (μM) per hr per mg of protein.

The Prevalent and Highly Conserved Cj0843c is Required for Ampicillin Resistance in Diverse *C. jejuni* Isolates

It's well known that the genome of *C. jejuni* species displayed considerable plasticity (de Boer et al., 2002; Poly et al., 2008; Duong and Konkel, 2009). In this study, a PCR survey was performed, demonstrating that the *Cj0843c* was present in 30 diverse *C. jejuni* isolates (data not shown). The representative isolates were listed in **Table 5**. Regardless of the level of β-lactamase activity and the level of ampicillin resistance, introduction of *Cj0843c* mutation into these isolates all resulted in the decrease of MIC of ampicillin by more than fourfold (**Table 5**).

In addition to this PCR survey, genome analysis also provided compelling evidence showing *Cj0843c* was highly conserved in *C. jejuni* and other closely related species. Specifically, *Cj0843c* was present in all 101 currently available *C. jejuni* genomes deposited in the database. Notably, the three-gene operon containing *Cj0843c* is also highly conserved in the genomes of different ε-proteobacteria, including 101 *C. jejuni*, 49 *C. coli*, and 298 *H. pylori* (Supplementary Figure S1 and detailed in Supplementary Table S1).

The multi-sequence alignment data show the percentage aa identity among *C. jejuni* strains ranges from 93 to 100%. The across-species alignment shows that the aa identity and homology between *C. jejuni* NCTC 11168 and *C. coli* RM2228 are 79 and 89%, respectively, and those between *C. jejuni* NCTC 11168 and *H. pylori* 26695 are 31 and 51%, respectively.

The Cj0843c is Localized in Periplasm

Based on annotation, Cj0843c is predicted to interact with the glycan strand of the periplasmic peptidoglycan. To confirm this, we first cloned *Cj0843c* into expression vector pET-28b and produced N-terminal 6xHis tagged recombinant Cj0843c (rCj0843c). Majority of rCj0843c is in the soluble fraction and was successfully purified by Ni-NTA affinity column (**Figure 2A**).

TABLE 5 | Cj0843c is prevalent and involved in intrinsic and acquired ampicillin resistance in different clinical *C. jejuni* isolates.

Strain	Source/host	*Cj0843c*[a]	β-Lactamase activity[b]	MIC (μg/ml)	
				Wild type	*Cj0843c::Tn5*
JL241	Human	+	−	16	4
JL36	Chicken	+	±	8	1
JL78	Human	+	−	4	0.25
JL81	Human	+	−	4	0.5
JL85	Human	+	−	2	0.25
JL90	Human	+	−	2	0.5
JL95	Ovine	+	+	16	2
JL100	Human	+	+	16	0.5
JL115	Human	+	++++	256	16
49	Chicken	+	−	4	0.25
Cj41	Chicken	+	±	8	1
SO40	Bovine	+	−	16	1
JL98	Human	+	+	8	2
86	Chicken	+	−	16	2

[a] *The prevalence of Cj0843c is detected by PCR using primer Cj0843c_F1 and Cj0843c_R1.*
[b] *The β-lactamase activity of each clinical isolate was measured using the cell lysate with the nitrocefin assay (Griggs et al., 2009). A yellow to red color change within 5 min at 37°C indicated a β-lactamase-positive reaction. +, positive β-lactamase activity; −, negative β-lactamase activity; ±, weak β-lactamase activity; ++++, red color developed immediately upon addition of substrate nitrocefin.*

The specific Cj0843c antiserum was successfully raised and was used for immunoblotting to determine localization of Cj0843c in *C. jejuni*. As shown in **Figure 2B**, Cj0843c is detected in the periplasm fraction but not in the spheroplast fraction of wild-type cells (left panel). The Cj0843c was not detected in the periplasm fraction of the isogenic Cj0843c mutant either (left panel in **Figure 2B**). As a control, CmeR, an intracellular regulator, is only detected in the spheroplast fractions in both wild type and *Cj0843c* mutants (right panel in **Figure 2B**). This immunoblotting analysis provides compelling evidence that that Cj0843c is localized in the periplasm, the place where peptidoglycan resides in Gram-negative bacteria.

Lytic Transglycosylase Activity of rCj0843c

The chloroform-treated *Cj0843c* mutant cells was used as cell wall substrates because the rCj0843c action sites on cell walls from this mutant are possibly intact. As shown in **Figure 2C**, the decrease in OD_{450nm} (ΔOD_{450nm}) in the reaction solution containing the rCj0843c is significantly larger than PBS control ($P < 0.05$), indicating the capability of rCj0843c as LT to hydrolyze cell wall.

Cj0843c is Required for *C. jejuni* Colonization

The role of Cj0843c in *in vivo* survival of *C. jejuni* was evaluated using chicken model system. As shown in **Figure 2D**, wild-type *C. jejuni* 81–176 could colonize chicken efficiently on days 6 and 10 post-challenge with colonization level as high as 10^9 CFU per gram of feces. In contrast, the isogenic *Cj0843c* mutant displayed significantly reduced colonization in the intestine ($P < 0.05$); the mutant was not detected in most of chickens. Complementation with the plasmid did not rescue the impaired colonization of the *Cj0843c* mutant, likely due to instability of the plasmid in the complemented strain. To test this, an *in vitro* plasmid stability assay was performed by subculturing complemented strain every 2–3 days in fresh antibiotic-free MH broth (1:400 dilution) for 10 days; by day 10, majority of the cells (85%) were observed to lose the complemented plasmid.

DISCUSSION

In this study, random transposon mutagenesis was used to identify novel genes contributing to beta-lactam resistance in *C. jejuni*, which led to the discovery of a putative LT Cj0843c that plays an important role in the intrinsic and acquired beta-lactam resistance in *C. jejuni*. Notably, the mutation of Cj0843c significantly reduced beta-lactamase activity and MIC for ampicillin (**Table 3** and **Figure 1**). The periplasmic Cj0843c was prevalent and highly conserved in *C. jejuni* and other ε-proteobacteria, such as *C. coli* and *H. pylori* (Supplementary Figure S1 and Supplementary Table S1), indicating the critically conserved role of Cj0843c in cell wall metabolism. Cj0843c is also required for *C. jejuni* colonization in the intestine (**Figure 2D**). Mutation of another cell wall metabolism-related gene pgp1 was also observed to impair *C. jejuni* colonization (Frirdich et al., 2012). However, at this stage, it is still premature to speculate how Cj0843c is involved in colonization. Mutation of Cj0843c may affect *C. jejuni* physiology and exert pleiotropic effects that are related to *C. jejuni in vivo* colonization.

The LT also have been observed to be involved in beta-lactam resistance in other bacteria. For instance, single (ΔMltB),

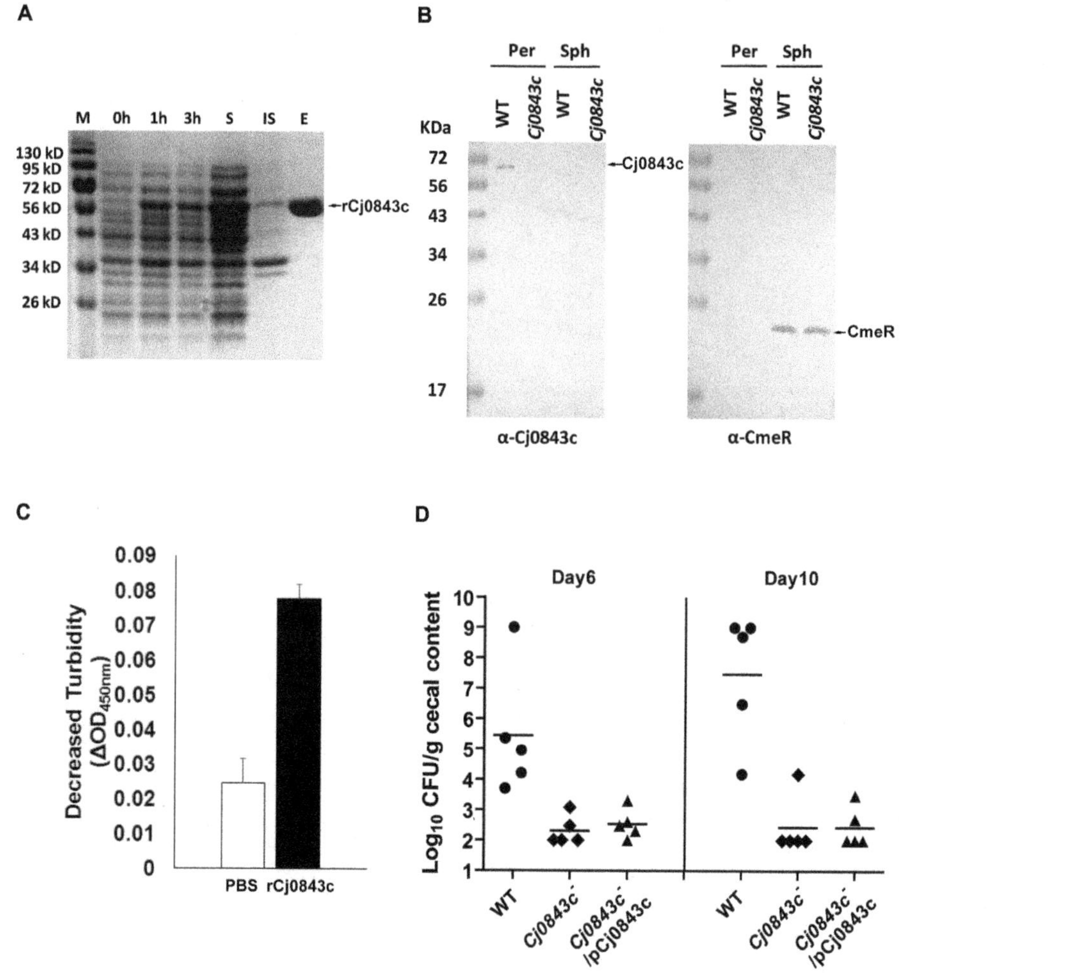

FIGURE 2 | Characterization of Cj0843c. (A) Expression and purification of rCj0843c. Cj0843 fragment was cloned into pET-28b vector. Expression of rCj0843c was induced in the presence of 0.5 mM IPTG. 0, 1 and 3 h, the cell lysates from pre-induction, 1 and 3 h induced cells; S, soluble fraction; IS, insoluble fraction; E, elution fraction. **(B)** Cj0843c is localized in periplasm. The intracellular regulator CmeR was used as cytoplasm control. Per, periplasm; Sph, spheroplast; WT, wild type. **(C)** Turbidimetric assay of rCj0843c. Chloroform-treated *Cj0843c*$^-$ mutant cells (crude cell walls) were mixed with rCj0843c or PBS control solution. The decrease of absorbance at 450 nm was measured after 2.5 h incubation. Each bar represents the mean ± SD from three independent measurements. **(D)** Critical role of Cj0843c in colonization of *C. jejuni* in chicken. The chickens in each group (10 birds) were inoculated with *C. jejuni* 81–176 (close circle), its isogenic *Cj0843c* mutant (diamond), and complementation strain (triangle) at dose of 10^5 CFU/chicken. At days 6 and 10 post-challenge, five chickens from each group were killed and cecal contents were collected for *C. jejuni* numeration. The detection limit is 10^2 CFU/gram fecal sample. Each horizontal line segment denotes the mean value of log transformed CFU of different strains at the indicated days post-inoculation. The detection limit is 10^2 CFU/gram fecal sample.

double (ΔMltA/ΔMltB; Kraft et al., 1999) or sextuple (Slt70, MltA, MltB, MltC, MltD, and EmtA; Korsak et al., 2005) LT mutants in an *E. coli* MC1061 displayed significantly decreased beta-lactamase activity. Specific inhibition of the LT Slt70 by bulgecin A suppressed the activity of beta-lactamase AmpC in *E. coli* (Kraft et al., 1999). Notably, not all PG-degrading enzymes are involved in beta-lactam resistance. For instance, the deletion of two amidases (cleaving the amide bond between *N*-acetylmuramic acid and L-Ala) and three DD-endopeptidases (acting on the peptide cross-links) had little effect on beta-lactam resistance (Korsak et al., 2005). In *C. jejuni*, inactivation of Pgp1, which is involved in cleaving monomeric tripeptides to dipeptides (Frirdich et al., 2012), did not affect beta-lactamase activity and the susceptibility of *C. jejuni* to ampicillin as shown in this study.

The LT-mediated beta-lactam resistance identified in this study indicates LT is a promising target for combinational antimicrobial chemotherapy in *C. jejuni*, even in ε-proteobacteria. Our genome survey suggested the three-gene operon containing Cj0843c is conserved across ε-proteobacteria. The LT-mediated beta-lactam resistance mechanism might be also prevalent in ε-proteobacteria. For example, the *H. pylori* homolog (Slt) shares high homology to the Cj0843c (31% aa identity and 51% aa similarity). Recently, Slt also has been found to contribute to amoxicillin resistance in *Helicobacter* (Bonis et al., 2012). Bulgecin A, the specific inhibitor of *H. pylori* Slt, could enhance the antimicrobial effect of amoxicillin (Bonis et al., 2012). Given amoxicillin is an important β-lactam component of the triple therapy to eradicate *H. pylori* infection in human (Tepes et al., 2012), LT inhibitor may serve as a good combination agent (e.g., together with beta-lactam/beta-lactamase inhibitors) to maximize the clinical efficacy of beta-lactam antibiotics.

The decreased β-lactamase activity in LT mutants might be correlated with altered metabolism of peptidoglycan (Kraft et al., 1999). In Gram-negative bacteria, the LT-degraded PG fragments, also called muropeptides, not only serve as cell wall recycling materials during cell growth, but also serve as a signal to turn on the production of β-lactamase through an intracellular transcriptional regulator (Jacobs et al., 1997; Boudreau et al., 2012; Zeng and Lin, 2013). Specifically, muropeptides was either transported into cytoplasm through inner membrane transport AmpG and bound by the regulator AmpR, or directly bound by response regulators of the BlrAB-like two-component regulatory system, to activate the expression of β-lactamase AmpC (Boudreau et al., 2012; Zeng and Lin, 2013). Mutation of the putative LT Cj0843c likely disrupt such intracellular signaling pathway, therefore interfering the induced expression of beta-lactamase and leading to significantly reduced beta-lactamase activity as well as ampicillin MIC observed in this study (**Figure 1**). This speculation needs to be examined in future studies.

AUTHOR CONTRIBUTIONS

JL is the project leader who oversights all the experiments described in this manuscript. XZ and JL contributed with the conception and design of the study. XZ and BG were involved in the collection of data. XZ and JL were involved in the analysis and interpretation of data; drafting and revision of the article; and final approval of the article.

ACKNOWLEDGMENTS

We thank Erin C. Gaynor (University of British Columbia, Canada) for providing genomic DNA of *pgp1* mutant, Dr. Patricia Guerry for providing *C. jejuni* BH-01-0142, and Samantha Brown for providing technical support. This work is supported by The University of Tennessee AgResearch.

REFERENCES

Alfredson, D. A., and Korolik, V. (2005). Isolation and expression of a novel molecular class D beta-lactamase, OXA-61, from *Campylobacter jejuni*. *Antimicrob. Agents Chemother.* 49, 2515–2518. doi: 10.1128/AAC.49.6.2515-2518.2005

Black, R. E., Levine, M. M., Clements, M. L., Hughes, T. P., and Blaser, M. J. (1988). Experimental *Campylobacter jejuni* infection in humans. *J. Infect. Dis.* 157, 472–479. doi: 10.1093/infdis/157.3.472

Bonis, M., Williams, A., Guadagnini, S., Werts, C., and Boneca, I. G. (2012). The effect of bulgecin A on peptidoglycan metabolism and physiology of *Helicobacter pylori*. *Microb. Drug Resist.* 18, 230–239. doi: 10.1089/mdr.2011.0231

Boudreau, M. A., Fisher, J. F., and Mobashery, S. (2012). Messenger functions of the bacterial cell wall-derived muropeptides. *Biochemistry* 51, 2974–2990. doi: 10.1021/bi300174x

Caldentey, J., and Bamford, D. H. (1992). The lytic enzyme of the *Pseudomonas* phage phi 6. Purification and biochemical characterization. *Biochim. Biophys. Acta* 1159, 44–50. doi: 10.1016/0167-4838(92)90073-M

Caldwell, D. B., Wang, Y., and Lin, J. (2008). Development, stability, and molecular mechanisms of macrolide resistance in *Campylobacter jejuni*. *Antimicrob. Agents Chemother.* 52, 3947–3954. doi: 10.1128/AAC.00450-08

de Boer, P., Wagenaar, J. A., Achterberg, R. P., Van Putten, J. P., Schouls, L. M., and Duim, B. (2002). Generation of *Campylobacter jejuni* genetic diversity in vivo. *Mol. Microbiol.* 44, 351–359. doi: 10.1046/j.1365-2958.2002.02930.x

Duong, T., and Konkel, M. E. (2009). Comparative studies of *Campylobacter jejuni* genomic diversity reveal the importance of core and dispensable genes in the biology of this enigmatic food-borne pathogen. *Curr. Opin. Biotechnol.* 20, 158–165. doi: 10.1016/j.copbio.2009.03.004

Elviss, N. C., Williams, L. K., Jorgensen, F., Chisholm, S. A., Lawson, A. J., Swift, C., et al. (2009). Amoxicillin therapy of poultry flocks: effect upon the selection of amoxicillin-resistant commensal *Campylobacter* spp. *J. Antimicrob. Chemother.* 64, 702–711. doi: 10.1093/jac/dkp277

Fibriansah, G., Gliubich, F. I., and Thunnissen, A. M. (2012). On the mechanism of peptidoglycan binding and cleavage by the endo-specific lytic transglycosylase MltE from *Escherichia coli*. *Biochemistry* 51, 9164–9177. doi: 10.1021/bi300900t

Frirdich, E., Biboy, J., Adams, C., Lee, J., Ellermeier, J., Gielda, L. D., et al. (2012). Peptidoglycan-modifying enzyme Pgp1 is required for helical cell shape and pathogenicity traits in *Campylobacter jejuni*. *PLoS Pathog* 8:e1002602. doi: 10.1371/journal.ppat.1002602

Fuda, C., Suvorov, M., Vakulenko, S. B., and Mobashery, S. (2004). The basis for resistance to beta-lactam antibiotics by penicillin-binding protein 2a of methicillin-resistant *Staphylococcus aureus*. *J. Biol. Chem.* 279, 40802–40806. doi: 10.1074/jbc.M403589200

Griggs, D. J., Peake, L., Johnson, M. M., Ghori, S., Mott, A., and Piddock, L. J. (2009). Beta-lactamase-mediated beta-lactam resistance in *Campylobacter* species: prevalence of Cj0299 (blaOXA-61) and evidence for a novel beta-Lactamase in *C. jejuni*. *Antimicrob. Agents Chemother.* 53, 3357–3364. doi: 10.1128/AAC.01655-08

Hamad, B. (2010). The antibiotics market. *Nat. Rev. Drug Discov.* 9, 675–676. doi: 10.1038/nrd3267

Hoang, K. V., Stern, N. J., Saxton, A. M., Xu, F., Zeng, X., and Lin, J. (2011). Prevalence, development, and molecular mechanisms of bacteriocin resistance in *Campylobacter*. *Appl. Environ. Microbiol.* 77, 2309–2316. doi: 10.1128/AEM.02094-10

Hoang, K. V., Wang, Y., and Lin, J. (2012). Identification of genetic loci that contribute to *Campylobacter* resistance to fowlicidin-1, a chicken host defense peptide. *Front. Cell Infect. Microbiol.* 2:32. doi: 10.3389/fcimb.2012.00032

Hoffmann, S., Batz, M. B., and Morris, J. G. Jr. (2012). Annual cost of illness and quality-adjusted life year losses in the United States due to 14 foodborne pathogens. *J. Food Prot.* 75, 1292–1302. doi: 10.4315/0362-028X.JFP-11-417

Hughes, R. A., and Cornblath, D. R. (2005). Guillain-barré syndrome. *Lancet* 366, 1653–1666. doi: 10.1016/S0140-6736(05)67665-9

Humphrey, T., O'brien, S., and Madsen, M. (2007). Campylobacters as zoonotic pathogens: a food production perspective. *Int. J. Food Microbiol.* 117, 237–257. doi: 10.1016/j.ijfoodmicro.2007.01.006

Iaconis, J. P., and Sanders, C. C. (1990). Purification and characterization of inducible beta-lactamases in *Aeromonas* spp. *Antimicrob. Agents Chemother.* 34, 44–51. doi: 10.1128/AAC.34.1.44

Jacobs, C., Frere, J. M., and Normark, S. (1997). Cytosolic intermediates for cell wall biosynthesis and degradation control inducible beta-lactam resistance in gram-negative bacteria. *Cell* 88, 823–832. doi: 10.1016/S0092-8674(00) 81928-5

Jacoby, G. A. (2009). AmpC beta-lactamases. *Clin. Microbiol. Rev.* 22, 161–182. doi: 10.1128/CMR.00036-08

Koningstein, M., Simonsen, J., Helms, M., Hald, T., and Molbak, K. (2011). Antimicrobial use: a risk factor or a protective factor for acquiring campylobacteriosis? *Clin. Infect. Dis.* 53, 644–650. doi: 10.1093/cid/cir504

Korfmann, G., and Wiedemann, B. (1988). Genetic control of beta-lactamase production in *Enterobacter cloacae. Rev. Infect. Dis.* 10, 793–799. doi: 10.1093/clinids/10.4.793

Korsak, D., Liebscher, S., and Vollmer, W. (2005). Susceptibility to antibiotics and beta-lactamase induction in murein hydrolase mutants of *Escherichia coli. Antimicrob. Agents Chemother.* 49, 1404–1409. doi: 10.1128/AAC.49.4.1404-1409.2005

Kraft, A. R., Prabhu, J., Ursinus, A., and Holtje, J. V. (1999). Interference with murein turnover has no effect on growth but reduces beta-lactamase induction in *Escherichia coli. J. Bacteriol.* 181, 7192–7198.

Lachance, N., Gaudreau, C., Lamothe, F., and Lariviere, L. A. (1991). Role of the beta-lactamase of *Campylobacter jejuni* in resistance to beta-lactam agents. *Antimicrob. Agents Chemother.* 35, 813–818. doi: 10.1128/AAC.35.5.813

Lin, J., Akiba, M., Sahin, O., and Zhang, Q. (2005). CmeR functions as a transcriptional repressor for the multidrug efflux pump CmeABC in *Campylobacter jejuni. Antimicrob. Agents Chemother.* 49, 1067–1075. doi: 10.1128/AAC.49.3.1067-1075.2005

Lin, J., and Martinez, A. (2006). Effect of efflux pump inhibitors on bile resistance and in vivo colonization of *Campylobacter jejuni. J. Antimicrob. Chemother.* 58, 966–972. doi: 10.1093/jac/dkl374

Lin, J., Michel, L. O., and Zhang, Q. (2002). CmeABC functions as a multidrug efflux system in *Campylobacter jejuni. Antimicrob. Agents Chemother.* 46, 2124–2131. doi: 10.1128/AAC.46.7.2124-2131.2002

Lin, J., Sahin, O., Michel, L. O., and Zhang, Q. (2003). Critical role of multidrug efflux pump CmeABC in bile resistance and in vivo colonization of *Campylobacter jejuni. Infect. Immun.* 71, 4250–4259. doi: 10.1128/IAI.71.8.4250-4259.2003

Lin, J., Wang, Y., and Hoang, K. V. (2009). Systematic identification of genetic loci required for polymyxin resistance in *Campylobacter jejuni* using an efficient in vivo transposon mutagenesis system. *Foodborne Pathog. Dis.* 6, 173–185. doi: 10.1089/fpd.2008.0177

Luo, N., Pereira, S., Sahin, O., Lin, J., Huang, S., Michel, L., et al. (2005). Enhanced in vivo fitness of fluoroquinolone-resistant *Campylobacter jejuni* in the absence of antibiotic selection pressure. *Proc. Natl. Acad. Sci. U.S.A.* 102, 541–546. doi: 10.1073/pnas.0408966102

Nachamkin, I., Allos, B. M., and Ho, T. (1998). *Campylobacter* species and Guillain-Barré syndrome. *Clin. Microbiol. Rev.* 11, 555–567.

Nikaido, H. (1998). Antibiotic resistance caused by gram-negative multidrug efflux pumps. *Clin. Infect. Dis.* 27(Suppl. 1), S32–S41. doi: 10.1086/514920

Nyati, K. K., and Nyati, R. (2013). Role of *Campylobacter jejuni* infection in the pathogenesis of Guillain-Barré syndrome: an update. *Biomed. Res. Int.* 2013:852195. doi: 10.1155/2013/852195

Parkhill, J., Wren, B. W., Mungall, K., Ketley, J. M., Churcher, C., Basham, D., et al. (2000). The genome sequence of the food-borne pathogen *Campylobacter jejuni* reveals hypervariable sequences. *Nature* 403, 665–668. doi: 10.1038/35001088

Poly, F., and Guerry, P. (2008). Pathogenesis of *Campylobacter. Curr. Opin. Gastroenterol.* 24, 27–31. doi: 10.1097/MOG.0b013e3282f1dcb1

Poly, F., Read, T. D., Chen, Y. H., Monteiro, M. A., Serichantalergs, O., Pootong, P., et al. (2008). Characterization of two *Campylobacter jejuni* strains for use in volunteer experimental-infection studies. *Infect. Immun.* 76, 5655–5667. doi: 10.1128/IAI.00780-08

Tepes, B., O'connor, A., Gisbert, J. P., and O'morain, C. (2012). Treatment of *Helicobacter pylori* infection 2012. *Helicobacter* 17(Suppl. 1), 36–42. doi: 10.1111/j.1523-5378.2012.00981.x

Vila, J., and Martinez, J. L. (2008). Clinical impact of the over-expression of efflux pump in nonfermentative Gram-negative bacilli, development of efflux pump inhibitors. *Curr. Drug Targets* 9, 797–807. doi: 10.2174/138945008785 747806

Wang, Y., and Taylor, D. E. (1990). Natural transformation in *Campylobacter* species. *J. Bacteriol.* 172, 949–955.

Yao, R., Alm, R. A., Trust, T. J., and Guerry, P. (1993). Construction of new *Campylobacter* cloning vectors and a new mutational cat cassette. *Gene* 130, 127–130. doi: 10.1016/0378-1119(93)90355-7

Zeng, X., Brown, S., Gillespie, B., and Lin, J. (2014). A single nucleotide in the promoter region modulates the expression of the beta-lactamase OXA-61 in *Campylobacter jejuni. J. Antimicrob. Chemother.* 69, 1215–1223. doi: 10.1093/jac/dkt515

Zeng, X., and Lin, J. (2013). Beta-lactamase induction and cell wall metabolism in Gram-negative bacteria. *Front. Microbiol.* 4:128. doi: 10.3389/fmicb.2013.00128

Zeng, X., Mo, Y., Xu, F., and Lin, J. (2013a). Identification and characterization of a periplasmic trilactone esterase, Cee, revealed unique features of ferric enterobactin acquisition in *Campylobacter. Mol. Microbiol.* 87, 594–608. doi: 10.1111/mmi.12118

Zeng, X., Xu, F., and Lin, J. (2013b). Specific TonB-ExbB-ExbD energy transduction systems required for ferric enterobactin acquisition in *Campylobacter. FEMS Microbiol. Lett.* 347, 83–91. doi: 10.1111/1574-6968.12221

Zeng, X., Xu, F., and Lin, J. (2009). Molecular, antigenic, and functional characteristics of ferric enterobactin receptor CfrA in *Campylobacter jejuni. Infect. Immun.* 77, 5437–5448. doi: 10.1128/IAI.00666-09

8

QnrS1- and Aac(6′)-Ib-cr-Producing *Escherichia coli* among Isolates from Animals of Different Sources: Susceptibility and Genomic Characterization

Daniela Jones-Dias [1,2], Vera Manageiro [1,2], Rafael Graça [1], Daniel A. Sampaio [3], Teresa Albuquerque [4], Patrícia Themudo [4], Luís Vieira [3], Eugénia Ferreira [1,2], Lurdes Clemente [4] and Manuela Caniça [1,2]*

[1] National Reference Laboratory of Antibiotic Resistances and Healthcare Associated Infections, Department of Infectious Diseases, National Institute of Health Dr. Ricardo Jorge, Lisbon, Portugal, [2] Centre for the Studies of Animal Science, Institute of Agrarian and Agri-Food Sciences and Technologies, Oporto University, Oporto, Portugal, [3] Innovation and Technology Unit, Human Genetics Department, National Institute of Health Dr. Ricardo Jorge, Lisbon, Portugal, [4] Instituto Nacional de Investigação Agrária e Veterinária, Lisboa, Portugal

***Correspondence:**
Vera Manageiro
vera.manageiro@insa.min-saude.pt

Salmonella enterica and *Escherichia coli* can inhabit humans and animals from multiple origins. These bacteria are often associated with gastroenteritis in animals, being a frequent cause of resistant zoonotic infections. In fact, bacteria from animals can be transmitted to humans through the food chain and direct contact. In this study, we aimed to assess the antibiotic susceptibility of a collection of *S. enterica* and *E. coli* recovered from animals of different sources, performing a genomic comparison of the plasmid-mediated quinolone resistance (PMQR)-producing isolates detected. Antibiotic susceptibility testing revealed a high number of non-wild-type isolates for fluoroquinolones among *S. enterica* recovered from poultry isolates. In turn, the frequency of non-wild-type *E. coli* to nalidixic acid and ciprofloxacin was higher in food-producing animals than in companion or zoo animals. Globally, we detected two *qnrS1* and two *aac(6′)-Ib-cr* in *E. coli* isolates recovered from animals of different origins. The genomic characterization of QnrS1-producing *E. coli* showed high genomic similarity (O86:H12 and ST2297), although they have been recovered from a healthy turtle dove from a Zoo Park, and from a dog showing symptoms of infection. The *qnrS1* gene was encoded in a IncN plasmid, also carrying bla_{TEM-1}-containing Tn*3*. Isolates harboring *aac(6′)-Ib-cr* were detected in two captive bottlenose dolphins, within a time span of two years. The additional antibiotic resistance genes of the two *aac(6′)-Ib-cr*-positive isolates (bla_{OXA-1}, bla_{TEM-1}, $bla_{CTX-M-15}$, *catB3, aac(3)-IIa,* and *tetA*) were enclosed in IncFIA plasmids that differed in a single transposase and 60 single nucleotide variants. The isolates could be assigned to the same genetic sublineage—ST131 *fimH*30-Rx (O25:H4), confirming clonal spread. PMQR-producing isolates were associated with symptomatic and asymptomatic hosts, which highlight the aptitude of *E. coli* to act as silent vehicles, allowing the accumulation of antibiotic resistance genes, mobile genetic elements and other relevant pathogenicity determinants. Continuous monitoring of health and sick animals toward the presence of PMQR should be strongly encouraged in order to restrain the clonal spread of these antibiotic resistant strains.

Keywords: pathogenicity, *E. coli*, clone, PMQR, multidrug resistance, veterinary

INTRODUCTION

Antibiotic resistance has been critically increasing over time and now constitutes one of the major health concerns worldwide. The uncontrolled use of antibiotics in human and veterinary practices, animal production and agriculture and the increasingly easiness in global transportation contributed to the dissemination of multidrug resistant pathogens that constitute a risk for humans, animals and the environment (Marshall and Levy, 2011; EFSA, 2015). Nowadays, antibiotic resistant *Salmonella enterica* and *Escherichia coli* are among the most problematic zoonotic bacteria, causing severe gastroenteritis in animals and humans (EFSA, 2015).

Fluoroquinolones constitute a group of broad spectrum antibiotics of critical importance, presenting applications in both human and veterinary medicines (Poirel et al., 2012). Therefore, resistance might easily emerge in animals and get transferred to humans through the food chain and direct or indirect contact. Several examples of such transmission have already been documented (Gomes-Neves et al., 2014; Damborg et al., 2015; Schmithausen et al., 2015). Fluoroquinolone resistance has emerged rapidly due to two main types of mechanisms: mutation of the chromosomal quinolone targets DNA gyrase and topoisomerase IV, and acquisition of the transferable plasmid-mediated quinolone resistance (PMQR) determinants *qnr*, *qepA*, *aac(6′)-Ib-cr*, and *oqxAB* (Veldman et al., 2011; Poirel et al., 2012). The alteration of chromosomal quinolone targets can lead to higher levels of resistance than PMQRs that are only able to guarantee low-level quinolone resistance. However, the ability of the latter to be spread by horizontal gene transfer constitutes a serious concern that should be addressed (Poirel et al., 2012). In fact, antibiotic resistance genes are frequently associated to mobile genetic elements such as insertion sequences (ISs), phages, transposons and plasmids, which enhance their ability to efficiently spread among different bacterial species (Stokes and Gillings, 2011). The most worrying mechanisms of resistance, which also show a transboundary spread between animals, humans and the environment, are, in fact, encoded by mobile antibiotic resistance genes. The occurrence of mobile genetic elements harboring multiple antibiotic resistance genes is also frequent, and enables the development of bacterial multidrug resistance, which may be responsible for therapeutic failures in animals or humans (Poirel et al., 2012).

In animals, as well as in humans, several factors can affect the progression and severity of an acute infection. The synchronized presence of antibiotic resistance genes, virulence factors, mobile genetic elements and other pathogenicity determinants, is ideal to the successful spread of these microorganisms in any environment (Cosentino et al., 2013).

In this study, PMQR-producing *E. coli* isolates were gathered from a collection of *S. enterica* and *E. coli* recovered from food-producing, companion and zoo animals, in the scope of their phenotypic and genotypic characterization. To further explore the genetic diversity of these isolates, as well as to understand the molecular features contributing to their spread and ability to cause infection, complete genomic sequencing was performed.

MATERIALS AND METHODS

Collection of bacterial Isolates

This study included 89 *S. enterica* isolates recovered from breeders ($n = 12$), broilers ($n = 33$), layers ($n = 33$), swine ($n = 6$), and food products of animal origin ($n = 5$) (**Table 1**). In poultry farms, samples were collected from feces and environment using sterile boots/sock swabs. Food products included uncooked fresh products such as minced meat, hamburgers, meat cuts, sausages, and table eggs, randomly recovered at a variety of retail stores. Samples from other animal species (pigeons, partridges, ducks, pets, and exotic animals) consisted of blood cultures and organs (lung, liver, spleen, kidneys, and intestine) collected during post-mortem examination. All samples were examined according to ISO norm 6579:2002 applied to *Salmonella* detection in food and animal feeding stuffs. After biochemical confirmation, *Salmonella* spp. isolates were sent to the *Salmonella* National Reference Laboratory (INIAV, Lisbon) in triple sugar iron slopes or SMID plates.

This study also included 91 *E. coli* isolates (**Table 1**) collected from food-producing animals [(bovine, swine and poultry), ($n =$

TABLE 1 | Distribution of the *S. enterica* ($n = 89$) and *E. coli* ($n = 91$) isolates.

Source	*S. enterica*			Source	*E. coli*
	Enteritidis	Other serotypes[a]	Total		
Breeders	12	0	12	Food	32
Layers	24	9	33	Companion	36
Broilers	32	1	33	Zoo	23
Swine	0	6	6		
Food of animal origin	3	2	5		
Total	71	18	89	Total	91

[a]*Salmonella 4,5:i:- (n = 1), Salmonella 6,7,14:-:1,2 (n = 1), Salmonella Bradenburg (n = 1), Salmonella Gallinarum (n = 1), Salmonella Give (n = 1), Salmonella Hadar (n = 1), Salmonella Heidelberg (n = 1), Salmonella IIIa 48:z10:- (n = 1), Salmonella Mbandaka (n = 1), Salmonella Rissen (n = 2), Salmonella Typhimurium (n = 3), Salmonella Virchow (n = 4).*

32)], pets [(dogs, cats, horses, and cage birds), ($n = 37$)] and zoo animals [(terrestrial and aquatic mammals, birds and reptiles), ($n = 22$)]. Samples consisted of swabs from organic fluids and cavities, fecal samples, urine samples, blood cultures, and organs collected during post-mortem examination and submitted for bacteriological analysis. Suspected *E. coli* colonies obtained in MacConkey agar plates were confirmed by API 20E strips (bioMérieux, Marcy-l'Étoile, France).

Serotypes of *S. enterica*

S. enterica isolates were serotyped by the slide agglutination method, using the method of Kauffmann-White scheme (Grimont and Weill, 2007).

Antibiotic Susceptibility Testing

Minimum inhibitory concentrations (MICs) were determined by agar dilution following standard recommendations, using a panel of 10 antimicrobial compounds: ampicillin, cefotaxime, nalidixic acid, ciprofloxacin, gentamicin, streptomycin, chloramphenicol, tetracycline, sulfamethoxazole, and trimethoprim (**Table 2**). Isolates harboring PMQR determinants were further studied by determination of the MICs to a larger panel of fluoroquinolones, which included moxifloxacin, gatifloxacin, levofloxacin, ofloxacin, enrofloxacin, and norfloxacin. To assess non-wild-type isolates, interpretation of results was performed according to the epidemiological cut-off values suggested by the European Committee on Antimicrobial Susceptibility Testing (EUCAST, http://mic.eucast.org/Eucast2/). For *Salmonella* spp., the cut-off value used for sulfamethoxazole was that for sulfonamides from Clinical Standards Laboratory Institute (http://clsi.org). MIC_{50} and MIC_{90} were calculated as reported elsewhere (Schwarz et al., 2010). *E. coli* ATCC 25922 was used as the quality control strain. Isolates were considered multidrug resistant (MDR) if they presented non-wild-type phenotypes against three or more structurally unrelated antibiotics (Magiorakos et al., 2011).

Molecular Characterization of Resistance

All isolates were evaluated regarding the presence of *qnrA*, *qnrB*, *qnrC*, *qnrD*, *qnrS*, *aac(6')-Ib-cr*, and *qepA* genes, using primers and conditions previously described (Jones-Dias et al., 2013), and *oqxAB* genes using primers and conditions first described in this study (oqxA-F, 5'-AGAGTTCAAAGCCACGCTG-3' and oqxb-R, 5'-CTCCTGCATCGCCGTCACCA-3'; initial denaturation of 94°C for 5 min; 94°C for 30 s, 64°C for 30 s and 72°C for 1 min, for 30 cycles; final step of extension of 72°C for 5 min). PMQR-producing isolates were also characterized regarding the production of β-lactamase-encoding genes and conventional Multilocus sequence typing (MLST), as described elsewhere (Jones-Dias et al., 2015).

Genomic Characterization of PMQR-Producing *E. coli*

The genomes of the four PMQR-producing *E. coli* (LV46221, LV46743, LV36464, and LV27950) were characterized. Genomic DNA was extracted using DNeasy Blood and Tissue Kit (Qiagen, Aarhus) and quantified using Qubit 1.0 Fluorometer (Invitrogen, Waltham). The Nextera XT DNA Sample Preparation Kit (Illumina, San Diego, CA) was used to prepare sequencing libraries from 1 ng of genomic DNA, according to the manufacturer's instructions. Paired-end sequencing of 150 bp reads was performed on a MiSeq (Illumina). Sequence reads were then trimmed and filtered according to quality criteria, and assembled *de novo* using CLC genomics workbench version 8.5.1 (QIAGEN, Aarhus). RAST (Rapid Annotation using Subsystem Technology) was used for subsystem annotation of the genomes (Aziz et al., 2012; Overbeek et al., 2014).

Identification of Pathogenicity-Related Genes

Pathogenicity-related genes were detected using a variety of online web tools. PathogenFinder 1.1, ResFinder 2.1, VirulenceFinder 1.4, SerotypeFinder 1.1, MLST 1.8, pMLST 1.4, and PHAST were used to estimate the pathogenicity determinants, acquired antibiotic resistance genes, virulence factors, serotypes, MLST, plasmid MLST and phage regions, respectively in the genomes of PMQR-producing *E. coli* (Zhou et al., 2011; Larsen et al., 2012; Zankari et al., 2012; Cosentino et al., 2013; Carattoli et al., 2014; Joensen et al., 2014, 2015). ISsaga was also used to detect and annotate insertion sequences in the draft genomes of the *E. coli* isolates (Varani et al., 2011). Specific analysis of antibiotic resistance genes and respective flanking regions was carried out with CLC genomics workbench version 8.5.1 (Qiagen, Aarhus). Contigs carrying antibiotic resistance genes were manually assembled whenever necessary and blasted against GenBank to identify their genetic location.

Nucleotide Sequence Genbank Accession Numbers

The draft genomes of isolates LV46221, LV46743, LV36464, and LV27950 have been deposited at DDBJ/EMBL/GenBank under the accessions LRXG00000000, LRXH00000000, LRXI00000000, and LRXJ00000000, respectively. The versions described in this paper are version LRXG01000000, LRXH01000000, LRXI01000000, and LRXJ01000000, respectively.

RESULTS

Serotypes of *Salmonella* spp.

S. enterica serotype Enteritidis is one of the most common serotype in humans (EFSA, 2015) and it was the most frequently detected among the 89 *S. enterica* isolates (71/89, 79.8%), being present in all food animals except swine. The remaining *Salmonella* serotypes were detected in a less extent and were comprised of *Salmonella* 4,5:i:- ($n = 1$), *Salmonella* 6,7,14:-:1,2 ($n = 1$), *Salmonella* Bradenburg ($n = 1$), *Salmonella* Gallinarum ($n = 1$), *Salmonella* Give ($n = 1$), *Salmonella* Hadar ($n = 1$), *Salmonella* Heidelberg ($n = 1$), *Salmonella* IIIa 48:z10:- ($n = 1$), *Salmonella* Mbandaka ($n = 1$), *Salmonella* Rissen ($n = 2$), *Salmonella* Typhimurium ($n = 3$), and *Salmonella* Virchow ($n = 4$).

Antimicrobial Susceptibility of *S. enterica* and *E. coli* Isolates

Susceptibility profiles of *S. enterica* and *E. coli* isolates differed with the animal group (**Table 2**). Although, high rates of non-wild-type *S. enterica* were detected for nalidixic acid (from 82

TABLE 2 | MIC_{50} and MIC_{90} for *S. enterica* ($n = 89$) and *E. coli* ($n = 91$) isolates.

Antibiotic	*S. enterica*				*E. coli*		
	Food animals				Food animals ($n = 32$)	Zoo Animals ($n = 23$)	Companion Animals ($n = 36$)
	Breeders ($n = 12$)	Broilers ($n = 33$)	Layers ($n = 33$)	Others[a] ($n = 11$)			
Na							
MIC_{50}	128	128	128	128	8	4	4
MIC_{90}	128	128	128	128	128	128	128
% Wt	0	12	6	18	59	77	78
%N-Wt	100	88	94	82	41	23	22
Cp							
MIC_{50}	0.25	0.25	0.25	0.25	0.03	0.015	0.015
MIC_{90}	0.25	0.25	0.25	0.5	8	8	8
% Wt	0	3	18	36	59	77	72
%N-Wt	100	97	82	64	41	23	28
A							
MIC_{50}	2	4	0.5	8	8	8	8
MIC_{90}	4	4	8	64	64	64	64
% Wt	100	100	94	64	53	50	53
%N-Wt	0	0	6	36	47	50	47
Ct							
MIC_{50}	0.125	0.06	0.125	0.125	≤0.06	0.06	≤0.06
MIC_{90}	0.125	0.125	0.125	2	0.125	0.125	0.125
% Wt	100	100	94	82	100	95	94
%N-Wt	0	0	6	18	0	5	6
G							
MIC_{50}	0.25	0.25	0.25	0.5	0.5	0.5	0.5
MIC_{90}	0.5	0.5	0.5	1	2	1	1
% Wt	100	100	100	100	91	91	100
%N-Wt	0	0	0	0	9	9	0
St							
MIC_{50}	2	2	4	32	4	4	4
MIC_{90}	8	4	128	64	256	256	128
% Wt	100	100	82	36	69	64	86
%N-Wt	0	0	18	64	31	36	14
T							
MIC_{50}	2	2	2	4	32	2	2
MIC_{90}	4	4	4	64	64	64	64
% Wt	92	100	91	55	47	59	75
%N-Wt	8	0	9	45	53	41	25
C							
MIC_{50}	8	4	8	8	4	8	8
MIC_{90}	8	8	8	16	64	8	16
% Wt	100	97	100	91	84	100	92
%N-Wt	0	3	0	9	16	0	8
Su							
MIC_{50}	128	128	128	128	16	32	16
MIC_{90}	128	128	128	>512	>512	>512	>512
% Wt	92	100	100	64	63	59	78
%N-Wt	8	0	0	36	38	41	22
Tp							
MIC_{50}	0.5	0.5	0.5	0.25	0.5	0.5	0.5
MIC_{90}	0.5	0.5	0.5	32	32	32	32
% Wt	92	100	100	73	81	68	81
%N-Wt	8	0	0	27	19	32	19

[a]*Others, pigs ($n = 6$) and food products of animal origin ($n = 5$).*

Na, nalidixic acid; Cp, ciprofloxacin; A, ampicillin; Ct, cefotaxime; G, gentamicin; St, streptomycin; T, tetracycline; C, chloramphenicol; Su, sulfamethoxazole; Tp, trimethoprim.

to 100%) and ciprofloxacin (from 64 to 100%) in all groups, they were particularly evident in poultry, and predominant in breeders. *S. enterica* isolates recovered from other sources (swine and food products, $n = 11$), showed higher non-wild-type phenotypes for ampicillin (36%), streptomycin (64%), tetracycline (45%), sulfamethoxazole (36%), and trimethoprim (27%) (**Table 2**). The poultry groups of breeders and broilers were mainly susceptible to ampicillin (100%), cefotaxime (100%), gentamicin (100%), and streptomycin (100%).

The frequency of non-wild-type isolates was globally higher for *E. coli* than for *S. enterica* against ampicillin (minimum value of 47 vs. 0%, respectively), tetracycline (minimum value of 25 vs. 0%, respectively), sulfamethoxazole (minimum value of 22 vs. 0%, respectively) and trimethoprim (minimum value of 19 vs. 0%, respectively). Although, no major discrepancies were noticed for *E. coli* in rates of non-wild-type isolates for the different animal groups, isolates recovered from food animals still presented more non-wild-type phenotypes than zoo or companion animals against nalidixic acid (41%), ciprofloxacin (41%), tetracycline (53%), and chloramphenicol (16%).

In *S. enterica* isolates from poultry, similar MIC_{50} and MIC_{90} values were observed for the majority of the antibiotics tested; major differences (≥3 fold dilutions) were observed for the group "others" for ampicillin (8 and 64 mg/L), tetracycline (4 and 64 mg/L), sulfamethoxazole (128 and >512 mg/L) and trimethoprim (0.25 and 32 mg/L). For *E. coli*, the most significant differences in MIC_{50} and MIC_{90} values were observed for nalidixic acid (4 and 128 mg/L), ampicillin (8 and 64 mg/L), streptomycin (4 and 128 mg/L), tetracycline (2 and 64 mg/L), sulfamethoxazole (16 and >512 mg/L) and trimethoprim (0.5–32 mg/L).

While for *S. enterica* only 9.0% (8/89) MDR isolates were detected, for *E. coli*, MDR was registered in 38.9% (35/90) of the isolates, which were distributed among 16/90 isolates from food-producing animals, 9/90 isolates from companion animals, and 10/90 isolates from zoo animals.

Molecular Characterization of *S. enterica* and *E. coli* Isolates

Overall, among the 180 isolates studied, we have detected and identified four PMQR determinants in *E. coli* isolates: two *qnrS1* were detected in isolates recovered from a captive turtle dove (LV46221) and a pet dog (LV46743), and two *aac(6')-Ib-cr* were isolated from *E. coli* recovered from captive bottlenose dolphins (LV36464 and LV27950). The detection of β-lactamase-encoding genes showed the presence of bla_{TEM-1}in isolates LV46221 and LV46743, and bla_{TEM-1}, bla_{OXA-1}, and $bla_{CTX-M-15}$ in LV36464 and LV27950. No other PMQR- or β-lactamase-encoding genes were identified in the collection of *E. coli* and *S. enterica* isolates.

Genomic Characterization of QnrS1-Producing *E. coli*

The assembly of the genome sequences of the two *qnrS1*-harboring *E. coli*, LV46221 and LV46743, yielded 200 and 199 contigs (each >200 bp long), which together comprised 4,799,985 bp and 4,801,518 bp, respectively. The average coverage of LV46221 was 135.9, while LV46743 displayed 114.1 fold. The maximum contig length obtained for these genomes was 398,205 bp and 333,601 bp, respectively (**Table 3**).

The automated annotation of the draft genomes showed that LV46221 (63%, 2879/4618) and LV46743 (63%, 2873/4609) presented a similar number of sequences attributed to specific subsystems (Figure S1). General annotation of both genomes showed 109 coding sequences associated with virulence, disease and defense, as well as 143 sequences coding for functions related with mobile genetic elements, such as phages, prophages, transposable elements, and plasmids. Globally, the proportion of each subsystem was equally represented in the genomes of the two isolates (Figure S1). According to RAST annotation system, LV46221 and LV46743 isolates carried 77 and 86 RNAs, respectively. The bioinformatics analysis of the genetic relatedness was carried out with regard to serotype and MLST: the serotypes of both isolates were defined as O86:H12, and they also shared the assigned MLST–ST2297 (**Table 4**).

In silico analysis of the antibiotic resistance genes (90% identity and 40% minimum length) confirmed the presence of a *qnrS1*, and identified bla_{TEM-1}gene in both isolates (**Table 4**). *qnrS1* was detected in a contig with an approximate length of 11,000 bp in both cases, showing 99% of homology with a resistance region from *S. enterica* subsp. *enterica* serovar Infantis pINF5 plasmid. By mapping all contigs against this plasmid, we detected bla_{TEM-1}-containing T*n3*, and a disrupted IS2-like element upstream of *qnrS1,* as well as IS*26* transposase downstream of the gene. Other contigs showed complementary regions, revealing the presence of a fragment encoding conjugation transfer genes upstream of Tn*3* that showed homology with *Salmonella* Virchow plasmid pVQS1 (99%).

LV46221 and LV46743 showed no additional PMQR or other acquired antibiotic resistance genes. Moreover, no mutations were detected in the quinolone resistance determining region (QRDR) of genes *gyrA*, *gyrB*, *parC,* and *parE,* which are known to confer high level resistance to fluoroquinolones (Veldman et al., 2011). The isolates were also characterized with regard to specific mobile genetic elements of different classes. The screening of typable plasmids (>98% homology) enabled the identification of IncN plasmids, which were further typed as ST1

TABLE 3 | Genome analysis of *E. coli* LV46221, LV46743, LV36464, and LV27950.

Isolates	LV46221	LV46743	LV36464	LV27950
Genome size (bp)	4,799,985	4,801,518	5,180,399	5,156,819
Number of contigs	200	199	136	209
Average coverage	135.9	114.1	178.7	150.1
N50 (bp)[a]	119,356	119,356	158,975	158,977
Maximum contig (bp)	398,205	333,601	399,998	369,918
Minimum contig (bp)	208	201	486	218
Protein-coding genes	4618	4609	5107	5069
RNAs	77	86	77	76

[a]*Minimum contig length of at least 50% of the contigs.*

TABLE 4 | General features of PMQR-harboring *E. coli* isolates recovered from animals of different sources.

Isolate	Origin	Year	Serotype	MIC (mg/L)								PMQR	Other resistance genes	Virulence factors	MLST	Plasmids	pMLST
				Mx	Cp	Ga	Le	Of	Ef	Na	Nx						
LV46221	Dove	2008	O86:H12	0.75	0.38	0.75	0.38	1	1.5	8	0.75	*qnrS1*	bla_{TEM-1}	*gad*, *iss*	ST2297	IncN	ST1
LV46743	Dog	2008	O86:H12	0.5	0.38	0.5	0.5	1.5	2	8	1.5	*qnrS1*	bla_{TEM-1}	*gad*	ST2297	IncN	ST1
LV36464	Dolphin	2009	O25:H4	>32	>32	8	>32	>32	>32	>256	>256	*aac(6')-Ib-cr*	*aac(3)-IIa*, $bla_{CTX-M-15}$ bla_{TEM-1}, bla_{OXA-1} *catB3*, *tetA*	*iss*, *sat*, *gad*	ST131	IncFIA, IncX	F-:A1:B-
LV27950	Dolphin	2011	O25:H4	12	>32	8	8	>32	>32	>256	>256	*aac(6')-Ib-cr*	*aac(3)-IIa*, $bla_{CTX-M-15}$ bla_{TEM-1}, bla_{OXA-1} *catB3*, *tetA*	*iss*, *sat*	ST131	IncFIA	F-:A1:B-

Mx, moxifloxacin; Cp, ciprofloxacin; Ga, gatifloxacin; Le, levofloxacin; Of, ofloxacin; Ef, enrofloxacin; Na, nalidixic acid; Nx, norfloxacin.
PMQR, Plasmid-mediated quinolone resistance.
MLST, Multilocus sequence typing.

by pMLST (**Table 4**). ISsaga allowed the specialized annotation of insertion sequences and revealed a different distribution of the same elements for LV46221 and LV46743: IS*1* (3.23 and 1.96%, respectively), IS*200*_IS*605* (3.23 and 3.92%, respectively), IS*21* (3.23 and 3.92%, respectively), IS*3* (24.19 and 21.57%, respectively), IS*4* (3.23 and 3.92%, respectively), IS*481* (1.61 and 1.96%, respectively), IS*5* (1.61 and 1.96%, respectively), IS6 (1.61 and 1.96%, respectively), IS*As1*(27.42 and 27.45%, respectively), IS*Kra4* (6.45 and 5.88%, respectively), IS*L3* (12.9 and 9.8%, respectively), ISNCY (9.68 and 11.76%, respectively), and finally Tn*3* (1.61 and 1.96%, respectively). IS*As1* was the most frequent element detected in both isolates, and IS*66* was exclusively detected in LV46743 (1.96%). Moreover, in LV46221 we identified 10 prophage regions among which three were questionable but seven were intact. The latter included prophage regions reaching up to 90.6Kb, containing 133 coding sequences (Table S1). In turn, in LV46743, 14 different prophages were detected that included one questionable, four incomplete and nine intact phage regions; intact zones ranged between regions of 10.4 Kb carrying 12 coding sequences, and 70.3 Kb with 88 protein coding DNA fragments. Overall, among the prophages showing higher scores for both genomes were serotype-converting *Shigella flexnerri* bacteriophage and Enterobacteria lambda phages (Table S1).

The total number of pathogenicity determinants, which according with PathogenFinder includes, for instance, virulence factors, antibiotic resistance genes and mobile genetic elements, detected a similar number of sequences in the genomes of *E. coli* LV46221 and LV46743: 607 and 611 different pathogenic families showed a 93.5% certainty of the isolates being human pathogens. Finally, the virulence factor glutamate decarboxylase (*gad*) was detected in both isolates, while the increased serum survival factor *iss* was exclusively identified in LV46221 (**Table 4**).

Genomic Characterization of Aac(6′)-ib-cr-Producing *E. coli*

The genome sequences of isolates LV36464 and LV27950, which were known to produce Aac(6′)-Ib-cr and CTX-M-15, were also compared. Their *de novo* assembly yielded 5,180,399 bp for LV36464 and 5,156,819 bp for LV27950 and displayed a mean coverage of 178.6 and 150.1 fold, respectively. Approximately, 136 and 209 contigs (each >200 bp long) were recovered for LV36464 and LV27950 with a maximum contig length of 399,998 and 369,918 bp, respectively (**Table 3**).

The automated annotation of the genomes showed a total number of coding sequences of 5107 for LV36464 and 5069 for LV27950, excluding 77 and 76 annotated RNA molecules. The distribution of the annotated coding sequences by subsystem showed an identical representation of functions in both isolates (LV36464: 368%, 3062/5107; LV27950: 61%, 3081/5069; Figure S2).

The serotypes of the LV36464 and LV27950 isolates obtained upon the analysis of *fliC*, *wzy*, and *wzx* genes, were defined as O25:H4. The epidemiology and diversity of *E. coli* isolates was also explored, assigning both of them to ST131 and to sublineage *fimH*30-Rx.

Globally, in isolates LV36464 and LV27950 seven different acquired antibiotic resistance genes were detected: *aac(6′)Ib-cr*, bla_{OXA-1}, bla_{TEM-1}, $bla_{CTX-M-15}$, *catB3*, *aac(3)-IIa*, and *tetA*. By mapping, the main difference between the plasmids carried by these isolates was the deletion of a 2400 bp sequence that displayed 99.7% homology with the transposase of Tn*5403*. Moreover, 60 single nucleotide variants have been detected between them. Both plasmids displayed an IncF plasmid from a ST131 *E. coli* isolate (JJ2434, unpublished) as its best blast hit. The comparative analysis with JJ2434 showed the absence of two regions of 9329 and 1740 bp that corresponded to deletions of genes coding for unknown functions, replication proteins, endonucleases, transcriptional regulators, and conjugation transfer proteins in LV36464 and LV27950 plasmids. The analysis of the QRDR of genes *gyrA* (from 67 to 106 aminoacids), *gyrB* (from 415 to 470 aminoacids), *parC* (from 47 to 133 aminoacids), and *parE* (from 450 to 528 aminoacids) revealed the presence of amino acid substitutions in *gyrA* (S83L and D87N) and *parC* (S80I and E84V) in both isolates.

A high number of mobile genetic elements was detected in the draft genomes of these isolates. Both harbored a plasmid (>98% homology) from incompatibility group IncFIA, which according to PlasmidFinder was classified as an IncFIA type 1. LV36464 accommodated an additional IncX plasmid. The distribution of insertion sequences present in LV36464 and LV27950 genomes was also globally similar: IS*1* (5.77 and 5.66%, respectively), IS*110* (3.85 and 1.89%, respectively), IS*1380* (1.92 and 1.89%, respectively), IS*200*_IS*605* (5.77 and 3.77%, respectively), IS*21* (3.85 and 3.77%, respectively), IS*3* (23.08 and 26.42%, respectively), IS*30* (1.92 and 3.77%, respectively), IS*4* (5.77 and 3.77%, respectively), IS*481* (3.85 and 3.77%, respectively), IS*6* (1.92 and 1.89%, respectively), IS*66* (11.54 and 11.32%, respectively), IS*As1* (1.92 and 1.89%, respectively), IS*L3* (19.23 and 18.87%, respectively) and IS*NCY* (9.62 and 9.43%, respectively). It is worth mentioning that the worldwide disseminated Tn*3* was only represented in the genome of LV36464 (3.39%), and IS*92* (1.89%) in LV27950. The specialized annotation of phage and prophages revealed that LV36464 harbored 17 regions: 8 intact, 6 incomplete and 4 questionable. These intact prophage regions ranged between 17.4 and 51.5 Kb, showing different numbers of coding sequences that varied between 24 and 88. In turn, LV27950 harbored 13 prophage regions: it displayed 10 intact regions spanning between 20.6 and 86.1 Kb. Globally, regions from five phages were present in the genomes of both and two were exclusive of each isolate (Table S1).

The detection of virulence factors in the genome of LV27950 revealed the presence of an increased serum survival factor provided by an ISS-encoding gene and a secreted autotransporter toxin denominated *sat* (**Table 4**). LV36464 shared the same virulence factors and, in addition, harbored a glutamate descarboxilase-encoding gene (*gad*). The overall estimation of pathogenicity factors present in the genome of the isolates, using known proteins with recognized involvement in pathogenicity as reference, enabled us to determine that the assembled contigs of LV36464 and LV27950 matched 553 and 544 pathogenic families, which resulted in the estimation of both isolates being human pathogens (93.1 and 93.3%), confirming their zoonotic potential.

DISCUSSION

The prevalence of antibiotic resistance genes in isolates from animal origin has been fairly assessed (Szmolka et al., 2011; Tamang et al., 2011; Bardon et al., 2013; Clemente et al., 2015). However, taking in account the current availability of genomic characterization tools, we are now able to proceed with more detailed characterizations of these genes, in a broader context. In this study, we characterized the genome of PMQR-producing *E. coli*. To understand the antibiotic susceptibility background of these specific isolates we have also evaluated the antibiotic susceptibility phenotypes of a collection of *S. enterica* and *E. coli* recovered from animals of different origins, in which the isolates were originally included.

The levels of non-wild type phenotypes revealed to be very distinct among *S. enterica* and *E. coli*. Non wild-type isolates for fluoroquinolones were particularly evident among poultry isolates recovered from *S. enterica*. Regarding *E. coli* isolates, the frequency of non-wild-type phenotypes to nalidixic acid and ciprofloxacin was higher in food-producing animals than in companion and zoo animals, which might be due to the high consumption of veterinary antibiotics in animal industrial units, particularly tetracyclines, sulphonamides, and fluoroquinolones (EFSA, 2015). Portugal still represents a European country with high antibiotic use in animals. This fact raises concerns regarding antibiotic resistance in veterinary settings (EMA, 2014). Different MIC_{50} and MIC_{90} (3-fold dilutions) were noted for some groups of each species: *E. coli* isolates for nalidixic acid, ciprofloxacin, ampicillin, streptomycin, tetracycline, sulfamethoxazole and trimethoprim, and *S. enterica* for ampicillin, cefotaxime, tetracycline, and trimethoprim.

Although, PMQR determinants are typically responsible by low level resistance, their presence has been increasingly reported in animals, resulting in an additional effect on the nonsusceptibility of fluoroquinolones (Ahmed and Shimamoto, 2013; Donati et al., 2014; Jamborova et al., 2015). The high MIC values of 128 mg/L against nalidixic acid and 8 mg/L against ciprofloxacin observed in some of the isolates of our collection may be associated with amino acid alterations in the quinolone resistance-determining region (QRDR). Indeed, although the fluoroquinolone non-susceptibility is frequently compromised by target modification, the PMQR-encoding genes have the potential to spread and promote co-selection of other antibiotic resistance genes (EMA, 2014). Late reports even suggest that the spread of PMQR may not be triggered by selection pressure, which justifies the low rates of these determinants in animals, despite the high use of fluoroquinolones (Veldman et al., 2011).

Considering the high level MICs, most likely caused by QRDR chromosomal mutations that might mask the presence of PMQR, we decided in this study to retrospectively search for these determinants in all isolates of the collection, regardless of the MIC value. We have detected four PMQR-encoding genes (4/180) (two *qnrS1* and two *aac(6′)-Ib-cr*) in *E. coli* LV46221, LV46743, LV36464, and LV27950 recovered from animals of different origins: a healthy turtle dove from a Zoo Park (2008), a diseased pet dog (2008), a bottlenose dolphin from a Zoo Park showing signs of respiratory infection (2009), and a second but healthy bottlenose dolphin from the same Zoo Park (2011) (**Table 4**).

The comparison of the genomes of QnrS1-producing *E. coli* revealed that isolates LV46221 and LV46743 were very similar in terms of their global pathogenicity potential, although they were recovered from animals of different classes and completely different backgrounds (**Table 4**). The absence of chromosomal mutations in the QRDR of isolates LV46221 and LV46743 corroborated the low fluoroquinolone MIC values obtained, which spanned between 0.38 mg/L for ciprofloxacin and 8 mg/L for nalidixic acid, highlighting the low level resistance conferred by QnrS1 determinants (Cavaco and Aarestrup, 2009). The plasmid region in which the *qnrS1* was enclosed in both isolates, that included the association with Tn*3*, has already been described in association with *qnrS1* genes in plasmids from *Shigella flexneri* recovered from food products, *Salmonella* Infantis from avian origin, and human clinical *Klebsiella pneumoniae* isolates, respectively (Hata et al., 2005; Chen et al., 2006; Kehrenberg et al., 2006). Moreover, we have previously detected other *qnrS1* from animals in Portugal, associated with a similar genetic environment, exclusively in food-producing animals (Jones-Dias et al., 2013). IncN plasmids harbored by LV46221 and LV46743 were assigned to ST1 by pMLST, which have also been associated with chickens and wild bird water in Czech Republic and the Netherlands, respectively (Ben Sallem et al., 2014).

Few genomic differences were noticed between the two *aac(6′)-Ib-cr-* and $bla_{CTX-M-15}$-harboring *E. coli.* In fact, the isolates could be assigned to the same genetic sublineage—ST131 *fimH*30-Rx, confirming clonal spread. Although, samples have been recovered within a reasonable time span of 2 years, their origin refers to two bottlenose dolphins of the same species held captive in the same Zoo Park. The presence of four chromosomal alterations in the QRDR region of isolates LV36464 and LV27950 was reflected in the high levels of fluoroquinolone MICs, which ranged between 8 and >256 mg/L. All antibiotic resistance genes detected in LV36464 and LV27950 [*aac(6′)Ib-cr*, bla_{OXA-1}, bla_{TEM-1}, $bla_{CTX-M-15}$, *catB3, aac(3)-IIa*, and *tetA*] could be traced back to a single multidrug resistance IncFIA plasmid that showed 99.9% of homology with a plasmid submitted this year to Genbank in U.S.A (JJ2434, unpublished). Although, 60 single nucleotide variants have been detected between the LV36464 and LV27950 plasmids, the main difference consisted of a single deletion that involved part of a transposase-encoding gene. The absence of a set of conjugation transfer proteins (*tra* genes), among other genes, highlighted the preponderance of clonal spread over horizontal gene transfer in ST131 *E. coli* (Nicolas-Chanoine et al., 2014). Although, several isoforms of identical plasmids have been detected worldwide, the simultaneous resistance to β-lactams, fluoroquinolones, aminoglycosides, chloramphenicol and tetracyclines has been a permanent feature, which reinforces the advantage that it confers (Boyd et al., 2004; Zhou et al., 2015). The detection of a ST131 *fimH*30-Rx *E. coli* in two dolphins, which are continuously in contact with a live audience, constitutes a public health concern. These clinically relevant multidrug resistant *E. coli* isolates have been on the rise for years (Nicolas-Chanoine et al., 2014). Initially restricted to clinical contexts, recent findings suggest that their prevalence in non-clinical settings is maintained by the constant exchange of isolates throughout the time, as verified in this study (Mathers et al., 2015).

Although, *E. coli* is a common inhabitant of the gastrointestinal tract of humans and animals, the detected transposons, plasmids and bacteriophages are essential to the acquisition of pathogenicity factors that enlarge their ability to adapt to new niches, allowing bacteria to increase the capacity to cause a broad spectrum of diseases (Bien et al., 2012). All isolates displayed genomic factors that may be critical to cause a zoonotic infection and that were reflected in high probabilities for the isolates to be human pathogens (>93%). Concerning virulence factors, we detected the presence of glutamate decarboxylase, increased serum survival gene and a secreted autotransporter toxin, irregularly distributed across the four isolates (**Table 3**), which did not denote any relation with the conditions of their respective hosts. These virulence factors confer resistance to extreme acid conditions of the intestines, enable the isolate to survive complement system and cause defined damage to kidney epithelium, being indicative of their ability to cause disease (Johnson et al., 2008; Becker Saidenberg et al., 2012). Indeed, *E. coli* isolates can frequently encode a number of virulence factors, which enable the bacteria to colonize the urinary tract and face highly effective host defenses (Bien et al., 2012).

Although, fluoroquinolones are consistently used in veterinary medicine, results presented in this study indicate that PMQR determinants occurred at a low frequency in these isolates (2.2%), as previously reported (Donati et al., 2014; Jamborova et al., 2015). However, the studied groups of animals should still be considered potential reservoirs for PMQR-producing isolates, especially because there is the inherent potential for transboundary dissemination. These isolates presented a set of genetic features essential to promote their own successful spread: multiple antibiotic resistance genes carried by well-known mobile genetic elements, virulence factors adequate to zoonotic transmission and numerous other pathogenicity factors.

The analysis of many bacterial genomic features showed us great genetic relatedness between the two *qnrS1-* and *aac(6′)-Ib-cr*-harboring isolates. The data gathered throughout this study illustrates two scenarios: the presence of the same strain in different hosts inhabiting remote locations and the persistence of a unique strain in a single niche during a long period of time. The strains were each associated with a case of symptomatic infection (LV46743 and LV36464) and with a report of microbiological control of an asymptomatic host (LV46221 and LV27950), which reinforces the ability of *E. coli* isolates to act as silent vehicles, allowing the accumulation of antibiotic resistance determinants, mobile genetic elements and other relevant pathogenicity determinants (Mathers et al., 2015). It is not certain whether these bacteria spread from humans to animals, between different animals or from the environment to animals. However, in the case of companion animals, but particularly zoo animals, surveillance is essential to prevent continuous dissemination. The contact between animals and owners, zookeepers, visitors, and handlers raises concerns, considering that these bacteria might easily spread to humans and to other animals (Veldman et al., 2011; Ewers et al., 2012).

Permanent surveillance of health and sick animals should be strongly encouraged, regardless of their origin, in order to monitor future trends in the dissemination of resistance to fluoroquinolones and other antibiotics. Furthermore, this genome project contains valuable scientific data which will certainly be helpful for molecular epidemiological surveys of ST131 *E. coli* clonal group.

AUTHOR CONTRIBUTIONS

DJD designed the study, acquired laboratory data, analyzed the data and wrote the manuscript. VM designed the study, analyzed the data and reviewed the manuscript. RG acquired laboratory data. DAS acquired laboratory data, TA, acquired laboratory or epidemiological data. PT acquired laboratory or epidemiological data. LV acquired laboratory data and reviewed the manuscript. EF acquired laboratory data and reviewed the manuscript. LC acquired laboratory or epidemiological data and reviewed the manuscript. MC designed the study and reviewed the manuscript. All authors read and approved the final manuscript.

FUNDING

These work was supported by Fundação para a Ciência e a Tecnologia (grant numbers PTDC/CVT/65713 and PEst-OE/AGR/UI0211/2011-2014). DJD has received research funding from Fundação para a Ciência e a Tecnologia (FCT, grant number SFRH/BD/80001/2011). VM was supported by FCT fellowship (grant SFRH/BPD/77486/2011), financed by the European Social Funds (COMPETE-FEDER) and national funds of the Portuguese Ministry of Education and Science (POPH-QREN).

REFERENCES

Ahmed, A. M., and Shimamoto, T. (2013). Molecular characterization of multidrug-resistant avian pathogenic *Escherichia coli* isolated from septicemic broilers. *Int. J. Med. Microbiol.* 303, 475–483. doi: 10.1016/j.ijmm.2013.06.009

Aziz, R. K., Devoid, S., Disz, T., Edwards, R. A., Henry, C. S., Olsen, G. J., et al. (2012). SEED servers: high-performance access to the SEED genomes, annotations, and metabolic models. *PLoS ONE* 7:e48053. doi: 10.1371/journal.pone.0048053

Bardon, J., Husičkova, V., Chromá, M., and Kolár, M. (2013). Prevalence and characteristics of *Escherichia coli* strains producing extended-spectrum β -lactamases in slaughtered animals in the Czech Republic. *J. Food Prot.* 76, 1773–1777. doi: 10.4315/0362-028X.JFP-13-114

Becker Saidenberg, A., Robaldo Guedes, N. M., Fernandes Seixas, G. H., Da Costa Allgayer, M., Pacífico De Assis, E., Fabio Silveira, L., et al. (2012). A survey for *Escherichia coli* virulence factors in asymptomatic free-ranging parrots. *ISRN Vet. Sci.* 2012:984813. doi: 10.5402/2012/984813

Ben Sallem, R., Ben Slama, K., Rojo-Bezares, B., Porres-Osante, N., Jouini, A., Klibi, N., et al. (2014). IncI1 plasmids carrying $bla_{CTX-M-1}$ or bla_{CMY-2} genes in *Escherichia coli* from healthy humans and animals in Tunisia. *Microb. Drug Resist.* 20, 495–500. doi: 10.1089/mdr.2013.0224

Bien, J., Sokolova, O., and Bozko, P. (2012). Role of uropathogenic *Escherichia coli* virulence factors in development of urinary tract infection and kidney damage. *Int. J. Nephrol.* 2012:681473. doi: 10.1155/2012/681473

Boyd, D. A., Tyler, S., Christianson, S., Mcgeer, A., Muller, M. P., Willey, B. M., et al. (2004). Complete nucleotide sequence of a 92-kilobase plasmid harboring the CTX-M-15 extended-spectrum β-lactamase involved in an outbreak in long-term-care facilities in Toronto, Canada. *Antimicrob. Agents Chemother.* 48, 3758–3764. doi: 10.1128/AAC.48.10.3758-3764.2004

Carattoli, A., Zankari, E., García-Fernández, A., Voldby Larsen, M., Lund, O., Villa, L., et al. (2014). *In silico* detection and typing of plasmids using PlasmidFinder and plasmid multilocus sequence typing. *Antimicrob. Agents Chemother.* 58, 3895–3903. doi: 10.1128/AAC.02412-14

Cavaco, L. M., and Aarestrup, F. M. (2009). Evaluation of quinolones for use in detection of determinants of acquired quinolone resistance, including the new transmissible resistance mechanisms *qnrA*, *qnrB*, *qnrS*, and *aac(6')Ib-cr*, in *Escherichia coli* and *Salmonella enterica* and determinations of wild-type distributions. *J. Clin. Microbiol.* 47, 2751–2758. doi: 10.1128/JCM.00456-09

Chen, Y. T., Shu, H. Y., Li, L. H., Liao, T. L., Wu, K. M., Shiau, Y. R., et al. (2006). Complete nucleotide sequence of pK245, a 98-kilobase plasmid conferring quinolone resistance and extended-spectrum β-lactamase activity in a clinical *Klebsiella pneumoniae* isolate. *Antimicrob. Agents Chemother.* 50, 3861–3866. doi: 10.1128/AAC.00456-06

Clemente, L., Manageiro, V., Jones-Dias, D., Correia, I., Themudo, P., Albuquerque, T., et al. (2015). Antimicrobial susceptibility and oxymino β-lactam resistance mechanisms in *Salmonella enterica* and *Escherichia coli* isolates from different animal sources. *Res. Microbiol.* 166, 574–583. doi: 10.1016/j.resmic.2015.05.007

Cosentino, S., Voldby Larsen, M., Møller Aarestrup, F., and Lund, O. (2013). PathogenFinder: distinguishing friend from foe using bacterial whole genome sequence data. *PLoS ONE* 8:e77302. doi: 10.1371/journal.pone.0077302

Damborg, P., Broens, E. M., Chomel, B. B., Guenther, S., Pasmans, F., Wagenaar, J. A., et al. (2015). Bacterial zoonoses transmitted by household pets: state-of-the-art and future perspectives for targeted research and policy actions. *J. Comp. Pathol.* doi: 10.1016/j.jcpa.2015.03.004. [Epub ahead of print].

Donati, V., Feltrin, F., Hendriksen, R. S., Svendsen, C. A., Cordaro, G., García-Fernández, A., et al. (2014). Extended-spectrum β-lactamases, AmpC β-lactamases and plasmid mediated quinolone resistance in *Klebsiella* spp. from companion animals in Italy. *PLoS ONE* 9:e90564. doi: 10.1371/journal.pone.0090564

EFSA (2015). EU Summary Report on antimicrobial resistance in zoonotic and indicator bacteria from humans, animals and food in 2013. *EFSA J.* 13:4036. doi: 10.2903/j.efsa.2015.4036

EMA (2014). *Sales of Veterinary Antimicrobial Agents in 26 EU/EEA Countries in 2012.* London: European Medicines Agency.

Ewers, C., Bethe, A., Semmler, T., Guenther, S., and Wieler, L. H. (2012). Extended-spectrum β-lactamase-producing and AmpC-producing *Escherichia coli* from livestock and companion animals, and their putative impact on public health: a global perspective. *Clin. Microbiol. Infect.* 18, 646–655. doi: 10.1111/j.1469-0691.2012.03850.x

Gomes-Neves, E., Antunes, P., Manageiro, V., Gärtner, F., Caniça, M., Da Costa, J. M., et al. (2014). Clinically relevant multidrug resistant *Salmonella enterica* in swine and meat handlers at the abattoir. *Vet. Microbiol.* 168, 229–233. doi: 10.1016/j.vetmic.2013.10.017

Grimont, P. A., and Weill, F. X. (2007). *Antigenic Formulae of the Salmonella Serovars, 9th Edn.* Paris: Institute Pasteur. WHO Collaborating Centre for Reference and Research on Salmonella.

Hata, M., Suzuki, M., Matsumoto, M., Takahashi, M., Sato, K., Ibe, S., et al. (2005). Cloning of a novel gene for quinolone resistance from a transferable plasmid in *Shigella flexneri* 2b. *Antimicrob. Agents Chemother.* 49, 801–803. doi: 10.1128/AAC.49.2.801-803.2005

Jamborova, I., Dolejska, M., Vojtech, J., Guenther, S., Uricariu, R., Drozdowska, J., et al. (2015). Plasmid-mediated resistance to cephalosporins and fluoroquinolones in various *Escherichia coli* sequence types isolated from rooks wintering in Europe. *Appl. Environ. Microbiol.* 81, 648–657. doi: 10.1128/AEM.02459-14

Joensen, K. G., Scheutz, F., Lund, O., Hasman, H., Kaas, R. S., Nielsen, E. M., et al. (2014). Real-time whole-genome sequencing for routine typing, surveillance, and outbreak detection of verotoxigenic *Escherichia coli. J. Clin. Microbiol.* 52, 1501–1510. doi: 10.1128/JCM.03617-13

Joensen, K. G., Tetzschner, A. M., Iguchi, A., Aarestrup, F. M., and Scheutz, F. (2015). Rapid and easy in silico serotyping of *Escherichia coli* isolates by use of whole-genome sequencing data. *J. Clin. Microbiol.* 53, 2410–2426. doi: 10.1128/JCM.00008-15

Johnson, T. J., Wannemuehler, Y. M., and Nolan, L. K. (2008). Evolution of the iss gene in *Escherichia coli. Appl. Environ. Microbiol.* 74, 2360–2369. doi: 10.1128/AEM.02634-07

Jones-Dias, D., Manageiro, V., Francisco, A. P., Martins, A. P., Domingues, G., Louro, D., et al. (2013). Assessing the molecular basis of transferable quinolone resistance in *Escherichia coli* and *Salmonella* spp. from food-producing animals and food products. *Vet. Microbiol.* 167, 523–531. doi: 10.1016/j.vetmic.2013.08.010

Jones-Dias, D., Manageiro, V., Martins, A. P., Ferreira, E., and Caniça, M. (2015). New class 2 integron In2-4 among IncI1-positive *Escherichia coli* isolates carrying ESBL and PMAβ genes from food animals in Portugal. *Foodborne Pathog. Dis.* 13, 36–39. doi: 10.1089/fpd.2015.1972

Kehrenberg, C., Friederichs, S., De Jong, A., Michael, G. B., and Schwarz, S. (2006). Identification of the plasmid-borne quinolone resistance gene *qnrS* in *Salmonella enterica* serovar Infantis. *J. Antimicrob. Chemother.* 58, 18–22. doi: 10.1093/jac/dkl213

Larsen, M. V., Cosentino, S., Rasmussen, S., Friis, C., Hasman, H., Marvig, R. L., et al. (2012). Multilocus sequence typing of total genome sequenced bacteria. *J. Clin. Microbiol.* 50, 1355–1361. doi: 10.1128/JCM.06094-11

Magiorakos, A. P., Srinivasan, A., Carey, R. B., Carmeli, Y., Falagas, M. E., Giske, C. G., et al. (2011). Multidrug-resistant, extensively drug-resistant and pandrug-resistant bacteria: an international expert proposal for interim standard definitions for acquired resistance. *Clin Microbiol. Infect.* 18, 268–281. doi: 10.1111/j.1469-0691.2011.03570.x

Marshall, B. M., and Levy, S. B. (2011). Food animals and antimicrobials: impacts on human health. *Clin. Microbiol. Rev.* 24, 718–733. doi: 10.1128/CMR.00002-11

Mathers, A. J., Peirano, G., and Pitout, J. D. (2015). The role of epidemic resistance plasmids and international high-risk clones in the spread of multidrug-resistant *Enterobacteriaceae. Clin. Microbiol. Rev.* 28, 565–591. doi: 10.1128/CMR.00116-14

Nicolas-Chanoine, M. H., Bertrand, X., and Madec, J. Y. (2014). *Escherichia coli* ST131, an intriguing clonal group. *Clin. Microbiol. Rev.* 27, 543–574. doi: 10.1128/CMR.00125-13

Overbeek, R., Olson, R., Pusch, G. D., Olsen, G. J., Davis, J. J., Disz, T., et al. (2014). The SEED and the Rapid Annotation of microbial genomes using Subsystems Technology (RAST). *Nucleic Acids Res.* 42, D206–D214. doi: 10.1093/nar/gkt1226

Poirel, L., Cattoir, V., and Nordmann, P. (2012). Plasmid-mediated quinolone resistance; interactions between Human, Animal, and Environmental Ecologies. *Front. Microbiol.* 3:24. doi: 10.3389/fmicb.2012.00024

Schmithausen, R. M., Schulze-Geisthoevel, S. V., Stemmer, F., El-Jade, M., Reif, M., Hack, S., et al. (2015). Analysis of transmission of MRSA and ESBL among pigs and farm personnel. *PLoS ONE* 10:e0138173. doi: 10.1371/journal.pone.0138173

Schwarz, S., Silley, P., Simjee, S., Woodford, N., Van Duijkeren, E., Johnson, A. P., et al. (2010). Editorial: assessing the antimicrobial susceptibility of bacteria obtained from animals. *J. Antimicrob. Chemother.* 65, 601–604. doi: 10.1093/jac/dkq037

Stokes, H. W., and Gillings, M. R. (2011). Gene flow, mobile genetic elements and the recruitment of antibiotic resistance genes into Gram-negative pathogens. *FEMS Microbiol. Rev.* 35, 790–819. doi: 10.1111/j.1574-6976.2011.00273.x

Szmolka, A., Fortini, D., Villa, L., Carattoli, A., Anjum, M. F., and Nagy, B. (2011). First report on IncN plasmid-mediated quinolone resistance gene qnrS1 in porcine *Escherichia coli* in Europe. *Microb. Drug Resist.* 17, 567–573. doi: 10.1089/mdr.2011.0068

Tamang, M. D., Nam, H. M., Kim, A., Lee, H. S., Kim, T. S., Kim, M. J., et al. (2011). Prevalence and mechanisms of quinolone resistance among selected nontyphoid *Salmonella* isolated from food animals and humans in Korea. *Foodborne Pathog. Dis.* 8, 1199–1206. doi: 10.1089/fpd.2011.0899

Varani, A. M., Siguier, P., Gourbeyre, E., Charneau, V., and Chandler, M. (2011). ISsaga is an ensemble of web-based methods for high throughput identification and semi-automatic annotation of insertion sequences in prokaryotic genomes. *Genome Biol.* 12:R30. doi: 10.1186/gb-2011-12-3-r30

Veldman, K., Cavaco, L. M., Mevius, D., Battisti, A., Franco, A., Botteldoorn, N., et al. (2011). International collaborative study on the occurrence of plasmid-mediated quinolone resistance in Salmonella enterica and *Escherichia coli* isolated from animals, humans, food and the environment in 13 European countries. *J. Antimicrob. Chemother.* 66, 1278–1286. doi: 10.1093/jac/dkr084

Zankari, E., Hasman, H., Cosentino, S., Vestergaard, M., Rasmussen, S., Lund, O., et al. (2012). Identification of acquired antimicrobial resistance genes. *J. Antimicrob. Chemother.* 67, 2640–2644. doi: 10.1093/jac/dks261

Zhou, K., Lokate, M., Deurenberg, R. H., Arends, J., Lo-Ten Foe, J., Grundmann, H., et al. (2015). Characterization of a CTX-M-15-producing *Klebsiella pneumoniae* outbreak strain assigned to a novel sequence type (1427). *Front. Microbiol.* 6:1250. doi: 10.3389/fmicb.2015.01250

Zhou, Y., Liang, Y., Lynch, K. H., Dennis, J. J., and Wishart, D. S. (2011). PHAST: a fast phage search tool. *Nucleic Acids Res.* 39, W347–352. doi: 10.1093/nar/gkr485

9

A Designed Experiments Approach to Optimizing MALDI-TOF MS Spectrum Processing Parameters Enhances Detection of Antibiotic Resistance in *Campylobacter jejuni*

Christian Penny[1]*, Beau Grothendick[2], Lin Zhang[2], Connie M. Borror[2], Duane Barbano[2], Angela J. Cornelius[3], Brent J. Gilpin[3], Clifton K. Fagerquist[4], William J. Zaragoza[4], Michele T. Jay-Russell[5], Albert J. Lastovica[6], Catherine Ragimbeau[7], Henry-Michel Cauchie[1] and Todd R. Sandrin[2]*

[1] Environmental Research and Innovation Department, Luxembourg Institute of Science and Technology, Esch-sur-Alzette, Luxembourg, [2] School of Mathematical and Natural Sciences, Arizona State University, Phoenix, AZ, USA, [3] Institute of Environmental Science and Research, Christchurch, New Zealand, [4] Agricultural Research Service, United States Department of Agriculture, Albany, CA, USA, [5] Western Center for Food Safety, University of California at Davis, Davis, CA, USA, [6] Department of Biotechnology, University of the Western Cape, Bellville, South Africa, [7] Epidemiological Surveillance of Infectious Diseases, Laboratoire National de Santé, Dudelange, Luxembourg

***Correspondence:**
Christian Penny
christian.penny@list.lu;
Todd R. Sandrin
todd.sandrin@asu.edu

MALDI-TOF MS has been utilized as a reliable and rapid tool for microbial fingerprinting at the genus and species levels. Recently, there has been keen interest in using MALDI-TOF MS beyond the genus and species levels to rapidly identify antibiotic resistant strains of bacteria. The purpose of this study was to enhance strain level resolution for *Campylobacter jejuni* through the optimization of spectrum processing parameters using a series of designed experiments. A collection of 172 strains of *C. jejuni* were collected from Luxembourg, New Zealand, North America, and South Africa, consisting of four groups of antibiotic resistant isolates. The groups included: (1) 65 strains resistant to cefoperazone (2) 26 resistant to cefoperazone and beta-lactams (3) 5 strains resistant to cefoperazone, beta-lactams, and tetracycline, and (4) 76 strains resistant to cefoperazone, teicoplanin, amphotericin, B and cephalothin. Initially, a model set of 16 strains (three biological replicates and three technical replicates per isolate, yielding a total of 144 spectra) of *C. jejuni* was subjected to each designed experiment to enhance detection of antibiotic resistance. The most optimal parameters were applied to the larger collection of 172 isolates (two biological replicates and three technical replicates per isolate, yielding a total of 1,031 spectra). We observed an increase in antibiotic resistance detection whenever either a curve based similarity coefficient (Pearson or ranked Pearson) was applied rather than a peak based (Dice) and/or the optimized preprocessing parameters were applied. Increases in antimicrobial resistance detection were scored using the jackknife maximum similarity technique following cluster analysis. From the first four groups of antibiotic resistant isolates, the optimized preprocessing parameters increased detection respective to the aforementioned groups by: (1) 5% (2) 9% (3) 10%, and (4) 2%. An additional second categorization was created from the collection consisting of 31 strains resistant to beta-lactams and 141 strains sensitive to beta-lactams. Applying optimal preprocessing parameters, beta-lactam resistance detection was increased by 34%. These results suggest that spectrum processing parameters, which are rarely optimized or adjusted, affect the performance of MALDI-TOF MS-based detection of antibiotic resistance and can be fine-tuned to enhance screening performance.

Keywords: MALDI-TOF MS, *Campylobacter jejuni,* antimicrobial resistance, antibiotic resistance, designed experiments, spectrum processing

INTRODUCTION

MALDI-TOF MS has revolutionized the field of molecular microbial diagnostics in recent years (Sauer and Kliem, 2010; Welker, 2011; Welker and Moore, 2011; Kliem and Sauer, 2012). This approach has been implemented in biomedical, veterinary and environmental routine procedures for bacterial identification at the genus, species, and sometimes at the subspecies level (e.g., Wieser et al., 2011; Croxatto et al., 2012; Koubek et al., 2012; Lartigue, 2013; Sandrin et al., 2013; Randall et al., 2015). While microbial identification using MALDI-TOF MS is rapid and reliable, the taxonomic resolution obtained from the mass spectra is not always sufficient, or the bioinformatics software pipeline is not optimized or adapted, for typing the candidate bacteria below the species level (Sandrin et al., 2013; Zhang et al., 2014). However, some studies have shown that categorization of strains of bacteria with respect to their membership in nucleic acid-based subgroups, pathogenicity traits or antimicrobial resistance (AMR) identification is indeed feasible, but depends on the level of variability inside a given taxon as well as on the precise identification of characteristic biomarkers using bioinformatics tools (Sandrin et al., 2013). Fine-tuning of mass spectrum analysis is evidently mandatory.

Rigorous analysis of spectra has permitted successful detection of AMR (e.g., Hrabák et al., 2013; Kostrzewa et al., 2013; Pulido et al., 2013), but further development is needed to render MALDI-based approaches a more routine, reliable, and effective alternative to traditional methods. As has been shown in several MALDI applications to discriminate bacterial strains (Mitchell et al., 2015), high reproducibility is required for reliable AMR detection. Although many portions of the MALDI-TOF MS workflow such as sample preparation and data acquisition have been optimized with regard to spectrum reproducibility and method performance (e.g., Freiwald and Sauer, 2009; Goldstein et al., 2013), no standardization for mass spectrum processing parameters has been proposed. Processing parameters are used to calculate, define, and resolve acquired spectra into interpretable data. Baseline subtraction, a common processing parameter, establishes a baseline from the spectrum, leaving a clearer picture of the remaining peaks. Another processing parameter, smoothing, reduces background noise, and increases signal-to-noise ratio. The manner in which the data are translated by processing parameters may affect the ability of MALDI-TOF MS-based fingerprinting to detect antibiotic resistance. In addition, different software packages that use distinct spectrum processing workflows and parameters are often used. Many of these programs do not offer the ability to alter and optimize spectrum processing parameters. Such optimization, though, may be necessary to enhance method performance, particularly with regard to resolving strain-level differences, such as AMR.

The issues regarding the ever-increasing bacterial resistance to large categories of antimicrobial compounds are particularly of public health concern for the world's leading bacterial gastroenteritis agent *Campylobacter* (World Health Organization [WHO], 2013). The species *Campylobacter jejuni* is recognized as the major food- and waterborne pathogen inside this taxon, and is a major threat to public health (Kaakoush et al., 2015; Wagenaar et al., 2015). AMR in *Campylobacter* is steadily increasing (e.g., Luangtongkum et al., 2009; Ge et al., 2013; Iovine, 2013; Wieczorek and Osek, 2013). Of particular concern is also the increasing incidence of AMR of *Campylobacter* spp. other than *C. jejuni*, whose disease potential is not fully appreciated at present (Lastovica, 2006; Lastovica et al., 2014). *Campylobacter* easily undergoes DNA transformation by foreign exogenous DNA resulting in many different antibiotic-resistant strains (Bae et al., 2014). Also, antibiotic resistance mutations in *C. jejuni* continue to develop (Iovine, 2013). For example, a single mutation in the gyrase subunit A (*gyr*A) gene, resulting in an amino acid substitution, is sufficient for conferring resistance to quinolones (Wang et al., 1993; Payot et al., 2006).

In diagnostic and clinical microbiology, as well as epidemiological surveillance, the need for implementation of early and precise information retrieval concerning AMR has been raised (Laxminarayan et al., 2013). This could greatly improve treatment of infectious diseases and help limit the spread of multiple resistant strains of harmful bacteria. In this context, the evolution toward microbial characterization, and more specifically AMR prediction through whole-genome sequencing (WGS) has been described in recent years including the identification of AMR-specific signatures in *Campylobacter* (e.g., Didelot et al., 2012; Zhao et al., 2016). But also, the potential of various MALDI-TOF MS applications for the prediction of AMR mechanisms has been identified (Hrabák et al., 2013; Kostrzewa et al., 2013). Most importantly, the use of mass spectrometry toolkits for the diagnosis of AMR in *Campylobacter* is emerging (Wieser et al., 2011; Lartigue, 2013; Schubert and Kostrzewa, 2015), and a new microbial typing method relying on mass spectrometry-based phyloproteomics (MSPP), permitting biomarker, and genetic features characterization in *Campylobacter*, has recently been published (Zautner et al., 2015). Still, the MALDI-TOF MS-based workflow remains in the need of optimization and simplification of robust, reliable and reproducible workflows, especially regarding data handling after automated routine acquisition of mass spectra.

Consequently, the overarching objective of this study was to determine whether MALDI-TOF mass spectrum processing parameters could be optimized to enhance the detection of antibiotic resistance in clinically relevant environmental, animal, and human isolates of *C. jejuni*. Therefore, 172 isolates of *C. jejuni* were collected from four continents, some of which share antibiotic resistances within four different groups (**Table 1**). Special emphasis was put on *C. jejuni* resistance to beta-lactams, as this antibiotics group is considered among the most important and widespread treatment with resistance issues (Wieser et al., 2011; Lartigue, 2013; Schubert and Kostrzewa, 2015). A designed experiments approach was employed (Zhang et al., 2014), in which spectrum processing parameters were varied to optimize detection of AMR. Translation of the genetic and phenotypic characteristics of *C. jejuni* might identify useful and straightforward information collection in a global One Health context (Maloy and Atlas, 2014). Our results suggest that a designed experiments approach allows optimization of mass spectrum analysis and enhances detection of AMR in *C. jejuni*.

MATERIALS AND METHODS

Campylobacter jejuni Strains and Culture Conditions

A collection of 16 *C. jejuni* isolates were used as a model system for the designed experiments and a total of 172 *C. jejuni* strains from various geographical and animal host origins were used in application of the model spectrum processing parameters (**Table 1**).

Antibiotic resistance profiles were established by a non-exhaustive series of phenotypic and genomic attribute tests of the *C. jejuni* isolate collection, depending on specific culture media used and availability of whole genome sequence data (WGS) of the strains. Genomics-based AMR potential of part of the

TABLE 1 | Characteristics of the *Campylobacter jejuni* isolates used in this study.

***C. jejuni* isolate collection**	
Number of strains	172
Geographic origin	Luxembourg, New Zealand, South Africa, USA
Sources	Alpaca, bovine, chicken, feral swine, goat, goose, human, milk product, ovine, raccoon, surface water, turkey, vole, wastewater, wildfowl
Antibiotic resistance profiles (phenotypically or genotypically confirmed resistances)	Group 1 (65 isolates): Cefoperazone Group 2 (26 isolates): Beta-lactams, cefoperazone Group 3 (5 isolates): Beta-lactams, cefoperazone, tetracycline Group 4 (76 isolates): Cefoperazone, teicoplanin, amphotericin B, cephalotin

collection was obtained through screening using the ResFinder bioinformatics platform[1] (Zankari et al., 2012).

For each strain, chocolate agar plates (Remel Microbiology Products, Lenexa, KS, USA) were inoculated with stock suspensions stored at −80°C in FBP medium (Gorman and Adley, 2004), and incubated for 40 ± 4 h at 42°C under microaerobic conditions in gastight jars (2.5 L, Remel) using CampyGen 2.5 L gaspacks (Remel). For biological replicates, the same stock suspension was streaked onto two to three separate chocolate agar plates on different days.

Sample Preparation

A previously described protein extraction sample preparation method was employed with minor modifications (Freiwald and Sauer, 2009). Briefly, cells from 40 ± 4 h cultures were pelleted by centrifugation (17,000 × *g* for 5 min) and washed with sterile double-distilled water (ddH_2O) (Millipore Corp.; Bedford, MA, USA). Cells were re-suspended in sterile ddH_2O, and the cell density of each suspension was adjusted to 0.8 ± 0.1 OD_{600}. Each 1 mL cell suspension was pelleted by centrifugation (17,000 × *g* for 5 min), and the supernatant was carefully removed. Cell pellets were inactivated by resuspension in 800 μL of absolute ethanol and 300 μL sterile ddH_2O. Inactivation was verified by streaking a loopful of the inactivated suspension onto chocolate agar and verification of absence of colony formation after 72 h of incubation under the conditions described above. Each sample was centrifuged (17,000 × *g* for 5 min), and the resulting supernatant was discarded. A washing step with 1 mL ddH_2O was performed on each cell pellet. Twenty-five microliters of 70% formic acid (Sigma–Aldrich, St. Louis, MO, USA) and 25 μL acetonitrile (Alfa Aesar, Ward Hill, MA, USA) were mixed with the pellet by vortexing thoroughly. Each sample was centrifuged (17,000 × *g* for 5 min), and the supernatant containing the protein extract was transferred into a sterile 1.5 mL microcentrifuge tube. Protein extract (1.0 μL) was pipetted onto a polished steel 96-well MALDI target plate (Bruker Daltonics, Billerica, MA, USA) and allowed to air-dry for 10 min. Samples were spotted onto predetermined, randomly distributed locations on the target plate. After the sample had dried, it was overlaid with 1.0 μL of α-cyano-4-hydroxycinnamic acid (ACROS, Fair Lawn, NJ, USA) matrix prepared in 50% acetonitrile and supplemented with 2.5% trifluoroacetic acid (ACROS, Fair Lawn, NJ, USA). Each isolate was spotted in three technical replicates per biological replicate.

MALDI-TOF MS Data Acquisition

MALDI-TOF MS analyses were performed using a Bruker Microflex LRF MALDI-TOF mass spectrometer (Bruker Daltonics) equipped with a nitrogen laser (λ = 337 nm) under the control of FlexControl software (v. 3; Bruker Daltonics). Each spectrum was obtained in a linear, positive ion mode and calibrated externally using ACTH (1–17) (2094.427 Da), ACTH (18–39) (2466.681 Da), insulin oxidized B (3494.651 Da), insulin (5734.518 Da), cytochrome C (12360.974 Da), and myoglobin (16952.306 Da). Data acquisition was performed automatically in

[1] https://cge.cbs.dtu.dk//services/ResFinder/

TABLE 2 | (A) Factors and levels used in the designed experiments for processing MALDI-TOF MS spectra of the *C. jejuni* collection.

Processing steps (factors)	Processing options (levels)
Baseline Subtraction 1: Binned Baseline	Binned Baseline, Monotone Minimum, Moving Bar, Rolling Disk
Smoothing: Kaiser Window	Gaussian, Kaiser window, Moving Average, Savitzky–Golay
Baseline Subtraction 2: Moving Bar	Binned Baseline, Monotone Minimum, Moving Bar, Rolling Disk
Similarity Coefficient	Dice, Pearson, Ranked Pearson

TABLE 2 | (B) Factors and levels used in the designed experiments approach with center points for highest scoring in predicted settings.

Processing options (factors)	Processing settings (levels)
Binned Baseline	Bin Size of 4, 77, 150
Kaiser Window	Window Size of 1, 21, or 40
Moving Bar	Bar Width of 3, 102, or 201

steps of 100 shots for a total of 500 shots. Laser power was set to the necessary minimum power for ionization of selected samples before starting the analyses. The signal-to-noise threshold was set at two, the minimum intensity threshold at 100, and the maximum number of peaks to 500. Peak width was set at 10 m/z and a height of 80%.

Spectrum Cluster Analysis

Mass spectra were exported from FlexAnalysis (version 3.0; Bruker Daltonics) as .txt files and imported into BioNumerics (version 7.1; Applied Maths, Sint-Martens-Latem, Belgium). Spectra were initially pre-processed using the default program settings (Baseline Subtraction, 1; Rolling Disk, 200). For cluster analysis, spectra were compared pairwise using the Pearson correlation coefficient. The Dice similarity coefficient, in which lists of peaks containing only binary values (present or absent) were generated from spectra, was also evaluated. A dendrogram was generated using the unweighted pair group method with an arithmetic mean (UPGMA) algorithm. Multidimensional scaling (MDS) analysis was performed as previously described to visualize the similarity between spectra (Goldstein et al., 2013). Jackknife analysis was performed as described previously using maximum similarities to quantify rates of correct classification with regard to AMR (Giebel et al., 2008).

Processing Steps and Settings Selection: Designed Experiments

Processing steps chosen as factors were based on those commonly cited in literature and an initial descriptive analysis of their effects on the response (jackknife score). These were found to be important in prior work in our lab, because of their ability to affect number of peaks and spectrum quality. The steps chosen were baseline subtraction, smoothing, and similarity coefficient. The levels, or different methods of baseline subtraction, smoothing, and similarity coefficient, were considered categorical variables, and each step was considered as a categorical variable (**Table 2A**). The highest scoring levels from each category were then selected and further optimized based on their numerical settings (**Table 2B**).

Statistical Analyses

Each of the two/three biological replicates contained three technical replicates. Each set of biological replicates was composed of sixty runs of calculations with varying processing step settings. All 180 experimental runs were carried out in 3 days in random order, and grouped into blocks by both day and biological replicate. Blocking, or grouping together, based on the aforementioned variables, helped to reduce sources of variability and increase precision (Montgomery, 2012). The datasets were subjected to analysis of main effects, interaction of factors, best, and worst combination of settings, significant factors affecting spectrum qualities, and *post hoc* tests on factors. Main effects and interactions of factors on reproducibility were analyzed based on analysis of variance (ANOVA) and *t*-tests using a 5% level of significance. *Post hoc* tests were performed using Tukey's test (Minitab Inc., PA, USA).

Parameter Optimization

An optimized setting for preprocessing parameters and similarity coefficient was determined using ANOVA. The optimized setting was applied to each dataset. The jackknife score (response) from each dataset was reported using either the default settings or optimized preprocessing settings with combinations of three different similarity coefficients: Dice, Pearson, and ranked Pearson. Jackknife analysis was used as described previously (Goldstein et al., 2013) to evaluate the extent to which MALDI-TOF MS profiles were assigned to particular AMR categories. Differences in spectrum quality and jackknife scores before and after optimization were identified using *t*-tests with a 5% level of significance. A second dendrogram and MDS were visualized following optimization. Both optimal and default preprocessing settings were applied to larger sets of *C. jejuni*. In addition, varying similarity coefficients, and jackknife scores were used to measure the effectiveness of each processing parameter combination.

RESULTS

A total of 172 different strains of *C. jejuni* were analyzed for this study. The sample collection was representative of diverse environments and hosts from four continents (**Table 1**). The MALDI-TOF MS profile of each strain was constituted using two sets of biological replicates, and each biological replicate was analyzed using three technical replicates (LX-32 is an exception due to the corruption of a single spectrum in biological replicate B2). Thus, the total number of spectra generated for this analysis was 1,031 spectra.

Within the strain collection, a model set of 16 *C. jejuni* isolates was used for optimizing spectrum preprocessing methods at levels below the species. Organisms for the model set were selected based on (i) their genetic fingerprints, considering six

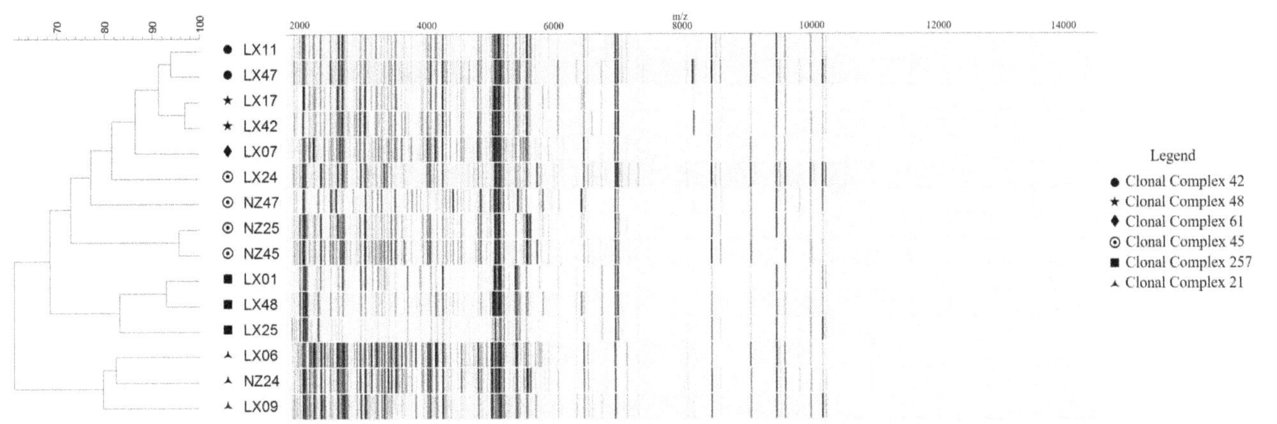

FIGURE 1 | MALDI-TOF MS spectra-based clustering of the *Campylobacter jejuni* reference strain collection conforming to the genetic fingerprints. Spectra are represented as pseudo-gels. Calculations and clustering were obtained using default settings in the BioNumerics 7.1. Genomic profiles are expressed as Clonal Complexes (CC) obtained through the standardized Multi-Locus Sequence Typing (MLST) method of Jolley and Maiden (2010).

TABLE 3 | Effect of MALDI-TOF MS spectrum processing parameters on AMR detection in strains of *C. jejuni.*

Antibiotic resistance group	Preprocessing	Similarity coefficient	Score
1	Default	Dice	89 ± 5
2	Default	Dice	87 ± 6
3	Default	Dice	73 ± 9
4	Default	Dice	93 ± 3
1	Default	Pearson	98 ± 1
2	Default	Pearson	97 ± 3
3	Default	Pearson	100 ± 5
4	Default	Pearson	100 ± 1
1	Default	Ranked	85 ± 14
2	Default	Ranked	73 ± 6
3	Default	Ranked	73 ± 28
4	Default	Ranked	98 ± 2
1	Optimized	Dice	92 ± 5
2	Optimized	Dice	88 ± 7
3	Optimized	Dice	80 ± 9
4	Optimized	Dice	96 ± 3
1	Optimized	Pearson	99 ± 0
2	Optimized	Pearson	98 ± 3
3	Optimized	Pearson	97 ± 5
4	Optimized	Pearson	100 ± 0
1	Optimized	Ranked	97 ± 3
2	Optimized	Ranked	97 ± 4
3	Optimized	Ranked	100 ± 0
4	Optimized	Ranked	100 ± 1

Scores represent mean (±SD) jackknife values calculated using maximum similarities.

major Clonal Complexes (CCs) obtained through MLST analysis and represented by one to four isolates each (with varying host sources and origins), and (ii) their respective MALDI-TOF MS spectrum profiles with regard to shared base peaks and varying degrees of peak intensity (**Figure 1**). For the model set, we utilized three biological replicates with three technical replicates each and generated a total of 144 spectra.

Relying on the example of the model set of isolates (excluding isolate LX-41 whose CC affiliation was not confirmed), it could be demonstrated that MALDI-TOF MS-based clustering of *C. jejuni*, based on peak mass and intensity ranges within the spectrum, was concordant with the genotype profiles expressed as CCs (**Figure 1**). All strains, except two isolates from CC-45, clustered together with their genetically closest neighbors from the same CC. Genetic diversity information on *Campylobacter* isolates could therefore be transcribed through MALDI-TOF MS fingerprinting profiles. This highlighted the potential of mass spectrometry for clonality prediction inside bacterial taxa. Then, characteristic traits such as AMR can individually be screened within each isolate, following optimization in the bioinformatics workflow for spectrum processing and MS-based clustering and typing.

In this context, we subsequently analyzed our model set of *C. jejuni* using the initial designed experiments approach for enhancing AMR detection and strain clustering into their respective groups of AMR (**Table 1**). The parameters for optimization were split into factors and then their individual components were referred to as levels (**Tables 2A,B**). The most optimal combination of the four parameters was found to be the following: (i) Binned Baseline (Bin Size of 77), (ii) Kaiser Window (Window Size of 33), (iii) Moving Bar (Bar Width of 129), and (iv) ranked Pearson similarity coefficient.

Following the model set analysis, these optimized parameters were applied to all spectra from the collection. Increases in rates of correct classification with regard to AMR, when switching from default settings to optimized settings, were observed (**Table 3**). Considering all four groupings of antibiotic-resistant *C. jejuni*, we observed a 5% increase in group 1, a 9% increase in group 2, a 10% increase in group 3, and finally, a 2% increase in group 4. Overall, use of optimized settings yielded a significant 7% increase (t-test, $p = 0.05$) in detection of AMR when compared to use of default settings. In each of the

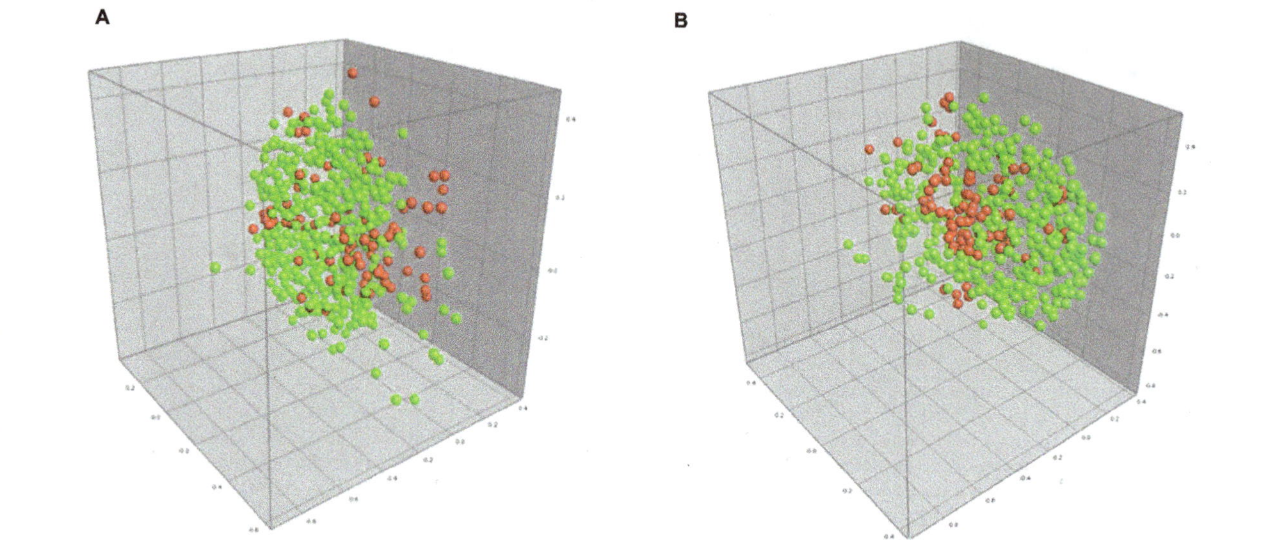

FIGURE 2 | Multidimensional scaling (MDS) representation of MALDI-TOF mass spectra of 172 isolates (516 spectra) of beta-lactam resistant (red) and sensitive (green) strains of *C. jejuni* using (A) default spectrum processing settings and (B) optimized processing settings defined in the designed experiments approach in this study. The ranked Pearson correlation coefficient was used to quantify similarity in both the default and optimized cases.

antibiotic resistance groups, the Pearson correlation coefficient outperformed the Dice similarity coefficient ($p = 0.0002$). In only one instance was there a decrease in the rate of correct classification when using optimized settings. When the settings for group 3 were swapped from default to optimal with the Pearson coefficient, we observed a decrease from 100 to 97% (**Table 3**).

We also performed a direct comparison between default processing settings and the optimized processing settings when applied to isolates exhibiting beta-lactam resistance (**Figure 2**; **Table 4**). The MDS representing optimized parameters shows tighter grouping compared to the default parameter MDS, thus representing an increase in AMR detection, and here specifically beta-lactam resistance. Use of optimized spectrum processing settings increased the rate of correct classification from 63.5 to 95.7%.

DISCUSSION

Workflows to rapidly characterize bacteria using MALDI-TOF MS typically include four components: (i) culturing, (ii) sample preparation, (iii) data acquisition, and (iv) data analysis (Sandrin et al., 2013). Each of the first three components of this common workflow have been shown previously to affect the ability of MALDI-TOF MS to reliably and accurately characterize bacteria at the strain level (Schumaker et al., 2012; Goldstein et al., 2013). Results presented here show clearly that the fourth component of this workflow, data analysis (spectrum processing parameters), affects the ability of MALDI-TOF MS to detect AMR in *C. jejuni*. To our knowledge, this work represents the first report of enhancing MALDI-TOF performance to detect AMR in *C. jejuni* through optimization of spectrum processing parameters.

Designed experiments have been used previously to enhance MALDI-TOF MS-based characterization of bacteria (Zhang et al., 2014). In that work, the third component of the MALDI-TOF MS workflow, data acquisition, was enhanced by systematically adjusting parameters (e.g., threshold base peak, S–N resolution, etc.) in an algorithm commonly used for automated spectrum acquisition. Similar to our work here applying designed experiments to data analysis, Zhang et al. (2014) reported increases in method performance (reproducibility) with optimization afforded by designed experiments. Furthermore, Zhang et al. (2014) reported that optimized data acquisition parameters obtained with one bacterium (*Pseudmonas aeruginosa*) were useful in increasing reproducibility of spectra of other bacteria (*Klebsiella pneumoniae* and *Serratia marcescens*). Further research is warranted to determine whether the optimized settings we identified here to enhance detection of AMR in *C. jejuni*, will enhance detection of AMR in other bacteria. Currently, the necessity for adapting the settings of variables and parameters for each individual microorganism or

TABLE 4 | Optimized spectrum preprocessing parameters enhance beta-lactam-resistance detection in *C. jejuni*.

Preprocessing	Similarity coefficient	Score
Default	Dice	86 ± 5
Default	Pearson	97 ± 3
Default	Ranked	74 ± 18
Optimized	Dice	89 ± 8
Optimized	Pearson	98 ± 2
Optimized	Ranked	98 ± 3

Scores represent mean (±SD) jackknife values calculated using maximum similarities.

taxon is rigorously being evaluated, but in that case optimization is facilitated with the use of the designed experiments approach described here.

Following spectrum processing (i.e., baseline subtraction, smoothing, etc.), the similarity of processed spectra is often quantified using previously described similarity coefficients including the Dice similarity coefficient, the Pearson correlation coefficient, or the ranked Pearson correlation coefficient (Dieckmann et al., 2008; Schmidt et al., 2009; Sandrin et al., 2013). Each of these coefficients has been used previously to compare spectra and characterize diverse bacteria using MALDI-TOF MS. Our work here suggests that the Dice correlation coefficient underperforms in comparison to Pearson correlation coefficients, particularly the ranked Pearson correlation coefficient. This is in accordance with our prior work with *Enterococcus* (Giebel et al., 2008), in which we reported the importance of considering peak intensity information, which is included in the Pearson correlation coefficient calculations but not the Dice coefficient. For this reason, future efforts to detect AMR using MALDI-TOF MS should use correlation coefficients that include peak intensity, such as the Pearson correlation coefficient.

Most likely in complement to current tools for *Campylobacter* fingerprinting, MALDI-TOF MS spectra indeed reflect the genetic diversity (Zautner et al., 2013), but more importantly reflect the actual genetic expression profile and AMR potential of the strain candidates upon isolation and culture. The designed experiments approach described here appears in this way as a convenient bioinformatics tool for the optimization of information retrieval from MALDI-TOF MS spectra. BioNumerics currently represents the most versatile and flexible routinely used software package for screening optimal processing variable values and parameters such as described in **Table 2**.

Within the next steps, further AMR profiling of *Campylobacter* based on MALDI-TOF MS should be undertaken, in order to obtain more complete AMR profiles in the future. Using extended bioinformatics and proteomics tools, AMR signature identification is likely to be pursued, e.g., by characterizing specific beta-lactamase biomarker(s) within the resistant *C. jejuni* mass spectra (Sparbier et al., 2012; Kostrzewa et al., 2013). Here, bottom-up and top-down proteomics approaches could be deployed in order to complement and supplement existing tools (e.g., Fagerquist et al., 2005, 2009; Sandrin et al., 2013). Also, further comparisons with AMR prediction through WGS data or MSPP phyloproteomics screening will certainly be fruitful (Zankari et al., 2012; Zautner et al., 2015).

The features and potential of MALDI-TOF MS will continue to contribute to significant scientific and technological advances in the fields of functional characterization and fingerprinting of microorganisms. As shown here, optimized bioinformatics workflows inside MALDI-TOF MS analysis will, among others, allow enhanced AMR detection for improved decision-making and healthcare through implementation in microbial subspecies typing and diagnostics. It would be interesting to adapt the analysis software inside the routine workflow by adding an AMR detection module fed with the optimized parameter settings for data acquisition, processing, and biomarker screening. Constitution of AMR profiles using *Campylobacter*-specific, sensitive and reproducible analysis parameters, such as those set-up here, will greatly add value to limiting the ongoing emergence of multi-drug resistances in *Campylobacter* sp.

AUTHOR CONTRIBUTIONS

CP, H-MC and TS designed the study. CP, BG, LZ, CB, DB, and TS were responsible for data acquisition and analysis. CP, AC, BG, AL, MJ-R, CR, CK, and WZ contributed to the *C. jejuni* strain collection set-up and the AMR profiling and genetic fingerprinting of the isolates. All authors contributed to the writing and/or critical reviewing of the manuscript, and have approved the manuscript.

ACKNOWLEDGMENTS

William G. Miller from USDA (USA), Stephen L.W. On from Lincoln University (NZ) and J. Mossong from the National Health Laboratory (LNS, Luxembourg) are acknowledged as facilitators of the project consortium constitution and strain collection assembling. We wish to acknowledge the assistance of Mary H. Chapman and Anna H. Bates from USDA. The authors warmly thank Cécile Walczak, Delphine Collard, Angela Tavares Furtado from LIST (Luxembourg) and Regina Diaz from ASU (USA) for technical and experimental support in the study.

REFERENCES

Bae, J., Oh, E., and Jeon, B. (2014). Enhanced transmission of antibiotic resistance in *Campylobacter jejuni* biofilms by natural transformation. *Antimicrob. Agents Chemother.* 58, 7573–7575. doi: 10.1128/AAC.04066-14

Croxatto, A., Prod'hom, G., and Greub, G. (2012). Applications of MALDI-TOF mass spectrometry in clinical diagnostic microbiology. *FEMS Microbiol. Rev.* 36, 380–407. doi: 10.1111/j.1574-6976.2011.00298.x

Didelot, X., Bowden, R., Wilson, D. J., Peto, T. E. A., and Crook, D. W. (2012). Transforming clinical microbiology with bacterial genome sequencing. *Nat. Rev. Genet.* 13, 601–612. doi: 10.1038/nrg3226

Dieckmann, R., Helmuth, R., Erhard, M., and Malorny, B. (2008). Rapid classification and identification of *Salmonellae* at the species and subspecies levels by whole-cell matrix-assisted laser desorption ionization-time of flight mass spectrometry. *Appl. Environ. Microbiol.* 74, 7767–7778. doi: 10.1128/AEM.01402-1408

Fagerquist, C. K., Garbus, B. R., Williams, K. E., Bates, A. H., Boyle, S., and Harden, L. A. (2009). Web-based software for rapid top-down proteomic identification of protein biomarkers, with implications for bacterial identification. *Appl. Environ. Microbiol.* 75, 4341–4353. doi: 10.1128/AEM.00079-79

Fagerquist, C. K., Miller, W. G., Harden, L. A., Bates, A. H., Vensel, W. H., Wang, G., et al. (2005). Genomic and proteomic identification of a DNA-binding protein used in the "fingerprinting" of *Campylobacter* species and strains by MALDI-TOF-MS protein biomarker analysis. *Anal. Chem.* 77, 4897–4907. doi: 10.1021/ac040193z

Freiwald, A., and Sauer, S. (2009). Phylogenetic classification and identification of bacteria by mass spectrometry. *Nat. Protoc.* 4, 732–742. doi: 10.1038/nprot.2009.37

Ge, B., Wang, F., Sjölund-Karlsson, M., and McDermott, P. F. (2013). Antimicrobial resistance in *Campylobacter*: susceptibility testing methods and resistance trends. *J. Microbiol. Methods* 95, 57–67. doi: 10.1016/j.mimet.2013.06.021

Giebel, R. A., Fredenberg, W., and Sandrin, T. R. (2008). Characterization of environmental isolates of *Enterococcus* spp. by matrix-assisted laser desorption/ionization time-of-flight mass spectrometry. *Water Res.* 42, 931–940. doi: 10.1016/j.watres.2007.09.005

Goldstein, J. E., Zhang, L., Borror, C. M., Rago, J. V., and Sandrin, T. R. (2013). Culture conditions and sample preparation methods affect spectrum quality and reproducibility during profiling of *Staphylococcus aureus* with matrix-assisted laser desorption/ionization time-of-flight mass spectrometry. *Lett. Appl. Microbiol.* 57, 144–150. doi: 10.1111/lam.12092

Gorman, R., and Adley, C. C. (2004). An evaluation of five preservation techniques and conventional freezing temperatures of -20°C and -85°C for long-term preservation of *Campylobacter jejuni*. *Lett. Appl. Microbiol.* 38, 306–310. doi: 10.1111/j.1472-765X.2004.01490.x

Hrabák, J., Chudáčková, E., and Walková, R. (2013). Matrix-assisted laser desorption ionization–time of flight (maldi-tof) mass spectrometry for detection of antibiotic resistance mechanisms: from research to routine diagnosis. *Clin. Microbiol. Rev.* 26, 103–114. doi: 10.1128/CMR.00058-12

Iovine, N. M. (2013). Resistance mechanisms in *Campylobacter jejuni*. *Virulence* 4, 230–240. doi: 10.4161/viru.23753

Jolley, K. A., and Maiden, M. C. (2010). BIGSdb: scalable analysis of bacterial genome variation at the population level. *BMC Bioinformatics* 11:595. doi: 10.1186/1471-2105-11-595

Kaakoush, N. O., Castaño-Rodríguez, N., Mitchell, H. M., and Man, S. M. (2015). Global epidemiology of *Campylobacter* infection. *Clin. Microbiol. Rev.* 28, 687–720. doi: 10.1128/CMR.00006-15

Kliem, M., and Sauer, S. (2012). The essence on mass spectrometry based microbial diagnostics. *Curr. Opin. Microbiol.* 15, 397–402. doi: 10.1016/j.mib.2012.02.006

Kostrzewa, M., Sparbier, K., Maier, T., and Schubert, S. (2013). MALDI-TOF MS: an upcoming tool for rapid detection of antibiotic resistance in microorganisms. *Proteomics Clin. Appl.* 7, 767–778. doi: 10.1002/prca.201300042

Koubek, J., Uhlik, O., Jecna, K., Junkova, P., Vrkoslavova, J., Lipov, J., et al. (2012). Whole-cell MALDI-TOF: rapid screening method in environmental microbiology. *Int. Biodeterior. Biodegrad.* 69, 82–86. doi: 10.1016/j.ibiod.2011.12.007

Lartigue, M.-F. (2013). Matrix-assisted laser desorption ionization time-of-flight mass spectrometry for bacterial strain characterization. *Infect. Genet. Evol.* 13, 230–235. doi: 10.1016/j.meegid.2012.10.012

Lastovica, A. J. (2006). Emerging *Campylobacter* spp.: the tip of the iceberg. *Clin. Microbiol. Newsl.* 28, 49–56. doi: 10.1016/j.clinmicnews.2006.03.004

Lastovica, A. J., On, S. L. W., and Zhang, L. (2014). "The Family Campylobacteraceae," in *The Prokaryotes*, eds E. Rosenberg, E. F. DeLong, S. Lory, E. Stackebrandt, and F. Thompson (Heidelberg:Springer), 307–335.

Laxminarayan, R., Duse, A., Wattal, C., Zaidi, A. K. M., Wertheim, H. F. L., Sumpradit, N., et al. (2013). Antibiotic resistance—the need for global solutions. *Lancet Infect. Dis.* 13, 1057–1098. doi: 10.1016/S1473-3099(13)70318-9

Luangtongkum, T., Jeon, B., Han, J., Plummer, P., Logue, C. M., and Zhang, Q. (2009). Antibiotic resistance in *Campylobacter*: emergence, transmission and persistence. *Future Microbiol.* 4, 189–200. doi: 10.2217/17460913.4.2.189

Maloy, S., and Atlas, R. M. (2014). *One Health: People, Animals, and The Environment*. Washington, DC: American Society of Microbiology. doi: 10.1128/9781555818432

Mitchell, M., Mali, S., King, C. C., and Bark, S. J. (2015). Enhancing MALDI time-of-flight mass spectrometer performance through spectrum averaging. *PLoS ONE* 10:e0120932. doi: 10.1371/journal.pone.0120932

Montgomery, D. C. (2012). *Design and Analysis of Experiments*, 8th Edn. Hoboken, NJ: John Wiley.

Payot, S., Bolla, J.-M., Corcoran, D., Fanning, S., Mégraud, F., and Zhang, Q. (2006). Mechanisms of fluoroquinolone and macrolide resistance in *Campylobacter* spp. *Microbes Infect.* 8, 1967–1971. doi: 10.1016/j.micinf.2005.12.032

Pulido, M. R., García-Quintanilla, M., Martín-Peña, R., Cisneros, J. M., and McConnell, M. J. (2013). Progress on the development of rapid methods for antimicrobial susceptibility testing. *J. Antimicrob. Chemother.* 68, 2710–2717. doi: 10.1093/jac/dkt253

Randall, L. P., Lemma, F., Koylass, M., Rogers, J., Ayling, R. D., Worth, D., et al. (2015). Evaluation of MALDI-ToF as a method for the identification of bacteria in the veterinary diagnostic laboratory. *Res. Vet. Sci.* 101, 42–49. doi: 10.1016/j.rvsc.2015.05.018

Sandrin, T. R., Goldstein, J. E., and Schumaker, S. (2013). MALDI TOF MS profiling of bacteria at the strain level: a review. *Mass Spectrom. Rev.* 32, 188–217. doi: 10.1002/mas.21359

Sauer, S., and Kliem, M. (2010). Mass spectrometry tools for the classification and identification of bacteria. *Nat. Rev. Microbiol.* 8, 74–82. doi: 10.1038/nrmicro2243

Schmidt, F., Fiege, T., Hustoft, H. K., Kneist, S., and Thiede, B. (2009). Shotgun mass mapping of *Lactobacillus* species and subspecies from caries related isolates by MALDI-MS. *Proteomics* 9, 1994–2003. doi: 10.1002/pmic.200701028

Schubert, S., and Kostrzewa, M. (2015). "Chapter 14 - MALDI-TOF mass spectrometry in the clinical microbiology laboratory; beyond identification," in *Methods in Microbiology*, Vol. 42, *Current and Emerging Technologies for the Diagnosis of Microbial Infections*, eds A. Sails and Y.-W. Tang (Cambridge, MA: Academic Press), 501–524.

Schumaker, S., Borror, C. M., and Sandrin, T. R. (2012). Automating data acquisition affects mass spectrum quality and reproducibility during bacterial profiling using an intact cell sample preparation method with matrix-assisted laser desorption/ionization time-of-flight mass spectrometry. *Rapid Commun. Mass Spectrom.* 26, 243–253. doi: 10.1002/rcm.5309

Sparbier, K., Schubert, S., Weller, U., Boogen, C., and Kostrzewa, M. (2012). Matrix-assisted laser desorption ionization–time of flight mass spectrometry-based functional assay for rapid detection of resistance against β-lactam antibiotics. *J. Clin. Microbiol.* 50, 927–937. doi: 10.1128/JCM.05737-5711

Wagenaar, J. A., Newell, D. G., Kalupahana, R. S., and Mughini-Gras, L. (2015). "*Campylobacter*: animal reservoirs, human infections, and options for control," in *Zoonoses - Infections Affecting Humans and Animals*, ed. A. Sing (Dordrecht: Springer), 159–177.

Wang, Y., Huang, W. M., and Taylor, D. E. (1993). Cloning and nucleotide sequence of the *Campylobacter jejuni* gyrA gene and characterization of quinolone resistance mutations. *Antimicrob. Agents Chemother.* 37, 457–463. doi: 10.1128/AAC.37.3.457

Welker, M. (2011). Proteomics for routine identification of microorganisms. *Proteomics* 11, 3143–3153. doi: 10.1002/pmic.201100049

Welker, M., and Moore, E. R. B. (2011). Applications of whole-cell matrix-assisted laser-desorption/ionization time-of-flight mass spectrometry in systematic microbiology. *Syst. Appl. Microbiol.* 34, 2–11. doi: 10.1016/j.syapm.2010.11.013

Wieczorek, K., and Osek, J. (2013). Antimicrobial resistance mechanisms among *Campylobacter*. *BioMed Res. Int.* 2013:e340605. doi: 10.1155/2013/340605

Wieser, A., Schneider, L., Jung, J., and Schubert, S. (2011). MALDI-TOF MS in microbiological diagnostics—identification of microorganisms and beyond (mini review). *Appl. Microbiol. Biotechnol.* 93, 965–974. doi: 10.1007/s00253-011-3783-3784

World Health Organization [WHO] (2013). *The Global View of Campylobacteriosis.* Available at: http://www.who.int/foodsafety/publications/campylobacteriosis/en/

Zankari, E., Hasman, H., Cosentino, S., Vestergaard, M., Rasmussen, S., Lund, O., et al. (2012). Identification of acquired antimicrobial resistance genes. *J. Antimicrob. Chemother.* 67, 2640–2644. doi: 10.1093/jac/dks261

Zautner, A. E., Masanta, W. O., Tareen, A. M., Weig, M., Lugert, R., Groß, U., et al. (2013). Discrimination of multilocus sequence typing-based *Campylobacter jejuni* subgroups by MALDI-TOF mass spectrometry. *BMC Microbiol.* 13:247. doi: 10.1186/1471-2180-13-247

Zautner, A. E., Masanta, W. O., Weig, M., Groß, U., and Bader, O. (2015). Mass spectrometry-based PhyloProteomics (MSPP): a novel microbial typing method. *Sci. Rep.* 5:13431. doi: 10.1038/srep13431

Zhang, L., Borror, C. M., and Sandrin, T. R. (2014). A designed experiments approach to optimization of automated data acquisition during characterization of bacteria with MALDI-TOF mass spectrometry. *PLoS ONE* 9:e92720. doi: 10.1371/journal.pone.0092720

Zhao, S., Tyson, G. H., Chen, Y., Li, C., Mukherjee, S., Young, S., et al. (2016). Whole-genome sequencing analysis accurately predicts antimicrobial resistance phenotypes in *Campylobacter* spp. *Appl. Environ. Microbiol.* 82, 459–466. doi: 10.1128/AEM.02873-15

10

Rapid Detection of *Acinetobacter baumannii* and Molecular Epidemiology of Carbapenem-Resistant *A. baumannii* in Two Comprehensive Hospitals of Beijing, China

Puyuan Li[1†], Wenkai Niu[1†], Huan Li[2†], Hong Lei[3], Wei Liu[2], Xiangna Zhao[2], Leijing Guo[1], Dayang Zou[2], Xin Yuan[1], Huiying Liu[1], Jing Yuan[2*] and Changqing Bai[1*]

[1] Department of Respiratory and Critical Care Diseases, 307th Hospital of Chinese People's Liberation Army, Beijing, China, [2] Institute of Disease Control and Prevention, Academy of Military Medical Sciences, Beijing, China, [3] Department of Clinical Laboratory, 309th Hospital of Chinese People's Liberation Army, Beijing, China

***Correspondence:**
*Changqing Bai,
Department of Respiratory and Critical Care Diseases, 307th Hospital of Chinese People's Liberation Army, No. 20 Dongda Street, Fengtai District, Beijing 100071, China
mlp1604@sina.com;
Jing Yuan,
Institute of Disease Control and Prevention, Academy of Military Medical Sciences, No. 20 Dongda Street, Fengtai District, Beijing 100071, China
yuanjing6216@163.com*

† These authors have contributed equally to this work.

Acinetobacter baumannii is an important opportunistic pathogen associated with a variety of nosocomial infections. A rapid and sensitive molecular detection in clinical isolates is quite needed for the appropriate therapy and outbreak control of *A. baumannii*. Group 2 carbapenems have been considered the agents of choice for the treatment of multiple drug-resistant *A. baumannii*. But the prevalence of carbapenem-resistant *A. baumannii* (CRAB) has been steadily increasing in recent years. Here, we developed a loop-mediated isothermal amplification (LAMP) assay for the rapid detection of *A. baumannii* in clinical samples by using high-specificity primers of the $bla_{\text{OXA-51}}$ gene. Then we investigated the OXA-carbapenemases molecular epidemiology of *A. baumannii* isolates in two comprehensive hospitals in Beijing. The results showed that the LAMP assay could detect target DNA within 60 min at 65°C. The detection limit was 50 pg/μl, which was about 10-fold greater than that of PCR. Furthermore, this method could distinguish *A. baumannii* from the homologous *A. nosocomialis* and *A. pittii*. A total of 228 positive isolates were identified by this LAMP-based method for *A. baumannii* from 335 intensive care unit patients with clinically suspected multi-resistant infections in two hospitals in Beijing. The rates of CRAB are on the rise and are slowly becoming a routine phenotype for *A. baumannii.* Among the CRABs, 92.3% harbored both the $bla_{\text{OXA-23}}$ and $bla_{\text{OXA-51}}$ genes. Thirty-three pulsotypes were identified by pulsed-field gel electrophoresis, and the majority belonged to clone C. In conclusion, the LAMP method developed for detecting *A. baumannii* was faster and simpler than conventional PCR and has great potential for both point-of-care testing and basic research. We further demonstrated a high distribution of class D carbapenemase-encoding genes, mainly OXA-23, which presents an emerging threat in hospitals in China.

Keywords: *Acinetobacter baumannii*, LAMP, rapid diagnosis, carbapenem resistance, molecular epidemiology

Introduction

Acinetobacter baumannii is an important opportunistic pathogen associated with a variety of nosocomial infections, such as ventilator-associated pneumonia, central line-associated bloodstream infections, urinary tract infections, surgical-site infections, and other types of wound infections, especially in intensive care units (ICUs; Peleg et al., 2008). This organism is well adapted to hospital environments, being capable of continually spreading to new patients and making itself a nosocomial pathogen of particular clinical concern and a public health threat (Dijkshoorn et al., 2007).

In recent years, multidrug-resistant *A. baumannii* (MDR-AB) isolates have been increasingly reported worldwide. MDR-AB strains are associated with an enhanced risk of mortality and prolonged durations of hospitalization (Kempf and Rolain, 2012; Antunes et al., 2014; Lemos et al., 2014). Carbapenems, mainly imipenem (IPM) and meropenem (MPM), have been used to treat MDR-AB infections (Perez et al., 2007). However, the incidence of carbapenem resistance in *A. baumannii* is growing steadily in China and many other countries (Poirel and Nordmann, 2006; Tiwari et al., 2012a,b). According to the CHINET 2010 year reports, the resistant to IPM and MPM in *A. baumannii* isolates was 62.3% and 63.8%, respectively (Xi et al., 2012). However, few data are available regarding the molecular epidemiology and antibiotic resistance of *A. baumannii* infections in hospitals in Beijing, China.

The accurate and rapid identification of *A. baumannii* is critical for appropriate infection control in hospital settings. To date, the most common and widespread detection methods include characterization via a phenotypic system and commercial phenotypic methods (e.g., the VITEK 2 system [Biomerieux] and the API 20 NE system) or DNA-based testing such as PCR (e.g., 16S rRNA gene amplification), which have been used to successfully identify most *Acinetobacter* species. However, there are some limitations in these methods (Janda and Abbott, 2007; Karah et al., 2011; Álvarez-Buylla et al., 2012). For example, several days are needed for incubation, and the laboratory diagnosis of *A. baumannii* is actually for that of the *A. calcoaceticus–A. baumannii* complex (ABC), which includes *A. calcoaceticus, A. baumannii, A. pittii* (three species), and *A. nosocomialis* (species 13TU; Peleg et al., 2008). These bacterial species are different in terms of symptomatology, dissemination patterns, mechanisms of antibiotic resistance, and epidemiology (Golanbar et al., 2011; Chiang et al., 2012).

The loop-mediated isothermal amplification (LAMP) method, which is based on autocycling strand displacement DNA synthesis in the presence of Bst DNA polymerase, can be used to amplify target DNA with high specificity (as four or six specific primers that recognize six or eight different sequences on the DNA target) under isothermal conditions in less than 60 min (Notomi et al., 2000). LAMP is highly sensitive and able to detect DNA at as few as six copies in the reaction mixture, and less prone to the presence of irrelevant DNA than PCR (Notomi et al., 2000). This novel method has been developed widely for the detection of numerous pathogens, including influenza A subtypes H1N1 (Nakauchi et al., 2011), H5N1 (Dinh et al., 2011), H7N9 (Nakauchi et al., 2014), as well as *Mycoplasma pneumoniae* (Gotoh et al., 2013), *Mycobacterium tuberculosis* (Kumar et al., 2014), severe acute respiratory syndrome virus coronavirus (Poon et al., 2004), and human immunodeficiency virus (Zeng et al., 2014).

In present study, we describe a LAMP method for the rapid detection of *A. baumannii* in clinical samples targeting the bla_{OXA-51} gene, which was based on visual testing. We also investigated molecular-epidemiology and antibiotic-resistance profiles, and detected several common oxacillinase genes from *A. baumannii* isolates obtained at two comprehensive hospitals in Beijing, China.

Materials and Methods

Bacterial Strains, Antimicrobial Susceptibility Testing, and Pulsed-Field Gel Electrophoresis (PFGE)

A total of 34 strains representing 9 *Acinetobacter* species (2 *A. baumannii* strains and 10 other *Acinetobacter* strains) and 22 non-*Acinetobacter* species used in this study to develop the LAMP assays. Three hundred and fifty-five clinical sputum samples and nasopharyngeal swabs were obtained from the ICU hospitalized patients with clinically suspected multi-resistant infections in 307th (Affiliated Hospital of Academy of Military Medical Sciences), and the 309th Hospital of PLA in China. Pertinent information and the source of all strains are listed in **Table 1**. The species identification were identified by the Vitek 2 system (Biomerieux Vitek, Inc., Hazelwood, MO, USA). *A. baumannii* bacteria were grown overnight at 37°C in Luria-Bertani (LB) broth, while non-*Acinetobacter* species were cultured at 37°C in brain heart infusion (BHI) broth overnight.

Antibiotic susceptibility testing was conducted by disk diffusion in accordance with the guidelines of the Clinical and Laboratory Standards Institute and was confirmed by the Vitek 2 System with the following antibiotics: ampicillin, ampicillin/sulbactam, aztreonam, ciprofloxacin, ceftazidime, ceftriaxone, cefepime, gentamycin, levofloxacin, IPM, MPM, piperacillin/tazobactam, piperacillin, tobramycin, and sulfamethoxazole. *Pseudomonas aeruginosa* ATCC 27853 was used as a control.

Genomic DNA was prepared in agarose plugs, and digested with the restriction enzyme *Apa*I (New England BioLabs, Beverly, MA, USA). The DNA restriction fragments were separated using a CHEF-DRIII apparatus (Bio-Rad Laboratories, Richmond, CA, USA). Gel images were analyzed using BioNumerics software, version 6.01 (Applied-Maths, Belgium). The interpretation of gels was performed by visual inspection using the criteria of Tenover et al. (1995).

Preparation of Isolated DNA

Genomic DNA from *Acinetobacter* species was prepared using the boiling method described by Olive and Bean (1999), with some modifications. Briefly, colonies of each isolate were picked from LB plates and suspended in 100 μl of ddH_2O. The bacterial

TABLE 1 | Bacteria strains used in this study.

Bacteria strains	Source	Strain type
***Acinetobacter* species**		
A. baumannii	CGMCC	Reference strain
A. baumannii ATCC 22933	CICC	Reference strain
A. calcoaceticus	CGMCC	Reference strain
A. nosocomialis	CGMCC	Reference strain
A. haemolyticus	CGMCC	Reference strain
A. Pittii	CICC	Reference strain
A. johnsonii	CGMCC	Reference strain
A. junii	CGMCC	Reference strain
A. calcoaceticus	The Microorganism Center[a]	Reference strain
A. lwoffii	The Microorganism Center (three strains)	Reference strain
Non-*Acinetobacter* species		
Bacillus megatherium 4623	The Microorganism Center	Reference strain
Beta-haemolytic streptococcus group A CMCC32213	The Microorganism Center	Reference strain
Bordetella pertussis ATCC 18530	The Microorganism Center	Reference strain
Brucella suis 3572	The Microorganism Center	Reference strain
Corynebacterium diphtheria CMCC38001	The Microorganism Center	Reference strain
Enteropathogenic Escherichia coli 2348	The Microorganism Center	Reference strain
Enterotoxigenic E. coli 44824	The Microorganism Center	Reference strain
E. coli ATCC25922	The Microorganism Center	Reference strain
Mycobacterium tuberculosis 8362	The Microorganism Center	Reference strain
Neisseria meningitides group B CMCC29022	The Microorganism Center	Reference strain
Pseudomonas aeruginosa ATCC27853	The Microorganism Center	Reference strain
Salmonella aberdeen 9264	The Microorganism Center	Reference strain
Salmonella enteritidis 50326-1	The Microorganism Center	Reference strain
Stenotrophomonas maltophilia 3859	The Microorganism Center	Reference strain
Shigella flexneri 4536	The Microorganism Center	Reference strain
Shigella sonnei 2531	The Microorganism Center	Reference strain
Staphylococcus aureus 2740	The Microorganism Center	Reference strain
Vibrio carchariae 5732	The Microorganism Center	Reference strain
Vibrio cholera 3802	The Microorganism Center	Reference strain
Vibrio parahaemolyticus 5474	The Microorganism Center	Reference strain
Yersinia enterocxolitica 1836	The Microorganism Center	Reference strain
Yersinia pestis 2638	The Microorganism Center	Reference strain

CGMCC, China General Microbiological Culture Collection Center; CICC, China Center of Industrial Culture Collection.
[a]*The Microorganism Center of the Institute of Disease Control and Prevention of the Academy of Military Medical Sciences.*

suspensions were boiled at 95°C for 15 min, centrifuged at 12,000 rpm for 5 min, and the supernatants were collected and transferred to fresh Eppendorf tubes as templates for use in LAMP and PCR assays. To determine the sensitivity and specificity of the LAMP assays, bacterial genomic DNA was extracted from *A. baumannii* using the Wizard® Genomic DNA Purification Kit A1125 (Promega, Madison, WI, USA). The DNA concentration was measured by using OD260 measurements (ND-1000 spectrophotometer, NanoDrop Technologies, Inc, Wilmington, DE, USA) and prepared by serial 10-fold dilutions to yield concentrations ranging from 500 ng/μl to 0.05 pg/μl.

Primer Design for LAMP Assay

The sequence of bla_{OXA-51} (GenBank No. DQ385606.1) was downloaded from the NCBI GenBank database and used to design bla_{OXA-51}-specific LAMP primers. The sequence was further analyzed by Primer Explorer software (version 4; http://www.primerexplorer.jp/lamp/), and five sets of primers were designed, including the outer forward primer (F3), the outer backward primer (B3), the forward inner primer (FIP), the backward inner primer (BIP), and additional loop primers (loops F and B), as shown in **Table 2**.

LAMP Reaction and Product Detection

LAMP reactions were performed in a total volume of 25 μl and contained 12.5 μl reaction mixtures (DNA Amplification Kit; Eiken Chemical Co., Ltd., Tochigi, Japan), 2.6 μl primer mixture (40 pmol for FIP and BIP, 20 pmol for LF and LB, and 5 pmol for F3 and B3), and 1 μl of *Bst* polymerase (eight units, New England BioLabs, Ipswich, MA, USA). Finally, 1-μl DNA of genomic template DNA (the concentration is above 50 ng/μl) was added to the reaction tubes. Reaction was performed in a LA-320CE instrument (Eiken Chemical Co., Ltd., Tochigi, Japan) at 65°C for 60 min and stopped by heating to 80°C for 5 min, according

TABLE 2 | Sequence of primers used for specific amplification of $bla_{OXA-51-like}$ and the OXA carbapenemases PCR detection.

Primer	Primer type	Sequence (5′–3′)
OXA-4F3	Forward outer	CTTATATAGTGACTGCTAATCCAA
OXA-4B3	Backward outer	ATTAAGCATTTTGAAGGTCGA
OXA-4FIP	Forward inner	ACCCGTAGTGTGTACTTCGTTAA ATTTTTACAGCGCTTCAAAATCTGA
OXA-4BIP	Backward inner	TTAGTTATCCAACAAGGCCAAACTT TTTAGCAGGTACATACTCGGTC
OXA-4LB	Loop forward	AAAGCTATGGTAATGATCTTGCTCG
$bla_{OXA-23-F}$	Forward	ATGAATAAATATTTTTACTTG
$bla_{OXA-23-R}$	Reverse	TTAAATAATATTCAGCTGTT
$bla_{OXA-24-F}$	Forward	ATGAAAAAAATTTATACTTCCT ATATTCAGC
$bla_{OXA-24-R}$	Reverse	TTAAATGATTCCAAGATTTTCTAGC
$bla_{OXA-51-like-F}$	Forward	TAATGCTTTGATCGGCCTTG
$bla_{OXA-51-like-R}$	Reverse	CTATAAAATACCTAATTKTTCTAA
$bla_{OXA-58-F}$	Forward	ATGAAATTATTAAAAATATTGAGT
$bla_{OXA-58-R}$	Reverse	ATAAATAATGAAAAACACCCAA

to the manufacturer's instructions. The LA-320CE instrument can monitor the turbidity of real-time LAMP products through spectrophotometric analysis by recording the optical density at 650 nm every 6 s with the help of a Loopamp real-time turbidimeter. In addition, a visual color-change detection method was employed. Briefly, 1 μl of fluorescence-detection reagent (Eiken Chemical Co., Ltd., Tochigi, Japan) was added to each 25 μl LAMP-reaction mixture prior to initiating the reactions. Positive reactions were identified by a green color change, while negative reactions remained orange in color. The color change could be observed by the naked eye under natural light, or with the aid of ultraviolet light excitation at 365 nm.

To compare the sensitivity and specificity of LAMP with PCR, normal PCR reactions were performed using the $bla_{OXA-51-like-F}$ and $bla_{OXA-51-like-R}$ primers (**Table 2**). The primers were synthesized commercially by Sangon Biotech Co., Ltd. (Beijing, China). PCR was performed as described previously (Kuo et al., 2012).

PCR Detection of Carbapenemase Genes

The class D OXA carbapenemases of *Acinetobacter* sp. are represented by 4 main phylogenetic subgroups: OXA-23-like, OXA-24-like, OXA-51-like, and OXA-58. The primers used for detecting these genes by PCR are listed in **Table 2**. PCR was performed in a 25-μl reaction mixtures containing 12.5 μl PCR Master Mix Reagent (Tiangen Biotech Co., Ltd., Beijing, China); 1 μl of forward primer (10 pmol), 1 μl of reverse primer (10 pmol), and 1 μl of DNA template. Reaction mixtures were initially heated to 94°C for 5 min, followed by 30 cycles at 94°C for 30 s, 55°C for 30 s, and 72°C for 90 s. The final extension step was performed at 72°C for 7 min. The PCR-amplified products were analyzed by 1% agarose gel electrophoresis and stained with ethidium bromide. Images were acquired using a Bio-Rad Gel Doc EQ imaging system.

Results

Optimization of the LAMP Assay Targeting $bla_{OXA-51-like}$

Five sets of different primers were initially tested for detection of the $bla_{OXA-51-like}$ gene, and the primers for *pga*D gene of *A. baumannii* were added as a control (Wang et al., 2013). Four of the five primer sets enabled successful amplification (**Figure 1**). The OXA-4 primer set amplified the target sequence within the shortest time and was, therefore, chosen as the optimal primer set (**Table 2**).

Reaction temperatures ranging from 55 to 69°C at a 2°C intervals were compared to determine optimal amplification conditions. The amplification efficiency was highest at 65°C (**Figure 2**) and was, therefore, used in subsequent experiments.

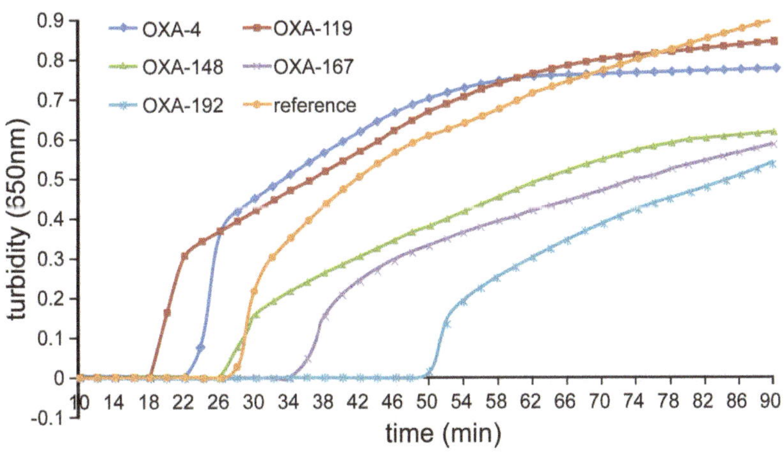

FIGURE 1 | Five sets of primers were used to amplify the indicated target genes of *Acinetobacter baumannii* under the same conditions. Turbidity was monitored using a Loopamp real-time turbidimeter by measuring the absorbance at 650 nm every 6 s. The OXA-4 primer set was chosen as the most appropriate primers for the rapid detection of *A. baumannii*.

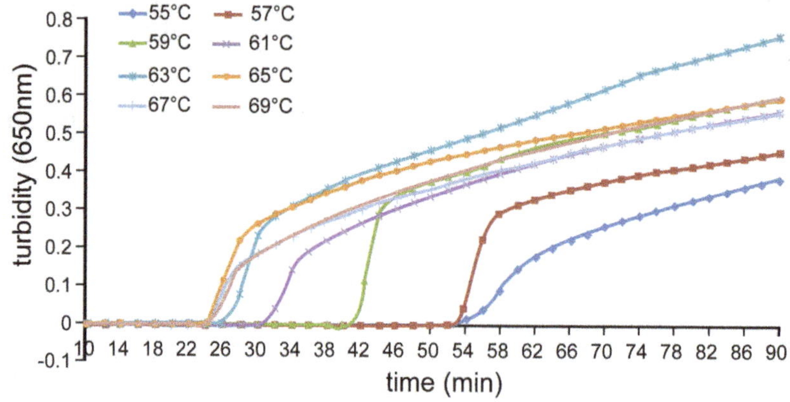

FIGURE 2 | Effect of differing temperatures on the efficiency of detection of *A. baumannii* by loop-mediated isothermal amplification (LAMP). Turbidity was monitored using a Loopamp real-time turbidimeter by measuring the absorbance at 650 nm every 6 s.

Specificity and Sensitivity of the LAMP Assay

To evaluate the specificity of LAMP detection for *A. baumannii*, genomic DNA was extracted from 2 *A. baumannii* strains, as well as other 7 *Acinetobacter* species (10 strains) and 22 non-*A. baumannii* reference strains, and tested using real-time turbidity or visual detection of color changes as readouts. Genomic *A. baumannii* DNA (ATCC 22933) and distilled water were used as positive and negative controls, respectively. As shown in **Figure 3**, both methods of analysis positively identified the *A. baumannii* isolates. All other strains (as well as the blank control) tested negatively, indicating that the LAMP assay was specific for *A. baumannii*. Interestingly, the LAMP assay could differentiate *A. baumannii* from other *Acinetobacter* species.

To compare the detection limit of traditional PCR with that of LAMP using either real-time turbidity or color-change measurements, 10-fold serial dilutions (50 ng/μl–5 pg/μl) were tested using genomic DNA extracted from *A. baumannii* ATCC 22933. As shown in **Figure 4**, the detection limits of real-time turbidity and visual detection were both 50 pg/μl, which was 10-fold more sensitive than traditional PCR assay.

Detection of *A. baumannii* in Clinical Samples

A total of 355 clinical sputum samples and nasopharyngeal swabs were collected for LAMP-based surveillance of $bla_{OXA-51-like}$ from ICU patients suspected of having multidrug-resistant infections in two hospitals in Beijing, China. Ten pairs of sputum samples and nasopharyngeal swabs from healthy people were collected as controls. All clinical samples were simultaneously analyzed by LAMP and PCR. Of the 355 clinical samples, the LAMP assay detected 228 positive samples and 127 negative samples, while the PCR assay detected 221 positive samples, and 134 negative samples. Then, *A. baumannii* was successfully cultured from all 228 samples that were positively identified by LAMP. Samples from the healthy control subjects all tested negatively by LAMP and PCR. The LAMP assay showed 100% specificity compared to 91.89% by PCR assay. Thus, the results

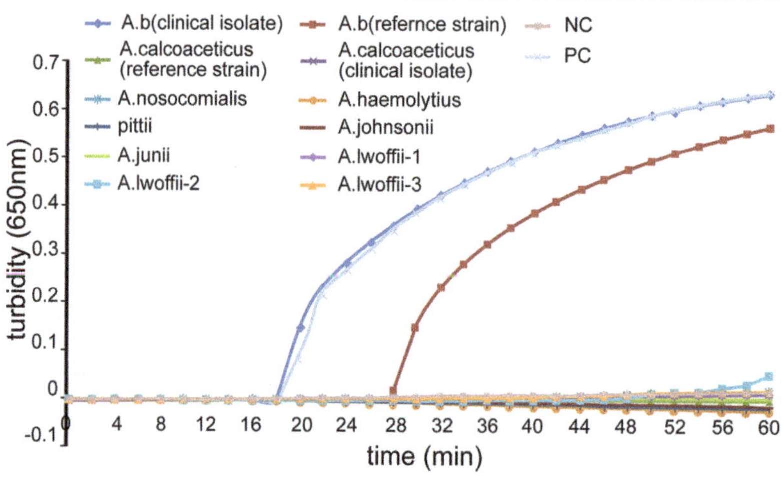

FIGURE 3 | Specificity of the LAMP reactions in detecting the $bla_{OXA-51-like}$ gene. Turbidity was monitored using a Loopamp real-time turbidimeter by measuring the absorbance at 650 nm every 6 s. Amplification was performed at 65°C for 60 min.

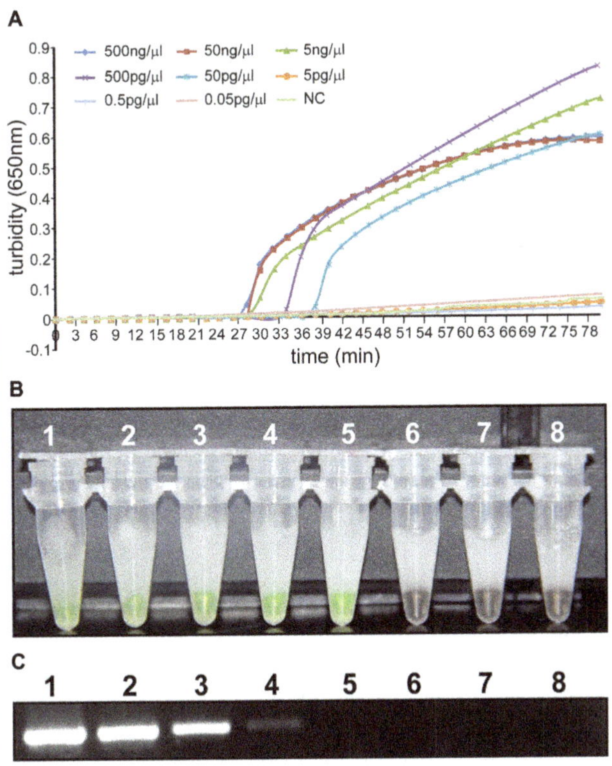

FIGURE 4 | Sensitivity of the LAMP reaction and PCR for detection of the *bla*$_{OXA-51-like}$ gene. Genomic DNA was diluted in a set of serial 10-fold dilutions. Both LAMP reactions **(A,B)** and PCR **(C)** were performed in duplicate for each dilution. Tubes and lanes: 1: 500 ng/µl, 2: 50 ng/µl, 3: 5 ng/µl, 4: 500 pg/µl, 5: 50 pg/µl, 6: 5 pg/µl, 7: 0.5 pg/µl, 8: 0.05 pg/µl. **(A)** Turbidity was monitored using a Loopamp real-time turbidimeter by measuring the absorbance at 650 nm every 6 s. **(B)** The direct visual method for the detection of LAMP. One microliter of fluorescent detection reagent was added to 25 µl of LAMP reaction mixture before the LAMP reactions were initiated. **(C)** PCR products were separated by 1% agarose gel electrophoresis and stained with ethidium bromide.

showed the LAMP assays were more sensitive and specific than PCR for the diagnosis of *A. baumannii* in clinical samples.

Antibiotic Susceptibility and Oxacillinase Distribution

A total of 228 clinical *A. baumannii* isolates were characterized by antibiotic susceptibility testing using both the VITEK®2 system and disk diffusion. Resistance rates were very high, with nearly 90% isolates being resistant to ampicillin, 68.2% being MDR-AB, 66.5% being resistant to IPM, and 63.6% being resistant to MPM.

Among all 145 isolates resistant to both IPM and MPM, 100% harbored the *bla*$_{OXA-51-like}$ gene, 92.3% (134 strains) co-occurred with the *bla*$_{OXA-23}$ gene, 1 isolate carrying both the *bla*$_{OXA-51-like}$ gene and *bla*$_{OXA-58}$ gene, and no isolate carried the *bla*$_{OXA-24}$ gene. Ten isolates were negative for the tested plasmid-mediated OXA-carbapenemase genes.

We also investigated the presence of the *bla*$_{OXA-51-like}$ gene in *A. baumannii* isolates susceptible to carbapenem treatment. All of these isolates harbored the naturally occurring *bla*$_{OXA-51-like}$ gene, making it an excellent candidate for the identification of *Acinetobacter* species.

Molecular Epidemiology of Carbapenem-Resistant *A. baumannii*

Forty-one out of 145 carbapenem-resistant *A. baumannii* isolates were analyzed by PFGE. Genomic DNA digested with *Apa*I showing similar patterns were designated as the same type, and those with 1–3 different bands compared with this type were designated as subtypes. Digested DNA with >3 different bands compared with one type were designated as other types. Bionumerisc software V6.01 was used to perform cluster analysis of these data.

A total of 33 PFGE-banding types were identified, suggesting a diverse population of *A. baumannii* rather than the spread of a specific clone. According to the dice similarity index (80%), these types could be clustered into eight distinct PFGE patterns (clones A–H), and clone C was the dominant clone with 24 isolates (**Figure 5**). Clinical isolates with PFGE-banding type 18 (PF-18) represented the dominant epidemic strain in the ICU during the testing period.

Discussion

Carbapenems including IPM and MPM are used as a last resort for treating MDR-AB. The incidence of carbapenem resistance in *A. baumannii* has increased steadily over the past decade and now represents a global problem. The Meropenem Yearly Susceptibility Test Information Collection program revealed a considerable worldwide increase in IPM and MPM resistance rates, which increased from 10 and 35% in 1999 to 47.9 and 57.4% in 2008, respectively (Rhomberg and Jones, 2009). Similarly, the SENTRY program documented an overall increase in IPM resistance from 34.5% in 2006 to 59.8% in 2009 (Gales et al., 2011). In the USA and Europe, carbapenem resistance accounted for 65% of *A. baumannii*-related pneumonia in 2012 (Farrell et al., 2014). In Asia, more than 60% of *A. baumannii* isolates causing hospital-acquired pneumonia were pan-resistant bacteria and resistant to carbapenem (Zarrilli et al., 2013; Tiwari and Moganty, 2014).

In this study, we observed that 66.5% (152 strains) or 63.6% (145 strains) of test isolates were resistant to IPM or MPM, respectively. The 228 clinical *A. baumannii* isolates were mainly collected from the ICUs of two hospitals; thus, the incidence of carbapenem resistance in *A. baumannii* was relatively high. Prolonged hospitalization, invasive medical procedures, and the prior use of broad-spectrum antibiotics (third-generation cephalosporins and fluoroquinolones) are risk factors for the acquisition of MDR-AB (Karageorgopoulos and Falagas, 2008). These findings indicated that treatment with carbapenem may potentially induce carbapenem resistance.

During PFGE analysis, 33 PFGE-banding patterns were identified and classified into 8 distinct clones, based on Tenover's criteria (Tenover et al., 1995). Clone C was the dominant clone, making it possibly responsible for the *A. baumannii* epidemic in the ICUs of the two comprehensive hospitals

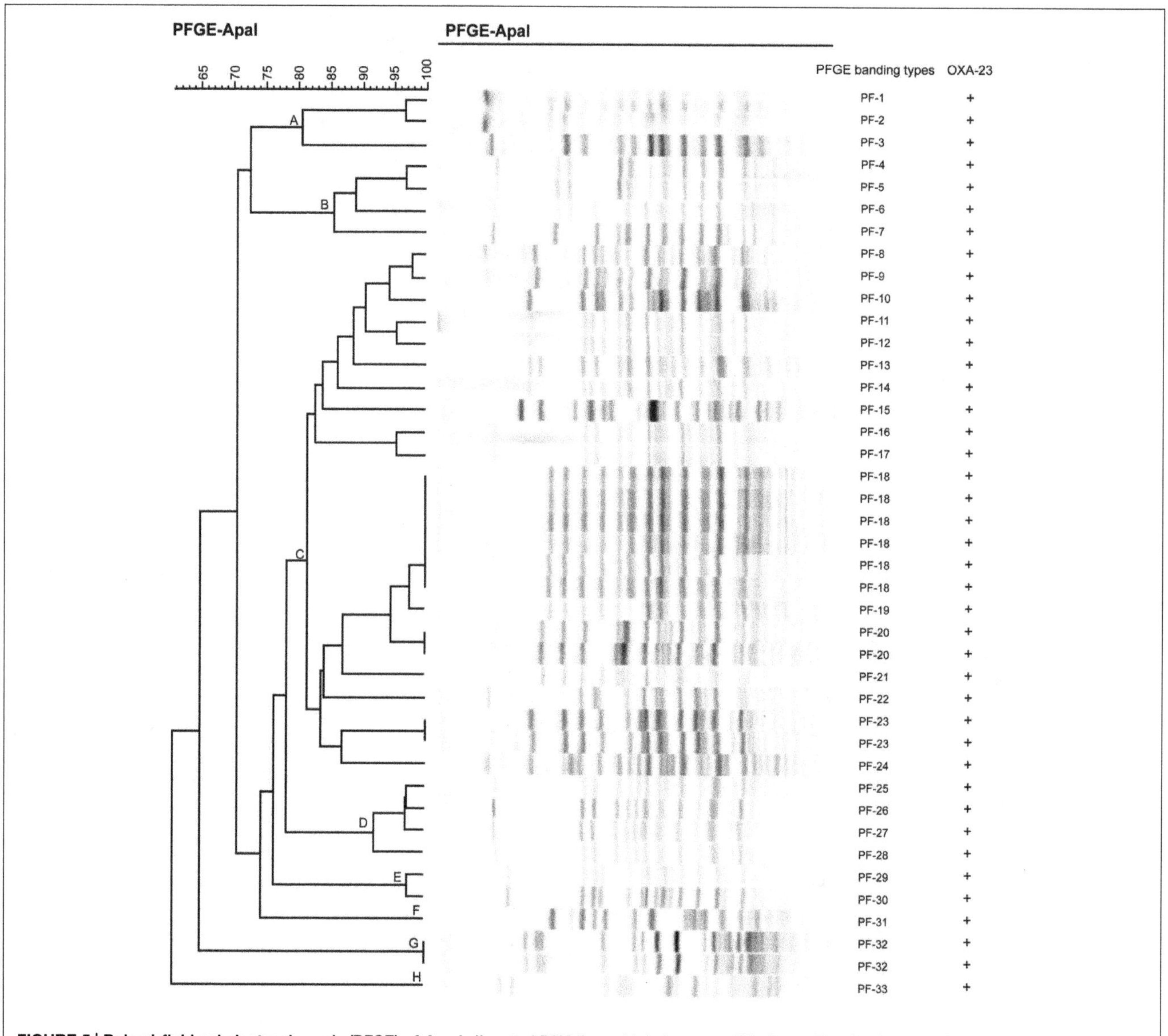

FIGURE 5 | Pulsed-field gel electrophoresis (PFGE) of *Apa* I-digested DNA from 41 *A. baumannii* isolates. The dendrogram shown was generated via the unweighted pair-group method using arithmetic averages approach, based on Dice similarity coefficients that were determined using BioNumerics software, V6.01.

from which we obtained the isolates. Clinical isolates of subtype PF-18 represented the main epidemic strain during the testing period. Previous results have demonstrated that carbapenem-resistant *A. baumannii* isolates showing the same PFGE patterns possess the same carbapenemase-associated genes (Yan et al., 2010; Park et al., 2012); however, our results were not consistent with these observations. Three isolates carrying only the $bla_{\text{OXA}-51-\text{like}}$ gene, but not the $bla_{\text{OXA}-23}$ gene, were grouped into different clones. However, isolates carrying both the $bla_{\text{OXA}-51-\text{like}}$ gene and the $bla_{\text{OXA}-23}$ gene were clustered into distinct clones, either. This may be due to the complicated resistance mechanism that underlies carbapenem resistance in *A. baumannii*.

Carbapenem susceptibility in *A. baumannii* is compromised by a variety of mechanisms. By far the most common mechanism are carbapenemases (Pogue et al., 2013). Carbapenem-hydrolyzing class D β-lactamases (CHDLs, Ambler class D), also known as oxacillinases, are the most common mediator of carbapenem resistance in *A. baumannii* (Poirel and Nordmann, 2006), although they are relatively inefficient compared with other types of carbapenemases, such as class B metallo-β-lactamases (MBLs; Ambler class B) represented by the VIM, IMP, SIM families, and the recently discovered New Delhi metallo-β-lactamase (NDM).

Among CHDLs in *A. baumannii*, there are four major distinct groups, including OXA-23, OXA-24, OXA-51-like, and OXA-58, which are encoded by the $bla_{\text{OXA}-23}$, $bla_{\text{OXA}-24}$, $bla_{\text{OXA}-51-\text{like}}$, and $bla_{\text{OXA}-58}$ genes, respectively (Poirel and Nordmann, 2006; Zavascki et al., 2010). The $bla_{\text{OXA}-23}$ gene has been reported in *A. baumannii* isolates worldwide and is mediated both by chromosomal integration and plasmids. The bla_{OXA-24} gene can also be localized to chromosomes or plasmids, appears to be less widespread than the bla_{OXA-23} gene, and is relatively rare in China (Poirel et al., 2010). The chromosomally located $bla_{OXA-51-like}$ gene is unique and naturally occurring in *A. baumannii*; thus, this gene is becoming an important genetic marker for the identification of organisms at the species level (Turton et al., 2006,). The plasmid-mediated bla_{OXA-58} gene has been reported in *Acinetobacter* sp. from many countries around the world, but is rare in China.

In this research, we found that in all the 145 CRAB isolates, the co-occurrence of $bla_{OXA-51-like}$ gene and bla_{OXA-23} gene could be detected in 134 isolates (92.3%). This result indicated that the plasmid-mediated transfer of bla_{OXA-23} gene might be the most common mechanism by which *A. baumannii* becomes carbapenem resistance in these two comprehensive military hospitals in Beijing. Although the bla_{OXA-58} gene and bla_{OXA-24} gene have been reported in many countries, but the prevalence of these two genes is relatively rare in China. That could be explained that only one isolate carried the bla_{OXA-58} gene and no bla_{OXA-24} gene was detected in the CRAB isolates. However, 10 isolates could detect none of the plasmid-mediated OXA-carbapenemase genes including bla_{OXA-23}, bla_{OXA-24} and bla_{OXA-58}, which indicated that these isolates might harbored other resistant genes such as MBLs against carbapenem. These data are consistent with other reports from China and other countries (Turton et al., 2006; Woodford et al., 2006; Zavascki et al., 2010; Tiwari et al., 2012a).

In the conventional PCR assay, the $bla_{OXA-51-like}$ gene could not be amplified from seven clinical isolates. We thought that the low bacterial contents and incorrect pathogen identification may account for the failure to amplify these samples. Thus, the seven strains were analyzed for the presence of the $bla_{OXA-51-like}$ gene by the LAMP method described here, yielding positive results in each case, which was confirmed using the Vitek 2 system. Our results showed that these clinical isolates were actually *A. baumannii*. These results suggest that occasionally the sensitivity of conventional PCR is not satisfactory and may introduce errors into diagnostic test results.

Compared with traditional methods for pathogen diagnosis, LAMP assays can generate results more easily and rapidly, with high sensitivity and specificity (Notomi et al., 2000). The LAMP reaction does not require temperature cycling, with just a temperature-controlled water bath or a constant-temperature environment being sufficient. LAMP primers are designed to match four or six of the six or eight independent target-sequence regions, so the specificity and sensitivity are enhanced greatly. Under optimum conditions, the LAMP reaction can be completed in 1 h. In this study, we described a LAMP assay based on the $bla_{OXA-51-like}$ gene for detecting *A. baumannii*. This LAMP method could detect the target DNA within 60 min at an isothermal temperature of 65°C. The detection limit of the LAMP assay was 50 pg/μl, which was about 10-fold greater than that of PCR. Furthermore, the LAMP method described here could distinguish *A. baumannii* from *A. nosocomialis* (genospecies 13TU), *A. pittii* (genospecies 3), and the *A. Baumannii* complex (*A. baumannii*, *A. nosocomialis*, *A. pittii*, and *A. calcoaceticus*). Previously, there were two reports on the use of an *A. baumannii* LAMP assay, based on targeting the 16S-23S rRNA intergenic spacer sequence (Soo et al., 2013) and the conserved regions of the *pga*D gene of *A. baumannii* (Wang et al., 2013). However, the former could not effectively distinguish *A. baumannii* from *A. nosocomialis*, and *A. pittii*, and the specificity of *A. baumannii* LAMP assay of the latter was only 75%.

Conclusion

A rapid, sensitive, specific, and effective LAMP assay was established for the detection of *A. baumannii*. The LAMP assay will be very useful for the rapid detection of pathogens in clinical samples. Meanwhile, this report provides some therapeutic recommendations for the treatment of *A. baumannii* infection and a warning that the growing emergence of carbapenem-resistant *A. baumannii* has led to an inadequacy of therapeutic choices in treating MDR-AB infections among patients in China. Our findings further emphasize that when investigating outbreaks caused by carbapenem-resistant *A. baumannii*, both the detection of carbapenemase-associated genes and PFGE are needed.

Author Contributions

Puyuan Li and Wenkai Niu wrote the main manuscript text. Puyuan Li, Huan Li, and Wei Liu prepared **Figures 1–4**. Leijing Guo prepared **Figure 5**. Puyuan Li, Wenkai Niu, Hong Lei, Xiangna Zhao, Dayang Zou, Xin Yuan, and Huiying Liu executed the experiments. Changqing Bai and Jing Yuan helped conceive the project and designed the experiments. All authors reviewed the manuscript.

Funding

This project was supported by the Beijing Natural Science Foundation (Grant No.7142118), a Translational Medicine Project from the Academy of Military Medical Science in 2013, Mega-projects of Science and Technology Research of China Grant 2013ZX10004-203, and Capital Characteristic Clinic project of Beijing (Z121107001012127).

Acknowledgments

We thank the 309th Hospital of PLA and Institute of Disease Control and Prevention, Academy of Military Medical Sciences for kindly providing clinical isolates and reference strains. We are grateful to Yin Xiuyun from the Department of Clinical Laboratory of the 307th Hospital of PLA for performing the collection of isolates. The analysis of PFGE by Wang Jian from the Institute of Disease Control and Prevention, Academy of Military Medical Sciences (Beijing, China) is gratefully appreciated. We also thank Wei Xiao, Cui Qian, Yang Zhan, Yan Xiabei, and Dong Derong for assistance during the course of this research.

References

Álvarez-Buylla, A., Culebras, E., and Picazo, J. J. (2012). Identification of *Acinetobacter* species: is Bruker biotyper MALDI-TOF mass spectrometry a good alternative to molecular techniques? *Infect. Genet. Evol.* 12, 345–349. doi: 10.1016/j.meegid.2012.01.002

Antunes, L., Visca, P., and Towner, K. J. (2014). *Acinetobacter baumannii*: evolution of a global pathogen. *Pathog. Dis.* 71, 292–301. doi: 10.1111/2049-632X.12125

Chiang, M.-C., Kuo, S.-C., Chen, S.-J., Yang, S.-P., Lee, Y.-T., Chen, T.-L., et al. (2012). Clinical characteristics and outcomes of bacteremia due to different genomic species of *Acinetobacter baumannii* complex in patients with solid tumors. *Infection* 40, 19–26. doi: 10.1007/s15010-011-0187-4

Dijkshoorn, L., Nemec, A., and Seifert, H. (2007). An increasing threat in hospitals: multidrug-resistant *Acinetobacter baumannii*. *Nat. Rev. Microbiol.* 5, 939–951. doi: 10.1038/nrmicro1789

Dinh, D. T., Le, M. T. Q., Vuong, C. D., Hasebe, F., and Morita, K. (2011). An updated loop-mediated isothermal amplification method for rapid diagnosis of H5N1 Avian Influenza Viruses. *Trop. Med. Health* 39, 3–7. doi: 10.2149/tmh.2010-21

Farrell, D. J., Sader, H. S., Flamm, R. K., and Jones, R. N. (2014). Ceftolozane/tazobactam activity tested against Gram-negative bacterial isolates from hospitalised patients with pneumonia in US and European medical centres (2012). *Int. J. Antimicrob. Agents* 43, 533–539. doi: 10.1016/j.ijantimicag.2014.01.032

Gales, A. C., Jones, R. N., and Sader, H. S. (2011). Contemporary activity of colistin and polymyxin B against a worldwide collection of Gram-negative pathogens: results from the SENTRY Antimicrobial Surveillance Program (2006–09). *J. Antimicrob. Chemother.* 66, 2070–2074. doi: 10.1093/jac/dkr239

Golanbar, G. D., Lam, C. K., Chu, Y.-M., Cueva, C., Tan, S. W., Silva, I., et al. (2011). Phenotypic and molecular characterization of *Acinetobacter* clinical isolates obtained from inmates of California correctional facilities. *J. Clin. Microbiol.* 49, 2121–2131. doi: 10.1093/jac/dkr239

Gotoh, K., Nishimura, N., Takeuchi, S., Hattori, F., Horiba, K., Isaji, M., et al. (2013). Assessment of the loop-mediated isothermal amplification assay for rapid diagnosis of *Mycoplasma pneumoniae* in pediatric community-acquired pneumonia. *Jpn. J. Infect. Dis.* 66, 539–542. doi: 10.1007/s10156-012-0388-5

Janda, J. M., and Abbott, S. L. (2007). 16S rRNA gene sequencing for bacterial identification in the diagnostic laboratory: pluses, perils, and pitfalls. *J. Clin. Microbiol.* 45, 2761–2764. doi: 10.1128/jcm.01228-07

Karageorgopoulos, D. E., and Falagas, M. E. (2008). Current control and treatment of multidrug-resistant *Acinetobacter baumannii* infections. *Lancet Infect. Dis.* 8, 751–762. doi: 10.1016/S1473-3099(08)70279-2

Karah, N., Haldorsen, B., Hegstad, K., Simonsen, G. S., Sundsfjord, A., Samuelsen, Ø, et al. (2011). Species identification and molecular characterization of *Acinetobacter* spp. blood culture isolates from Norway. *J. Antimicrob. Chemother.* 66, 738–744. doi: 10.1093/jac/dkq521

Kempf, M., and Rolain, J.-M. (2012). Emergence of resistance to carbapenems in *Acinetobacter baumannii* in Europe: clinical impact and therapeutic options. *Int. J. Antimicrob. Agents* 39, 105–114. doi: 10.1016/j.ijantimicag.2011.10.004

Kumar, P., Pandya, D., Singh, N., Behera, D., Aggarwal, P., and Singh, S. (2014). Loop-mediated isothermal amplification assay for rapid and sensitive diagnosis of tuberculosis. *J. Infect.* 69, 607–615. doi: 10.1016/j.jinf.2014.08.017

Kuo, H. Y., Chang, K. C., Kuo, J. W., Yueh, H. W., and Liou, M. L. (2012). Imipenem: a potent inducer of multidrug resistance in *Acinetobacter baumannii*. *Int. J. Antimicrob. Agents* 39, 33–38. doi: 10.1016/j.ijantimicag.2011.08.016

Lemos, E., de la Hoz, F., Einarson, T., McGhan, W., Quevedo, E., Castañeda, C., et al. (2014). Carbapenem resistance and mortality in patients with *Acinetobacter baumannii* infection: systematic review and meta-analysis. *Clin. Microbiol. Infect.* 20, 416–423. doi: 10.1111/1469-0691.12363

Nakauchi, M., Takayama, I., Takahashi, H., Tashiro, M., and Kageyama, T. (2014). Development of a reverse transcription loop-mediated isothermal amplification assay for the rapid diagnosis of avian influenza A (H7N9) virus infection. *J. Virol. Methods* 204, 101–104. doi: 10.1016/j.jviromet.2014.03.028

Nakauchi, M., Yoshikawa, T., Nakai, H., Sugata, K., Yoshikawa, A., Asano, Y., et al. (2011). Evaluation of reverse transcription loop-mediated isothermal amplification assays for rapid diagnosis of pandemic influenza A/H1N1 2009 virus. *J. Med. Virol.* 83, 10–15. doi: 10.1002/jmv.21934

Notomi, T., Okayama, H., Masubuchi, H., Yonekawa, T., Watanabe, K., Amino, N., et al. (2000). Loop-mediated isothermal amplification of DNA. *Nucleic Acids Res.* 28, E63. doi: 10.1093/nar/28.12.e63

Olive, D. M., and Bean, P. (1999). Principles and applications of methods for DNA-based typing of microbial organisms. *J. Clin. Microbiol.* 37, 1661–1669.

Park, Y. K., Jung, S.-I., Park, K.-H., Kim, S. H., and Ko, K. S. (2012). Characteristics of carbapenem-resistant *Acinetobacter* spp. other than *Acinetobacter baumannii* in South Korea. *Int. J. Antimicrob. Agents* 39, 81–85. doi: 10.1016/j.ijantimicag.2011.08.006

Peleg, A. Y., Seifert, H., and Paterson, D. L. (2008). *Acinetobacter baumannii*: emergence of a successful pathogen. *Clin. Microbiol. Rev.* 21, 538–582. doi: 10.1128/CMR.00058-07

Perez, F., Hujer, A. M., Hujer, K. M., Decker, B. K., Rather, P. N., and Bonomo, R. A. (2007). Global challenge of multidrug-resistant *Acinetobacter baumannii*. *Antimicrob. Agents Chemother.* 51, 3471–3484. doi: 10.1128/aac.01464-06

Pogue, J. M., Mann, T., Barber, K. E., and Kaye, K. S. (2013). Carbapenem-resistant *Acinetobacter baumannii*: epidemiology, surveillance and management. *Expert Rev. Anti Infect. Ther.* 11, 383–393. doi: 10.1586/eri.13.14

Poirel, L., Naas, T., and Nordmann, P. (2010). Diversity, epidemiology, and genetics of class D beta-lactamases. *Antimicrob. Agents Chemother.* 54, 24–38. doi: 10.1128/AAC.01512-08

Poirel, L., and Nordmann, P. (2006). Carbapenem resistance in *Acinetobacter baumannii*: mechanisms and epidemiology. *Clin. Microbiol. Infect.* 12, 826–836. doi: 10.1111/j.1469-0691.2006.01456.x

Poon, L. L., Leung, C. S., Tashiro, M., Chan, K. H., Wong, B. W., Yuen, K. Y., et al. (2004). Rapid detection of the severe acute respiratory syndrome (SARS) coronavirus by a loop-mediated isothermal amplification assay. *Clin. Chem.* 50, 1050–1052. doi: 10.1373/clinchem.2004.032011

Rhomberg, P. R., and Jones, R. N. (2009). Summary trends for the meropenem yearly susceptibility test information collection program: a 10-year experience in the United States (1999–2008). *Diagn. Microbiol. Infect. Dis.* 65, 414–426. doi: 10.1016/j.diagmicrobio.2009.08.020

Soo, P.-C., Tseng, C.-C., Ling, S.-R., Liou, M.-L., Liu, C.-C., Chao, H.-J., et al. (2013). Rapid and sensitive detection of *Acinetobacter baumannii* using loop-mediated isothermal amplification. *J. Microbiol. Methods* 92, 197–200. doi: 10.1016/j.mimet.2012.11.020

Tenover, F. C., Arbeit, R. D., Goering, R. V., Mickelsen, P. A., Murray, B. E., Persing, D. H., et al. (1995). Interpreting chromosomal DNA restriction patterns produced by pulsed-field gel electrophoresis: criteria for bacterial strain typing. *J. Clin. Microbiol.* 33, 2233–2239.

Tiwari, V., Kapil, A., and Moganty, R. R. (2012a). Carbapenem-hydrolyzing oxacillinase in high resistant strains of *Acinetobacter baumannii* isolated from India. *Microb. Pathog.* 53, 81–86. doi: 10.1016/j.micpath.2012.05.004

Tiwari, V., Vashistt, J., Kapil, A., and Moganty, R. R. (2012b). Comparative proteomics of inner membrane fraction from carbapenem-resistant *Acinetobacter baumannii* with a reference strain. *PLoS ONE* 7:e39451. doi: 10.1371/journal.pone.0039451

Tiwari, V., and Moganty, R. R. (2014). Conformational stability of OXA-51 β-lactamase explains its role in carbapenem resistance of *Acinetobacter baumannii*. *J. Biomol. Struct. Dyn.* 32, 1406–1420. doi: 10.1080/07391102.2013.819789

Turton, J. F., Woodford, N., Glover, J., Yarde, S., Kaufmann, M. E., and Pitt, T. L. (2006). Identification of *Acinetobacter baumannii* by detection of the blaOXA-51-like carbapenemase gene intrinsic to this species. *J. Clin. Microbiol.* 44, 2974–2976. doi: 10.1128/jcm.01021-06

Wang, Q., Zhou, Y., Li, S., Zhuo, C., Xu, S., Huang, L., et al. (2013). Real-time fluorescence loop mediated isothermal amplification for the detection of *Acinetobacter baumannii*. *PLoS ONE* 8:e66406. doi: 10.1371/journal.pone.0066406

Woodford, N., Ellington, M. J., Coelho, J. M., Turton, J. F., Ward, M. E., Brown, S., et al. (2006). Multiplex PCR for genes encoding prevalent OXA carbapenemases in *Acinetobacter* spp. *Int. J. Antimicrob. Agents* 27, 351–353. doi: 10.1016/j.ijantimicag.2006.01.004

Xi, H., Xu, Y., Zhu, D., Wang, F., Ni, Y., Sun, J., et al. (2012). CHINET 2010 surveillance of antibiotic resistance in *Acinetobacter baumannii* in China. *Chin. J. Infect. Chemother.* 2, 006.

Yan, Z.-Q., Shen, D.-X., Cao, J.-R., Chen, R., Wei, X., Liu, L.-P., et al. (2010). Susceptibility patterns and molecular epidemiology of multidrug-resistant *Acinetobacter baumannii* strains from three military hospitals in China. I. *J. Antimicrob. Agents* 35, 269–273. doi: 10.1016/j.ijantimicag.2009.10.016

Zarrilli, R., Pournaras, S., Giannouli, M., and Tsakris, A. (2013). Global evolution of multidrug-resistant *Acinetobacter baumannii* clonal lineages. *Int. J. Antimicrob. Agents* 41, 11–19. doi: 10.1016/j.ijantimicag.2012.09.008

Zavascki, A. P., Carvalhaes, C. G., Picão, R. C., and Gales, A. C. (2010). Multidrug-resistant *Pseudomonas aeruginosa* and *Acinetobacter baumannii*: resistance mechanisms and implications for therapy. *Expert Rev. Anti Infect. Ther.* 8, 71–93. doi: 10.1586/eri.09.108

Zeng, Y., Zhang, X., Nie, K., Ding, X., Ring, B. Z., Xu, L., et al. (2014). Rapid quantitative detection of Human immunodeficiency virus type 1 by a reverse transcription-loop-mediated isothermal amplification assay. *Gene* 541, 123–128. doi: 10.1016/j.gene.2014.03.015

11

Complete Nucleotide Sequence of pGA45, a 140,698-bp IncFII Plasmid$_Y$ Encoding *bla*$_{IMI-3}$-Mediated Carbapenem Resistance, from River Sediment

Bingjun Dang[1,2], Daqing Mao[1]* and Yi Luo[2]*

[1] School of Environmental Science and Engineering, Tianjin University, Tianjin, China, [2] Ministry of Education Key Laboratory of Pollution Processes and Environmental Criteria, College of Environmental Science and Engineering, Nankai University, Tianjin, China

***Correspondence:**
Daqing Mao
mao@tju.edu.cn;
Yi Luo
luoy@nankai.edu.cn

Plasmid pGA45 was isolated from the sediments of Haihe River using *Escherichia coli* CV601 (*gfp*-tagged) as recipients and indigenous bacteria from sediment as donors. This plasmid confers reduced susceptibility to imipenem which belongs to carbapenem group. Plasmid pGA45 was fully sequenced on an Illumina HiSeq 2000 sequencing system. The complete sequence of plasmid pGA45 was 140,698 bp in length with an average G + C content of 52.03%. Sequence analysis shows that pGA45 belongs to IncFII$_Y$ group and harbors a backbone region which shares high homology and gene synteny to several other IncF plasmids including pNDM1_EC14653, pYDC644, pNDM-Ec1GN574, pRJF866, pKOX_NDM1, and pP10164-NDM. In addition to the backbone region, plasmid pGA45 harbors two notable features including one *bla*$_{IMI-3}$-containing region and one type VI secretion system region. The *bla*$_{IMI-3}$-containing region is responsible for bacteria carbapenem resistance and the type VI secretion system region is probably involved in bacteria virulence, respectively. Plasmid pGA45 represents the first complete nucleotide sequence of the *bla*$_{IMI}$-harboring plasmid from environment sample and the sequencing of this plasmid provided insight into the architecture used for the dissemination of *bla*$_{IMI}$ carbapenemase genes.

Keywords: carbapenem resistance, plasmid, pGA45, T6SS, antibiotic resistance

INTRODUCTION

The overuse and misuse of antibiotics have contributed to the emergence and spread of antibiotic resistance genes (ARGs) and multidrug resistance pathogens (Zhang and Zhang, 2011; He et al., 2014). Now ARGs have been recognized as a new type of pollutants (Pruden et al., 2006). Among various ARGs, carbapenem resistance genes, especially plasmid mediated carbapenem resistance genes, have raised worldwide concern, leading to the extensive research on some of these genes and related plasmid architecture(McGann et al., 2012; Tiwari et al., 2012; Villa et al., 2012, 2013; Lo et al., 2013; Tiwari and Moganty, 2014). Acquired carbapenem resistance can be resulted from carbapenemases of Amber class A (IMI, GES and KPC), Amber class B (metallo β-lactamases including IMP, VIM and NDM) or Amber class D (OXA-48 and OXA-181) (Nordmann et al.,

2012). The bla_{KPC} gene of Amber class A and the metallo β-lactamase genes have been the research focus but there is rare reports about the other carbapenem resistance genes especially little is known about the bla_{IMI} genes and the plasmid architecture involved in the dissemination of this type of genes (Aubron et al., 2005; Yu et al., 2006; Rojo-Bezares et al., 2012; Teo et al., 2013; Chen et al., 2015).

The bla_{IMI-1} gene was first identified in 1996 and found to be located in the chromosome of *Enterobacter cloacae* isolates whereas bla_{IMI-2} was first identified in 2005 in *Enterobacter asburiae* isolates and found to be related to plasmids (Rasmussen et al., 1996; Aubron et al., 2005). In 2009, a new variant of bla_{IMI-1}, bla_{IMI-3}, was identified in Hong Kong in *Enterobacter cloacae* isolates (Chu et al., 2011). The bla_{IMI-3} was also located in the conjugative plasmids. The bla_{IMI}-mediated carbapenem resistance is an infrequent mechanism but it has been reported both in clinical strains and environmental bacteria from rivers. Horizontal transfer may occur between environmental bacteria and clinical strains. With the horizontal transfer, the bla_{IMI} genes would broaden their hosts and inevitably pose serious risks to the public health. For further research on the dissemination of bla_{IMI} genes, the full sequence of bla_{IMI}-related plasmid is needed. Here we report the first complete nucleotide sequence of bla_{IMI}-carrying conjugative plasmid from the environment sample.

MATERIALS AND METHODS

Studying Sites and Sample Collection

Sediment sample was collected under JinGang Bridge of Haihe River. JinGang Bridge was located in densely populated urban areas with frequent human activities. Sediment sample was collected with a grab sampler and then put into sterile containers. The sample was immediately taken to the laboratory and stored in −20°C for subsequent experiments after sampling was completed.

Isolation of the Conjugative Plasmids Conferring Resistance to Imipenem

In order to obtain conjugative plasmids which confer resistance to imipenem, amipicillin resistant plasmids were first isolated by filter mating assays and these ampicillin resistant plasmids were then subjected to antibiotic susceptibility testing against imipenem and other antibiotics. The filter mating assays were applied using *Escherichia coli* CV601 (*gfp*-tagged, kanamycin and rifampicin resistant) as recipients and sediment samples as donors (Heuer et al., 2002). Transconjugants were selected by Mueller-Hinton agar plates supplemented with ampicillin (100 mg L^{-1}), kanamycin (50 mg L^{-1}), rifampicin (50 mg L^{-1}) and cycloheximide (100 mg L^{-1}). *E. coli* CV601 recipient culture was plated on the same selective plates as controls. The procedure used for filter mating assays was described by Heuer et al. (2002) with slight modification. Briefly, the sediment samples from which the indigenous bacteria were used as donors were doubled to 2 g and the Luria-Bertani (LB) broth used for resuspending the sediment samples was accordingly doubled to 18 ml. After incubation for 2 days, transconjugants were determined by green fluorescence which is resulted from green fluorescence protein (GFP) gene. All the ampicillin resistant transconjugants were then streaked on the ampicillin selective plates. Overnight culture of these transconjugants were stored in −80°C for further study.

Antibiotic Susceptibility Testing of the Ampicillin Resistant Transconjugants

Kirby-Bauer disk diffusion method was applied to determine which ampicillin resistant transconjugants confer resistance to imipenem. According to the criteria of the Clinical and Laboratory Standards Institute (CLSI), the disks used in this study are as follows: imipenem (10 μg), ampicillin (10 μg), gentamicin (10 μg), streptomycin (10 μg), tetracycline (30 μg), ciprofloxacin (5 μg), sulfamethoxazole (300 μg) and erythromycin (15 μg). *E. coli* ATCC25922 was used as quality control strain. In this study, one transconjugant designated GA45 was found to confer resistance to imipenem and ampicillin. The conjugative plasmid harbored by GA45 was named pGA45 and stored for further analysis.

Conjugative Transfer Experiments and the Role Determination of pGA45 in Recipient Strains

To assess the conjugative frequency of plasmid pGA45, liquid mating assays were employed using *E. coli* CV601 (pGA45) as donor strains and *E. coli* J53 (azide and nalidixic acid resistance) as recipient strains. For liquid mating assay, overnight cultures of donor and recipient strains were centrifuged, washed and adjusted to the optical density of 0.6 at the wavelength of 600 nm (OD_{600}) with LB broth. Then 0.5 ml cultures of each donor and recipient strains were mixed and make up to the volume of 5 ml with LB broth. After incubation of 16 h in 37°C, transconjugants were selected on LB plates containing azide (200 mg L^{-1}), nalidixic acid (20 mg L^{-1}) and ampicillin (100 mg L^{-1}). Conjugative frequency was determined by the following formula: conjugative frequency = transconjugants (CFU/ml)/recipients (CFU/ml). The *E. coli* J53 transconjugants were then tested against imipenem to confirm the role of pGA45 in recipient strains. The results showed that pGA45 also conferred resistance to imipenem in recipient strains.

Plasmid Sequencing and Bioinformatics

Plasmid DNA from the *E. coli* J53 transconjugants was extracted using a Qiagen plasmid midikit (Qiagen, Inc). The plasmid DNA was sequenced on an Illumina HiSeq 2000 sequencing system. Sequencing reads were *de novo* assembled into contigs using the SOAPdenovo 2.04 software (Li et al., 2008, 2010). Gaps between contigs were closed by PCR with standard Sanger sequencing. Glimmer 3.02 was used to predict putative open reading frames (ORFs) (Salzberg et al., 1998; Delcher et al., 1999, 2007). All ORFs were translated and aligned with different protein databases including NR (version: 20121005), KEGG (version: 59), COG (version: 20090331), SwissProt (version: 201206) and GO (version: 1.419).

Nucleotide Sequence Accession Number

The complete nucleotide sequence of pGA45 was deposited in GenBank under accession no. KT780723.

RESULTS

Sequencing of plasmid pGA45 generated 237,937,000 reads in total. Reads either of low quality or representing the host chromosome contamination through comparison with the sequence of reference strain *E. coli* MG1655 were filtered. In the end, 34 contigs were obtained and then assembled into 10 scaffolds. Through PCR and Sanger sequencing, gaps between contigs and scaffolds were closed. The complete sequence of plasmid pGA45 was 140,698 bp in length with an average G + C content of 52.03% (**Figure 1**). Analysis of the sequence identified 157 ORFs, 64 of which were transcribed in the opposite direction. The backbone of this plasmid included the replication region, stability region 1, and transfer region (51524 bp), making up 36.6% of the total sequence. This backbone region shared high homology and gene synteny to several other IncF plasmids including pNDM1_EC14653 (Wu et al., 2015), pYDC644 (GenBank accession no.: KR351290), pNDM-Ec1GN574 (GenBank accession no.: KJ812998), pRJF866 (Qu et al., 2015), pKOX_NDM1 (Huang et al., 2013) (86% query coverage and 97% nucleotide identity, NCBI database) and pP10164-NDM (Sun et al., 2015) (86% query coverage and 94% nucleotide identity, NCBI database). Notably, all these plasmids were recently sequenced and four of them were found in China. Thus, to our best of knowledge, pGA45 and other recently sequenced plasmids represent a new IncF subtype and this type of plasmids exhibit a high prevalence in China. By contrast, the rest parts of pGA45 [including the variable region, the stability region 2 and the type VI secretion system (T6SS) region] showed no significant similarities with other sequenced plasmids in GenBank.

The replication region (1,431 bp) of pGA45 (positions 75496–76926), including the replication initiation protein gene *repA* and replication regulatory protein gene *repA2*, shared 93% nucleotide similarity with the six IncF plasmids mentioned above with 100% query coverage. Plasmid pGA45 was further assigned to the IncFII$_Y$ incompatibility group through sequence queries against the plasmid MLST databases[1].

Plasmid pGA45 contained one transfer region (position 42643–73867 bp) that comprised 21 *tra* genes, 3 *trb* genes (ordered as follows: *traM, traY, traA, traL, traE, traK, traB, traV, traP, traC, trbI, traW, traU, trbC, traN, traF, traQ, trbB, traH, traG, traT, traD, traI, traX*) and *finO*. Mating out experiments demonstrated that this region made pGA45 self-transmissible at a relatively high frequency of $(7.81 \pm 7.15) \times 10^{-3}$ transconjugants per recipient between *E. coli* CV601 and *E. coli* J53.

The genes on plasmid pGA45 that are responsible for plasmid stability and maintenance included *umuC-umuD* genes which confer resistance to UV light, *relE-relB* genes encoding a toxin-antitoxin system, *ardA* gene with antirestriction function, *parA-parB* genes for partition, *psiA-psiB* genes involved in the bacterial SOS inhibition and *ssb* gene involved in recombination and repair.

The variable region of plasmid pGA45 contained two resistance genes including one ARG bla_{IMI-3} and one copper resistance gene *copC* (with 54% coverage and 94% amino acid identity to *Klebsiella pneumoniae* subsp. pneumoniae DSM 30104, NCBI database). Plasmid pGA45 also harbored a T6SS region (position 82987–114739bp) which may be related to bacterial pathogenesis.

DISCUSSION

The bla_{IMI-3} gene from the variable region was the only ARG harbored by pGA45. The bla_{IMI-3}-containing region (position 58145–74139 bp) was bracketed by one copy of insertion sequence IS*Ec36*[2] and one copy of insertion sequence highly similar to IS*Ecl1*[2] (with 100% coverage and 94% nucleotide identity to IS*Ecl1*) in the same orientation (**Figure 2**). IS*Ec36* was first identified in a bla_{IMI-2}-bearing *E. coli* W635 strain (Rojo-Bezares et al., 2012). In this strain, bla_{IMI-2} was detected upstream the IMI-2R gene. However, in plasmid pGA45, bla_{IMI-3} and IMI-3R changed positions with each other and IMI-3R was located upstream the bla_{IMI-3} gene. Another well characterized bla_{IMI}-containing structure was from *Enterobacter cloacae* plasmid pT103 (GenBank accession no.: NG_036022.1) (Yu et al., 2006). In this partially sequenced plasmid, the bla_{IMI}-containing region comprises two IS*Ec13*[2] (one is partial) elements flanking the bla_{IMI-3} and bla_{IMI-3R} genes in the opposite directions and one partial IS*Ec36* located downstream of this region. In all these characterized bla_{IMI}-containing regions, bla_{IMI} genes have close relationships with insertion sequence IS*Ec36*. Therefore, IS*Ec36* may play an essential role in the dissemination of bla_{IMI} genes between different plasmids. It is also noteworthy to point out that the six plasmids mentioned above similar to pGA45 in backbones mainly have two different bacterial hosts, *Klebsiella pneumoniae* and *Enterobacter cloacae*. In addition, the identified bla_{IMI} genes were mostly from *Enterobacter* species. In view of this, the most probable hosts for plasmid pGA45 were *Enterobacter* species.

Another notable feature harbored by pGA45 was the T6SS region. Compared to other similar IncFII plasmids, the T6SS region was unique to pGA45. This region was most closely related to the T6SS system of plant pathogen *Erwinia amylovora* not only in nucleotide identity (71% coverage and 82% nucleotide identity) but also in gene organization. Previous studies showed that bla_{IMI-2} and bla_{IMI-3} genes were located on plasmids with sizes ranging from 48.5 to 80 kb (one of these plasmids had been identified to belong to IncF group). In this study, pGA45 was much bigger than these plasmids. This perhaps resulted from the

[1]http://pubmlst.org/plasmid

[2]https://www-is.biotoul.fr//

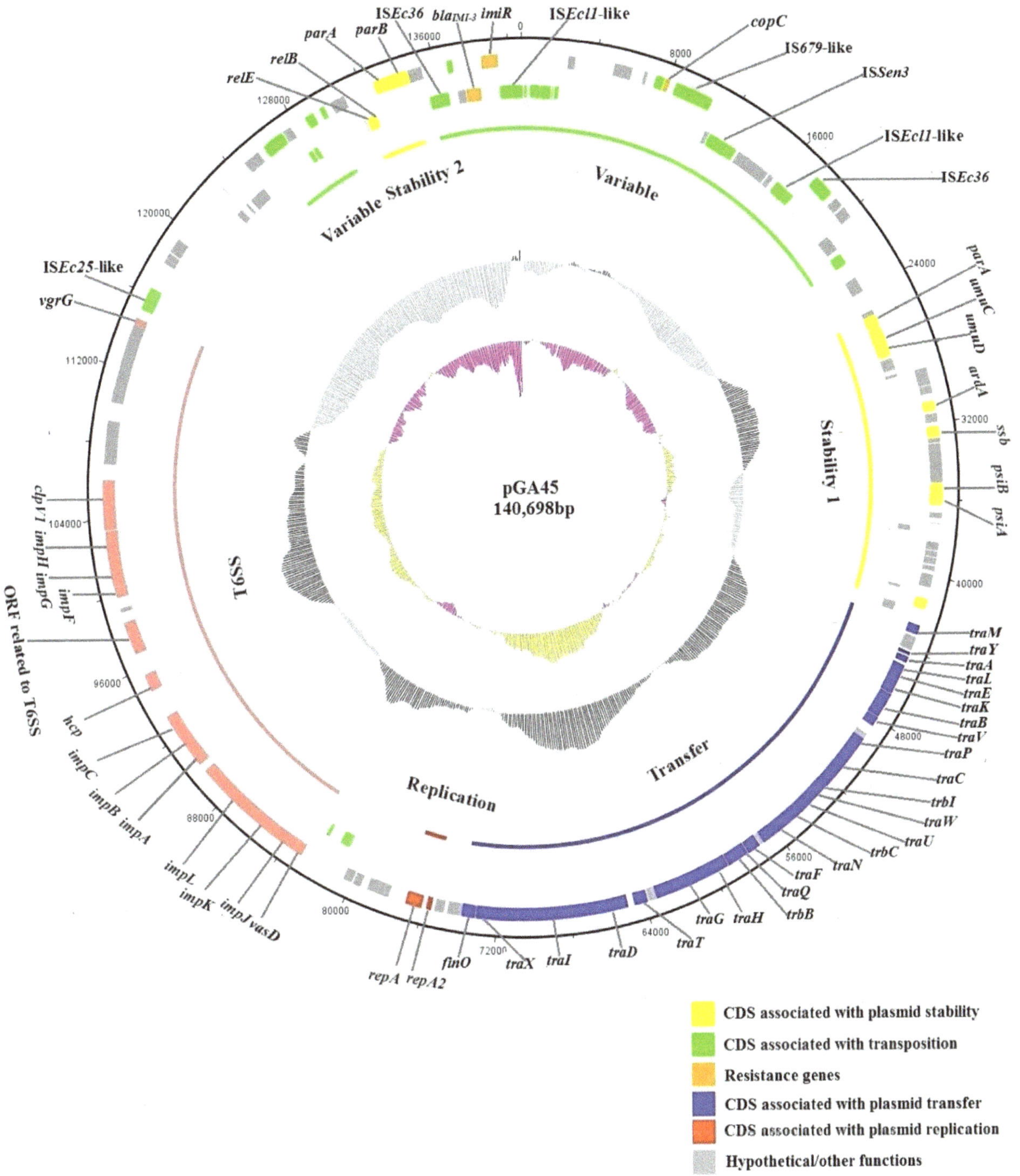

FIGURE 1 | Circular map of plasmid pGA45 (GenBank KT780723). The rings show from outside to inside (i) position of predicted coding sequences in the clockwise direction, (ii) position of predicted coding sequences in the counterclockwise direction, (iii) different regions of plasmid pGA45, (iv) GC plot in a 10,000-bp window, (v) GC skew in a 10,000-bp window. Each predicted coding sequence is color-coded by its function as shown in the figure.

integration of this T6SS region (31753 bp). The T6SS region of plasmid pGA45 was flanked by a copy of IS*Ec25*-like element (with 100% coverage and 85% nucleotide identity to IS*Ec25*) downstream and two transposase genes (with weak amino acid identity to known transposase) upstream. The T6SS region of plasmid pGA45 comprised 14 T6SS-related genes including *vasD* (with 93% coverage and 64.46% amino acid identity to *Erwinia amylovora* ATCC 49946, KEGG database),

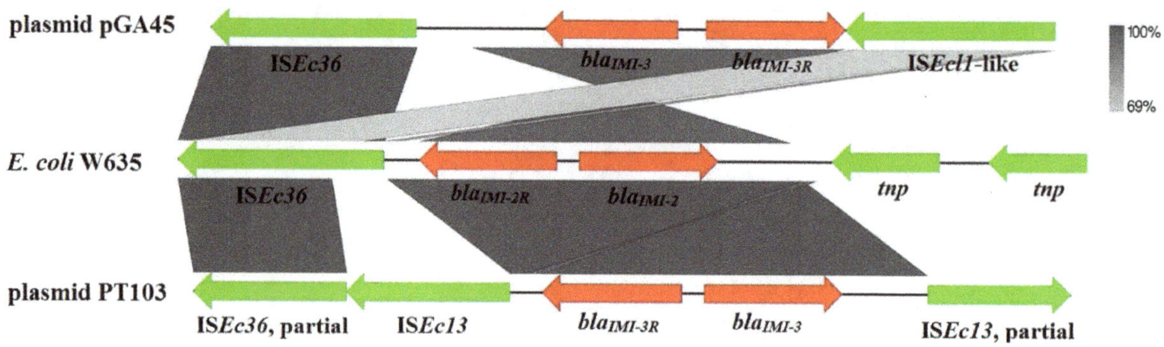

FIGURE 2 | Schematic representation and comparison of *bla*$_{IMI}$-containing genetic structures. Gray shading represents shared regions among three *bla*$_{IMI}$-containing structures. Genes and mobile elements are color-coded based on their functions. Mobile elements are displayed using green arrows while antibiotic resistance genes are shown by red arrows. GenBank accession no.: plasmid pGA45, KT780723; *E. coli* W635, JN412066.1; plasmid pT103, NG_036022.1.

impJ (with 100% coverage and 82.55% amino acid identity to *Erwinia pyrifoliae* Ep1/96, KEGG database), *impK* (with 99% coverage and 84.26% amino acid identity to *Erwinia pyrifoliae* Ep1/96, KEGG database), *impL* (with 100% coverage and 84.38% amino acid identity to *Erwinia tasmaniensis*, KEGG database), *impA* (with 99% coverage and 77.45% amino acid identity to *Erwinia amylovora* ATCC 49946, KEGG database), *impB* (with 97% coverage and 86.52% amino acid identity to *Erwinia amylovora* ATCC 49946, KEGG database), *impC* (with 100% coverage and 94.99% amino acid identity to *Erwinia billingiae*, KEGG database), *hcp* (with 99% coverage and 86.79% amino acid identity to *Enterobacter cloacae subsp. cloacae* ATCC 13047, KEGG database), an ORF encoding a FHA-domain containing protein (with 97% coverage and 70.38% amino acid identity to *Erwinia pyrifoliae* Ep1/96, KEGG database), *impF* (with 99% coverage and 85.03% amino acid identity to *Erwinia amylovora* ATCC 49946, KEGG database), *impG* (with 100% coverage and 87.5% amino acid identity to *Erwinia pyrifoliae* Ep1/96, KEGG database), *impH* (with 99% coverage and 76.95% amino acid identity to *Erwinia tasmaniensis*, KEGG database), *clpV* (with 99% coverage and 89.64% amino acid identity to *Erwinia amylovora* ATCC 49946, KEGG database) and *vgrG* (with 100% coverage and 96.92% amino acid identity to *Kosakonia radicincitans* DSM 16656, NR database).

The T6SS was a recently discovered phage-like secretion apparatus. First reported in *Vibrio cholerae* and *Pseudomonas aeruginosa*, T6SS was likely to be involved in bacterial pathogenesis through acting like a potential nano-syringe for the translocation of effector proteins into the host cell (Pukatzki et al., 2006; Sarris et al., 2011). The Hcp (haemolysin co-regulated protein) and VgrG (valine-glycine repeat G protein) proteins are putative effectors for T6SS (Russell et al., 2014) and the genes encoding these two proteins are also found to be located in the T6SS region of plasmid pGA45. T6SS-related genes are harbored by many kinds of Gram-negative bacterial pathogens which can result in human or animal diseases. In this study, plasmid pGA45 was isolated from river sediment which was collected from urban section of Haihe River. This area was densely populated and strongly affected by human activities. In previous published literatures, most of the *bla*$_{IMI}$ isolates were from in clinical settings. Therefore, the occurrence of T6SS and *bla*$_{IMI-3}$-containing plasmid pGA45 in the river environment are a potential risk for human health and the horizontal transfer of this plasmid between *Enterobacteriaceae* bacteria may aggravate this situation.

CONCLUSION

This report demonstrated the complete nucleotide sequence of the *bla*$_{IMI}$-harboring plasmid. The sequencing of this plasmid provided insight into the architecture used for the dissemination of *bla*$_{IMI}$ carbapenemase genes. In addition to the *bla*$_{IMI}$ gene, plasmid pGA45 also harbored a T6SS cluster probably involved in bacteria virulence. Notably, this plasmid was isolated from environment sample, which will increase the risks of obtaining infections resulted from various types of pathogens carrying this plasmid.

AUTHOR CONTRIBUTIONS

DM and YL designed experiments; BD carried out experiments and analyzed experimental results; BD wrote the manuscript.

ACKNOWLEDGMENTS

We are greatly thankful to Professor Holger Heuer (Julius Kühn-Institut) for providing *E. coli* CV601 and *E. coli* J53. This work was supported by the National Natural Science Foundation of China (Grants 41473085 and 31470440, 31270542), the Ministry of Education, People's Republic of China as an innovative research team project (grant No. IRT13024).

REFERENCES

Aubron, C., Poirel, L., Ash, R. J., and Nordmann, P. (2005). Carbapenemase-producing Enterobacteriaceae, U.S. rivers. *Emerg. Infect. Dis.* 11, 260–264. doi: 10.3201/eid1102.030684

Chen, Z., Li, H., Feng, J., Li, Y., Chen, X., Guo, X., et al. (2015). NDM-1 encoded by a pNDM-BJ01-like plasmid p3SP-NDM in clinical *Enterobacter aerogenes*. *Front. Microbiol.* 6:294. doi: 10.3389/fmicb.2015.00294

Chu, Y. W., Tung, V. W., Cheung, T. K., Chu, M. Y., Cheng, N., Lai, C., et al. (2011). Carbapenemases in enterobacteria,Hong Kong, China, 2009. *Emerg. Infect. Dis.* 17, 130–132. doi: 10.3201/eid1701.101443

Delcher, A. L., Bratke, K. A., Powers, E. C., and Salzberg, S. L. (2007). Identifying bacterial genes and endosymbiont DNA with Glimmer. *Bioinformatics* 23, 673–679. doi: 10.1093/bioinformatics/btm009

Delcher, A. L., Harmon, D., Kasif, S., White, O., and Salzberg, S. L. (1999). Improved microbial gene identification with GLIMMER. *Nucleic Acids Res.* 27, 4636–4641. doi: 10.1093/nar/27.23.4636

He, L.-Y., Liu, Y.-S., Su, H.-C., Zhao, J.-L., Liu, S.-S., Chen, J., et al. (2014). Dissemination of antibiotic resistance genes in representative broiler feedlots environments: identification of indicator ARGs and correlations with environmental variables. *Environ. Sci. Technol.* 48, 13120–13129. doi: 10.1021/es5041267

Heuer, H., Krögerrecklenfort, E., Wellington, E., Egan, S., Van Elsas, J., Van Overbeek, L., et al. (2002). Gentamicin resistance genes in environmental bacteria: prevalence and transfer. *FEMS Microbiol. Ecol.* 42, 289–302. doi: 10.1111/j.1574-6941.2002.tb01019.x

Huang, T. W., Wang, J. T., Lauderdale, T. L., Liao, T. L., Lai, J. F., Tan, M. C., et al. (2013). Complete sequences of two plasmids in a blaNDM-1-positive *Klebsiella oxytoca* isolate from Taiwan. *Antimicrob. Agents Chemother.* 57, 4072–4076. doi: 10.1128/AAC.02266-12

Li, R., Li, Y., Kristiansen, K., and Wang, J. (2008). SOAP: short oligonucleotide alignment program. *Bioinformatics* 24, 713–714. doi: 10.1093/bioinformatics/btn025

Li, R., Zhu, H., Ruan, J., Qian, W., Fang, X., Shi, Z., et al. (2010). De novo assembly of human genomes with massively parallel short read sequencing. *Genome Res.* 20, 265–272. doi: 10.1101/gr.097261.109

Lo, W. U., Cheung, Y. Y., Lai, E., Lung, D., Que, T. L., and Ho, P. L. (2013). Complete sequence of an IncN plasmid, pIMP-HZ1, carrying blaIMP-4 in a *Klebsiella pneumoniae* strain associated with medical travel to China. *Antimicrob. Agents Chemother.* 57, 1561–1562. doi: 10.1128/AAC.0 2298-12

McGann, P., Hang, J., Clifford, R. J., Yang, Y., Kwak, Y. I., Kuschner, R. A., et al. (2012). Complete sequence of a novel 178-kilobase plasmid carrying bla(NDM-1) in a *Providencia stuartii* strain isolated in Afghanistan. *Antimicrob. Agents Chemother.* 56, 1673–1679. doi: 10.1128/AAC.05604-11

Nordmann, P., Dortet, L., and Poirel, L. (2012). Carbapenem resistance in Enterobacteriaceae: here is the storm! *Trends Mol. Med.* 18, 263–272. doi: 10.1016/j.molmed.2012.03.003

Pruden, A., Pei, R., Storteboom, H., and Carlson, K. H. (2006). Antibiotic resistance genes as emerging contaminants: studies in northern Colorado. *Environ. Sci. Technol.* 40, 7445–7450. doi: 10.1021/es060413l

Pukatzki, S., Ma, A. T., Sturtevant, D., Krastins, B., Sarracino, D., Nelson, W. C., et al. (2006). Identification of a conserved bacterial protein secretion system in *Vibrio cholerae* using the *Dictyostelium* host model system. *Proc. Natl. Acad. Sci. U.S.A.* 103, 1528–1533. doi: 10.1073/pnas.0510322103

Qu, H., Wang, X., Ni, Y., Liu, J., Tan, R., Huang, J., et al. (2015). NDM-1-producing Enterobacteriaceae in a teaching hospital in Shanghai, China: IncX3-type plasmids may contribute to the dissemination of blaNDM-1. *Int. J. Infect. Dis.* 34, 8–13. doi: 10.1016/j.ijid.2015.02.020

Rasmussen, B. A., Bush, K., Keeney, D., Yang, Y. J., Hare, R., O'gara, C., et al. (1996). Characterization of IMI-1 β-lactamase, a class A carbapenem-hydrolyzing enzyme from *Enterobacter cloacae*. *Antimicrob. Agents Chemother.* 40, 2080–2086.

Rojo-Bezares, B., Martin, C., Lopez, M., Torres, C., and Saenz, Y. (2012). First detection of blaIMI-2 gene in a clinical *Escherichia coli* strain. *Antimicrob. Agents Chemother.* 56, 1146–1147. doi: 10.1128/AAC.05478-11

Russell, A. B., Peterson, S. B., and Mougous, J. D. (2014). Type VI secretion system effectors: poisons with a purpose. *Nat. Rev. Microbiol.* 12, 137–148. doi: 10.1038/nrmicro3185

Salzberg, S. L., Delcher, A. L., Kasif, S., and White, O. (1998). Microbial gene identification using interpolated Markov models. *Nucleic Acids Res.* 26, 544–548. doi: 10.1093/nar/26.2.544

Sarris, P. F., Zoumadakis, C., Panopoulos, N. J., and Scoulica, E. V. (2011). Distribution of the putative type VI secretion system core genes in *Klebsiella* spp. *Infect. Genet. Evol.* 11, 157–166. doi: 10.1016/j.meegid.2010.09.006

Sun, F., Yin, Z., Feng, J., Qiu, Y., Zhang, D., Luo, W., et al. (2015). Production of plasmid-encoding NDM-1 in clinical Raoultella ornithinolytica and *Leclercia adecarboxylata* from China. *Front. Microbiol.* 6:458. doi: 10.3389/fmicb.2015.00458

Teo, J. W., La, M. V., Krishnan, P., Ang, B., Jureen, R., and Lin, R. T. (2013). *Enterobacter cloacae* producing an uncommon class A carbapenemase, IMI-1, from Singapore. *J. Med. Microbiol.* 62, 1086–1088. doi: 10.1099/jmm.0.053363-0

Tiwari, V., Kapil, A., and Moganty, R. R. (2012). Carbapenem-hydrolyzing oxacillinase in high resistant strains of *Acinetobacter baumannii* isolated from India. *Microb. Pathog.* 53, 81–86. doi: 10.1016/j.micpath.2012.05.004

Tiwari, V., and Moganty, R. R. (2014). Conformational stability of OXA-51 β-lactamase explains its role in carbapenem resistance of *Acinetobacter baumannii*. *J. Biomol. Struct. Dyn.* 32, 1406–1420. doi: 10.1080/07391102.2013.819789

Villa, L., Carattoli, A., Nordmann, P., Carta, C., and Poirel, L. (2013). Complete sequence of the IncT-type plasmid pT-OXA-181 carrying the blaOXA-181 carbapenemase gene from *Citrobacter freundii*. *Antimicrob. Agents Chemother.* 57, 1965–1967. doi: 10.1128/AAC.01297-12

Villa, L., Poirel, L., Nordmann, P., Carta, C., and Carattoli, A. (2012). Complete sequencing of an IncH plasmid carrying the blaNDM-1, blaCTX-M-15 and qnrB1 genes. *J. Antimicrob. Chemother.* 67, 1645–1650. doi: 10.1093/jac/dks114

Wu, W., Feng, Y., Carattoli, A., and Zong, Z. (2015). The emergence of *Enterobacter cloacae* producing both KPC and NDM carbapenemases: characterization by whole genome sequencing. *Antimicrob. Agents Chemother.* AAC.1275-15. doi: 10.1128/AAC.01275-15

Yu, Y. S., Du, X. X., Zhou, Z. H., Chen, Y. G., and Li, L. J. (2006). First isolation of blaIMI-2 in an *Enterobacter cloacae* clinical isolate from China. *Antimicrob. Agents Chemother.* 50, 1610–1611. doi: 10.1128/AAC.50.4.1610-1611.2006

Zhang, X. X., and Zhang, T. (2011). Occurrence, abundance, and diversity of tetracycline resistance genes in 15 sewage treatment plants across China and other global locations. *Environ. Sci. Technol.* 45, 2598–2604. doi: 10.1021/es103672x

12

Effect of Photodynamic Therapy on the Virulence Factors of *Staphylococcus aureus*

Maria Bartolomeu[1], Sónia Rocha[1], Ângela Cunha[1], M. G. P. M. S. Neves[2], Maria A. F. Faustino[2]* and Adelaide Almeida[1]*

[1] Departamento de Biologia and Centro de Estudos do Ambiente e do Mar, University of Aveiro, Aveiro, Portugal,
[2] Departamento de Química and Unidade de Investigação em Química Orgânica, Produtos Naturais e Agroalimentares, University of Aveiro, Aveiro, Portugal

***Correspondence:**
Adelaide Almeida
aalmeida@ua.pt;
Maria A. F. Faustino
faustino@ua.pt

Staphylococcus aureus is a Gram-positive bacterium that is present in the human microbiota. Nevertheless, these bacteria can be pathogenic to the humans. Due to the increasing occurrence of antibiotic-resistant *S. aureus* strains, new approaches to control this pathogen are necessary. The antimicrobial photodynamic inactivation (PDI) process is based in the combined use of light, oxygen, and an intermediary agent (a photosensitizer). These three components interact to generate cytotoxic reactive oxygen species that irreversibly damage vital constituents of the microbial cells and ultimately lead to cell death. Although PDI is being shown to be a promising alternative to the antibiotic approach for the inactivation of pathogenic microorganisms, information on effects of photosensitization on particular virulence factors is strikingly scarce. The objective of this work was to evaluate the effect of PDI on virulence factors of *S. aureus* and to assess the potential development of resistance of this bacterium as well as the recovery of the expression of the virulence factors after successive PDI cycles. For this, the photosensitizer 5,10,15,20-tetrakis(1-methylpyridinium-4-yl)porphyrin tetra-iodide (Tetra-Py^{+}-Me) and six strains of *S. aureus* [one reference strain, one strain with one enterotoxin, two strains with three enterotoxins and two methicillin resistant strains (MRSA) – one with five enterotoxins and the other without enterotoxins] were used. The effect of photosensitization on catalase activity, beta hemolysis, lipases, thermonuclease, enterotoxins, coagulase production, and resistance/susceptibility to methicillin was tested. To assess the development of resistance after successive cycles of treatment, three strains of *S. aureus* (ATCC 6538, 2065 MA, and SA 3 MRSA) were used. The surviving colonies of a first cycle of PDI were collected from the solid medium and subjected to further nine consecutive cycles of PDI. The results indicate that the expression of some external virulence factors is affected by PDI and enterotoxin producing strains were more susceptible to PDI than non-toxigenic strains. The surviving bacteria did not develop resistance. PDI, contrarily to traditional antibiotics, inhibited the expression of virulence factors, efficiently inactivating either highly virulent strains and low virulent *S. aureus* strains, inactivating also antibiotic susceptible and resistant strains, without development of photoresistance after at least 10 consecutive cycles of treatment, and so this therapy may become a strong promising alternative to antibiotics to control pathogenic microorganisms.

Keywords: *Staphylococcus aureus*, photodynamic inactivation (PDI), virulence factors, coagulase, enterotoxins, antibiotic/methicillin resistance

INTRODUCTION

Staphylococcus aureus is a Gram-positive bacterium that resides on the surface of the skin and on mucous membranes of warm-blooded animals (Morikawa et al., 2001; Costa A.R. et al., 2013) as a commensal microorganism, asymptomatically colonizing the host (Bronner et al., 2004). Nevertheless, due to its invasiveness and taking advantage of host immune weaknesses, *S. aureus* is able to cause a wide spectrum of infections affecting different organs (Bronner et al., 2004; Baptista et al., 2015), from infections of superficial lesions to intoxications and life threatening systemic conditions (Bien et al., 2011). This opportunistic bacterium is a major human pathogen not only associated with community-acquired bacteremia but also nosocomial bacteremia (Morikawa et al., 2001; Cheung et al., 2004; Bien et al., 2011), being readily able to acquire antibiotic resistance (Morikawa et al., 2001). Its ability to survive under stressful conditions, such as those imposed by host immune system, is due to the activation of stress response mechanisms (Morikawa et al., 2001; Bronner et al., 2004; Cheung et al., 2004). These mechanisms involve the action of an interactive regulatory network that includes the accessory gene regulator (*agr*) and staphylococcal accessory element (*sae*) (Bronner et al., 2004; Novick and Geisinger, 2008; Costa A.R. et al., 2013). These two components of the regulatory system regulate the expression of several exoproteins and cell wall-associated proteins related to virulence (Costa A.R. et al., 2013). The regulatory network also includes the staphylococcal accessory regulator A (*sarA*) and its homologs that regulate the expression of some virulence factors; the sigma factors (σ), as the primary sigma factor, σ^A, that may function in living process through the housekeeping genes expression and the alternative sigma factor σ^B, which may participate on the bacterial response to stress conditions by regulating the expression of several genes involved on stress response (Morikawa et al., 2001; Cheung et al., 2004; Costa A.R. et al., 2013).

The *S. aureus* pathogenicity involves a wide array of cell wall and extracellular components orderly expressed during the different stages of infection: colonization, avoidance, or invasion of the host immune defense, growth, and cellular division culminating in bacterial dissemination, causing toxic effects to the host (Cheung et al., 2004; Bien et al., 2011; Costa A.R. et al., 2013; Ebrahimi et al., 2014). Some of the cell wall components are responsible for the recognition of adhesive matrix molecules, such as the clumping factor proteins (Clf) that mediates the adherence to fibrinogen (Costa A.R. et al., 2013) and the carotenoid pigment staphyloxanthin that acts as virulence factor once it is able to perform an antioxidant action against oxidant-based reactions (Clauditz et al., 2006; Liu and Nizet, 2009; Costa A.R. et al., 2013). The extracellular components include the superantigen molecules such as the staphylococcal enterotoxins (SE), a family of a single chain proteins with small molecular-weight (24–30 kDa; Johnson et al., 1991; Baptista et al., 2015); the cytolytic β-hemolysin, the clotting factor coagulase, besides more exoenzymes as lipases and nucleases, in which their main function is to disrupt the host cells/tissue and the inactivation of host immune mechanisms of defense (Costa A.R. et al., 2013).

Additionally to the virulence factors already described, *S. aureus* has a notorious capacity to acquire antibiotic resistance (Guillemot, 1999; Morikawa et al., 2001; Ito et al., 2003; Chambers and DeLeo, 2009; Costa A.R. et al., 2013; Theuretzbacher, 2013), by a bacterial gene mutation and horizontal transfer of resistance genes from external sources (Ito et al., 2003; Chambers and DeLeo, 2009). The resistance to penicillin emerged in the mid-1940s, only a few years after the introduction of this antibiotic in the clinical practice (Chambers and DeLeo, 2009; Costa A.R. et al., 2013). Later, in 1959, the semi-synthetic antibiotic methicillin was introduced for the treatment of infections caused by penicillin-resistant *S. aureus* (Enright et al., 2002; Costa A.R. et al., 2013). Yet, in 1961 the first cases of methicillin-resistant *S. aureus* (MRSA) isolates (Chambers and DeLeo, 2009; Costa A.R. et al., 2013) were reported and currently, only few compounds are still effective in the treatment of MRSA infections (Chambers and DeLeo, 2009; Theuretzbacher, 2011).

With the knowledge that the development of new classic antibiotics is not likely to solve the resistance drug problem for too long (Chambers and DeLeo, 2009), non-traditional antimicrobial approaches to treat MRSA infections will be needed. Ideally, the new antimicrobial methods should be non-invasive and non-toxic to the hosts, but efficient and with fast action, avoiding the development of resistance (Calin and Parasca, 2009; Kossakowska et al., 2013; Alves et al., 2014; Almeida et al., 2015). In this context, the photodynamic inactivation (PDI) arises as a photo chemotherapeutic approach with forthcoming applications as antimicrobial therapy (Almeida et al., 2009, 2015; Carvalho et al., 2009; Costa et al., 2012; Alves et al., 2013, 2014, 2015b; Melo et al., 2013). This technology has already proved to be effective against Gram-positive and Gram-negative bacteria, viruses, fungi, and parasites (Almeida et al., 2011, 2015; Costa et al., 2012). The photodynamic effect is based on the use of visible light and an agent (photosensitizer, PS) capable to absorb energy from light and transfer it to molecular oxygen, originating highly cytotoxic species, namely reactive oxygen species (ROS) as singlet oxygen ($^1O_2$), hydrogen peroxide (H_2O_2), peroxide anion radical ($O_2^{\bullet-}$), and hydroxyl radical ($OH^\bullet$; Alves et al., 2008, 2013, 2014; Calin and Parasca, 2009; Melo et al., 2013). These reactive cytotoxic species can cause irreversible damages to molecular cell constituents or even its destruction (Alves et al., 2014). Initially, the PS adheres to the microbial external structures and later, during the irradiation process, the PDI is initiated and cellular components, such as proteins and lipids will be exposed to oxidizing reactions which will alter their structure and, subsequently, affect the biological function in which they are involved (Alves et al., 2014).

As PDI acts *via* ROS, a high number of microbial targets are simultaneously affected, thus preventing the development of resistance (Costa et al., 2008; Tavares et al., 2010), and allowing the inactivation of a broad-spectrum of microorganisms, independently of their resistance profiles to classic antimicrobials (Tavares et al., 2010; Arrojado et al., 2011; Costa et al., 2011; Almeida et al., 2014). In addition, PDI affects the expression of virulence factors, also causing their degradation (Kömerik et al., 2000; Tubby et al., 2009; Kossakowska et al., 2013). The effects of PDI on virulence factors is of extreme importance as they may be present during the infection process, when the microorganism is present, but they can also be present when the microorganism is not present already, such as in the case of intoxications, causing severe damage to the host.

Clinical trials using light based therapies to evaluate the potential use of photodynamic therapy in the clinical field have been conducted along the last years, with positive results, including studies against viral infections, such as the ones caused by human papilloma virus, with systemic and topical applications (Bujia et al., 1993; Shikowitz et al., 1998) and to treat herpes simplex lesions, with topical applications (Moore et al., 1972). Non-viral infections by *Propionibacterium acnes*, a natural porphyrin producer, were already efficiently inactivated (Kawada et al., 2002; Elman et al., 2003), among others, as acne vulgaris (Ormond and Freeman, 2013). Nowadays the miniaturization of the light devices such as low-power lasers, light emitting diodes, or conventional lamps able to activate the antimicrobial molecules place this technology closer to be use in clinical application. Superficial skin infections like wounds and burns can be easily treated (Ebrahimi et al., 2014). Using fiber-optic technology, most regions of the anatomy are also accessible. *Loci* of infection could be managed endoscopically, allowing local application both of the PS agent and light (Dai et al., 2010; Kharkwal et al., 2011). Even for deep-seated infections a transcutaneous needle could deliver both drug and light via fibers.

Some *in vitro* studies showed that the biological activity of lipopolysaccharides from *Escherichia coli* and proteases from *Pseudomonas aeruginosa* were successfully reduced by toluidine blue (TBO)-mediated PDI (Tubby et al., 2009). Additionally, light-activated methylene blue (MB) showed to inhibit the expression of staphylococcal V8 protease, alpha-hemolysin and sphingomyelinase (Tubby et al., 2009). However, the information about the effects of PDI on virulence factor is still scarce. The objectives of this work were the evaluation of the effect of PDI on some virulence factors of *S. aureus* – catalase activity, beta hemolysis, lipases, thermonuclease, enterotoxins, coagulase – and the assessment of development of resistance to PDI treatment. For that, a cationic porphyrin 5,10,15,20-tetrakis(1-methylpyridinium-4-yl)porphyrin tetra-iodide (Tetra-Py$^+$-Me) was used as PS against on six *S. aureus* strains – ATCC 6538, 2153 MA, 2065 MA, 2095 M1A1, DSM 25693 MRSA, and SA 3 MRSA.

MATERIALS AND METHODS

Experimental Design

An experimental procedure was established in order to study the effects of PDI on some virulence factors expression/activity of *S. aureus* strains and to test the potential development of resistance to PDI by *S. aureus* strains after successive photodynamic cycles of treatment, testing also the recovery of the expression/activity of the virulence factors after the successive photodynamic cycles of treatment. Six different strains of *S. aureus*, including methicillin resistant and susceptible strains, as well as, enterotoxin and non-enterotoxin producing strains were tested. The effect of PDI on the expression/activity of virulence factors was tested in all strains. The potential development of resistance to PDI and the recovery of the expression/activity of the virulence factors after the successive cycles of treatment were tested only in three of the strains. For each of these three strains, a total of ten cycles of treatments were performed.

Characterization of Bacterial Strains and Culture Conditions

Six strains of *S. aureus* were used in this study: ATCC 6538, a non-enterotoxic strain; 2153 MA, the only strain used that does not ferment mannitol (Baptista et al., 2015), producing SE A; 2065 MA, with SE A, G, I, and *S. aureus* 2095 M1A1 with SE C, G and I – the three strains isolated from food products and characterized in the Centre of Biotechnology and Fine Chemistry of the Faculty of Biotechnology of the Catholic University, Porto, Portugal; *S. aureus* DSM 25693, a methicillin-resistant (MRSA) strain, positive for SE A, C, H, G, and I; and a staphylococcal strain isolated from a biological sample from the lower respiratory tract of an hospitalized individual, a non-enterotoxic MRSA strain (SA 3 MRSA; Gonçalves et al., 2014).

All the strains were grown in Brain-Heart Infusion (BHI, Liofilchem, Italy) at 37°C for 18 h at 170 rpm, in order to reach the stationary phase, corresponding approximately to a concentration of 10^8–10^9 colony forming units per mL (CFU mL^{-1}). Before each PDI assay, a colony of *S. aureus* was transferred to 30 mL of BHI and incubated as previously described. Subsequently, an aliquot was transferred to fresh medium, and grown in the same conditions. This procedure was repeated twice.

Photosensitizer

The PS 5,10,15,20-tetrakis(1-methylpyridinium-4-yl)porphyrin tetra-iodide (Tetra-Py$^+$-Me) used in this study was prepared according to the literature (Carvalho et al., 2010). Their ^{1}H NMR and UV–vis spectra were consistent with the literature data. Their purity was confirmed by thin layer chromatography and ^{1}H NMR. ^{1}H NMR (DMSO-d_6): -3.12 (s, 2H, *N*H), 4.73 (s, 12H, CH_3), 9.00 (d, $J = 6.5$ Hz, 8H, Py-o-H), 9.22 (s, 8H, β-H), 9.49 (d, $J = 6.5$ Hz, 8H, Py-m-H). UV–vis (DMSO) λ_{max} (log ε): 425 (5.43), 516 (4.29), 549 (3.77), 588 (3.84), 642 (3.30) nm. The stock solutions (500 μM) of this porphyrin were prepared using the polar aprotic solvent dimethyl sulfoxide (DMSO).

Antimicrobial Photodynamic Therapy (PDI) Treatments

Bacterial cultures in stationary phase were 10-fold diluted in phosphate buffered saline (PBS) and this bacterial suspension was distributed in sterilized glass beakers. The appropriate quantity of the PS Tetra-Py$^+$-Me was added to achieve a final concentration of 5.0 μM. The total volume of final solution was 10 mL per beaker. During the experiments, light and dark controls were also performed: in the light control the beaker without Tetra-Py$^+$-Me was exposed to light; in the dark control the beaker containing 5.0 μM Tetra-Py$^+$-Me was protected from light with aluminum foil during the experiment. During the pre-irradiation period, the samples were incubated for 10 min with stirring, at room temperature, in order to promote the binding of the porphyrin to *S. aureus* cells. The samples were exposed to an artificial white light (PAR radiation, 13 OSRAM 21 lamps of 18 W each, 380–700 nm) with an irradiance of 40 W m^{-2} for 60 min, under stirring. During the experiment, aliquots of treated and control samples were collected at times 0, 5, 10, 15, 30, and 60 min.

Enumeration of Viable Cells

From each treated and control samples 10-fold serial dilutions were prepared in sterile PBS (10^{-1} to 10^{-6}). Aliquots of 100 μL were pour-plated, in duplicate, in Plate Count Agar medium (PCA, Liofilchem, Italy). The plates were incubated at 37°C for 48 h and the number of colonies was counted. Three independent assays were performed.

PDI Resistance Assays

In order to verify the development of resistance to PDI treatment with Tetra-Py^{+}-Me, ten cycles of PDI were performed. After each cycle of a total irradiation time of 60 min, a new set of bacterial cultures were prepared from an isolated colony, surviving to the previous cycle of PDI (at 37°C, 18 h, 170 rpm). The PDI treatment was repeated under similar conditions. Three independent assays were performed.

Virulence Factors, Mannitol Fermentation, and Methicillin Susceptibility

To assess if PDI treatments affected the virulence factors of *S. aureus*, treated and controls samples were tested for the presence or activity of virulence factors, according to literature (Baptista et al., 2015). One typical colony of *S. aureus* was selected from each strain. The β-hemolysin activity was detected by streaking Blood Agar Plates (Sheep Blood 7%; BAP, Liofilchem, Italy) and observing the development of a clear/yellow zone surrounding *S. aureus* colonies. Lipase and lecithinase activities were assessed by streaking Baird Park Agar (BPA, Liofilchem, Italy) in which *S. aureus* colonies appear in black, with an opaque precipitation zone (lipase activity) and a clear zone surrounding it (lecithinase activity). The mannitol fermentation was evaluated using Mannitol Salt Agar (MSA, Liofilchem, Italy), being the positive results detected by a change of color of the medium from pink to yellow. Catalase activity was assessed using Catalase/Oxy Test (Liofilchem, Italy), interpreting the formation of gas bubbles as a positive result. The activity of bound coagulase (clumping factor) was determined using Pastorex Staph Plus (Bio-Rad, USA) and the activity of free coagulase was detected using BBL Coagulase Plasma Rabbit (BD, USA). For this, 1.0 mL of supernatant of treated and non-treated samples was collected by centrifugation at 13,000 × *g* for 10 min, at 4°C, and 0.5 mL of BBL Coagulase Plasma reagent was added and the mixture was incubated at 37°C for 24 h. The results were considered positive when the agglutination occurred. The rate of clot formation was evaluated according to the manufacturer's instruction. Thermonuclease activity was determined by D.N.A. Toluidine Blue Agar (Bio-Rad, USA) and positive results were detected as a change of color of the halos from blue to pink. The presence of SE was determined using SET-RPLA Kit Toxin Detection Kit (Thermo Scientific, UK), a kit based on reversed passive latex agglutination technique, according to the manufacturer's instruction. Treated and non-treated samples were centrifuged at 900 × *g* for 20 min at 4°C. The presence of enterotoxins H, G, and I was not tested since SET-RPLA Kit Toxin Detection Kit only covers SE A, B, C, and D, which are the most common enterotoxins of *S. aureus* (Baptista et al., 2015). The susceptibility to methicillin was determined using the cefoxitin disk screen test, accordingly to the Clinical and Laboratory Standards Institute [CLSI] (2013). Cultures with halos ≥22 mm were considered methicillin susceptible and cultures with halos ≤21 were classified as methicillin resistant (Clinical and Laboratory Standards Institute [CLSI], 2013). Carotenoid pigments (staphyloxanthin) were determined using a protocol adapted from Morikawa et al. (2001). Each strain was cultured in BHI medium at 37°C for 72 h. Twenty milliliters of the culture were harvested by centrifugation (10,000 × *g*, 10 min) and washed with purified water. The cells were suspended in 5.0 mL of methanol and heated in a bath at 55°C for 15 min, until visible pigments have been extracted. Cellular debris was removed by centrifugation at 15,000 × *g* for 10 min. The absorbance at 465 nm of the methanol extracts were measured in a quartz cuvette in a spectrophotometer (Dynamica Halo DB-20, UK).

The β-hemolysis, lipase and lecithinase, catalase, bound coagulase and thermonuclease activities, mannitol fermentation and methicillin susceptibility were tested in the PDI surviving cells, after plating and incubation at 37°C. Methicillin susceptibility was inferred from the diameter of the inhibition zone around cefoxitin disks, and the results represent the average of the inhibition zones from three independent tests. Free coagulase and SE A and C activities were assessed in the supernatant of treated samples and controls after PDI assays.

The effect of PDI on the isolated toxins was also individually assessed. Purified SE A and C (available on SET-RPLA Kit Toxin Detection Kit as SE A and C controls) were subjected to the PDI treatment. The concentration of the PS was the same used before: 5.0 μM; the amount of SE used was 63 μL from the reconstituted control reagents (the kit control solution contains 25 ng of purified enterotoxin reconstituted in 0.5 mL of diluent from the kit as showed in Figure in section "Quantity of Enterotoxins (ng) Per Kit" of the Supplementary Material), and PBS was added to make up a total volume of 2.0 mL of solution, which was irradiated. Light and dark controls were included. At times 0, 5, 10, 15, 30, and 60 min aliquots of 25 μL were collected and the activity of the SE was tested using the SET-RPLA Kit Toxin Detection Kit.

RESULTS

Bacterial Inactivation by PDI

Cells suspensions of *S. aureus* strains were subjected to 60 min of PDI treatments (5.0 μM of Tetra-Py^{+}-Me and an irradiance

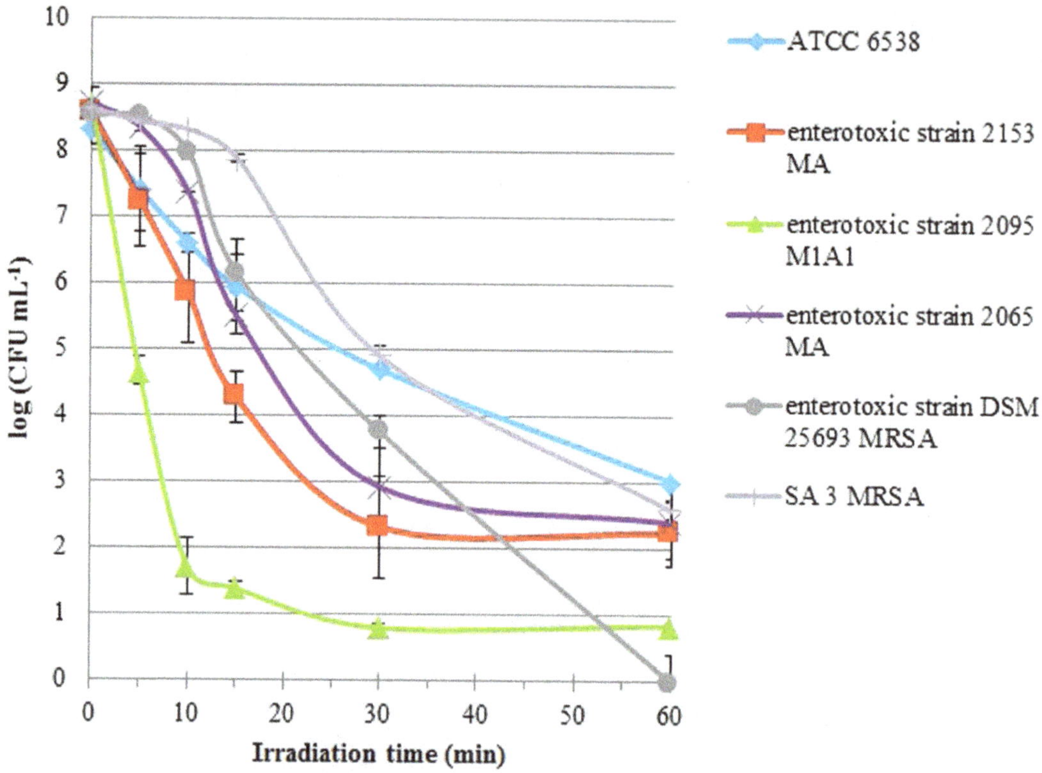

FIGURE 1 | Survival curves of six *S. aureus* strains (ATCC 6538, enterotoxic strains 2153 MA, 2095 M1A1, 2065 MA, and DSM 25693 MRSA and SA 3 MRSA) incubated with 5.0 μM of Tetra-Py$^+$-Me and irradiated with white light (380–700 nm) with an irradiance of 40 W m^{-2} for 60 min. Lines representing light (LC) and dark (DC) controls viability were omitted, since cell viability in the controls was not affected. Values represent the mean of three independent experiments with two replicates each; error bars indicate the standard deviation.

of 40 W m^{-2}), and aliquots were taken before (0 min) and after 5, 10, 15, 30, and 60 min of treatment. All the strains were efficiently inactivated by PDI (**Figure 1**). After 60 min of treatment under the tested conditions reductions higher than 5 log CFU mL^{-1} were observed for all the tested strains. However, in general, the pattern of photoinactivation was different among the *S. aureus* strains as showed by the log10 reduction rates (**Figure 1**).

The enterotoxic strains were more efficiently inactivated than the non-enterotoxic ones. The toxigenic *S. aureus* strain 2095 M1A1 was particularly susceptible to PDI showing a reduction of 7 log within the first 10 min of irradiation. With equivalent irradiation time, the enterotoxic strain 2153 MA showed a reduction of only 2.5 log and all the other strains were inactivated less than 2 log. For DSM 25693 MRSA strain, also an enterotoxic, a linear decrease was observed after 15 min of treatment, reaching complete inactivation after 60 min of treatment (8.5 log). After 60 min of treatment, the inactivation factors for the other strains were 5.3 log for ATCC 6538, 6.0 log for SA 3 MRSA, 6.3 log for 2065 MA, 6.3 log for 2153 MA, and 7.8 log for 2095 M1A1. In the controls, the concentration of viable cells did not vary, indicating that the viability of bacterial cells was neither affected by light alone (light control), nor by the direct toxicity of the PS (dark control).

Development of Resistance after Repeated PDI Cycles and Recovery of Viability Between Cycles

Three *S. aureus* strains (ATCC 6538, 2065 MA, and SA 3 MRSA) were subjected to ten consecutive PDI cycles (**Figure 2**). The authors decide to test 10 cycles having into account previous results of the research group (Tavares et al., 2010; Costa et al., 2011). The PDI efficiency of photosensitization with Tetra-Py$^+$-Me was not affected during the sequence of 10 PDI cycles.

Effect of PDI on *S. aureus* Virulence Factors, Methicillin Susceptibility, and Mannitol Fermentation

After each PDI assay, the activity and presence of virulence factors, mannitol fermentation, and methicillin susceptibility were tested (**Table 1**).

The surviving cells to PDI treatments retained the capacity to express all the virulence factors and to ferment mannitol. However, the activity of the extracellular virulence factors free coagulase and enterotoxins, assessed in the supernatant of treated samples, was affected (see section "Testing the Presence of Free Coagulase" of Supplementary Material and **Table 1**). For the test of free coagulase, the BBL Coagulase Plasma reagent was

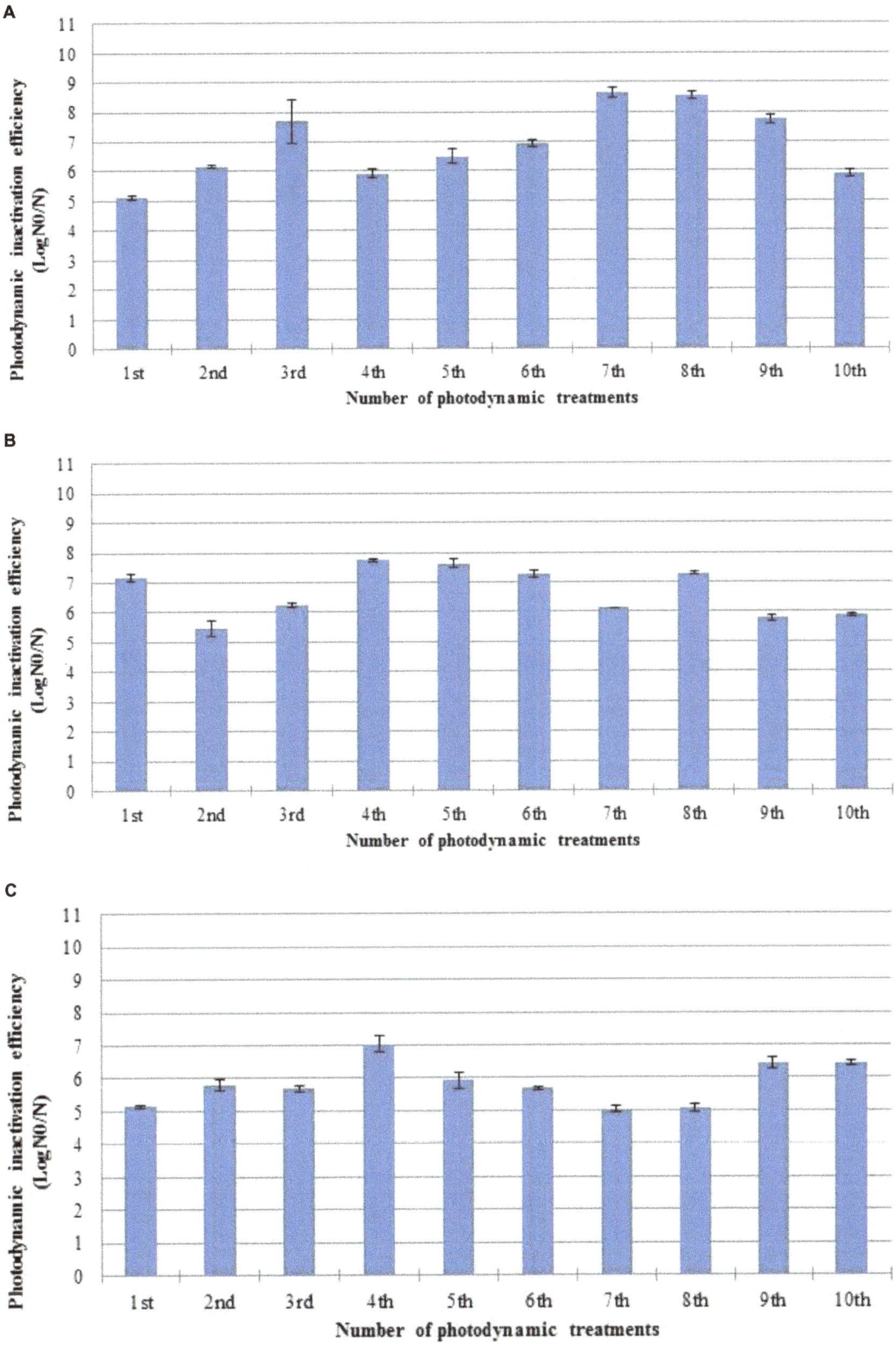

FIGURE 2 | Photodynamic inactivation efficiency of ten consecutive cycles of *S. aureus* ATCC 6538 (A), 2065 MA (B), and SA 3 MRSA (C) by 5.0 μM of Tetra-Py$^+$-Me after 60 min of irradiation with white light (40 W m^{-2}). N_0 represents the plaque counts of bacterial cells before the irradiation; N represents the plaque counts after the cycle treatment; error bars indicate the standard deviation.

TABLE 1 | The activity of the virulence factors, mannitol fermentation, and susceptibility to methicillin were tested, after PDI treatments, in presence of 5.0 μM of Tetra-Py$^+$-Me and irradiated with white light (380–700 nm) with an irradiance of 40 W m^{-2} for 60 min.

Staphylococcus aureus strains	Samples	Surviving cells							Supernatant		
		β-Hemolysis	Lipase and lecithinase	Mannitol fermentation	Catalase	Bound Coagulase	Thermonuclease	Susceptibility to methicillin (mm)	Free coagulase	SEs A	SEs C
ATCC 6538	S	+	+	+	+	+	+	30	–	#	#
	LC	+	+	+	+	+	+	29	4^+	#	#
	DC	+	+	+	+	+	+	29	4^+	#	#
2153 MA	S	+	+	–	+	+	+	25	–	–	#
	LC	+	+	–	+	+	+	26	3^+	+	#
	DC	+	+	–	+	+	+	26	3^+	+	#
2065 MA	S	+	+	+	+	+	+	28	–	–	#
	LC	+	+	+	+	+	+	28	3^+	+	#
	DC	+	+	+	+	+	+	28	3^+	+	#
2095 M1A1	S	+	+	+	+	+	+	27	–	#	–
	LC	+	+	+	+	+	+	26	3^+	#	+
	DC	+	+	+	+	+	+	27	3^+	#	+
DSM 25693 MRSA	S	+	+	+	+	+	+	<21	–	–	–
	LC	+	+	+	+	+	+	<21	3^+	+	+
	DC	+	+	+	+	+	+	<21	3^+	+	+
SA 3 MRSA	S	+	+	+	+	+	+	<21	–	#	#
	LC	+	+	+	+	+	+	<21	4^+	#	#
	DC	+	+	+	+	+	+	<21	4^+	#	#

These tests were performed in three independent assays for each strain. Cardinal symbol in the "Supernatant, SE" columns means that such tests have not been performed for the respective strains once these strains do not produce the mentioned virulence factors.

added to an aliquot of supernatant and the resulting samples was incubated for 24 h. Clot formation was not detected in photosensitized samples. The SE test, performed in the supernatant of photosensitized cells by the SET-RPLA Kit Toxin Detection Kit test, revealed the formation of a tight button, interpreted as absence of SE or presence at a concentration below the detection limit. These two virulence factors persisted in light and dark controls.

Susceptibility of Staphylococcal Isolated Enterotoxins to PDI

The isolated enterotoxins A and C were directly treated by PDI [see section "Purified SE A (A) and C (B) Subjected to Photodynamic Treatment" of Supplementary Material and **Table 2**]. The positive result corresponds to agglutination, leading to the formation of a lattice structure and negative correspond to the formation of a tight button, which occurs if SE are absent or present in a concentration bellow the detection level (TD0900, SET-RPLA, 2015). Before the treatment, enterotoxins A and C were still detected (formation of a lattice structure). During the PDI, the formation of the lattice structure decreases (as seen in the first well of 15 and 30 min test, see section "Purified SE A (A) and C (B) Subjected to Photodynamic Treatment" of Supplementary Material) and the formation of a tight button (as seen in the first well of 60 min test), begins to occur, indicating the shift to a negative result. After 60 min of irradiation, the inactivation was >68% for both SE [SE A and C; see section "Calculating the Decrease (%) of Enterotoxins After PDI Assays" of Supplementary Material].

TABLE 2 | The purified SE A and C were subjected to PDI for 60 min.

Irradiation time		Isolated and purified SEs	
		A	C
0	S	+	+
	LC	+	+
	DC	+	+
60	S	–	–
	LC	+	+
	DC	+	+

The SE activity was assessed before (0 min), during (5, 10, 15, and 30 min) and after 60 min of treatment for treated (S) and non-treated samples (light control, LC; dark control, DC). Three independent assays were performed.

Carotenoid Pigments Content

Carotenoid pigments were detected in all the tested strains. The strains SA 3 MRSA with an absorbance at 465 nm of 0.995 ± 0.001 and the 2065 MA with an absorbance of 0.911 ± 0.017, display the highest concentration of pigments, followed by DSM 25693 MRSA (Abs of 0.788 ± 0.021), ATCC

6538 (Abs of 0.701 ± 0.005), 2153 MA (Abs of 0.480 ± 0.002), and 2095 M1A1 (Abs of 0.411 ± 0.013).

DISCUSSION

According to literature, the susceptibility of *S. aureus* to PDI is strain-dependent and MRSA strains seem to have a lower susceptibility to PDI than methicillin-sensitive counterparts (Grinholc et al., 2008). The lower susceptibility of MRSA strains to PDI has been attributed to slime production by the MRSA strains used (Grinholc et al., 2008).

In this study, all the strains tested were susceptible to PDI, with a survival reduction above 5 log CFU mL^{-1}, which according to American Society of Microbiology is higher than the minimum required (reduction > 3 log CFU mL^{-1}) for a new approach to be termed as antimicrobial (ASM, 2015). However, as observed in previous studies, a strain-dependent efficiency of inactivation was observed (Grinholc et al., 2008). Nonetheless PDI does not seem to be antibiotic-susceptible dependent, since DSM 25693, an MRSA and enterotoxic strain, was the only strain that was inactivated to the limit of detection of the method, with a survival reduction of 8.5 log. Another MRSA strain, SA 3 MRSA, was not as efficiently inactivated, but the inactivation profile was similar to that of the reference, ATCC 6538 strain. The four enterotoxic strains were more efficiently inactivated that the two non-enterotoxic strains (see **Figure 1**), which could suggest that the enterotoxic strains are more susceptible to PDI. However, as showing the log10 reduction rates differences in PDI inactivation between enterotoxic strains were observed, which means that other cell factors may contribute to these differences in PDI efficiency. Whereby, further studies should be performed exploiting the factors which may contribute to the difference in PDI susceptibility among the bacterial strain.

Carotenoid pigment content is related with the resistance of *S. aureus* to several stress factors, such as external oxidative stress. Several studies have shown that mutant strains that are unable to produce carotenoids are more susceptible to those stress factors (Liu et al., 2005; Clauditz et al., 2006; Cebrián et al., 2007). In an attempt to verify if carotenoid pigments were able to attenuate oxidative damages and consequent cellular inactivation, the pigment content of each strain was measured. Although a direct relation between carotenoids content and PDI efficiency was not observed for all the strains, the least susceptible strains to PDI (ATCC 6538 and SA 3 MRSA) show a high relative concentration of this pigment, with absorbances of 0.701 and 0.995, respectively.

Once the photodynamic action occurs through ROS generation (formed along the irradiation process), the damages (through oxidative process) can affect a variety of cellular components with great importance in the maintenance of bacterial stability, such as molecular components (proteins and lipids) of external structures, and enzymes (Alves et al., 2014; Almeida et al., 2015). The majority of virulence factors of *S. aureus* are proteins or enzymes that are prone to photodynamic oxidative damage. The results of this study show that the phenotypic expression of the of β-hemolysin, lipase, lecithinase, catalase and bound coagulase by surviving cells cultivated on PCA medium for 48 h at 37°C was not affected by PDI. Mannitol uptake and fermentation also persisted. Previous proteomic analysis showed that the oxidative damage caused by PDI treatment affects the expression of functional proteins involved in cell division, metabolic activities, oxidative stress responses, and sugar uptake (Alves et al., 2014, 2015a). However, the mentioned studies were performed in treated cells. Since the detection of virulence factors activity in our study was performed in the surviving cells after a period of recovery, it would be expected that the bacteria, even if injured during PDI treatments, would be able to continue producing those virulence factors and other enzymes.

Antioxidant enzymes such as superoxide dismutase, catalase, and peroxidase can give protection against some ROS but not against singlet oxygen. So, according to the literature porphyrinic compounds (Almeida et al., 2011), namely the tetracationic porphyrin Tetra-Py^+-Me used in this study, exert their photodynamic action by a type II mechanism and consequently singlet oxygen is the main ROS (Tavares et al., 2011; Costa L. et al., 2013). Moreover, has been shown that singlet oxygen is able to inactivate these enzymes, namely the catalase enzyme (Kim et al., 2001). However, no effect of the PDI process was observed for this enzyme, once that in this study, the catalase activity was only determined after a recovery period of the persistent cells, and not during the PDI treatment – condition in which could be detected some changes in the activity of catalase. Further studies are needed to clarify whether the ROS produced by the Tetra-Py^+-Me during PDI treatments affect catalase enzyme and even other enzymes when they are outside the cells.

Nevertheless, some of these virulence factors are released to the extracellular compartment, becoming more exposed to the effects of the PDI process suffering a greater damage.

In this study, the presence/activity of two external virulence factors (free coagulase and enterotoxins A and C) in the supernatant of PDI treatment samples was assessed. The results show that both virulence factors are affected by PDI. This represents an advantage relatively to traditional antibiotics, which act only on bacterial cell and not on extracellular virulence factors. These results are in accordance with those observed in the previous studies by Kömerik et al. (2000) and Tubby et al. (2009).

The response of one of the most important *S. aureus* virulence factors, the SE which are the staphylococcal food poisoning causative agents, was also assessed after PDI treatment in order to confirm the effect of PDI on extracellular virulence factors. Two isolated enterotoxins, SE A and C, were treated by PDI. The porphyrin Tetra-Py^+-Me at a concentration of 5.0 μM reduced at least in 68% the amount of active SE A and C. This discovery is of great importance since it is known that this family of proteins covers very stable, resistant to heat and to degrading enzymes molecules (Schelin et al., 2011). These results demonstrate that PDI is not only effective in the inactivation of microorganisms but also in the degradation of released external virulence factors.

One of the main advantages of PDI is that because of the nature of the photoinactivation process, development of resistance is very unlikely (Tavares et al., 2010; Costa et al., 2011). The results obtained in this study do not show evidence of resistance development in the three strains subjected to ten PDI cycles, which corroborates literature conclusions. Considerable reduction in the efficiency of photosensitization of *S. aureus* strains ATCC 6538, enterotoxic 2065 MA and SA 3 MRSA after ten consecutive photosensitization sessions of 60 min with 5.0 μM of Tetra-Py$^+$-Me was not observed. As in this study, the viable bacterial colonies have been aseptically removed from the plate and suspended in PBS after each PDI cycle, the cellular density obtained after the colony resuspension could be different. To avoid differences in the PDI efficiency due to different bacterial densities, this parameter was controlled in all the experiments by measuring the optical density of the bacteria suspension before each assay.

CONCLUSION

Overall, it can be concluded that (1) although the efficiency of PDI to inactivate *S. aureus* is strain-dependent, all the strains can be effectively inactivated, namely the enterotoxic strains; (2) PDI process is not only effective in the inactivation of microorganisms but also in the degradation of their external virulence factors after their release to the exterior; and (3) *S. aureus* strains do not develop resistance to PDI treatment.

The research conducted so far, allowed the development of very promising and successful *in vitro* photoinactivation protocols for enterotoxigenic and non-enterotoxigenic strains of *S. aureus*. However, their evaluation *in vivo*, along with validation of their feasibility according to different sample settings and different enterotoxigenic and non-enterotoxigenic strains of *S. aureus*, as well as on biofilms developed by these bacteria, are now required. Bacterial biofilms are not only more difficult to inactivate than planktonic bacteria, but bacteria in a biofilm-mode are also much more prone to become resistant to antimicrobial agents or strategies (Beirão et al., 2014). In fact, some mechanisms, such as horizontal gene transfer and quorum sensing, occur only in a biofilm-state (Madsen et al., 2012; Solano et al., 2014).

AUTHOR CONTRIBUTIONS

MB did the experimental work and drafted the manuscript. SR participated in the experimental work. AA has been involved in the coordination, conception, design of the study and helped to draft the manuscript. ÂC, MF, and MN participated in the design of the study, acquisition and interpretation of data, and also helped.

ACKNOWLEDGMENTS

The authors are thankful to the University of Aveiro, to FCT/MEC for the financial support to the QOPNA research Unit (FCT UID/QUI/00062/2013) and Centre for Environmental and Marine Studies (CESAM) unit (project Pest-C/MAR/LA0017/2013), through national founds and, where applicable, co-financed by the FEDER, within the PT2020 Partnership Agreement, and also to the Portuguese NMR Network.

REFERENCES

Almeida, A., Cunha, A., Faustino, M. A. F., Tomé, A. C., and Neves, M. G. P. M. S. (2011). "Porphyrins as antimibrobial photosensitizing agents," in *Photodynamic Inactivation of Microbial Pathogens: Medical and Environmental Applications*, eds M. R. Hamblin and G. Jori (Cambridge: Royal Society of Chemistry), 83–160.

Almeida, A., Cunha, A., Gomes, N. C. M., Alves, E., Costa, L., and Faustino, M. A. F. (2009). Phage therapy and photodynamic therapy: low environmental impact approaches to inactivate microorganisms in fish farming plants. *Mar. Drugs* 7, 268–313. doi: 10.3390/md7030268

Almeida, A., Faustino, M. A. F., and Tomé, J. P. C. (2015). Photodynamic inactivation of bacteria: finding the effective targets. *Future Med. Chem.* 7, 1221–1224. doi: 10.4155/fmc.15.59

Almeida, J., Tomé, J. P. C., Neves, M. G. P. M. S., Tomé, A. C., Cavaleiro, J. A. S., Cunha, A., et al. (2014). Photodynamic inactivation of multidrug-resistant bacteria in hospital wastewaters: influence of residual antibiotics. *Photochem. Photobiol. Sci.* 13, 626–633. doi: 10.1039/c3pp50195g

Alves, E., Carvalho, C. M. B., Tomé, J. P. C., Faustino, M. A. F., Neves, M. G. P. M. S., Tomé, A. C., et al. (2008). Photodynamic inactivation of recombinant bioluminescent *Escherichia coli* by cationic porphyrins under artificial and solar irradiation. *J. Ind. Microbiol. Biotechnol.* 35, 1447–1454. doi: 10.1007/s10295-008-0446-2

Alves, E., Esteves, A. C., Cunha, A., Faustino, M. A. F., Neves, M. G. P. M. S., and Almeida, A. (2015a). Protein profiles of *Escherichia coli* and *Staphylococcus warneri* are altered by photosensitization with cationic porphyrins. *Photochem. Photobiol. Sci.* 14, 1169–1178. doi: 10.1039/C4PP00194J

Alves, E., Faustino, M. A. F., Neves, M. G. P. M. S., Cunha, A., Nadais, H., and Almeida, A. (2015b). Potential applications of porphyrins in photodynamic inactivation beyond the medical scope. *J. Photochem. Photobiol. C Photochem. Rev.* 22, 34–57. doi: 10.1016/j.jphotochemrev.2014.09.003

Alves, E., Faustino, M. A. F., Neves, M. G. P. M. S., Cunha, A., Tomé, J. P. C., and Almeida, A. (2014). An insight on bacterial cellular targets of photodynamic inactivation. *Future Med. Chem.* 6, 141–164. doi: 10.4155/fmc.13.211

Alves, E., Santos, N., Melo, T., Maciel, E., Dória, M. L., Faustino, M. A. F., et al. (2013). Photodynamic oxidation of *Escherichia coli* membrane phospholipids: new insights based on lipidomics. *Rapid Commun. Mass Spectrom.* 27, 2717–2728. doi: 10.1002/rcm.6739

Arrojado, C., Pereira, C., Tomé, J. P. C., Faustino, M. A. F., Neves, M. G. P. M. S., Tomé, A. C., et al. (2011). Applicability of photodynamic antimicrobial chemotherapy as an alternative to inactivate fish pathogenic bacteria in aquaculture systems. *Photochem. Photobiol. Sci.* 10, 1691–1700. doi: 10.1039/c1pp05129f

ASM (2015). *Antimicrobial Agents and Chemotherapy, Instructions to Authors, 1.* Available at: http://aac.asm.org/site/misc/journal-ita_abb.xhtml#04

Baptista, I., Queirós, R. P., Cunha, A., Saraiva, J. A., Rocha, S. M., and Almeida, A. (2015). Inactivation of enterotoxic and non-enterotoxic *Staphylococcus aureus* strains by high pressure treatments and evaluation of its impact on virulence factors. *Food Control* 57, 252–257. doi: 10.1016/j.fm.2014.09.016

Beirão, S., Fernandes, S., Coelho, J., Faustino, M. A. F., Tomé, J. P., Neves, M. G. P. M. S., et al. (2014). Photodynamic inactivation of bacterial and yeast biofilms with a cationic porphyrin. *Photochem. Photobiol.* 60, 1387–1396. doi: 10.1111/php.12331

Bien, J., Sokolova, O., and Bozko, P. (2011). Characterization of virulence factors of *Staphylococcus aureus*: novel function of known virulence factors that are implicated in activation of airway epithelial proinflammatory response. *J. Pathog.* 2011, 13. doi: 10.4061/2011/601905

Bronner, S., Monteil, H., and Prévost, G. (2004). Regulation of virulence determinants in *Staphylococcus aureus*: complexity and applications. *FEMS Microbiol. Rev.* 28, 183–200. doi: 10.1016/j.femsre.2003.09.003

Bujia, J., Feyh, J., and Kastenbauer, E. (1993). Photodynamic therapy with derivatives from hemotoporphyrines for recurrent laryngeal papillomatosis of the children. Early results. *An. Otorrinolaringol. Ibero Am.* 20, 251–259.

Calin, M. A., and Parasca, S. V. (2009). Light sources for photodynamic inactivation of bacteria. *Lasers Med. Sci.* 24, 453–460. doi: 10.1007/s10103-008-0588-5

Carvalho, C. M. B., Alves, E., Costa, L., Tomé, J. P. C., Faustino, M. A. F., Neves, M. G. P. M. S., et al. (2010). Functional cationic nanomagnet – porphyrin hybrids for the photoinactivation of microorganisms. *ACS Nano* 4, 7133–7140. doi: 10.1021/nn1026092

Carvalho, C. M. B., Tomé, J. P. C., Faustino, M. A. F., Neves, M. G. P. M. S., Tomé, A. C., Cavaleiro, J. A. S., et al. (2009). Antimicrobial photodynamic activity of porphyrin derivatives: potential application on medical and water disinfection. *J. Porphyr. Phthalocyanines* 13, 574–577. doi: 10.1142/S1088424609000528

Cebrián, G., Sagarzazu, N., Pagán, R., Condón, S., and Mañas, P. (2007). Heat and pulsed electric field resistance of pigmented and non-pigmented enterotoxigenic strains of *Staphylococcus aureus* in exponential and stationary phase of growth. *Int. J. Food Mocrobiol.* 118, 304–311. doi: 10.1016/j.ijfoodmicro.2007.07.051

Chambers, H. F., and DeLeo, F. (2009). Waves of resistance: *Staphylococcus aureus* in the antibiotic Era. *Nat. Rev. Microbiol.* 7, 629–641. doi: 10.1038/nrmicro2200

Cheung, A. L., Bayer, A. S., Zhang, G., Gresham, H., and Xiong, Y. Q. (2004). Regulation of virulence determinants in vitro and in vivo in *Staphylococcus aureus*. *FEMS Immunol. Med. Microbiol.* 40, 1-9. doi: 10.1016/S0928-8244(03)00309-2

Clauditz, A., Resch, A., Wieland, K. P., Peschel, A., and Gotz, F. (2006). Staphyloxanthin plays a role in the fitness of *Staphylococcus aureus* and its ability to cope with oxidative stress. *Infect. Immun.* 74, 4950–4953. doi: 10.1128/IAI.00204-06

Clinical and Laboratory Standards Institute [CLSI] (2013). *Performance Strandards for Antimicrobial Susceptibility Testing. CLSI Approved Standard M100-S23.* Wayne, PA: Clinical and Laboratory Standards Institute.

Costa, A. R., Batistão, D. W. F., Ribas, R. M., Sousa, A. M., Pereira, O., and Botelho, C. M. (2013). "*Staphylococcus aureus* virulence factors and disease," in *Microbial Pathogens and Strategies for Combating Them: Science, Technology and Education*, ed. A. Méndez-Vilas (Badajoz: Formatex Research Center), 702–710.

Costa, L., Alves, E., Carvalho, C. M. B., Tomé, J. P. C., Faustino, M. A. F., Neves, M. G. P. M. S., et al. (2008). Sewage bacteriophage photoinactivation by cationic porphyrins: a study of charge effect. *Photochem. Photobiol. Sci.* 7, 415–422. doi: 10.1039/b712749a

Costa, L., Faustino, M. A. F., Neves, M. G. P. M. S., Cunha, A., and Almeida, A. (2012). Photodynamic inactivation of mammalian viruses and bacteriophages. *Viruses* 4, 1034–1074. doi: 10.3390/v4071034

Costa, L., Faustino, M. A. F., Tomé, J. P. C., Neves, M. G. P. M. S., Tomé, A. C., Cavaleiro, J. A. S., et al. (2013). Involvement of type I and type II mechanisms on the photoinactivation of non-enveloped DNA and RNA bacteriophages. *J. Photochem. Photobiol. B Biol.* 120, 10–16. doi: 10.1016/j.jphotobiol.2013.01.005

Costa, L., Tomé, J. P. C., Neves, M. G. P. M. S., Tomé, A. C., Cavaleiro, J. A. S., Faustino, M. A. F., et al. (2011). Evaluation of resistance development and viability recovery by a non-enveloped virus after repeated cycles of aPDT. *Antiviral Res.* 91, 278–282. doi: 10.1016/j.antiviral.2011.06.007

Dai, T., Huang, Y.-Y., and Hamblin, M. R. (2010). Photodynamic therapy for localized infections – state of the art. *Photodiagnosis Photodyn. Ther.* 6, 170–188. doi: 10.1016/j.pdpdt.2009.10.008

Ebrahimi, A., Ghasemi, M., and Ghasemi, B. (2014). Some virulence factors of staphylococci isolated from wound and skin infections in Shahrekord, IR Iran. *Jundishapur J. Microbiol.* 7:e9225. doi: 10.5812/jjm.9225

Elman, M., Slatkine, M., and Harth, Y. (2003). The effective treatment of acne vulgaris by a high-intensity, narrow band 405-420 nm light source. *J. Cosmet. Laser Ther.* 5, 111–117. doi: 10.1080/14764170310001276

Enright, M. C., Robinson, D. A., Randle, G., Feil, E. J., Grundmann, H., and Spratt, B. G. (2002). The evolutionary history of methicillin-resistant *Staphylococcus aureus* (MRSA). *Proc. Natl. Acad. Sci. U.S.A.* 99, 7687–7692. doi: 10.1073/pnas.122108599

Gonçalves, M., Eira, D., Tomé, R., Mendes, F., Valado, A., Armando, C., et al. (2014). Prevalence of the Panton-Valentine Leukocidin in *Staphylococcus aureus* associated with upper respiratory tract infections. *Int. J. Med. Med. Sci.* 1, 8–13.

Grinholc, M., Szramka, B., Kurlenda, J., Graczyk, A., and Bielawski, K. P. (2008). Bactericidal effect of photodynamic inactivation against methicillin-resistant and methicillin-susceptible *Staphylococcus aureus* is strain-dependent. *J. Photochem. Photobiol. Biol.* 90, 57–63. doi: 10.1016/j.jphotobiol.2007.11.002

Guillemot, D. (1999). Antibiotic use in humans and bacterial resistance. *Curr. Opin. Microbiol.* 2, 494–498. doi: 10.1016/S1369-5274(99)00006-5

Ito, T., Okuma, K., Ma, X. X., Yuzawa, H., and Hiramatsu, K. (2003). Insights on antibiotic resistance of *Staphylococcus aureus* from its whole genome: genomic island SCC. *Drug Resist. Updat.* 6, 41–52. doi: 10.1016/S1368-7646(03)00003-7

Johnson, H. M., Russell, J. K., and Pontzer, C. H. (1991). Staphylococcal enterotoxin microbial superantigens. *FASEB J.* 5, 2706–2712.

Kawada, A., Aragane, Y., Kameyama, H., Sangen, Y., and Tezuka, T. (2002). Acne phototherapy with a high-intensity, enhanced, narrow-band, blue light source: an open study and in vitro investigation. *J. Dermatol. Sci.* 30, 129–135. doi: 10.1016/S0923-1811(02)00068-3

Kharkwal, G. B., Sharma, S. K., Huang, Y.-Y., Dai, T., and Hamblin, M. R. (2011). Photodynamic therapy for infections: clinical applications. *Lasers Surg. Med.* 43, 755–767. doi: 10.1002/lsm.21080

Kim, S. Y., Kwon, O. J., and Park, J. W. (2001). Inactivation of catalase and superoxide dismutase by singlet oxygen derived from photoactivated dye. *Biochimie* 83, 437–444. doi: 10.1016/S0300-9084(01)01258-5

Kömerik, N., Wilson, M., and Poole, S. (2000). The effect of photodynamic action on two virulence factors of gram-negative bacteria. *Photochem. Photobiol.* 72, 676–680. doi: 10.1562/0031-8655(2000)072<0676:TEOPAO>2.0.CO;2

Kossakowska, M., Nakonieczna, J., Kawiak, A., Kurlenda, J., Bielawski, K. P., and Grinholc, M. (2013). Discovering the mechanisms of strain-dependent response of *Staphylococcus aureus* to photoinactivation: oxidative stress toleration, endogenous porphyrin level and strain's virulence. *Photodiagnosis Photodyn. Ther.* 10, 348–355. doi: 10.1016/j.pdpdt.2013.02.004

Liu, G. Y., Essex, A., Buchanan, J. T., Datta, V., Hoffman, H. M., Bastian, J. F., et al. (2005). *Staphylococcus aureus* golden pigment impairs neutrophil killing and promotes virulence through its antioxidant activity. *J. Exp. Med.* 202, 209–215. doi: 10.1084/jem.20050846

Liu, G. Y., and Nizet, V. (2009). Color me bad: microbial pigments as virulence factors. *Trends Microbiol.* 17, 406–413. doi: 10.1016/j.tim.2009.06.006

Madsen, J. S., Burmølle, M., Hansen, L. H., and Sørensen, S. J. (2012). The interconnection between biofilm formation and horizontal gene transfer. *FEMS Immunol. Med. Microbiol.* 65, 183–195. doi: 10.1111/j.1574-695X.2012.00960.x

Melo, T., Santos, N., Lopes, D., Alves, E., Maciel, E., Faustino, M. A. F., et al. (2013). Photosensitized oxidation of phosphatidylethanolamines monitored by electrospray tandem mass spectrometry. *J. Mass Spectrom.* 48, 1357–1365. doi: 10.1002/jms.3301

Moore, C., Wallis, C., Melnick, J. L., and Kuns, M. D. (1972). Photodynamic treatment of herpes keratitis. *Infect. Immun.* 5, 169–171.

Morikawa, K., Maruyama, A., Inose, Y., Higashide, M., Hayashi, H., and Ohta, T. (2001). Overexpression of sigma factor, sigma(B), urges *Staphylococcus aureus* to thicken the cell wall and to resist beta-lactams. *Biochem. Biophys. Res. Commun.* 288, 385–389. doi: 10.1006/bbrc.2001.5774

Novick, R. P., and Geisinger, E. (2008). Quorum sensing in staphylococci. *Annu. Rev. Genet.* 42, 541–564. doi: 10.1146/annurev.genet.42.110807.091640

Ormond, A., and Freeman, H. (2013). Dye sensitizers for photodynamic therapy. *Materials* 6, 817–840. doi: 10.3390/ma6030817

Schelin, J., Wallin-Carlquist, N., Cohn, M. T., Lindqvist, R., and Barker, G. C. (2011). The formation of *Staphylococcus aureus* enterotoxin in food environments and advances in risk assessment. *Virulence* 2, 580–592. doi: 10.4161/viru.2.6.18122

Shikowitz, M. J., Abramson, A. L., Freeman, K., Steinberg, B. M., and Nouri, M. (1998). Efficacy of DHE photodynamic therapy for respiratory Papillomatosis: immediate and long-term results. *Laryngoscope* 108, 962–967. doi: 10.1097/00005537-199807000-00002

Solano, C., Echeverz, M., and Lasa, I. (2014). Biofilm dispersion and quorum sensing. *Curr. Opin. Microbiol.* 18, 96–104. doi: 10.1016/j.mib.2014.02.008

Tavares, A., Carvalho, C. M. B., Faustino, M. A. F., Neves, M. G. P. M. S., Tomé, J. P. C., Tomé, A. C., et al. (2010). Antimicrobial photodynamic therapy: study of bacterial recovery viability and potential development of resistance after treatment. *Mar. Drugs* 8, 91–105. doi: 10.3390/md8010091

Tavares, A., Carvalho, C. M. B., Faustino, M. A. F., Neves, M. G. P. M. S., Tomé, J. P. C., Tomé, A. C., et al. (2011). Mechanisms of photoinactivation of Gram-negative recombinant bioluminescent bacteria by cationic porphyrins. *Photochem. Photobiol. Sci.* 10, 1659–1669. doi: 10.1039/c1pp05097d

TD0900, SET-RPLA (2015). *Toxin Detection Kit SET-RPLA Staphylococcal Enterotoxins, OXOID.* Available at: http://www.oxoid.com/uk/blue/prod_detail/prod_detail.asp?pr=TD0900&org=153&c=uk&lang=en (accessed April 13, 2015).

Theuretzbacher, U. (2011). Resistance drives antibacterial drug development. *Curr. Opin. Pharmacol.* 11, 433–438. doi: 10.1016/j.coph.2011.07.008

Theuretzbacher, U. (2013). Global antibacterial resistance: the never-ending story. *J. Glob. Antimicrob. Resist.* 1, 63–69. doi: 10.1016/j.jgar.2013.03.010

Tubby, S., Wilson, M., and Nair, S. P. (2009). Inactivation of staphylococcal virulence factors using a light-activated antimicrobial agent. *BMC Microbiol.* 9:211. doi: 10.1186/1471-2180-9-211

13

Salmonella Enteritidis Isolate Harboring Multiple Efflux Pumps and Pathogenicity Factors, Shows Absence of O Antigen Polymerase Gene

Daniela Jones-Dias [1,2†], Lurdes Clemente [3†], Conceição Egas [4], Hugo Froufe [4], Daniel A. Sampaio [5], Luís Vieira [5], Maria Fookes [6], Nicholas R. Thomson [6], Vera Manageiro [1,2] and Manuela Caniça [1]*

[1] National Reference Laboratory of Antibiotic Resistances and Healthcare Associated Infections, Department of Infectious Diseases, National Health Institute Doutor Ricardo Jorge (INSA), Lisbon, Portugal, [2] Centre for the Studies of Animal Science, Institute of Agrarian and Agri-Food Sciences and Technologies, University of Porto, Porto, Portugal, [3] Microbiology and Mycology Laboratory, Instituto Nacional de Investigação Agrária e Veterinária, Lisbon, Portugal, [4] Biocant, Parque Tecnológico de Cantanhede, Cantanhede, Portugal, [5] Innovation and Technology Unit, Human Genetics Department, National Health Institute Doutor Ricardo Jorge (INSA), Lisbon, Portugal, [6] Wellcome Trust Sanger Institute, Wellcome Trust Genome Campus, Hinxton, UK

Keywords: *Salmonella* Enteritidis, omphalitis, *wzy* deletion, epidemiology, pathogenicity factors, MGE, metal tolerance

Correspondence:
Vera Manageiro
vera.manageiro@insa.min-saude.pt

† These authors have contributed equally to this work.

BACKGROUND

Salmonella enterica is one of the most important causes of gastrointestinal infection in humans, being the great majority of infections related to the consumption of poultry meat and eggs (Foley and Lynne, 2008; EFSA/ECDC, 2015).

In animals, infections caused by serotype Enteritidis are rarely responsible for severe disease with animals frequently becoming asymptomatic carriers, except in the case of young chicks and poults, where outbreaks exhibiting clinical disease are often accompanied by high mortality rates (Foley et al., 2008, 2013). Indeed, *S. enterica* subsp. *enterica* serovar Enteritidis (*S.* Enteritidis) has been responsible for severe disease in industrial poultry farming facilities worldwide, posing a potential hazard for public health (Lutful Kabir, 2010).

In order to be infectious, *Salmonella* needs to adapt to different niches and conditions, where virulence and heavy-metal-tolerance factors play an important role, through co-selection events and the formation of pathogenicity islands, respectively (Hensel, 2004; Medardus et al., 2014). Furthermore, antibiotic resistance determinants can also facilitate their survival, with ubiquitous chromosomally encoded efflux mechanisms, playing an important role in both intrinsic, and acquired multidrug resistance. Other resistance mechanisms, such as changes in the membrane permeability, enzymatic modification, and target alterations may increase the levels of bacterial resistance, contributing to the success of the infection (Poole, 2004; Delmar et al., 2014; Li et al., 2015).

Both antibiotic susceptibility determination and serotyping constitute very useful tools for the epidemiologic classification of *S. enterica* isolates. Indeed, in *S. enterica*, the resistance rates fluctuate according to the serotype and with the antibiotic (Clemente et al., 2015). Classically, serotyping is based on the antigenic reactivity of lipolysaccharide (O antigen) and flagellar proteins (H antigen), followed by a designation using names or formulas (Grimont and Weill, 2007). In this study, we aimed to analyze the genome of a *S.* Enteritidis isolate responsible for omphalitis in chicks, exploring the molecular features associated with antibiotic resistance and pathogenicity, as well as the ability to spread the respective determinants.

METHODS

Bacterial Isolate, Antibiotic Susceptibility Testing, and Serotyping

The isolate (LV60) was recovered from a sample collected from the yolk sac of a chick with omphalitis, under the scope of the "*Salmonella* National Control Programme in food-producing animals and food of animal origin for bacteriological diagnosis, serotype identification and antibiotic susceptibility testing." The guidelines of the Commission Decision (CD), 2007/407/EC were followed. LV60 was tested for its antimicrobial resistance through the determination of minimum inhibitory concentrations (MICs) using the agar dilution method, as previously described (Clemente et al., 2013) and according to the European Committee on Antimicrobial Susceptibility Testing (EUCAST) guidelines (http://www.eucast.org/). Briefly, a panel of 11 antibiotic compounds was tested in a 2-fold concentration series over the following ranges: ampicillin and tetracycline (0.5–64 μg/mL), gentamicin and trimethoprim (0.25–32 μg/mL), ciprofloxacin (0.008–8 μg/mL), cefotaxime (0.06–8 μg/mL), nalidixic acid and streptomycin (2–512 μg/mL), chloramphenicol (2–256 μg/mL), florfenicol (1–128 μg/mL) and sulphamethoxazole (8–1024 μg/mL). The epidemiological cut-off values recommended by EUCAST to *Salmonella* spp. were

TABLE 1 | Single nucleotide variants that represent amino acid substitutions in *S.* Enteritidis LV60 using *S.* Enteritidis strain p125109 as the reference genome.

Reference Position	Reference	Allele	Gene (Product)	Amino acid change	Coverage
40158	C	T	SEN_RS00180 (arylsulfatase)	Pro92Ser	155
55278	C	A	*ileS* (isoleucine-tRNA ligase)	Ala557Glu	144
93979	G	A	SEN_RS00415 (hypothetical protein)	Ala96Thr	127
156264	G	A	SEN_RS00685 (peptidase M23)	Gly299Asp	123
353437	T	C	SEN_RS01600 (isopropylmalate isomerase)	Val454Ala	119
357149	A	T	SEN_RS01625 (hypothetical protein)	Leu1Met	177
401018	C	A	*prpE* (acetyl-CoA synthetase)	Arg9Ser	132
411602	T	G	SEN_RS01845 (hypothetical protein)	Trp209Gly	58
561577	T	C	SEN_RS02560 (MFS transporter)	Ser333Pro	68
659902	T	G	*dpiB* (sensor histidine kinase)	Tyr3Asp	52
988620	G	C	SEN_RS04610 (hypothetical protein)	Ala89Pro	130
1044895	G	T	*helD* (DNA helicase IV)/Mobile element	Ala204Ser	75
1156702	G	C	*sirA* (virulence gene transcriptional regulator)	Val181Leu	112
1325689	A	G	SEN_RS06450 (hydrogenase-1 operon protein HyaF)	Tyr209His	93
1427037	T	A	SEN_RS06930 (diguanylate phosphodiesterase)	Asp16Glu	92
1787654	A	G	SEN_RS08735 (transporter)	Arg348Gly	79
1807289	G	A	SEN_RS08820 (lipoprotein)	Ala14Val	79
1931818	C	T	SEN_RS09505 (NAD-dependent deacetylase)	Met37Ile	82
2115337	C	T	SEN_RS10585 (cobalamin biosynthesis protein CbiB)	Gly167Ser	104
2419980	G	A	SEN_RS11950 (NADH:ubiquinone oxidoreductase subunit M)	Leu474Phe	130
2426844	A	G	SEN_RS11980 (NADH dehydrogenase subunit G)	Val610Ala	125
2463887	T	C	SEN_RS12170 (amino acid transporter)	Ile452Val	34
2647060	G	A	SEN_RS12985 (outer membrane protein RatA)	Pro459Ser	108
2647626	G	T	SEN_RS12985 (outer membrane protein RatA)	Ala270Glu	111
2672592	A	C	SEN_RS13070 (hypothetical protein)	Ile313Ser	61
2956057	C	A	SEN_RS14420 (2-C-methyl-D-erythritol 4-phosphate cytidylyltransferase)	Arg53Leu	123
3185834	C	A	SEN_RS15495 (D-mannonate oxidoreductase)	Asn151Lys	81
3659470	G	T	SEN_RS17815 (membrane protein)	Gln71Lys	122
3802073	G	A	*coaD* (phosphopantetheine adenylyltransferase)	Val116Ile	127
4051393	T	C	SEN_RS19620 (DNase TatD)	Ser141Pro	150
4059155	G	A	*fadB* (3-ketoacyl-CoA thiolase)	Ala395Val	84
4348398	A	G	SEN_RS20980 (membrane protein)/ Salmonella Pathogenicity Island 4	Asn2902Asp	158
4402123	C	T	SEN_RS21190 (sugar:sodium symporter)	Ala350Val	77
4476625	T	C	SEN_RS21580 (hypothetical protein)	Lys76Glu	170
4555382	C	T	SEN_RS21985 (DNA polymerase III subunit chi)	Asp10Asn	110

used for the interpretation of susceptibility testing results. Quality control was performed using the *Escherichia coli* ATCC 25922 strain. LV60 isolate was then serotyped by the slide agglutination method for its O and H antigens using the method of Kauffman-White scheme (Grimont and Weill, 2007).

Whole Genome Sequencing (WGS), Assembly, and Annotation

Genomic DNA was extracted using DNeasy Blood and Tissue Kit (Qiagen), and DNA quantification was performed by Qubit Fluorometric Quantitation (Life Technologies), according to with the manufacturer's instructions. The genome was sequenced using a double strategy of 454 (Roche) and MiSeq (Illumina) sequencing.

Five hundred nanograms of bacterial DNA were fragmented by nebulization, followed by adaptor ligation to create double stranded DNA libraries and sequenced on a 454 GS FLX Titanium according to the standard manufacturer's instructions (Roche-454 Life Sciences). The second genome library was prepared from 1 ng of genomic DNA using the Nextera XT DNA Sample Preparation Kit (Illumina) and sequenced on the Illumina MiSeq sequencer (Illumina) using paired-end 2 × 150 bp reads.

First quality evaluation of raw read sequences and their corresponding quality values were assigned by the FastQC software. Reads were then trimmed and filtered according to quality criteria, and *de novo* assembled with Ray, version 2.3.1 (Boisvert et al., 2010). Contigs were searched for identity through blastn (http://blast.ncbi.nlm.nih.gov/Blast.cgi) against the nr/nt NCBI database to identify the closest bacterial genome and/or plasmid. Therefore, LV60 genome was mapped against the bacterial genome of S. Enteritidis strain p125109 and its plasmid (NC_011294 and HG970000, respectively) using GS Mapper version 2.9 (Roche). Additionally SNV (single nucleotide variants) and structural variants were also detected with the GS Mapper (Roche, version 2.9).

Structural and functional annotation was performed using PGP (Prokaryotic Genome Prediction) (Egas et al., 2014), an in-house developed pipeline. Taxonomy identification was performed by BLASTP search against the NCBI GenBank non-redundant (nr) database of the 16s rRNA sequence gene, identified in the previous step and confirmed using RNAmmer v1.2 (Lagesen et al., 2007).

The final data was submitted in the DDBJ/EMBL/GenBank databases, using the Sequin software tool (http://www.ncbi.nlm.nih.gov/Sequin/). This dataset, which includes files in Genbank (LIHI01.1.gbff.gz), Fasta (LIHI01.1.fsa_nt.gz), and ASN.1 (LIHI01.1.bbs.gz) formats, can be accessed and/or reused at http://www.ncbi.nlm.nih.gov/nuccore/LIHI00000000.

In silico Analyses

CLC genomics workbench 8.0 (QIAGEN, Aarhus), PathogenFinder 1.1, ResFinder 2.1, PlasmidFinder 1.3, and MLST 1.8 (MultiLocus Sequence Typing) were used to estimate the number of pathogenicity determinants, acquired antibiotic resistance genes, plasmids and the MLST using the S. Enteritidis genome (Larsen et al., 2012; Zankari et al., 2012; Cosentino et al., 2013; Carattoli et al., 2014). SeqSero tool was used for *Salmonella* serotyping by whole genome sequencing (Zhang et al., 2015).

PHAST search web tool was applied to detect, identify and annotate prophage sequences (Zhou et al., 2011). ISsaga was used for the high throughput identification and semiautomatic annotation of insertion sequences in the genome (Varani et al., 2011). The presence of molecular determinants of antimicrobial resistance was predicted based on homology and SNP models using the Comprehensive Antibiotic Resistance Database (CARD; https://card.mcmaster.ca/analyze/rgi), through Resistance Gene Identifier software (RGI; McArthur et al., 2013).

RESULTS

LV60 isolate was serotyped as S. Enteritidis, using the method of Kauffman-White scheme, and found to be wild-type to all the antibiotics tested, except tetracycline.

The *de novo* assembly yielded 4.977 Mbp distributed in 83 contigs (largest contig with 970,921 bp) with a N50 of 491,005 bp. Overall, the structural and functional annotation with PGP detected 97 tRNA genes, 7 rRNA genes and identified 4656 mRNA genes.

From mapping against the bacterial genome of S. Enteritidis strain p125109, the main difference between the two genomes was the absence of the O-antigen polymerase gene *wzy* in the LV60 isolate, which in S. Enteritidis is located outside the O antigen gene cluster (Liu et al., 2014). The coding sequence of *wzy* gene was searched against the assembled genome using blastn, confirming its absence. The flanking regions of *wzy* gene, which coded for a disrupted membrane and a hypothetical protein, were also absent. The *wzy* gene is involved in the Wzx/Wzy-dependent pathway, which constitutes the predominant pathway for O-antigen production in Gram-negative bacteria, specifically in *Salmonella* (Hong et al., 2015).

However, in this study, the absence of the *wzy* gene did not compromised the use of a high-throughput genome sequencing serotype determination method (Zhang et al., 2015), which corroborated the result obtained by the gold standard method. Indeed, this method, based on the detection of O and H antigens encoding genes, predicted an antigenic profile 9:g,m:- based on the O-9,46 *wba*V gene, which encodes to the O-antigen tyvelosyl transferase. Furthermore, the S. Enteritidis serotype was confirmed by the presence of *sdf* gene (*Salmonella* difference fragment virulence gene), a characteristic marker of commonly circulating S. *enterica* serovar Enteritidis (Agron et al., 2001).

Sixty-one SNVs were detected between LV60 and the S. Enteritidis strain p125109. The SNVs that resulted in amino acid substitutions are represented in **Table 1**. *In silico* analysis with ResFinder tool did not reveal the presence of any acquired antibiotic resistance genes (90% identity and 40% minimum length) or plasmids (95% identity). However, the RGI analysis, using the *perfect algorithm*, showed the presence of a *Salmonella*-specific MerR-like gold (Au) sensor- GolS—involved in Au resistance (Pontel et al., 2007). This constitutes a matter of concern since antibacterial biocides and metals can contribute

TABLE 2 | Perfect and strict best hit results, by predicted gene, obtained using the Resistance Gene Identifier (RGI).

Predicted gene	e-value	Identity (%)	Contig	Average coverage	Start	Stop	RGI Cut-off	RGI Protein Model_type	Antibiotic Resistance Ontology (ARO) category
golS	1.41E–108	100	4	147.97	80575	81039	Perfect	homolog	efflux pump conferring AR; chloramphenicol RG; beta-lactam RG; gene modulating antibiotic efflux
acrF	0	99	4	147.97	73608	76775	Strict	homolog	efflux pump conferring AR; beta-lactam RG; fluoroquinolone RG
sdiA	0	99	2	127.7	1179091	1179813	Strict	homolog	chloramphenicol RG; gene modulating antibiotic efflux; fluoroquinolone RG; efflux pump conferring AR; tetracycline RG; rifampin RG; beta-lactam RG
crp	1.30E–151	99	7	160.37	388833	389465	Strict	homolog	efflux pump conferring AR; macrolide RG; beta-lactam RG; gene modulating antibiotic efflux; fluoroquinolone RG
mdsA	0	98	4	147.97	76772	77977	Strict	homolog	efflux pump conferring AR; chloramphenicol RG; beta-lactam RG
mdsC	0	98	4	147.97	72134	73624	Strict	homolog	efflux pump conferring AR; chloramphenicol RG; beta-lactam RG
aac(6')-Iy	2.36E–101	97	2	127.7	808040	808477	Strict	homolog	antibiotic inactivation enzyme; aminoglycoside RG
cpxR	1.24E–160	97	3	152.34	67603	68301	Strict	homolog	efflux pump conferring AR; aminocoumarin RG; aminoglycoside RG; gene modulating antibiotic efflux
bacA	0	97	14	155.64	142061	142882	Strict	homolog	peptide AR gene; gene conferring AR via molecular bypass
cpxA	0	96	3	152.34	66233	67606	Strict	homolog	efflux pump conferring AR; aminocoumarin RG; aminoglycoside RG; gene modulating antibiotic efflux
baeR	5.11E–165	96	2	127.7	107261	107983	Strict	homolog	efflux pump conferring AR; aminocoumarin RG; aminoglycoside RG; gene modulating antibiotic efflux
emrY	0	95	8	158.13	93935	95473	Strict	homolog	efflux pump conferring AR; tetracycline RG
marA	1.35E–82	95	2	127.7	702301	702690	Strict	homolog	chloramphenicol RG; gene modulating antibiotic efflux; gene modulating permeability to antibiotic; fluoroquinolone RG; efflux pump conferring AR; tetracycline RG; rifampin RG; beta-lactam RG
H-NS	9.89E–75	94	2	127.7	965098	965511	Strict	homolog	gene modulating antibiotic efflux; macrolide RG; fluoroquinolone RG; efflux pump conferring AR; tetracycline RG; beta-lactam RG
mexD	0	94	5	135.43	37513	40626	Strict	homolog	chloramphenicol RG; trimethoprim RG; macrolide RG; fluoroquinolone RG; efflux pump conferring AR; beta-lactam RG
phoP	6.18E–151	93	2	127.7	417112	417786	Strict	homolog	efflux pump conferring AR; polymyxin RG; macrolide RG; gene modulating antibiotic efflux; gene altering cell wall charge conferring AR
emrR	7.58E–115	93	8	158.13	92089	92619	Strict	homolog	efflux pump conferring AR; gene modulating antibiotic efflux; fluoroquinolone RG
mexD	0	93	4	147.97	209028	212177	Strict	homolog	chloramphenicol RG; trimethoprim RG; macrolide RG; fluoroquinolone RG; efflux pump conferring AR; beta-lactam RG
mdtH	0	92	2	127.7	349496	350704	Strict	homolog	efflux pump conferring AR
mdtK	0	92	2	127.7	607306	608679	Strict	homolog	efflux pump conferring AR; fluoroquinolone RG
mexN	0	92	2	127.7	113873	116995	Strict	homolog	efflux pump conferring AR; chloramphenicol RG

(Continued)

TABLE 2 | Continued

Predicted gene	e-value	Identity (%)	Contig	Average coverage	Start	Stop	RGI Cut-off	RGI Protein Model_type	Antibiotic Resistance Ontology (ARO) category
mexN	0	91	2	127.7	110792	113872	Strict	homolog	efflux pump conferring AR; chloramphenicol RG
emrD	0	90	7	160.37	11534	12718	Strict	homolog	efflux pump conferring AR
mdtG	0	90	2	127.7	339682	340896	Strict	homolog	efflux pump conferring AR
pmrA	1.77E–143	90	9	160.96	119082	119750	Strict	homolog	polymyxin RG; gene altering cell wall charge conferring AR
emrA	0	89	8	158.13	92719	93918	Strict	homolog	efflux pump conferring AR; fluoroquinolone RG
pmrE	0	89	2	127.7	174573	175739	Strict	homolog	polymyxin RG; gene altering cell wall charge conferring AR
baeS	0	89	2	127.7	107980	109383	Strict	homolog	efflux pump conferring AR; aminocoumarin RG; aminoglycoside RG; gene modulating antibiotic efflux
tolC	0	89	14	155.64	163404	164879	Strict	homolog	chloramphenicol RG; macrolide RG; fluoroquinolone RG; efflux pump conferring AR; aminocoumarin RG; tetracycline RG; rifampin RG; beta-lactam RG
acrE	0	88	1	155.02	4223	5380	Strict	homolog	efflux pump conferring AR; beta-lactam RG; fluoroquinolone RG
mexD	0	88	1	155.02	1098	4211	Strict	homolog	chloramphenicol RG; trimethoprim RG; macrolide RG; fluoroquinolone RG; efflux pump conferring AR; beta-lactam RG
mdfA	0	87	13	131.07	105101	106333	Strict	homolog	efflux pump conferring AR
pmrF	0	87	5	135.43	231615	232598	Strict	homolog	polymyxin RG; gene altering cell wall charge conferring AR
mdtM	0	86	11	163.1	148308	149549	Strict	homolog	efflux pump conferring AR
ramA	1.93E–71	86	4	147.97	311233	311622	Strict	homolog	chloramphenicol RG; gene modulating antibiotic efflux; gene modulating permeability to antibiotic; fluoroquinolone RG; efflux pump conferring AR; tetracycline RG; rifampin RG; beta-lactam RG
mdtD	0	86	2	127.7	109383	110795	Strict	homolog	efflux pump conferring AR
acrA	0	85	4	147.97	212200	213393	Strict	homolog	chloramphenicol RG; fluoroquinolone RG; efflux pump conferring AR; tetracycline RG; rifampin RG; beta-lactam RG
phoQ	0	85	2	127.7	415649	417112	Strict	homolog	efflux pump conferring AR; polymyxin RG; macrolide RG; gene modulating antibiotic efflux; gene altering cell wall charge conferring AR
pmrB	0	85	9	160.96	118002	119081	Strict	homolog	polymyxin RG; gene altering cell wall charge conferring AR
mdtA	0	82	2	127.7	116995	118332	Strict	homolog	efflux pump conferring AR; aminocoumarin RG
pmrC	0	82	9	160.96	119747	121390	Strict	homolog	polymyxin RG; gene altering cell wall charge conferring AR
acrR	1.83E–124	82	4	147.97	213535	214188	Strict	variant	chloramphenicol RG; gene modulating antibiotic efflux; fluoroquinolone RG; efflux pump conferring AR; antibiotic resistant gene variant or mutant; tetracycline RG; rifampin RG; beta-lactam RG
robA	0	81	11	163.1	77518	78387	Strict	homolog	chloramphenicol RG; gene modulating antibiotic efflux; fluoroquinolone RG; efflux pump conferring AR; tetracycline RG; rifampin RG; beta-lactam RG
arnA	0	79	5	135.43	229636	231618	Strict	homolog	polymyxin RG; gene altering cell wall charge conferring AR

(Continued)

TABLE 2 | Continued

Predicted gene	e-value	Identity (%)	Contig	Average coverage	Start	Stop	RGI Cut-off	RGI Protein Model_type	Antibiotic Resistance Ontology (ARO) category
mdtL	0	77	16	156.65	44691	45878	Strict	homolog	efflux pump conferring AR
rosB	0	74	4	147.97	230248	231924	Strict	homolog	polymyxin RG
rosA	0	71	4	147.97	232128	233348	Strict	homolog	efflux pump conferring AR; polymyxin RG
rpoB	0	58	19	154.2	4220	8248	Strict	variant	rifampin RG; antibiotic resistant gene variant or mutant
katG	0	56	3	152.34	121560	123740	Strict	variant	antibiotic resistant gene variant or mutant; isoniazid RG
gyrB	0	55	16	156.65	54369	56783	Strict	homolog	aminocoumarin RG; antibiotic resistant gene variant or mutant
macB	0	50	13	131.07	143618	145564	Strict	homolog	efflux pump conferring AR; macrolide RG
vanG	8.15E–81	38	4	147.97	113335	114447	Strict	homolog	glycopeptide RG; AR gene cluster, cassette, or operon; gene conferring AR via molecular bypass
macA	2.30E–51	35	13	131.07	142503	143621	Strict	homolog	efflux pump conferring AR; macrolide RG

RG, resistance gene; AR, antibiotic resistance.

to the development and maintenance of antibiotic resistance in bacterial communities through mechanisms of cross- or co-resistance (Baker-Austin et al., 2006; Lemire et al., 2013; Pal et al., 2015).

Furthermore, the RGI strict algorithm, which detects previously unknown variants of known antimicrobial resistance genes, identified 52 genes involved in efflux, transport, and permeability, which might justify the low-level tetracycline resistance identified by phenotypic methods (**Table 2**). Resistance to additional classes of antibiotics such as fluoroquinolones, aminoglycosides, and chloramphenicol were bioinformatically predicted. Indeed, efflux pumps are often associated with discrete decreases in antibiotic susceptibility that may not necessarily reflect an alteration in interpretation categories (Fernández and Hancock, 2012). Genes responsible for the intrinsic resistance to benzylpenicillin, glycopeptides, macrolides, and rifampicin were also detected.

The total number of pathogenicity determinants present in the genome of *S.* Enteritidis LV60, matching 1164 pathogenic families, showed a 94.1% certainty of the isolate being a human pathogen. Here we highlight the presence of *Salmonella* Pathogenicity Island 4, which usually encodes a non-fimbrial adhesion and the cognate type 1 secretion system (Gerlach et al., 2007).

The use of complementary web tools assigned this isolate to ST11, which according with MLST data (http://mlst.warwick.ac.uk/) is commonly found among CTX-M-14 and CTX-M-15-producing *S.* Enteritidis human isolates (Kim et al., 2011; Bado et al., 2012). In this study, the identification of ST11 in an isolate of animal origin, together with other pathogenicity determinants may suggest its zoonotic potential.

We also identified 6 prophage regions, among which three were incomplete and three were intact. The last included prophage regions reaching the lengths of 64.3, 49.2, and 31.7 Kb, and encoding 42, 78, and 66 DNA coding sequences, respectively.

Overall, 33 different IS were detected within the genome, which were distributed as follows: 27.03% of IS*3* family, 18.92% of IS*256* family, 13.51% of IS unclassified elements, 10.81% of IS*200*/IS*605* complex, and of IS*L3* family, 8.11% of IS*481* family, 5.41% of IS*630* family, and 2.7% of IS*1* and IS*110* families. All identified structures (pathogenicity island, prophages, ISs) constitute a multiplicity of pathogenicity factors in LV60 *S.* Enteritidis isolate and contribute for the fitness of the isolate in different environments; its presence may also suggest the possibility of acquisition of other factors by different mechanisms, including resistance genes e.g., by horizontal gene transfer, contributing to its biological diversity and genetic evolution.

CONCLUSION

The detection of an avian *S.* Enteritidis isolate harboring multiple efflux pumps, pathogenicity factors, a variety of mobile genetic elements and heavy-metal-tolerance genes raises concerns regarding the dissemination of infection in birds and potential risk of zoonotic transmission.

This study demonstrated the added value of WGS as a routine tool for surveillance programs directed to food-producing animals, which might complement sanitary measures, essential to prevent the spread of *Salmonella* infections among animals. It also proved to have an added value as a complementary typing method. Moreover, the simultaneous detection of putative Au resistance, intrinsic antibiotic resistant genes, and mobile genetic elements, underline this method as a helpful resource to follow the spread and evolution of antibiotic resistance in this species by genomic comparison studies.

AUTHOR CONTRIBUTIONS

DJ designed the study, performed molecular experiments, analyzed the data and wrote the manuscript. LC performed the microbiological experiments and reviewed the manuscript. CE, HF performed 454 Roche genome sequencing experiments and analyze the data; DS, LV performed Illumina genome sequencing experiments. MF, NT analyzed the data. VM designed the study, analyzed the data and reviewed the manuscript. MC designed the study, reviewed and edited the manuscript. All authors read and approved the final manuscript.

FUNDING

DJ has received research funding from Fundação para a Ciência e a Tecnologia (FCT, grant number SFRH/BD/80001/2011). VM was supported by FCT fellowship (grant SFRH/BPD/77486/2011), financed by the European Social Funds (COMPETE-FEDER) and national funds of the Portuguese Ministry of Education and Science (POPH-QREN). We thank the support of FCT grant number PEst-OE/AGR/UI0211/2011-2014 and UID/MULTI/00211/2013.

REFERENCES

Agron, P. G., Walker, R. L., Kinde, H., Sawyer, S. J., Hayes, D. C., Wollard, J., et al. (2001). Identification by subtractive hybridization of sequences specific for *Salmonella enterica* serovar Enteritidis. *Appl. Environ. Microbiol.* 67, 4984–4991. doi: 10.1128/AEM.67.11.4984-4991.2001

Bado, I., García-Fulgueiras, V., Cordeiro, N. F., Betancor, L., Caiata, L., Seija, V., et al. (2012). First human isolate of *Salmonella enterica* serotype Enteritidis harboring $bla_{CTX-M-14}$ in South America. *Antimicrob. Agents Chemother.* 56, 2132–2134. doi: 10.1128/AAC.05530-11

Baker-Austin, C., Wright, M. S., Stepanauskas, R., and McArthur, J. V. (2006). Co-selection of antibiotic and metal resistance. *Trends Microbiol.* 14, 176–182. doi: 10.1016/j.tim.2006.02.006

Boisvert, S., Laviolette, F., and Corbeil, J. (2010). Ray: simultaneous assembly of reads from a mix of high-throughput sequencing technologies. *J. Comput. Biol.* 17, 1519–1533. doi: 10.1089/cmb.2009.0238

Carattoli, A., Zankari, E., García-Fernández, A., Voldby Larsen, M., Lund, O., Villa, L., et al. (2014). *In silico* detection and typing of plasmids using PlasmidFinder and plasmid multilocus sequence typing. *Antimicrob. Agents Chemother.* 58, 3895–3903. doi: 10.1128/AAC.02412-14

Clemente, L., Manageiro, V., Ferreira, E., Jones-Dias, D., Correia, I., Themudo, P., et al. (2013). Occurrence of extended-spectrum β-lactamases among isolates of *Salmonella enterica* subsp. *enterica* from food-producing animals and food products, in Portugal. *Int. J. Food Microbiol.* 167, 221–228. doi: 10.1016/j.ijfoodmicro.2013.08.009

Clemente, L., Manageiro, V., Jones-Dias, D., Correia, I., Themudo, P., Albuquerque, T., et al. (2015). Antimicrobial susceptibility and oxymino-β-lactam resistance mechanisms in *Salmonella enterica* and *Escherichia coli* isolates from different animal sources. *Res. Microbiol.* 166, 574–583. doi: 10.1016/j.resmic.2015.05.007

Cosentino, S., Voldby Larsen, M., Møller Aarestrup, F., and Lund, O. (2013). PathogenFinder-distinguishing friend from foe using bacterial whole genome sequence data. *PLoS ONE* 8:e77302. doi: 10.1371/journal.pone.0077302

Delmar, J. A., Su, C. C., and Yu, E. W. (2014). Bacterial multidrug efflux transporters. *Annu. Rev. Biophys.* 43, 93–117. doi: 10.1146/annurev-biophys-051013-022855

Egas, C., Barroso, C., Froufe, H. J., Pacheco, J., Albuquerque, L., and Da Costa, M. S. (2014). Complete genome sequence of the radiation-resistant bacterium *Rubrobacter radiotolerans* RSPS-4. *Stand. Genomic Sci.* 9, 1062–1075. doi: 10.4056/sigs.5661021

European Food Safety Authority/European Center Disease Control (EFSA/ECDC) (2015). EU Summary Report on antimicrobial resistance in zoonotic and indicator bacteria from humans, animals and food in 2013. *EFSA J.* 13:4036. doi: 10.2903/j.efsa.2015.4036

Fernández, L., and Hancock, R. E. W. (2012). Adaptive and mutational resistance: role of porins and efflux pumps in drug resistance. *Clin. Microbiol. Rev.* 25, 661–681. doi: 10.1128/CMR.00043-12

Foley, S. L., Johnson, T. J., Ricke, S. C., Nayak, R., and Danzeisen, J. (2013). *Salmonella* pathogenicity and host adaptation in chicken-associated serovars. *Microbiol. Mol. Biol. Rev.* 77, 582–607. doi: 10.1128/MMBR.00015-13

Foley, S. L., and Lynne, A. M. (2008). Food animal-associated *Salmonella* challenges: pathogenicity and antimicrobial resistance. *J. Anim. Sci.* 86, E173–E187. doi: 10.2527/jas.2007-0447

Foley, S. L., Lynne, A. M., and Nayak, R. (2008). *Salmonella* challenges: prevalence in swine and poultry and potential pathogenicity of such isolates. *J. Anim. Sci.* 86, E149–E162. doi: 10.2527/jas.2007-0464

Gerlach, R. G., Jäckel, D., Stecher, B., Wagner, C., Lupas, A., Hardt, W. D., et al. (2007). *Salmonella* Pathogenicity Island 4 encodes a giant non-fimbrial adhesin and the cognate type 1 secretion system. *Cell Microbiol.* 9, 1834–1850. doi: 10.1111/j.1462-5822.2007.00919.x

Grimont, P. A., and Weill, F. X. (2007). *Antigenic Formulae of the Salmonella Serovars, 9th Edn.* Paris: Institute Pasteur; WHO Collaborating Centre for Reference and Research on *Salmonella*.

Hensel, M. (2004). Evolution of pathogenicity islands of *Salmonella enterica*. *Int. J. Med. Microbiol.* 294, 95–102. doi: 10.1016/j.ijmm.2004.06.025

Hong, Y., Morcilla, V. A., Liu, M. A., Russell, E. L., and Reeves, P. R. (2015). Three Wzy polymerases are specific for particular forms of an internal linkage in otherwise identical O units. *Microbiology* 161, 1639–1647. doi: 10.1099/mic.0.000113

Kim, Y., Bae, I. K., Jeong, S. H., Lee, C. H., Lee, H. K., Ahn, J., et al. (2011). Occurrence of IncFII plasmids carrying the $bla_{CTX-M-15}$ gene in *Salmonella enterica* serovar Enteritidis sequence type 11 in Korea. *Diagn. Microbiol. Infect. Dis.* 71, 171–173. doi: 10.1016/j.diagmicrobio.2011.05.004

Lagesen, K., Hallin, P. F., Rødland, E., Stærfeldt, H. H., Rognes, T., and Ussery, D. W. (2007). RNammer: consistent annotation of rRNA genes in genomic sequences. *Nucleic Acids Res.* 35, 3100–3108. doi: 10.1093/nar/gkm160

Larsen, M. V., Cosentino, S., Rasmussen, S., Friis, C., Hasman, H., Marvig, R. L., et al. (2012). Multilocus sequence typing of total-genome-sequenced bacteria. *J. Clin. Microbiol.* 50, 1355–1361. doi: 10.1128/JCM.06094-11

Lemire, J. A., Harrison, J. J., and Turner, R. J. (2013). Antimicrobial activity of metals: mechanisms, molecular targets and applications. *Nat. Rev. Microbiol.* 11, 371–384. doi: 10.1038/nrmicro3028

Li, X.-Z., Plésiat, P., and Nikaido, H. (2015). The challenge of efflux-mediated antibiotic resistance in gram-negative bacteria. *Clin. Microbiol. Rev.* 28, 337–418. doi: 10.1128/CMR.00117-14

Liu, B., Knirel, Y. A., Feng, L., Perepelov, A. V., Senchenkova, S. N., Reeves, P. R., et al. (2014). Structural diversity in *Salmonella* O antigens and its genetic basis. *FEMS Microbiol. Rev.* 38, 56–89. doi: 10.1111/1574-6976.12034

Lutful Kabir, S. M. (2010). Avian colibacillosis and salmonellosis: a closer look at epidemiology, pathogenesis, diagnosis, control and public health concerns. *Int. J. Environ. Res. Public Health* 7, 89–114. doi: 10.3390/ijerph7010089

McArthur, A. G., Waglechner, N., Nizam, F., Yan, A., Azad, M. A., Baylay, A. J., et al. (2013). The comprehensive antibiotic resistance database. *Antimicrob. Agents Chemother.* 57, 3348–3357. doi: 10.1128/AAC.00419-13

Medardus, J. J., Molla, B. Z., Nicol, M., Morrow, W. M., Rajala-Schultz, P. J., Kazwala, R., et al. (2014). In-feed use of heavy metal micronutrients in U.S. Swine production systems and its role in persistence of multidrug-resistant salmonellae. *Appl. Environ. Microbiol.* 80, 2317–2325. doi: 10.1128/AEM.04283-13

Pal, C., Bengtsson-Palme, J., Kristiansson, E., and Larsson, D. G. (2015). Co-occurrence of resistance genes to antibiotics, biocides and metals reveals novel insights into their co-selection potential. *BMC Genomics* 16:964. doi: 10.1186/s12864-015-2153-5

Pontel, L. B., Audero, M. E. P., Esparíz, M., Checa, S. K., and Soncini, F. C. (2007). GolS controls the response to gold by the hierarchical induction of *Salmonella*-specific genes that include a CBA efflux-coding operon. *Mol. Microbiol.* 66, 814–825. doi: 10.1111/j.1365-2958.2007.05963.x

Poole, K. (2004). Efflux-mediated multiresistance in Gram-negative bacteria. *Clin. Microbiol. Infect.* 10, 12–26. doi: 10.1111/j.1469-0691.2004.00763.x

Varani, A. M., Siguier, P., Gourbeyre, E., Charneau, V., and Chandler, M. (2011). ISsaga is an ensemble of web-based methods for high throughput identification and semi-automatic annotation of insertion sequences in prokaryotic genomes. *Genome Biol.* 12, R30. doi: 10.1186/gb-2011-12-3-r30

Zankari, E., Hasman, H., Cosentino, S., Vestergaard, M., Rasmussen, S., Lund, O., et al. (2012). Identification of acquired antimicrobial resistance genes. *J. Antimicrob. Chemother.* 67, 2640–2644. doi: 10.1093/jac/dks261

Zhang, S., Yin, Y., Jones, M. B., Zhang, Z., Deatherage Kaiser, B. L., Dinsmore, B. A., et al. (2015). *Salmonella* serotype determination utilizing high-throughput genome sequencing data. *J. Clin. Microbiol.* 53, 1685–1692. doi: 10.1128/JCM.00323-15

Zhou, Y., Liang, Y., Lynch, K. H., Dennis, J. J., and Wishart, D. S. (2011). PHAST: a fast phage search tool. *Nucleic Acids Res.* 39, W347–W352. doi: 10.1093/nar/gkr485

14

Enhanced Biocide Mitigation of Field Biofilm Consortia by a Mixture of D-Amino Acids

Yingchao Li[1], Ru Jia[2], Hussain H. Al-Mahamedh[3], Dake Xu[4] and Tingyue Gu[2]**

[1] College of Mechanical Engineering and Applied Electronics Technology, Beijing University of Technology, Beijing, China, [2] Department of Chemical and Biomolecular Engineering, Institute for Corrosion and Multiphase Technology, Ohio University, Athens, OH, USA, [3] Saudi Basic Industries Corporation, Jubail, Saudi Arabia, [4] Institute of Metal Research, Chinese Academy of Sciences, Shenyang, China

***Correspondence:**
Tingyue Gu
gu@ohio.edu;
Dake Xu
xudake@imr.ac.cn

Microbiologically influenced corrosion (MIC) is a major problem in the oil and gas industry as well as in many other industries. Current treatment methods rely mostly on pigging and biocide dosing. Biocide resistance is a growing concern. Thus, it is desirable to use biocide enhancers to improve the efficacy of existing biocides. D-Amino acids are naturally occurring. Our previous work demonstrated that some D-amino acids are biocide enhancers. Under a biocide stress of 50 ppm (w/w) hydroxymethyl phosphonium sulfate (THPS) biocide, 1 ppm D-tyrosine and 100 ppm D-methionine used separately successfully mitigated the *Desulfovibrio vulgaris* biofilm on carbon steel coupons. The data reported in this work revealed that 50 ppm of an equimolar mixture of D-methionine, D-tyrosine, D-leucine, and D-tryptophan greatly enhanced 50 ppm THPS biocide treatment of two recalcitrant biofilm consortia containing sulfate reducing bacteria (SRB), nitrate reducing bacteria (NRB), and fermentative bacteria, etc., from oil-field operations. The data also indicated that individual D-amino acids were inadequate for the biofilm consortia.

Keywords: biocide, biocide enhancer, D-amino acid, biofilm consortium, microbiologically influenced corrosion

INTRODUCTION

Microbiologically influenced corrosion (MIC) was first reported over 100 years ago (Gaines, 1910). It has become a major problem in the oil and gas industry in recent years because water injection is practiced more frequently than ever to increase well pressure. In this process, microbes and nutrients are introduced into the reservoirs and they subsequently show up in the pipelines, leading to MIC. MIC was suspected as a major contributing factor in the pipeline leak caused by a 0.25″ × 0.5″ hole at the bottom of a pipe in the Trans-Alaska Pipeline in 2006 (Jacobson, 2007). In a separate reported case, an 8″ diameter pipeline carrying oil and produced water failed in only 8 months due to MIC (Bhat et al., 2011). A recent pipeline failure case was published suggesting that MIC was likely the culprit in the leak of a 24″ CO_2 gathering line 2 years after commissioning, after ruling out other corrosion mechanisms (Hinkson et al., 2013). Skovhus and Eckert (2014) discussed several MIC cases and pointed out that MIC is becoming more prevalent nowadays due to aging equipment and increased awareness.

In the MIC caused by biofilms of sulfate reducing bacteria (SRB), elemental iron (Fe^0) in carbon steel serves as an electron donor. Xu and Gu (2014) designed an SRB starvation experiment to support this hypothesis. They found that under carbon source starvation, MIC pitting accelerated despite the fact that the biofilm lost some cell mass due to the starvation.

SRB switched to Fe^0 as electron donor for energy production to help their survival. Rajala et al. (2015) suggested that the presence of carbon steel benefited the microbial community in a nutrient-deficient anaerobic environment. In this kind of MIC, cross-cell wall electron transport is required for SRB to utilize extracellular electrons released by Fe^0 oxidation in their cytoplasm for sulfate reduction, meaning that the biofilm must be electrogenic (Gu, 2012). Recent studies further suggested that electron transfer is a bottleneck in SRB MIC against carbon steel and 304 stainless steel (Li et al., 2015; Zhang et al., 2015). MIC by acid-producing bacteria (APB) belongs to a different type of MIC because the oxidant (proton) is reduced outside the cells on the steel surface rather than in the cytoplasm (Gu, 2012). Underneath an APB biofilm, the local pH is much more acidic than in the bulk-fluid pH, leading to organic acid attacks. In both types of MIC discussed above, biofilms are responsible. Thus, biofilm mitigation is a key to MIC mitigation.

In the field, microbes form synergistic biofilm consortia. It is well known that biofilm cells (sessile cells) are far more recalcitrant than planktonic cells. Through several different mechanisms, a biofilm protects inner sessile cells from harmful factors. In one way, a biofilm can slow down the diffusion of antimicrobial agents (Mah and O'Toole, 2001; Stewart and Costerton, 2001). Furthermore, it can slow down the metabolic rate to reduce the intake of antimicrobial agents. Tuomanen et al. (1986) found that the increased resistance to antibacterial agents was accompanied by a low growth rate or no growth. Biofilms also preserve persister cells when they are under attack. These persister cells quickly rebound when the environment becomes less hostile (Lewis, 2001). Sessile cells in biofilms can also use efflux pumps to prevent antimicrobial agents from entering the cells. They can upregulate resistant genes to break down antimicrobial agents (Lewis, 2001). These anti-microbial mechanisms make the mitigation of biofilm consortia difficult. It is said that as a rule of thumb, a ten times or higher biocide concentration may be required to treat biofilms

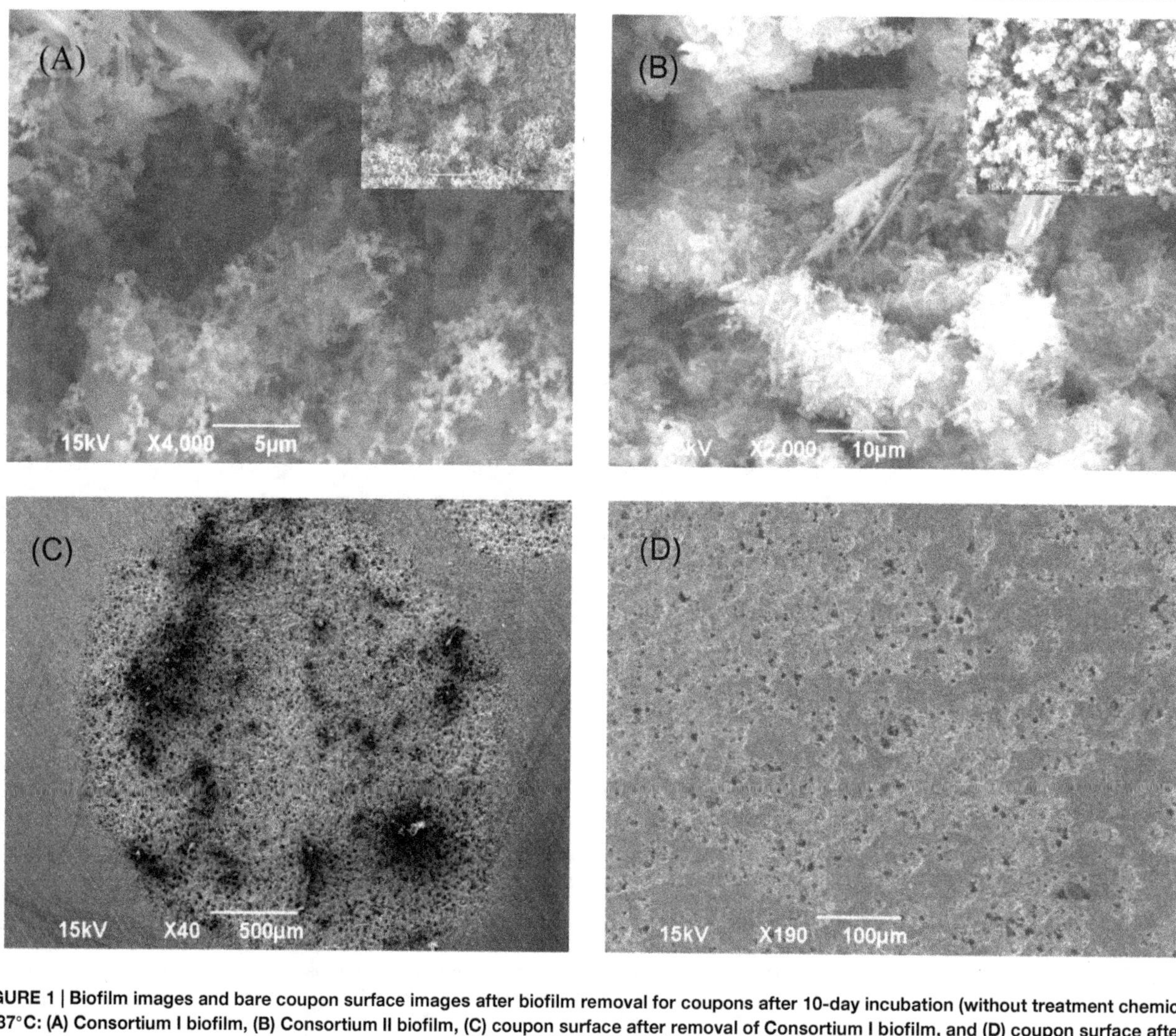

FIGURE 1 | Biofilm images and bare coupon surface images after biofilm removal for coupons after 10-day incubation (without treatment chemicals) at 37°C: (A) Consortium I biofilm, (B) Consortium II biofilm, (C) coupon surface after removal of Consortium I biofilm, and (D) coupon surface after removal of Consortium II biofilm.

compared with that needed for the treatment of planktonic cells (Nickel et al., 1985; Videla, 1996; Vance and Thrasher, 2005).

Pigging and biocides are two primary ways to mitigate problematic biofilms (Videla, 2002). Biocide applications can be performed during pigging by placing a biocide "plug" in a pipeline between two pigs. However, some pipelines are not piggable due to complicated elbows and other devices (Tiratsoo, 2013). Since pigging cannot completely remove biofilms, it is likely that the residual sessile cells can bounce back quickly. A biocide is needed to delay the recovery of biofilms. Tetrakis hydroxymethyl phosphonium sulfate (THPS) is one of the widely used biocides in the oil and gas industry because it is biodegradable and effective against a broad spectrum of microorganisms. THPS is designated by the US Environmental Protection Agency (EPA) as a green chemical (United States Environmental Protection Agency, 1997). It disrupts the disulphide bond in proteins and enzymes in microbes (Denyer, 1995; Russell, 2002; Ballantyne and Jordan, 2004; Greene et al., 2006). In field operations, repeated use of the same biocide will inevitably cause dosage escalation because of the selective promotion of resistant microbes over time. In some field operations, THPS dosage is so high such that the sulfate introduced by THPS precipitates with barium in the drilling fluid causing problematic scale formation downhole. High doses of biocides also raise environmental concerns in addition to increased cost. More effective uses of existing biocides are highly desirable.

Despite continued research in new biocides, it is unlikely that a blockbuster biocide will replace THPS or glutaraldehyde (another popular green biocide for large-scale applications) in oilfield applications any time soon. Thus, it is desirable to use biocide enhancers to make existing biocides such as THPS more effective. D-Amino acids were reported to enhance the efficacy of THPS in the mitigation of the *Desulfovibrio vulgaris* biofilm (Xu et al., 2012a,b, 2014). Most recently, Jia et al. (2016) demonstrated that D-amino acids enhanced two other biocides, namely alkyldimethylbenzylammonium chloride and tributyl tetradecyl phosphonium chloride against a biofilm consortium. Although previously considered rare in nature, D-amino acids are now considered ubiquitous due to the advancement of analytical techniques and the increased interests in their biological functions. They are found in microorganisms, food, plants, animals, and even in humans (Konno et al., 2009). While the biological functions of D-amino acids are not fully understood, it is believed that they could serve as a signal molecule. Lam et al. (2009) stated that the synthesis of D-amino acids might be a common way of self-adjustment of cells to the changing environment. Kolodkin-Gal et al. (2010) found that D-methionine (D-met), D-tyrosine (D-tyr), D-leucine (D-leu), and D-tryptophan (D-trp) triggered the *Bacillus subtilis* biofilm's disassembly. They also tested an equimolar mixture of four D-amino acids. Xu and Liu (2011) confirmed that 100 ppm (w/w) D-tyr triggered the biofilm dispersal in their test using activated sludge on membrane filters. Xu et al. (2012a, 2014) found that D-tyr and D-met were effective against the *D. vulgaris* biofilm on carbon steel coupons.

In this work, the efficacies of THPS combined with a mixture of D-amino acids against two oil-field biofilm consortia (labeled as Consortium I and Consortium II) were investigated. An equimolar mixture of four D-amino acids (D-met, D-tyr, D-leu, and D-trp) were tested with 50 ppm THPS. Individual D-met and D-tyr were also tested with THPS for comparison.

MATERIALS AND METHODS

Bacterium, Nutrient Medium, Biofilm Growth Substratum, and Chemicals

In this work, two biofilm consortia collected from an oil field were used to investigate the efficacy of 50 ppm THPS in combination with D-amino acids. The consortia were collected from oilfield operations in the form of planktonic cells in liquids in glass jars. The liquid samples were used to inoculate the ATCC 1249

TABLE 1 | Metabolic assignments of dominant bacterial species (%).

Species	Consortium I	Consortium II	Trait
Bacillus sp.	< 1	6.0	Biosurfactant producing; Varies
Bacterioides sp.	2.9	1.4	Fermenting bacteria
Garciella sp.	27.7	78.8	NRB; Sulfidogen; TRB
Salmonella enterica	61.5	0	SRB; TRB
Soehngenia sp.	4.1	0	Fermenting bacteria
Tepidibacter sp.	2.7	13.6	Biodeg (HC)

TABLE 2 | SRB sessile cell counts of Consortia I and II after 7-day biofilm prevention test using D-tyr and D-met.

Biofilm	Treatment	MPN sessile cell count (cells/cm^2)
Consortium I	No treatment chemical (control)	10^7
	50 ppm THPS	10^7
	50 ppm THPS + 100 ppm D-met	10^6
	50 ppm THPS + 1 ppm D-tyr	10^5
	50 ppm THPS + 10 ppm D-tyr	10^5
Consortium II	No treatment chemical (control)	10^7
	50 ppm THPS	10^7
	50 ppm THPS + 100 ppm D-met	10^6
	50 ppm THPS + 1 ppm D-tyr	10^6
	50 ppm THPS + 10 ppm D-tyr	10^6

TABLE 3 | SRB sessile cell counts of Consortium I biofilm after 7-day biofilm prevention test using a D-amino acid mixture.

Treatment	MPN sessile cell count (cells/cm^2)
No treatment chemical (control)	10^7
50 ppm THPS	10^7
50–500 ppm D-mix	10^5
50 ppm THPS + 50 ppm D-mix	10^3

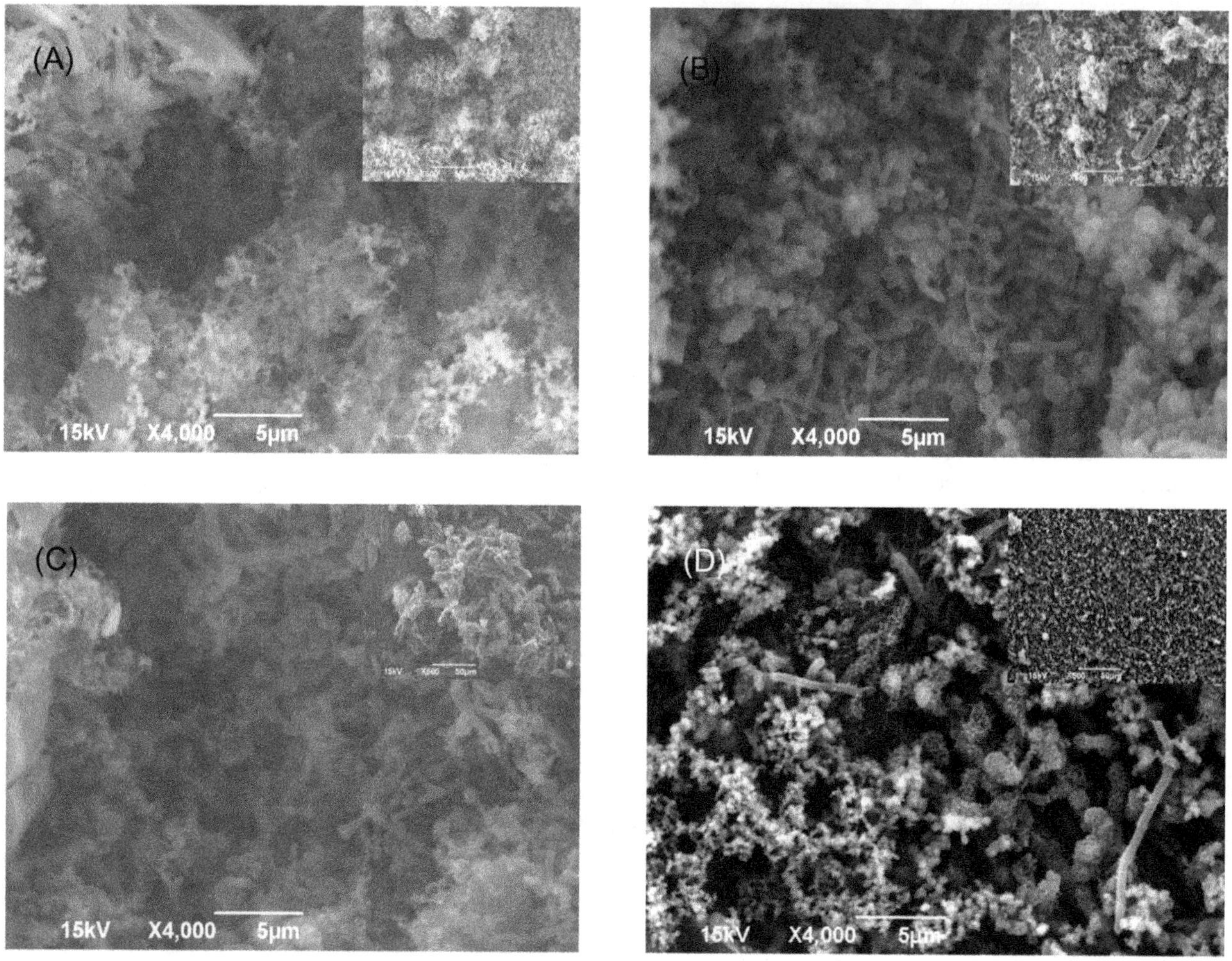

FIGURE 2 | SEM images of Consortium I biofilm after 7-day incubation in the biofilm prevention test with: (A) no treatment chemical (control), (B) 50 ppm THPS, (C) 50 ppm D-mix, and (D) 50 ppm THPS + 50 ppm D-mix. The scale bar in the inserted small image is 50 μm.

medium that is a modified Baar's medium. L-Cysteine at 100 ppm was added to the medium as an oxygen scavenger to eliminate any possible oxygen ingress.

Coin-shaped C1018 (UNS G10180) carbon steel coupons were used to grow biofilms. The composition of C1018 was (wt%): C 0.14–0.20, Mn 0.60–0.90, P 0.04, S 0.05, Si 0.15–0.30, and Fe balance. For each coupon, only the 1.2 cm^2 top surface was exposed to the culture medium, and the remainder was painted with Teflon. Coupons were polished with 180, 400, and 600 grit sandpapers, sequentially. They were cleaned with isopropanol and dried under UV light for 20 min.

D-Amino acids, THPS, and all chemicals used in the culture medium were purchased from Sigma–Aldrich (St Louis, MO, USA) or Fisher Scientific (Pittsburgh, PA, USA). In the 50 ppm equimolar D-amino acid mixture (D-mix), the concentrations of D-met and D-trp in the mixture were much less than the concentration of each D-amino acid which was needed to enhance 50 ppm THPS in the mitigation of the *D. vulgaris* biofilm on carbon steel (Xu et al., 2012a, 2014).

Biofilm Prevention and Biofilm Removal Tests

In order to evaluate the efficacies of the cocktails of THPS + D-amino acid(s), both biofilm prevention and biofilm removal tests were carried out in the lab. Before the operation, the culture medium, anaerobic vials, pipettes, and tweezers were sterilized in an autoclave at 121 °C for 20 min before use. D-Amino acids were not autoclaved due to possible oxidation at a high temperature. Their stock solutions were filter-sterilized. The culture medium and solutions containing the biocide treatment chemicals were sparged with filtered N_2 for 45 min to remove O_2. In the biofilm prevention test, two duplicate coupons, 100 ml medium, treatment chemicals, and 1 ml biofilm consortium seed culture were put into each 125 ml anaerobic vial in an anaerobic chamber. The initial planktonic cell concentration right after inoculation was 10^6 cells/ml. The anaerobic chamber was sparged with filtered N_2 for 45 min to remove oxygen before use. After the vials were sealed, they were placed in a 37°C incubator. After 7-day incubation, coupons were taken out for further measurement

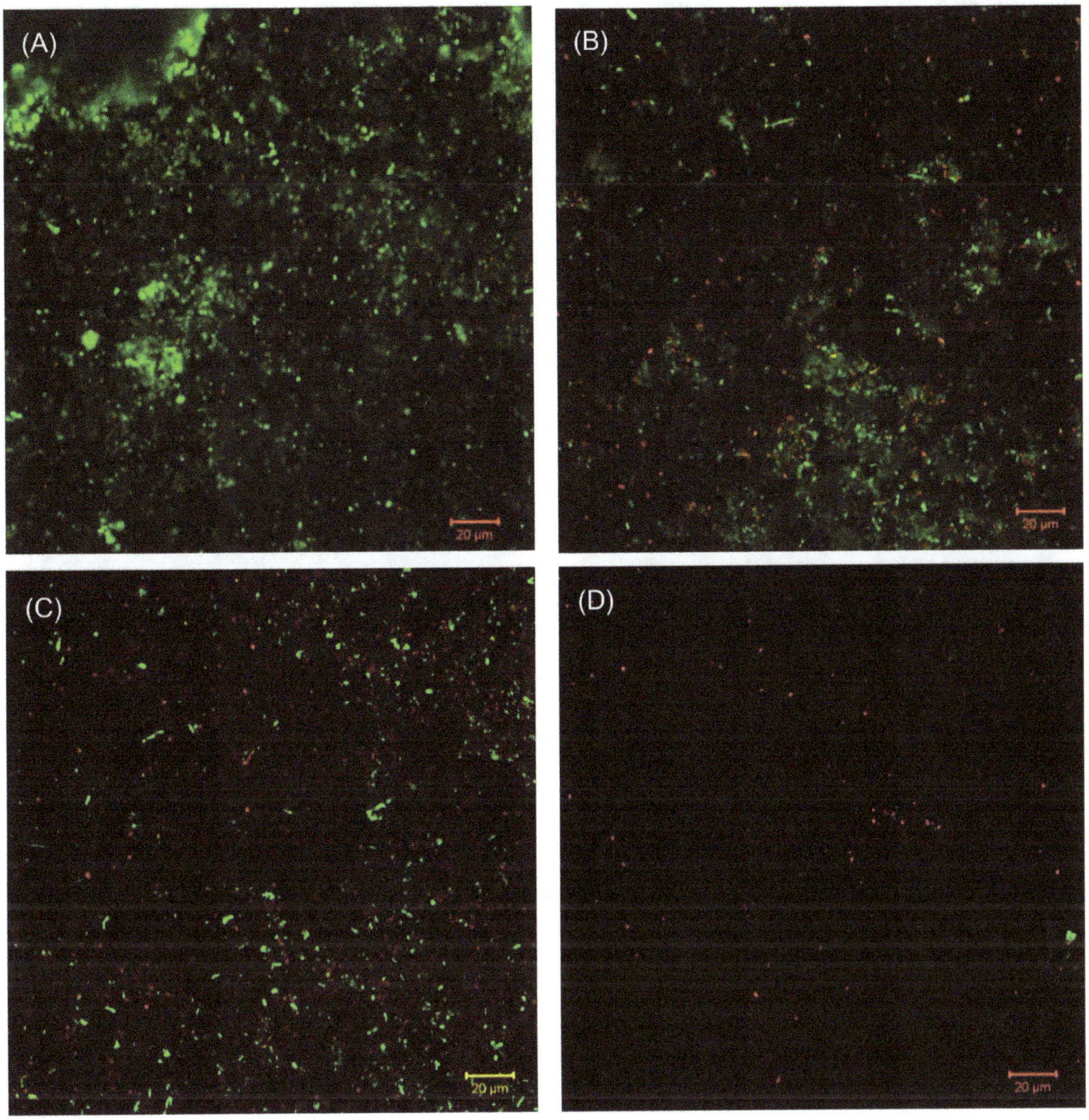

FIGURE 3 | CLSM images of biofilms after 7-day incubation in the biofilm prevention test with: (A) no treatment chemical (control), (B) 50 ppm THPS, (C) 50 D-mix, and (D) 50 ppm THPS + 50 ppm D-mix.

and observation. In the biofilm removal test, biofilms were first grown on coupons without treatment chemicals for 3 days to achieve maturity. Coupons covered by the mature biofilm were taken out and put into a phosphate-buffered saline (PBS) solution (pH 7.4) with treatment chemicals in a Petri dish for 3 h in the anaerobic chamber at room temperature. Coupons were taken out for analysis afterwards. Each test was repeated twice and triplicate coupons were used for each test condition.

TABLE 4 | SRB sessile cell counts of Consortium I after 3-h biofilm removal test.

Treatment	MPN sessile cell count (cells/cm^2)
No treatment chemical (control)	10^7
50 ppm THPS	10^7
50–500 ppm D-mix	10^5
50 ppm THPS + 50 ppm D-mix	10^3

Enumeration of Sessile Cells

The Biosan Sani-Check SRB test kit (Sani-Check® Product #100, Biosan Laboratories, Warren, MI, USA) was used for the most probable number (MPN) cell counts. The biofilm consortium on the coupon surface was removed with the small brush that was a part of the test kit. The brush was then inserted into the test kit's vial containing a solid SRB culture medium for incubation at 37°C. The time it took to show the black color (FeS) reflected the

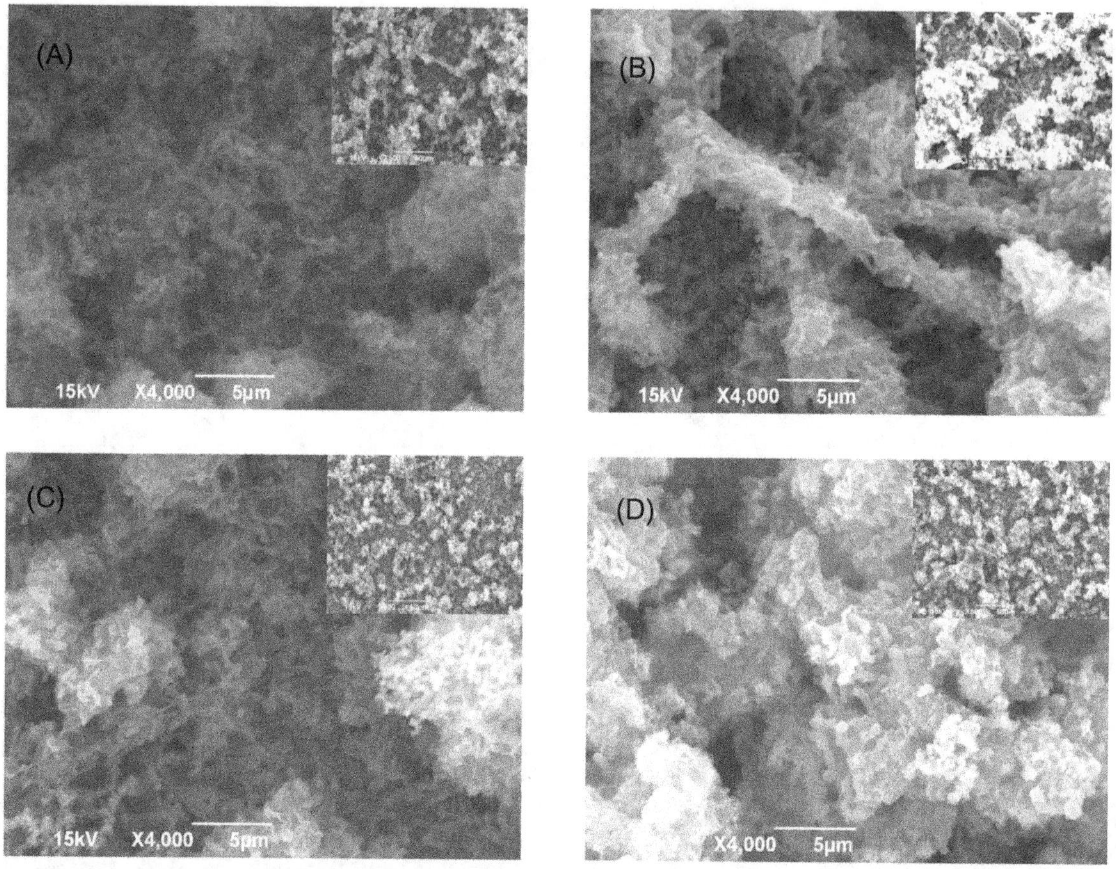

FIGURE 4 | SEM images of Consortium I biofilm after 3-h treatment in PBS buffer containing: (A) no treatment chemical (control), (B) 50 ppm THPS, (C) 100 ppm D-mix, and (D) 50 ppm THPS + 50 ppm D-mix, in the biofilm removal test. The scale bar in the inserted small images is 50 μm.

SRB cell concentration based on vendor's calibration (Xu et al., 2012a,b, 2014).

Scanning Electron Microscope (SEM) for Biofilm Observation

Scanning electron microscope observation with a Model JSM-6390 SEM (JEOL Ltd., Tokyo, Japan) was used to observe the biofilm morphology. The coupons for SEM observation of biofilms were first submerged in 4% (w/w) glutaraldehyde for 2 h and then dehydrated in 25, 50, 75, and 100% (v/v) isopropanol sequentially for 5 min total. And then, the biofilms were dehydrated in a critical point dryer using CO_2. Finally, biofilms covered coupons were coated with palladium to provide conductivity (Xu et al., 2012a,b, 2014). It should be noted that SEM images should not be used for quantitative cell counting because of uneven distribution of sessile cells.

Confocal Laser Scanning Microscopy (CLSM) for Biofilm Observation

Confocal laser scanning microscopy using Model LSM 510 microscope (Carl Zeiss, Jena, Germany) was used to detect living and dead cells in biofilms. The dyes used to stain the biofilms were in the L7012 Live/Dead® BacLight™ Bacterial Viability Kit (Life Technologies, Grand Island, NY, USA), in which SYTO 9 is a green-fluorescent stain and propidium iodide a red-fluorescent stain. Thus, living cells appear as green color at an excitation wavelength of 488 nm and dead cells red at 559 nm. Before being put into the dye solution for 15 min in a dark condition, coupons were washed with the PBS buffer for 15 s three times to wash away the culture medium, biocide residue, and planktonic cells (Mah et al., 2003; Turonova et al., 2015).

RESULTS

Oil-Field Biofilm Consortia

Biofilm Consortia I and II were supplied by an oil and gas company. **Figure 1** shows that both biofilm consortia formed robust biofilms on coupons after incubation in the culture medium for 10 days at 37°C. The images also reveal that the sessile cells in both biofilm consortia appeared to have different morphologies, indicating that they were mixed-culture consortia. Since the ATCC 1249 culture medium is designed for SRB, the dominant sessile population observed was likely SRB. After the biofilms were removed, pits underneath the biofilms resembled

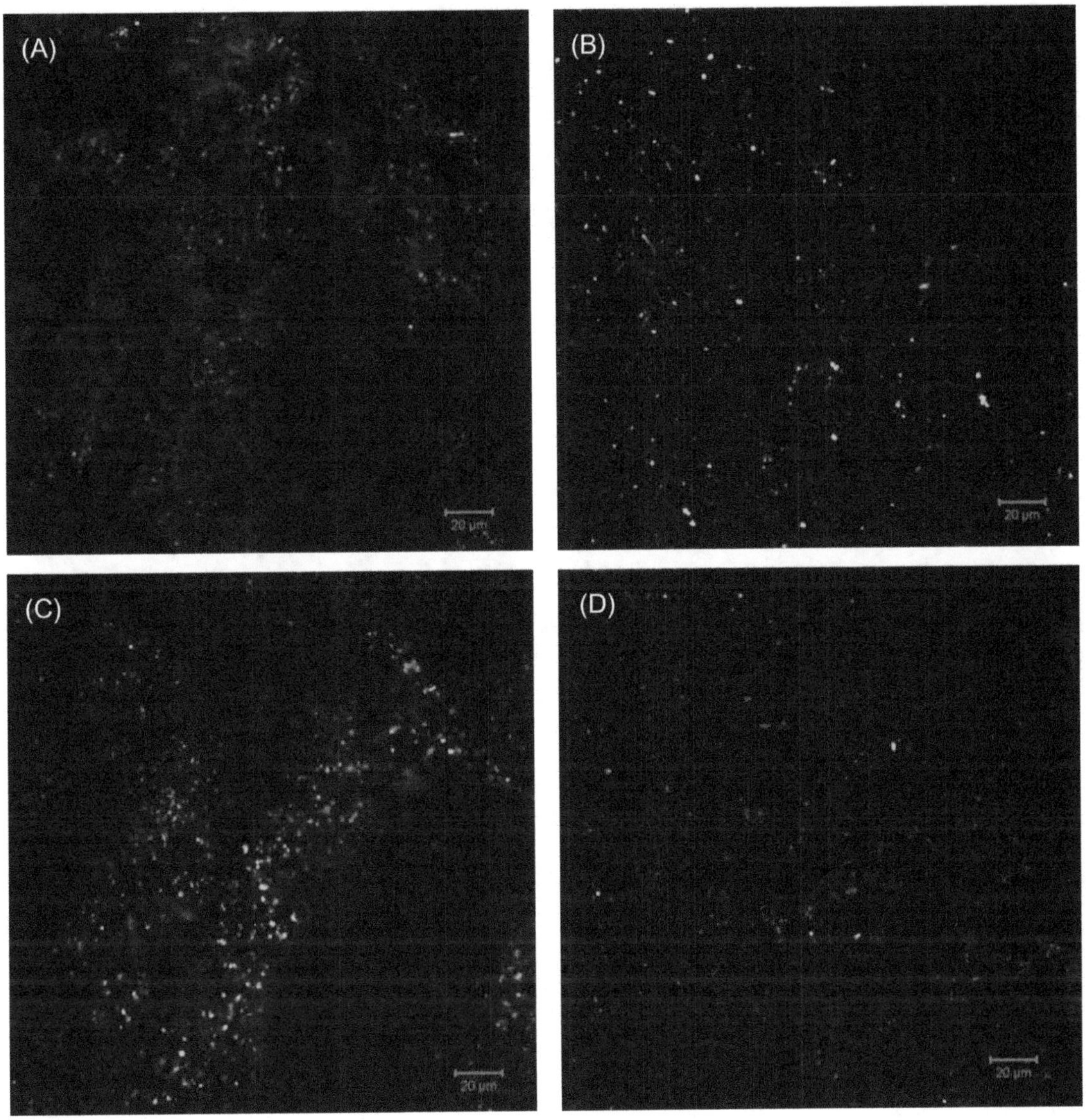

FIGURE 5 | CLSM images of biofilms in the 3-h treatment in PBS buffer with: (A) no treatment chemical (control), (B) 50 ppm THPS, (C) 50 ppm D-mix, and (D) 50 ppm THPS + 50 ppm D-mix.

TABLE 5 | SRB sessile cell counts of Consortium II after 7-day biofilm prevention test.

Treatment	MPN sessile cell count (cells/cm^2)
No treatment chemical (control)	10^7
50 ppm THPS	10^7
50–500 ppm D-mix	10^6
50 ppm THPS + 50 ppm D-mix	10^4

TABLE 6 | SRB sessile cell counts of Consortium II after 3-h biofilm removal test.

Treatment	MPN sessile cell count (cells/cm^2)
No treatment chemical (control)	10^7
50 ppm THPS	10^7
50–500 ppm D-mix	10^6
50 ppm THPS + 50 ppm D-mix	10^4

characteristic MIC pits (**Figure 1**). The specific weight losses of the coupons were 0.0047 and 0.0058 g/cm^2 for Consortium I and Consortium II, respectively. Both values were much larger than the 0.0018 g/cm^2 caused by pure-strain *D. vulgaris* incubated under the same conditions.

The phylogenetic identification of Consortia I and II shown in **Table 1** was carried out by Ecolyse, Inc. (College Station, TX, USA). Ecolyzed used the bacterial tag-encoded FLX amplicon pyrosequencing (bTEFAP) method with 515F-GTGCCAGCMGCCGCGGTAA and

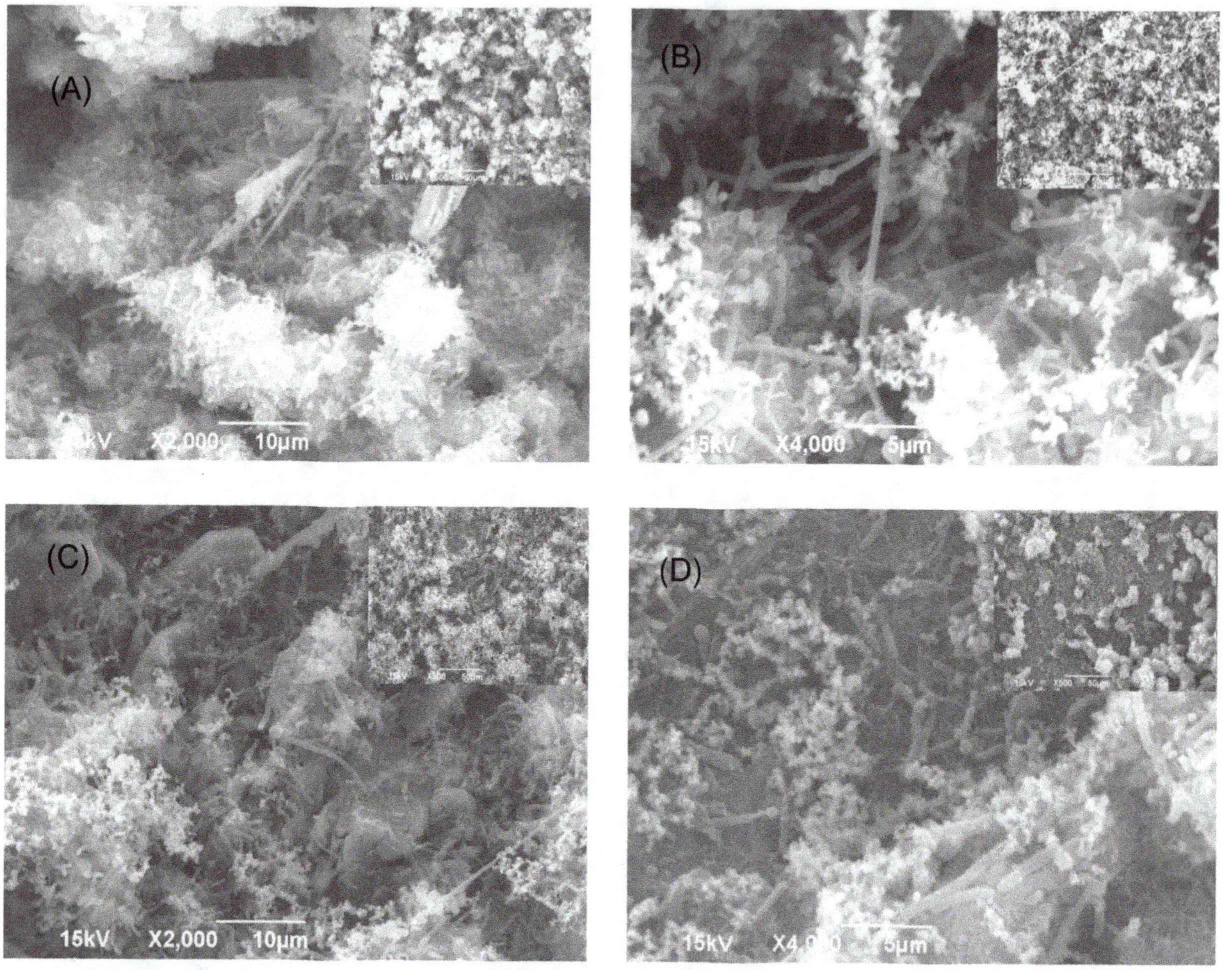

FIGURE 6 | SEM images of Consortium II biofilm after 7-day incubation in the biofilm prevention test with: (A) no treatment chemical (control), (B) 50 ppm THPS, (C) 100 ppm D-mix, and (D) 50 ppm THPS + 50 ppm D-mix in the biofilm prevention test. The scale bar in the inserted small images is 50 μm.

806R-TAATCTWTGGGVHCATCAGG as primers for DNA analysis. A forward primer and a reverse fusion primer were used for sample amplification. The amplified product was processed to create single-stranded DNA using the Ion PGM protocols by Life Technologies (Carlsbad, CA, USA). Sequencing was performed using the Ion PGM semiconductor sequencing method by Life Technologies.

In **Table 1**, "Sulfidogens" are bacteria that reduce sulfur and produce sulfide. "Biodeg," abbreviated from biodegradation, refers to bacteria utilizing substrates or compounds that cannot be used by most of the other bacteria. "HC" means hydrocarbon. The metagenomics data reveal that *Bacillus* sp., *Bacterioides* sp., *Garciella* sp., *Salmonella enterica*, *Soehngenia* sp., and *Tepidibacter* sp. were detected in Consortia I. Consortium II contained all these species, except *Salmonella enterica* and *Soehngenia* sp. The MIC caused by *Bacillus* sp. were studied since 1990s (Jack et al., 1992). *Bacteroides* sp. are normally found in mammals (Huang et al., 2011). *Bacteroides* sp. secret organic acids which are able to cause Type II MIC (Zhu et al., 2003). *Garciella* sp. and *Soehngenia* sp. were collected from the oil and gas field (Miranda-Tello et al., 2003; Kano et al., 2009; Naranjo-Briceño et al., 2012). *Garciella* sp. may cause MIC by producing hydrogen sulfide from the thiosulfate reduction (Miranda-Tello et al., 2003). *Salmonella* sp. and *Soehngenia* sp. are related to MIC because they produce hydrogen sulfide in their metabolisms (Barrett and Clark, 1987; Parshina et al., 2003). *Tepidibacter* sp. were found in oil fields (Tan et al., 2012).

Individual D-Amino Acids as Biocide Enhancers in the Mitigation of Field Biofilm Consortia

In our previous tests, the cocktails of 50 ppm THPS + 100 ppm D-met and 50 ppm THPS + 1 ppm D-tyr both achieved 5 log reduction of the SRB sessile cell count against *D. vulgaris* on carbon steel coupons (Xu et al., 2012a, 2014). However, the data in **Table 2** illustrate that in the biofilm prevention tests against Consortia I and II, the same cocktails only achieved 1 or 2 log reduction of the SRB sessile cell count, much less than 5 for *D. vulgaris*. The data presented in **Table 2**

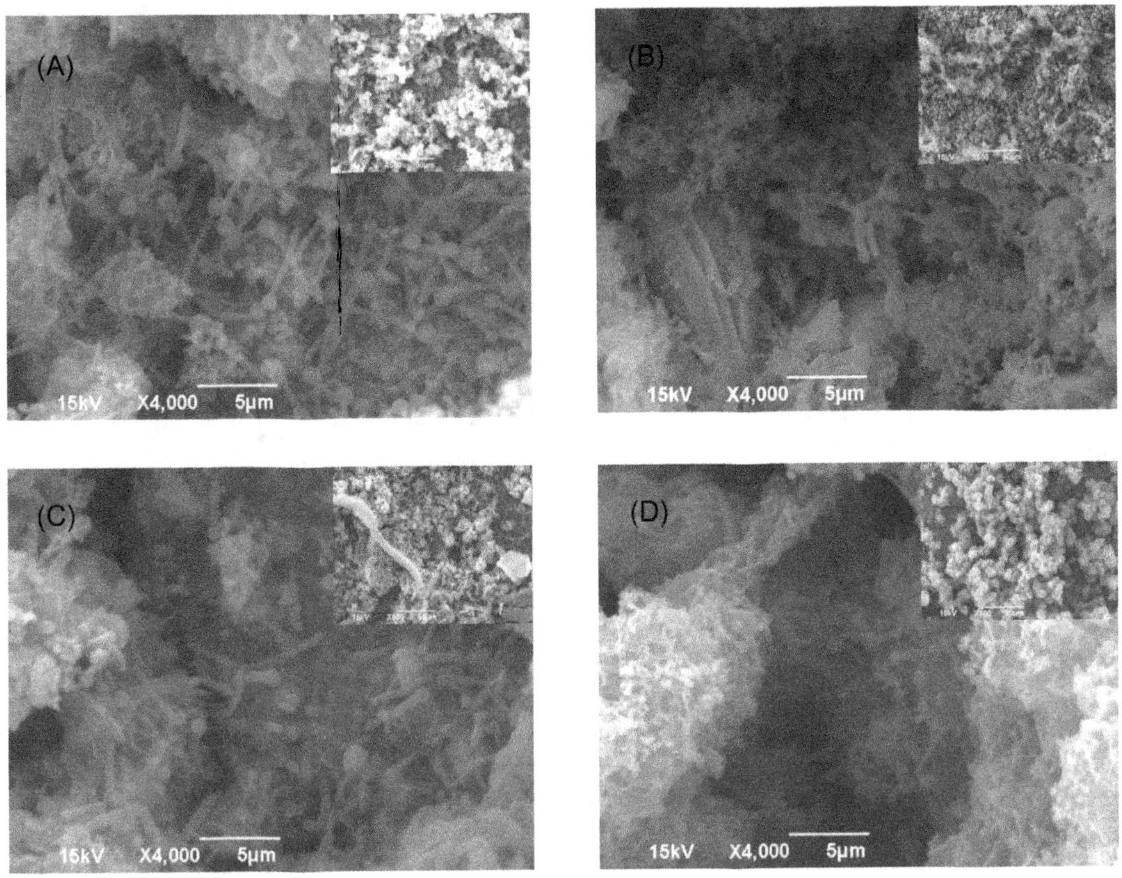

FIGURE 7 | SEM images of Consortium II biofilm after 3-h treatment in PBS buffer containing: (A) no treatment chemical (control), (B) 50 ppm THPS, (C) 100 ppm D-mix, and (D) 50 ppm THPS + 50 ppm D-mix in biofilm removal test. The scale bar in the inserted small images is 50 μm.

also show that increasing D-tyr from 1 to 10 ppm did not improve the outcome. All these data suggest that the field biofilm consortia were much more recalcitrant than the pure-strain *D. vulgaris*.

D-Amino Acid Mixture as Biocide Enhancer Against Consortium I

For the mitigation of the biofilm Consortium I, **Table 3** data reveal that 50 ppm D-mix enhanced 50 ppm THPS in both biofilm prevention and biofilm removal tests. In the biofilm prevention test, 50 ppm THPS without enhancement did not reduce the SRB sessile cell count on the coupon surface compared with the control without treatment. While the treatment with 500 ppm D-mix without THPS achieved 2 log reduction of the SRB sessile cell count. The data in **Table 3** show that the combination of 50 ppm THPS + 50 ppm D-mix was able to achieve 4 log reduction of the SRB sessile cell count. This demonstrated that the 50 ppm D-mix enhanced 50 ppm THPS in the biofilm prevention test for biofilm Consortium I considerably.

The SEM images of the biofilm Consortium I after a 7-day biofilm prevention test in **Figure 2** are consistent with the results in **Table 3**. Different cell shapes in the biofilm image confirmed that this was a mixed-culture biofilm. Sessile cells were easily found on coupons treated with either 50 ppm THPS or 500 ppm D-mix alone. However, with the 50 ppm THPS + 50 ppm D-mix cocktail treatment, the amount of sessile cells was much less than the amount of sessile cells after treatment with either 50 ppm THPS or 500 ppm D-mix. The CLSM images support the cell count data and are consistent with the SEM images. On the control coupon surface in **Figure 3A**, abundant living cells can be seen. In the treatments of 50 ppm THPS alone and 50 ppm D-mix alone in **Figures 3B,C**, dead cells as are seen but living cells are far more abundant. In **Figure 3D**, the amounts of both living and dead cells are much less and most cells were dead cells. It should be noted that although sessile cells were found on the SEM image in **Figure 2D**, they were dead cells that had not yet detached from the coupon according to the CLSM image in **Figure 3D**.

Similar efficacies were obtained in the biofilm removal test for biofilm Consortium I. The data provided in **Table 4** illustrate that the separate applications of 50 ppm THPS and 500 ppm D-mix had limited effects on Consortium I. It was found that 50 ppm THPS achieved no reduction of the SRB sessile cell count and 500 ppm D-mix achieved only 2 log reduction of the SRB sessile cell count. While the cocktail of 50 ppm THPS + 50 ppm D-mix

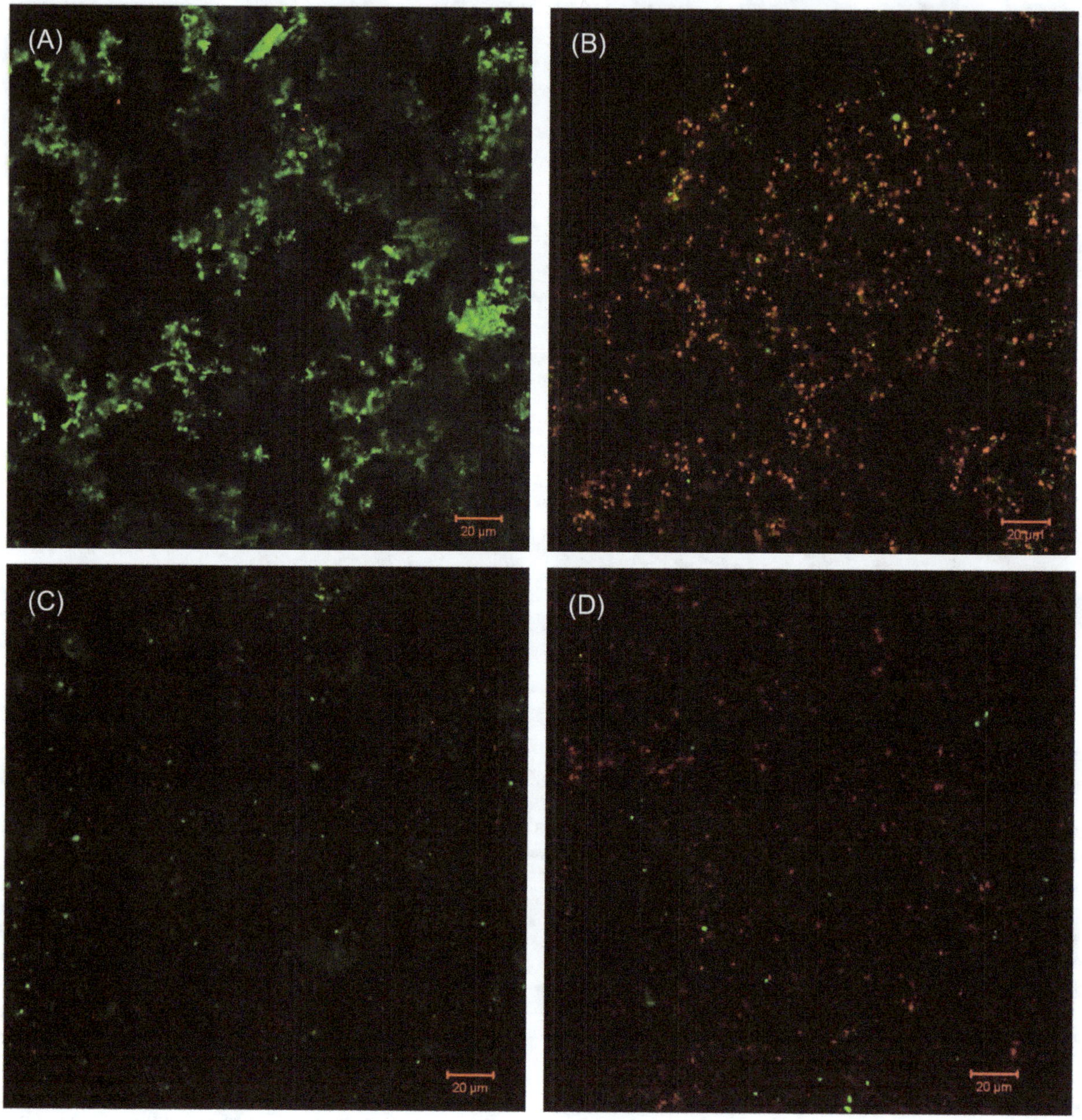

FIGURE 8 | CLSM images of Consortium II biofilm after 7-day incubation in the biofilm prevention test with: (A) no treatment chemical (control), (B) 50 ppm THPS, (C) 50 ppm D-mix, and (D) 50 ppm THPS + 50 ppm D-mix in the biofilm prevention test.

provided a 4 log reduction of the SRB sessile cell count after the 3-h biofilm removal test and the SEM images support the reduction of the sessile cells (**Figure 4**). **Figure 4** shows that sessile cells were present in the biofilm of Consortium I after treatment with either 50 ppm THPS or 100 ppm D-mix alone. The same trend was observed in the CLSM images (**Figure 5**) showing that more living cells were found on the control coupon surface than on the coupon surfaces treated with 50 ppm THPS and 50 ppm D-mix alone. On the coupon surface treated with 50 ppm THPS + 50 ppm D-mix, more dead cells and less living cells were found than on the coupon surface in the other three treatments.

D-Amino Acid Mixture as Biocide Enhancer Against Consortium II

Similar treatment outcomes were obtained for Consortium II. It was found that 50 ppm D-mix enhanced 50 ppm THPS in both biofilm prevention and biofilm removal tests. Comparable to the mitigation of Consortium I, 50 ppm THPS alone had no effect on the SRB sessile cell count in both biofilm prevention and biofilm removal tests for Consortium II compared with the untreated control (**Tables 5** and **6**). The cocktail of 50 ppm THPS + 50 ppm D-mix achieved 3 log reduction of the SRB

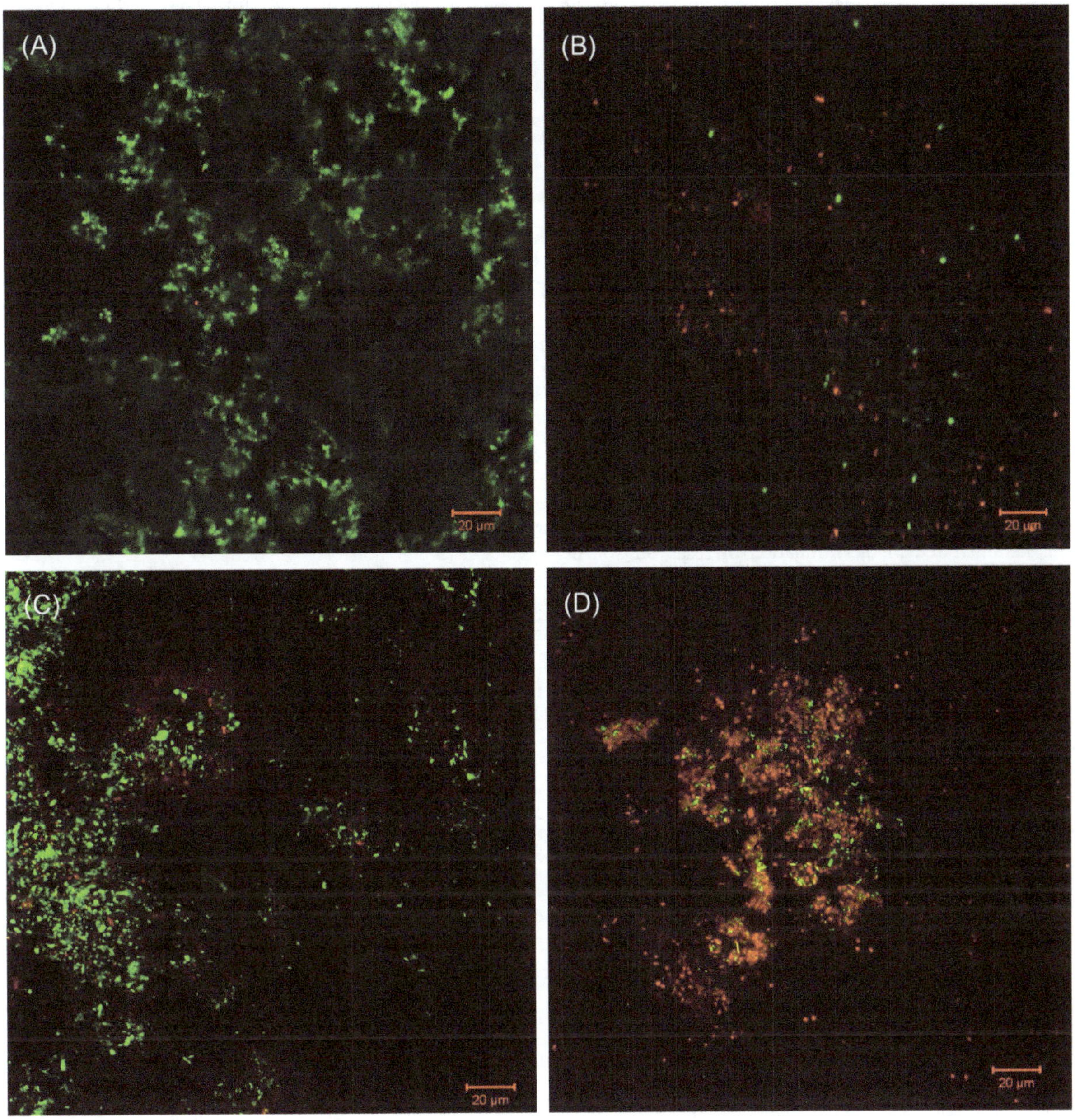

FIGURE 9 | CLSM images of Consortium II biofilm after 3-h treatment in PBS buffer containing: (A) no treatment chemical (control), (B) 50 ppm THPS, (C) 50 ppm D-mix, and (D) 50 ppm THPS + 50 ppm D-mix in the biofilm removal test.

sessile cell count in both biofilm prevention and biofilm removal tests for biofilm Consortium II. In **Figures 6** and **7**, sessile cells are easily seen on the following: the control coupon (no treatment), the coupon treated with 50 ppm THPS, and the coupon treated with 500 ppm D-mix. Although sessile cells are still noticeable on the surface of coupons treated with 50 ppm THPS + 50 ppm D-mix, they are less abundant. Moreover, according to the CLSM images in **Figures 8** and **9**, on the coupon surfaces treated with 50 ppm THPS + 50 ppm D-mix (**Figures 8D** and **9D**), most cells were dead cells. The data suggest that the binary combination of 50 ppm THPS and 50 ppm D-mix had an excellent efficacy against Consortium II owing to the enhancement of the D-mix.

DISCUSSION

The exact mechanism of how D-amino acids enhance biofilm mitigation is not completely understood. It was hypothesized that D-amino acids trigger biofilm disassembly by replacing the D-alanine terminus in peptidoglycans that exist in all bacterial cell walls (Kolodkin-Gal et al., 2010). Kolodkin-Gal et al. (2010)

and Xu et al. (2014) found that adding a high concentration of D-alanine (D-ala) rendered D-met ineffective. It was also suggested that D-amino acids may modify the synthesis of peptidoglycans (Lam et al., 2009). Cava et al. (2011) suggested that D-amino acids were necessary in the remodeling of the cell wall structure. Leiman et al. (2013) pointed out that D-tyr, D-leu, and D-trp inhibited the formation of the *B. subtilis* biofilm because these D-amino acids interfered with protein synthesis. Their data suggested that D-tyr acted as a growth inhibitor toward *B. subtilis*. It is highly possible that specific D-amino acids are effective for specific bacteria. Sarkar and Pires (2015) tested millimolar concentrations of several D-amino acids against some bacteria and found no inhibition of biofilm formation. This is consistent with the view proposed in Xu et al.'s (2012a,b, 2014) work that a biocide stress is needed.

It is not a surprise that the combination of THPS and D-amino acid mixtures showed a synergetic effect in the mitigation of field biofilm consortia. The synergy between biocides and other agents, such as the injection of nitrate, has been demonstrated in the mitigation of reservoir souring (Xue and Voordouw, 2015). The results above proved the hypothesis that a D-amino acid mixture instead of an individual D-amino acid would be needed in the mitigation of a biofilm consortium. The cocktail of 50 ppm THPS + 50 ppm D-mix achieved a better efficacy (1 log more reduction) for Consortium I than for Consortium II, suggesting that biofilm Consortium II might be more recalcitrant. It was also possible that a different D-amino acid mixture may work better for Consortium II. Different microbial species in the biofilm consortia probably required different D-amino acids as the biofilm dispersal factor. It is reasonable that in the mitigation of other biofilm consortia, the particular D-amino acid mixture in this work may need adjustments. Optimization is likely needed to decide a cost-efficient D-amino acid mixture that offers a good efficacy.

The comparison of SEM and CLSM biofilm images in this work suggests that SEM images could give a false impression that sessile cells were abundant while in reality the cells might be mostly dead cells. This should not be a problem if a biofilm is already detached from a coupon surface. Unlike CLSM, SEM can be used to show different cell shapes in a mixed-culture biofilm.

Hence, this lab work showed that 100 ppm D-met and 1 ppm D-tyr individually did not enhance or only slightly enhanced 50 ppm THPS in the mitigation of two field biofilm consortia on C1018 coupon surfaces although they worked very well for the pure-strain *D. vulgaris* biofilm. This work demonstrated that an equimolar mixture at a total concentration of 50 ppm consisting of D-met, D-tyr, D-leu, and D-trp greatly enhanced 50 ppm THPS in the mitigation of the biofilm consortia. It was found that the cocktail achieved extra 4 log reduction of the SRB sessile cell counts in both the biofilm prevention and biofilm removal tests for biofilm Consortium I compared with the treatment with 50 ppm THPS alone, while for Consortium II it was extra 3 log.

AUTHOR CONTRIBUTIONS

YL, RJ, and HA-M designed the experiments and conducted the data analysis. YL, DX, and TG wrote and edited the manuscript. All authors participated in discussion about the results and the manuscript.

ACKNOWLEDGMENT

We gratefully acknowledge the financial support from the US DOT-PHMSA CAAP program, TOTAL and SABIC. This paper was partially based on CORROSION/2015 Conference Paper No. 2015-5522. We thank NACE International (Houston, TX, USA) for granting the permission to publish in a journal.

REFERENCES

Ballantyne, B., and Jordan, S. L. (2004). "Biocides," in *Pesticide Toxicology and International Regulation*, eds T. C. Marrs and B. Ballantyne (New York, NY: John Wiley & Sons), 365–409.

Barrett, E. L., and Clark, M. A. (1987). Tetrathionate reduction and production of hydrogen sulfide from thiosulfate. *Microbiol. Rev.* 51, 192–205.

Bhat, S., Sharma, V. K., Thomas, S., Anto, P. F., and Singh, S. K. (2011). Failure of a new 8-in pipeline from group gathering station to central tank farm. *Mater. Perform.* 50, 50–53.

Cava, F., Lam, H., de Pedro, M., and Waldor, M. (2011). Emerging knowledge of regulatory roles of D-amino acids in bacteria. *Cell Mol. Life Sci.* 68, 817–831. doi: 10.1007/s00018-010-0571-8

Denyer, S. P. (1995). Mechanisms of action of antibacterial biocides. *Int. Biodeter. Biodegr.* 36, 227–245. doi: 10.1016/0964-8305(96)00015-7

Gaines, H. A. (1910). Bacterial activity as a corrosion induced in the soil. *J. Engineer. Ind. Chem.* 2, 128–130. doi: 10.1021/ie50016a003

Greene, E. A., Brunelle, V., Jenneman, G. E., and Voordouw, G. (2006). Synergistic inhibition of microbial sulfide production by combinations of the metabolic inhibitor nitrite and biocides. *Appl. Environ. Microbiol.* 72, 7897–7901. doi: 10.1128/AEM.01526-06

Gu, T. (2012). Can acid producing bacteria be responsible for very fast MIC pitting. *Paper presented at NACE Corrosion/2012, Paper No. C2012-0001214*, Salt Lake City, UT.

Hinkson, D., Wheeler, C., and Oney, C. (2013). MIC in a CO_2 gathering line? A field case study of microbiologically influenced corrosion. *Paper presented at Corrosion/2013, Paper number: C2013-0002276*, Orlando, FL.

Huang, J. Y., Lee, S. M., and Mazmanian, S. K. (2011). The human commensal *Bacteroides fragilis* binds intestinal mucin. *Anaerobe* 17, 137–141. doi: 10.1016/j.anaerobe.2011.05.017

Jack, R. F., Ringelberg, D. B., and White, D. C. (1992). Differential corrosion rates of carbon steel by combinations of *Bacillus* sp., *Hafnia alvei* and *Desulfovibrio gigas* established by phospholipid analysis of electrode biofilm. *Corros. Sci.* 33, 1843–1853. doi: 10.1016/0010-938X(92)90188-9

Jacobson, G. A. (2007). Corrosion at Prudhoe Bay : a lesson on the line. *Mater. Perform.* 46, 26–34.

Jia, R., Yang, D., Li, Y., Al-Mahamedh, H. H., and Gu, T. (2016). Enhancement of alkyldimethylbenzylammonium chloride and tributyl tetradecyl phosphonium chloride biocides using D-amino acids against a field biofilm consortium. *Paper presented at Corrosion/2016, Paper number: C2016-7279*, Vancouver, BC.

Kano, S., Mukaidani, T., Hattori, Y., Fujiwara, K., Miyagawa, Y., Takabayashi, K., et al. (2009). Diversity of indigenous anaerobes and methane conversion system from reservoir oil by indigenous anaerobes in depleted oil fields. *J. Jpn Petrol. Inst.* 52, 297–306. doi: 10.1627/jpi.52.297

Kolodkin-Gal, I., Romero, D., Cao, S., Clardy, J., Kolter, R., and Losick, R. (2010). D-amino acids trigger biofilm disassembly. *Science* 328, 627–629. doi: 10.1126/science.1188628

Konno, R., Bruckner, H., D'Aniello, A., Fisher, G. H., and Fujii, N. (2009). *D-Amino Acids Practical Methods and Protocols: Analytical Methods for D-Amino Acids.* New York, NY: Nova Science Publishers.

Lam, H., Oh, D. C., Cava, F., Takacs, C. N., Clardy, J., de Pedro, M. A., et al. (2009). D-amino acids govern stationary phase cell wall remodeling in bacteria. *Science* 325, 1552–1555. doi: 10.1126/science.1178123

Leiman, S. A., May, J. M., Lebar, M. D., Kahne, D., Kolter, R., and Losick, R. (2013). D-amino acids indirectly inhibit biofilm formation in *Bacillus subtilis* by interfering with protein synthesis. *J. Bacteriol.* 195, 5391–5395. doi: 10.1128/JB.00975-13

Lewis, K. (2001). Riddle of biofilm resistance. *Antimicrob. Agents Chemother.* 45, 999–1007. doi: 10.1128/AAC.45.4.999-1007.2001

Li, Y., Zhang, P., Xu, D., Xu, C., and Gu, T. (2015). D-amino acids enhanced biocide mitigation of field biofilm consortia in lab tests. *Paper presented at Corrosion/2015, Paper number: C2015-5522*, Dallas, TX.

Mah, T. F. C., and O'Toole, G. A. (2001). Mechanisms of biofilm resistance to antimicrobial agents. *Trends Microbiol.* 9, 34–39. doi: 10.1016/S0966-842X(00)01913-2

Mah, T. F. C., Pitts, B., Pellock, B., Walker, G. C., Stewart, P. S., and O'Toole, G. A. (2003). A genetic basis for *Pseudomonas aeruginosa* biofilm antibiotic resistance. *Nature* 426, 306–310. doi: 10.1038/nature02122

Miranda-Tello, E., Fardeau, M. L., Sepúlveda, J., Fernández, L., Cayol, J. L., Thomas, P., et al. (2003). *Garciella nitratireducens* gen. nov., sp. nov., an anaerobic, thermophilic, nitrate- and thiosulfate-reducing bacterium isolated from an oilfield separator in the Gulf of Mexico. *Int. J. Syst. Evol. Microbiol.* 53, 1509–1514. doi: 10.1099/ijs.0.02662-0

Naranjo-Briceño, L., de Sisto, A., García, D., Duque, Z., Freites-Sibada, M., Rojas, D., et al. (2012). "Metagenomics tools and SEM applied to identify a pool of corrosive sulfate-reducing bacteria (SRB) from naphtha transporting pipelines of Venezuelan Oil Industries," in *Proceedings of the BIT's 3rd Annual World Congress of Petromicrobiology; Xi'an, PRC*, Huixian.

Nickel, J. C., Ruseska, I., Wright, J. B., and Costerton, J. W. (1985). Tobramycin resistance of *Pseudomonas aeruginosa* cells growing as a biofilm on urinary catheter material. *Antimicrob. Agents Chemother.* 27, 619–624. doi: 10.1128/AAC.27.4.619

Parshina, S. N., Kleerebezem, R., Sanz, J. L., Lettinga, G., Nozhevnikova, A. N., Kostrikina, N. A., et al. (2003). *Soehngenia saccharolytica* gen. nov., sp. nov. and *Clostridium amygdalinum* sp. nov., two novel anaerobic, benzaldehyde-converting bacteria. *Int. J. Syst. Evol. Microbiol.* 53, 1791–1799. doi: 10.1099/ijs.0.02668-0

Rajala, P., Carpén, L., Vepsäläinen, M., Raulio, M., Sohlberg, E., and Bomberg, M. (2015). Microbially induced corrosion of carbon steel in deep groundwater environment. *Front. Microbiol.* 6:647. doi: 10.3389/fmicb.2015.00647

Russell, A. D. (2002). Antibiotic and biocide resistance in bacteria: introduction. *J. Appl. Microbiol.* 92, 1S–3S. doi: 10.1046/j.1365-2672.92.5s1.14.x

Sarkar, S., and Pires, M. M. (2015). D-amino acids do not inhibit biofilm formation in *Staphylococcus aureus*. *PLoS ONE* 10:e0117613. doi: 10.1371/journal.pone.0117613

Skovhus, T., and Eckert, R. (2014). Practical aspects of MIC detection, monitoring and management in the oil and gas industry. *Paper presented Corrosion/2014, Paper number: C2014-3920*, San Antonio, TX.

Stewart, P. S., and Costerton, W. (2001). Antibiotic resistance of bacteria in biofilms. *Lancet* 358, 135–138. doi: 10.1016/S0140-6736(01)05321-1

Tan, H. Q., Wu, X. Y., Zhang, X. Q., Wu, M., and Zhu, X. F. (2012). *Tepidibacter mesophilus* sp. nov., a mesophilic fermentative anaerobe isolated from soil polluted by crude oil, and emended description of the genus *Tepidibacter*. *Int. J. Syst. Evol. Microbiol.* 62, 66–70. doi: 10.1099/ijs.0.027409-0

Tiratsoo, J. (2013). *The Ultimate Guide to Unpiggable Pipelines.* Available at: http://pipelinesinternational.com/shop/the_ultimate_guide_to_unpiggable_pipelines/081249/

Tuomanen, E., Durack, D. T., and Tomasz, A. (1986). Antibiotic tolerance among clinical isolates of bacteria. *Antimicrob. Agents Chemother.* 30, 521–527. doi: 10.1128/AAC.30.4.521

Turonova, H., Briandet, R., Rodrigues, R., Hernould, M., Hayek, N., Stintzi, A., et al. (2015). Biofilm spatial organization by the emerging pathogen *Campylobacter jejuni*: comparison between NCTC 11168 and 81-176 strains under microaerobic and oxygen-enriched conditions. *Front. Microbiol.* 6:709. doi: 10.3389/fmicb.2015.00709

United States Environmental Protection Agency (1997). *THPS Biocides: A New Class of Antimicrobial Chemistry. (1997 Designing Greener Chemicals Award).* Available at: http://www2.epa.gov/greenchemistry/1997-designing-greener-chemicals-award

Vance, I., and Thrasher, D. R. (2005). "Reservoir souring: mechanisms and prevention," in *Petroleum Microbiology*, eds B. Ollivier and M. Magot (Washington, DC: ASM Press), 123–142.

Videla, H. A. (1996). "Biofilms and biofouling," in *Manual of Biocorrosion*, ed. H. A. Videla (Boca Raton, FL: CRC Lewis Publisher), 47–71.

Videla, H. A. (2002). Prevention and control of biocorrosion. *Int. Biodeter. Biodegr.* 49, 259–270. doi: 10.1016/S0964-8305(02)00053-7

Xu, D., and Gu, T. (2014). Carbon source starvation triggered more aggressive corrosion against carbon steel by the *Desulfovibrio vulgaris* biofilm. *Int. Biodeter. Biodegr.* 91, 74–81.

Xu, D., Li, Y., and Gu, T. (2012a). A synergistic D-tyrosine and tetrakis hydroxymethyl phosphonium sulfate biocide combination for the mitigation of an SRB biofilm. *World J. Microbiol. Biotechnol.* 28, 3067–3074. doi: 10.1007/s11274-012-1116-0

Xu, D., Li, Y., and Gu, T. (2014). D-Methionine as a biofilm dispersal signaling molecule enhanced tetrakis hydroxymethyl phosphonium sulfate mitigation of *Desulfovibrio vulgaris* biofilm and biocorrosion pitting. *Mater. Corros.* 65, 837–845. doi: 10.1002/maco.201206894

Xu, D., Wen, J., Fu, W., Gu, T., and Raad, I. (2012b). D-amino acids for the enhancement of a binary biocide cocktail consisting of THPS and EDDS against an SRB biofilm. *World J. Microb. Biotechnol.* 28, 1641–1646. doi: 10.1007/s11274-011-0970-5

Xu, H., and Liu, Y. (2011). D-Amino acid mitigated membrane biofouling and promoted biofilm detachment. *J. Membrane Sci.* 376, 266–274. doi: 10.1016/j.memsci.2011.04.030

Xue, Y., and Voordouw, G. (2015). Control of microbial sulfide production with biocides and nitrate in oil reservoir simulating bioreactors. *Front. Microbiol.* 8:1387. doi: 10.3389/fmicb.2015.01387

Zhang, P., Xu, D., Li, Y., Yang, K., and Gu, T. (2015). Electron mediators accelerate the microbiologically influenced corrosion of 304 stainless steel by the *Desulfovibrio vulgaris* biofilm. *Bioelectrochemistry* 101, 14–21. doi: 10.1016/j.bioelechem.2014.06.010

Zhu, X. Y., Lubeck, J., and Kilbane, J. J. (2003). Characterization of microbial communities in gas industry pipelines. *Appl. Environ. Microbiol.* 69, 5354–5363. doi: 10.1128/AEM.69.9.5354-5363.2003

15

Downregulation of Host Tryptophan–Aspartate Containing Coat (TACO) Gene Restricts the Entry and Survival of *Leishmania donovani* in Human Macrophage Model

Venkateswara Reddy Gogulamudi[1,2], Mohan Lal Dubey[1], Deepak Kaul[3], Venkata Subba Rao Atluri[4] and Rakesh Sehgal[1]**

[1] Department of Parasitology, Postgraduate Institute of Medical Education and Research, Chandigarh, India, [2] Department of Physiology, Tulane University School of Medicine, New Orleans, LA, USA, [3] Department of Experimental Medicine and Biotechnology, Postgraduate Institute of Medical Education and Research, Chandigarh, India, [4] Department of Immunology, Herbert Wertheim College of Medicine, Florida International University, Miami, FL, USA

***Correspondence:**
Rakesh Sehgal,
Department of Parasitology,
Postgraduate Institute of Medical Education and Research,
Chandigarh – 160012, India
sehgalpgi@gmail.com;
Venkateswara Reddy Gogulamudi,
Department of Physiology, Tulane University School of Medicine,
New Orleans, LA-70112, USA
gvrmicro@gmail.com

Leishmania are obligate intracellular protozoan parasites of mammalian hosts. Promastigotes of *Leishmania* are internalized by macrophages and transformed into amastigotes in phagosomes, and replicate in phagolysosomes. Phagosomal maturation arrest is known to play a crucial role in the survival of pathogenic *Leishmania* within activated macrophages. Recently, tryptophan–aspartate containing coat (TACO) gene has been recognized as playing a central role in the survival of *Mycobacterium tuberculosis* within human macrophages by arresting the phagosome maturation process. We postulated that a similar association of TACO gene with phagosomes would prevent the vacuole from maturation in the case of *Leishmania*. In this study we attempted to define the effect of TACO gene downregulation on the entry/survival of *Leishmania donovani* intracellularly, by treatment with Vitamin D_3 (Vit.D_3)/Retinoic acid (RA) and chenodeoxycholic acid (CDCA)/RA combinations in human THP-1 macrophages (*in vitro*). Treatment with these molecules downregulated the TACO gene in macrophages, resulting in reduced parasite load and marked reduction of disease progression in *L. donovani* infected macrophages. Taken together, these results suggest that TACO gene downregulation may play a role in subverting macrophage machinery in establishing the *L. donovani* replicative niche inside the host. Our study is the first to highlight the important role of the TACO gene in *Leishmania* entry, survival and to identify TACO gene downregulation as potential drug target against leishmaniasis.

Keywords: leishmaniasis, TACO gene, Coronin-1A, host–parasite interactions, intracellular parasite, vitamin D, retinoic acid, chenodeoxycholic acid

Introduction

Leishmaniasis is a major public health issue in many parts of the world, affecting over 20 million people worldwide. About 350 million people are at risk of being infected with leishmaniasis, and 1.5-2 million children and adults develop the disease each year (Desjeux, 2004). This disease is caused by a parasite, which belongs to the genus *Leishmania*. All species of the genus *Leishmania* are obligate intracellular parasites that pass their life cycle in two hosts: the mammalian host, and the insect vector, the female sandfly. In human and other mammalian hosts, they multiply within macrophages, in which they occur exclusively in the amastigote form. Intracellular parasites have evolved through diverse mechanisms to enhance their survival and replication within host cells (Hackstadt, 2000). These mechanisms greatly involve adaptations for survival in different intracellular compartments that permit the parasites to avoid lysosomal killing. Although functions of most of these strategies remain unclear, the majority is expressed early on infectious process, suggesting that manipulation of the vacuole is critical to the outcome of the host-parasite interaction.

Tryptophan–aspartate containing coat (TACO) protein (a coat protein of phagosomes), also known as Coronin 1A, was shown to restrict the delivery of *Mycobacteria* to lysosomes (Ferrari et al., 1999). TACO/Coronin-1A belongs to the tryptophan–aspartate (WD) repeat containing family proteins (Neer et al., 1994; Suzuki et al., 1995), some of which are implicated in cytoskeletal organization, signal transduction, motility (Burrows et al., 1995), cytokinesis and vesicle formation (Pryer et al., 1993). Specifically, TACO is a 57 kDa polypeptide that binds to actin and is involved in cytoskeletal modulation (Gatfield et al., 2005), cytokinesis and intracellular membrane transport (Rybakin and Clemen, 2005). TACO is present on the cytoplasmic face of the plasma membrane and is retained by vacuoles carrying mycobacteria through phagocytosis, results in shielding of the mycobacteria within phagosomes of the host molecule by inhibiting its fusion with any other organelle, including lysosomes (Ferrari et al., 1999). Therefore, the active retention of TACO around the mycobacterial phagosome prevents the delivery of this machinery, and the pathogen continues to survive and replicate within the TACO armored phagosome. Several lines of evidence have been developed to show that TACO becomes activated in *Mycobacterium tuberculosis* infected cells, and this contributes to disease pathogenesis. Recent studies have shown that the downregulation of TACO leads to the suppression of mycobacteria infectivity and multiplication rate (Anand and Kaul, 2005).

However, the possible contribution of TACO in the inhibition of fusion of *Leishmania donovani*-containing phagosomes was not studied. Both *Mycobacterium* and *Leishmania* are intracellular organisms with macrophages as their primary target cells. These interference mechanisms are the main focus of this study. Dermine et al. (2000) suggested that it would be of interest to validate whether this TACO protein is also coupled with *Leishmania*-containing phagosomes. In addition to their limited availability, anti-leishmanial drugs have disadvantages such as toxicity, required prolonged treatment, challenge of drug resistance and high cost (Sundar et al., 2007). Attempts to develop newer synthetic compounds have met with a limited success. Thus, there is an urgent need to develop better anti-leishmanial drugs to supplement those in present use. Simple compounds like vitamins have not yet been explored as sources for possible anti-leishmanial agents. Vitamin D_3 (Vit.D3), retinoic acid (RA), and chenodeoxycholic acid (CDCA) have been explored against *M. tuberculosis*; however, no scientific data is available on the utility of these endogenous molecules with regard to their anti-leishmanial activity *in vitro* or *in vivo*.

Taking all these findings into consideration, the aim of this study was to assess the effect of downregulation of TACO gene expression on entry and survival of *L. donovani* in human macrophages. The present study was designed to explore the inherent capacity of isoprenoid (CDCA, derived from mevalonate pathway) and vitamins to regulate TACO gene transcription, and their effect on entry and survival of *Leishmania* intracellularly. Based upon its previously described effects, this study has been designed to address these significant gaps in evidence that downregulation of TACO gene expression will lead to inhibition of *Leishmania* entry and survival in host macrophages. Such approach may help in the development of new, safe, effective, and inexpensive drug molecules, which can act at preventive and therapeutic levels against *Leishmania* infection.

Materials and Methods

Parasites

The standard strain of *L. donovani*: MHOM/IN/80/DD8 being maintained in the Department of Parasitology, PGIMER, Chandigarh, by serial *in vitro* culture and passaged through BALB/c mice for maintenance of virulence was used in the study.

Macrophage Cell Line

THP-1, a human monocytic leukemia cell line was procured from NCCS, Pune, India. THP-1 monocytic cells were cultured in complete culture medium containing RPMI-1640 and HEPES (Invitrogen) supplemented with 10% fetal calf serum and 1% Penicillin (5000 U/ml)-streptomycin (5000 μg/ml; Sigma-Aldrich). The cells were kept in a humidified atmosphere at 37°C and 5% CO_2. Cells were seeded in six-well plates (1×10^7 cells/ml) in the complete medium. The cells were incubated with 30 nM/ml Phorbol 12-myristate 13-acetate (PMA, Sigma-Aldrich) for 72 h (Tsuchiya et al., 1982; Verstraelen et al., 2008), which induced differentiation of these cells into adherent macrophages. Plates were washed twice with pre-warmed RPMI-1640 to remove PMA, and 2000 μl of complete RPMI-1640 medium was then added. Differentiated cells were maintained until experiments were conducted.

Conventional RT-PCR

After differentiation of THP-1 cells into macrophages as explained above, culture medium was aspirated and cells were rinsed with PBS. These cells were processed for total RNA extraction using TRI Reagent solution (Ambion, USA) based on acid guanidinium thiocyanate-phenol-chloroform method (Chomczynski and Sacchi, 1987). Quantity and quality of RNA were determined by reading absorbance at 260 and 280 nm. First-strand cDNA was synthesized from 1.5 μg of total cellular RNA using random hexamer primers and Moloney murine leukemia virus (M-MuLV) reverse transcriptase (RT) in a 20 μl reaction volume. Reagents were obtained from RevertAid™ first strand cDNA synthesis kit (Fermentas, USA). 1 μl of cDNA was used as a template in each PCR reaction. cDNA of each sample was amplified using primers specific for TACO gene and carried out using glyceraldehyde phosphate dehydrogenase (GAPDH) as a control for RT efficiency. PCR reagents were obtained from MBI Fermentas and specific primers were obtained from MWG-Biotech. PCR was performed in a 25 μl reaction volume containing 1x PCR buffer, 2.5 mM $MgCl_2$, 0.2 mM of each dNTP, 0.5 μM of each primer and 0.625 U of Taq (*Thermus aquaticus*) DNA polymerase. The primer sequences are described below. TACO (512 bp) Forward: 5′-CCAGTGCTATGGGATGTGCGCG-3′ Reverse: 5′-GACACGACTCGCTTGTCACGGC-3′ GAPDH (270 bp) Forward: 5′-AAGGCACAGACATGGTTGGT-3′ Reverse: 5′-TGGAAAGCAAACTGCCCTGA-3′.

TACO Gene Sequencing

Polymerase chain reaction amplicons were detected by electrophoresis using 1.5% agarose gels and visualized using ethidium bromide. The amplified TACO gene PCR product of the expected size 512 bp was extracted from the agarose gel with a Mini Gel Extraction Kit (Qiagen). The PCR products were purified using Microspin columns (Amersham Pharmacia) prior to sequencing. Sequencing was done using specific primers and ABI PRISM Big Dye Terminator cycle sequencing ready reaction kit. The sequences were analyzed on an ABI PRISM 3730 DNA analyzer (Applied Biosystems, Foster City, CA, USA). The sequence of amplicon was confirmed by single direction using TACO primers.

Determination of TACO mRNA Level

GAPDH gene was used as a control. The relative levels of TACO gene mRNA in Vit.D_3/RA and CDCA/RA treated cells were determined by real-time PCR. The concentrations of molecules showing the maximum gene downregulation were used in further studies.

After treating the THP-1 cells with PMA as explained above, culture medium was aspirated and cells were rinsed with PBS. At the end of the incubation, the cells were incubated for 24 h in the presence of various stimuli: one set of cultures were pre-treated with Vit.D_3/RA (Sigma–Aldrich, USA) at two doses (0.5/0.5, 1.0/1.0 μM), and another set were pre-treated with CDCA/RA in a dose dependent manner (25, 50, 75, and 100 μM of CDCA) in the constant presence of RA at 0.5 μM for 24 h at 37°C in 5% CO_2. After 24 h of incubation at 37°C, real time PCR (relative quantification) was performed using LightCycler 480 SYBR Green I master mix (Roche) detection method to confirm the quantitative expression of TACO gene. GAPDH was used as internal control. Reaction mixture containing 1 μl (20-30 ng) of purified cDNA, 10 μl of 2X master mix (SYBR Greenl Dye), 10 picomoles of each primer of TACO and GAPDH genes was prepared and total volume was made up to 20 μl in nuclease free water. The cDNA synthesis reaction was performed with RNA along with all the other components but without RT enzyme. A "no-RT" control would yield a PCR product in case of genomic DNA contamination of the RNA sample. In order to nullify the variation in samples, we have presented the data of our quantitative analysis as ΔCp (ΔCp = Cp Target gene - Cp GAPDH). Cp (crossing point) value is inversely proportional to the gene level, thus Cp has an indirect relationship with the relative levels of the target gene; the greater the value, the lower the expression level.

Relative gene expression of TACO mRNA was performed by real-time PCR using SYBR Green-I master detection method using specific primers. To minimize the loading variations, GAPDH, an internal control gene, was run in all the samples from different groups. The real-time PCR analysis of transcripts for GAPDH in the Vit.D_3/RA and CDCA/RA in different doses showed similar amplification and dissociation curves. In order to nullify the due variation in samples, the data was normalized to GAPDH, which served as internal control (ΔCp = Cp Target gene - Cp GAPDH), then again normalized to control ($\Delta\Delta Cp = \Delta Cp$ Test sample - ΔCp Control sample), and final data was presented in the form of relative fold change by $2^{-\Delta\Delta Cp}$.

Western Blot Analysis

After differentiation of THP-1 cells into macrophages as explained above, culture medium was aspirated and cells were rinsed with PBS. Adhered macrophages were detached by adding 1 ml acutase (PAA Laboratories, UK) at 37°C for 10 min. The cells were pelleted and the supernatant was discarded. The cells were washed gently by resuspending in 1 ml of PBS, and pelleted at low speed. Cell pellet was lysed in 1 ml of lysis buffer [50 mM Tris-HCl, pH 7.6, 150 mM NaCl, 5 mM EDTA, 1 mM ethylene glycol-bis (β-aminoethyl ether) *N, N, N′, N′*-tetraacetic acid (EGTA), 0.1% Triton X-100, 0.3% w/v β-mercaptoethanol, 0.28 TIU/ml aprotinin, 2 mM phenylmethylsulphonyl fluoride (PMSF), leupeptin 0.5 mg/ml and containing 100 μl protease inhibitor cocktail (Roche, Mannheim, Germany)] for 3 min at 4°C. Western blotting was carried out using a Mini Trans-blot electrophoretic transfer assembly (Bio-Rad Laboratories, USA; Towbin et al., 1979). After the transfer, PVDF membrane was blocked with 5% PBS-skimmed milk for 2 h and incubated with primary antibody (Novus Biologicals, USA) diluted in 5% PBS-skimmed milk overnight at 4°C. The membrane was then washed twice with PBST, once with PBS and incubated with Horseradish peroxidase (HRP)-conjugated secondary antibodies (Santa Cruz Biotechnology, Inc., USA) diluted in 5% PBS-skimmed milk, against the respective primary antibodies for 2 h. Protein bands were visualized by enhanced chemiluminescence (ECL) plus detection system with UV-Pro Transilluminator.

Immunofluoroscence Assay

For the localization of TACO protein, immunofluoroscence was done on THP-1 cells by growing cells on cover slips and exposing them to PMA for 48 h at 37°C and in the presence of 5% CO_2 to permit cell differentiation into macrophages. Two sets of cells were fixed with 4% (w/v) paraformaldehyde (PFA) in PBS for 20 min, permeabilized and blocked with 0.2% (w/v) BSA/0.1% (w/v) saponin in PBS (blocking solution) for 20 min. The cells were subsequently incubated with rabbit Coronin 1A antibody (Novus biological, USA) for 60 min at room temperature. After washing three times with PBST, cells were incubated with goat anti rabbit IgG FITC- conjugated secondary antibody (Immunology Consultants Laboratory, Inc., USA), for 60 min at 37°C. After incubation, cells were washed thrice with PBS and immediately examined by fluorescence microscopy (Olympus BX51, Japan) equipped with a UV filter system. Images were obtained with a CCD camera (Olympus, model no.E330-ADU1.2X, Japan).

Effect of Macrophage TACO Gene Downregulation on *L. donovani* Infection *In Vitro*

Once the maximal downregulation dose of TACO mRNA was determined by treatment with the above molecules, the same dose was applied during the parasite infection study. One set of THP-1 macrophages were treated with the maximal downregulating dose of Vit.D_3/RA and another set with CDCA/RA. After 24 h of treatment, the cells were washed two times with plain medium. Infection of macrophage was carried out using a virulent strain (DD8) of *L. donovani* grown in axenic culture. These promastigotes were added to macrophages at a ratio of 10:1. This culture was incubated for 1 h at 37°C in 5% CO_2 incubator. Non-adherent cells were washed out and macrophages were cultivated in complete culture medium supplemented with 10% heat inactivated FBS, streptomycin (200 ug/ml), benzyl penicillin (200 U/ml) and gentamicin (40 ug/ml). Parasite load and replication rate was determined at different time intervals: early (2 and 4 h), middle (24 and 48 h) and late (72 and 96 h) stages. Infected macrophages on the cover slips were fixed and stained with Giemsa. Parasite loads were examined microscopically by counting at least 500 target macrophages for each cover slip. Efficacy of the molecules was determined by calculating the number of amastigotes per 100 macrophages at each time point.

Statistical Analysis

Data was expressed as the mean ± SD values of triplicate samples. The statistical significance of the differences between and within groups was determined by analysis of variance (ANOVA) to define the multiple comparisons amongst different groups. The statistical analyses were performed using SPSS software. Differences were considered statistically significant for $p < 0.05$.

Results

Optimum Concentration of PMA for Differentiation of THP-1 Monocytes to Macrophages

According to the results presented in **Figure 1**, monocytes in suspension were converted to matured macrophages in 72 h after treatment with PMA. Treatment with 30 nM/ml PMA for 72 h induced changes in morphology; their rounded shape became elongated and flattened. However, attachment of cells at 20 nM/ml was unstable, and the cells were easily detached by washing. This indicated that the concentrations below 30 nM/ml PMA were not enough to differentiate the THP-1 cells stably. Hence, the minimal concentration of PMA for stable differentiation was determined to be 30 nM/ml. Cell adhesion and spreading, which are hallmarks of macrophages, were then examined under a microscope. Macrophage cells grew in a distinct morphological pattern, showing a significant raise in adhesion and spreading patterns to the growth substratum.

Infectivity of *L. donovani* Promastigotes in Differentiated THP-1 Macrophages and TACO Gene Expression

Differentiated THP-1 macrophages were infected with virulent *L. donovani* promastigotes for 24 h. As demonstrated in **Figure 2**, the *L. donovani* promastigotes exhibited a marked infectivity to macrophages 24 h after infection. The uptake of parasites by mammalian cells was determined by Giemsa staining.

In order to determine the expression of TACO gene expression in *Leishmania* infected macrophages, RT-PCR was performed using specific primers with equal concentration of cDNAs. The house-keeping gene GADPH was amplified and used as a loading control. Gels containing RT-PCR products were photographed by UV-Pro Transilluminator camera and bands were analyzed (**Figure 3**). This assay confirmed the 512 bp TACO gene

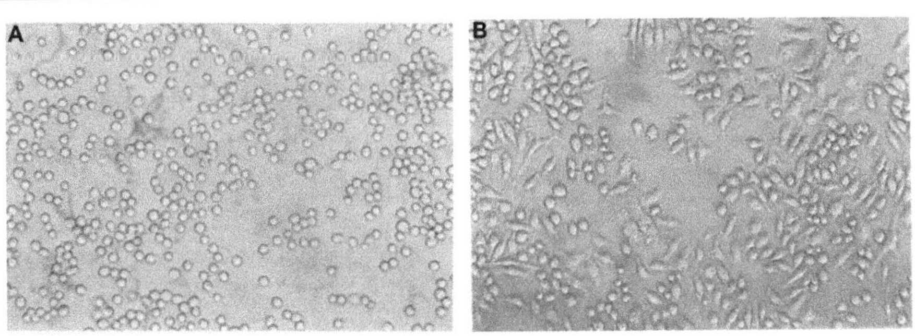

FIGURE 1 | Phase contrast micrographs of THP-1 cells in culture induced by PMA. THP-1 cells were incubated with PMA (30 nM/ml) for 72 h. Morphological changes in THP-1 (40X) on **(A)** Day 1 **(B)** Day 3 are shown. Their morphology changed from a rounded shape to elongated and flattened.

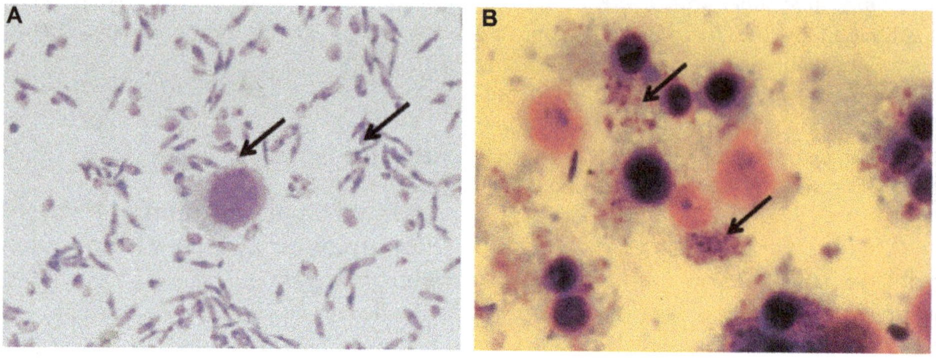

FIGURE 2 | Giemsa stained micrograph showing human macrophage cell line (THP-1) infected with *L. donovani* promastigotes. (A) Promastigotes and Macrophages; **(B)** Macrophages showing intracellular parasite converted to amastigotes after internalization (100X; indicated by arrowheads).

expression, when the PCR product showing ethidium bromide-stained bands obtained after electrophoresis along with the marker (**Figure 3**) and 240 bp of GAPDH gene.

Sequencing of PCR product of TACO gene (512 bp band) from agarose gel electrophoresis and BLAST search for homologous nucleotides in the database showed that 512 bp of TACO gene expression showed the highest (100%) homology to other TACO mRNAs in many organisms including humans. This confirmed that the PCR amplified gene was the exact product of TACO/Coronin 1A. This TACO gene sequence has been deposited in GenBank under the accession number GQ2141031.

Localization and Expression of TACO in THP-1 Macrophages

TACO protein localization in human THP-1 macrophages were determined by indirect immunofluoroscence using an affinity-purified antibody. Strong punctuate staining of TACO protein was observed in the cytoplasmic face of activated macrophages (**Figure 4**). Observation of this assay showed TACO protein localization on the cytoplasmic face of plasma membranes of activated THP-1 human macrophages.

Expression of TACO protein in human macrophages was confirmed by Western blot analysis using a specific antibody. Results showed that in lysates of THP-1 macrophages (**Figure 5**), anti-TACO/Coronin 1A antibody recognized a single 57 kDa protein in Western blots, confirming the expression of TACO protein.

Vitamin D_3/Retinoic Acid Regulates TACO Gene Expression in THP-1 Macrophages

During this phase, to study the transcriptional regulation of TACO gene by Vit.D_3/RA and CDCA/RA, experiments were designed to determine the optimum dose of molecules used

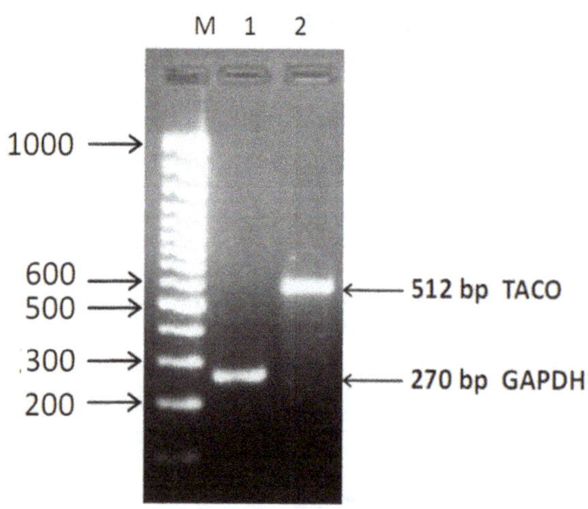

FIGURE 3 | Agarose gel photograph showing ethidium bromide stained bands of RT-PCR products of TACO and GAPDH genes. Lane M: 100 bp DNA ladder. Lane 1: GAPDH gene; Lane2: TACO gene.

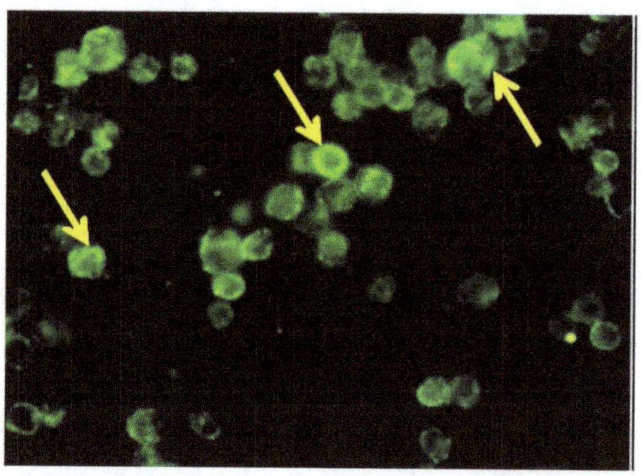

FIGURE 4 | Localization of TACO/Coronin1A in differentiated THP-1 macrophages. Monocytes cultured on glass coverslips were differentiated into macrophages in the presence of PMA, fixed, permeabilized and stained with primary antibody, TACO/Coronin 1A Antibody, for 2 h followed by FITC labeled secondary antibody. Cells were observed under fluorescent microscope equipped with a UV filter system using 100X; indicated by arrowheads.

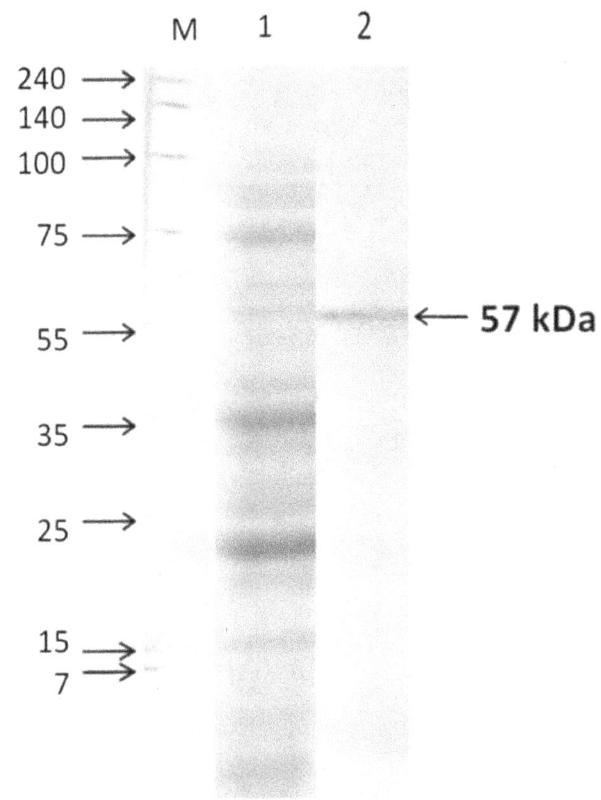

FIGURE 5 | Western blot analysis of TACO protein in THP-1 cells. Cells were harvested after differentiation with PMA (30 nM/ml) for 72 h. Whole cell extracts were prepared and separated by SDS-PAGE on 10% gels, and Western blot assay was performed using TACO/Coronin-1A Antibody and goat anti-rabbit IgG-HRP antibody. Lane M: Marker; Lane1: SDS PAGE Profile; Lane 2: Western Blot showing the TACO protein of 57 kDa. Results are representative of at least three separate experiments that gave similar results.

for downregulation of TACO mRNA. Compounds from two different categories, i.e., isoprenoids derived from mevalonate pathway and vitamins (A, D), were evaluated for their effect on TACO gene expression. Exposure of THP-1 differentiated macrophages to Vit.D_3 and RA for 24 h resulted in significant dose dependent downregulation of TACO mRNA expression. TACO mRNA level was significantly downregulated by 0.686 fold ($p < 0.0001$) in cells treated with 0.5 μM/0.5 μM Vit.D_3/RA compared to controls. Whereas cells treated with a dose of 1.0 μM/1.0 μM Vit.D_3/RA, mRNA level was highly downregulated by 0.949 fold ($p < 0.0001$) when compared to control groups. The effective dose on TACO mRNA downregulation of this combination was 1.0 μM/1.0 μM as compared with control groups (**Figures 6A,B**).

Chenodeoxycholic Acid/Retinoic Acid Regulates TACO Gene Expression in a Dose Dependent Manner

Further, exposure of THP-1 macrophages to a combination of CDCA 0–100 μM and RA (0.5 μM) caused a further reduction in TACO mRNA expression levels (**Figure 6C**). Surprisingly, a combined dose of 25 μM CDCA 0.5 μM RA resulted in moderate upregulation by 0.33 fold ($p = 0.132$) of TACO mRNA compared to control groups (**Figure 6D**). In additional doses, TACO mRNA expression was downregulated at the doses of 50 μM/0.5 μM by 0.165 fold ($p = 0.498$), 75 μM/0.5 μM by 0.441 fold ($p < 0.002$) and 100 μM/0.5 μM by 0.717 fold ($p < 0.0001$) as compared to control cells. In this combination of molecules (CDCA/RA) 100 μM/0.5 μM dose was most effective in downregulation of TACO gene as compared to control groups (**Figure 6D**).

Vitamin D_3/Retinoic Acid and Chenodeoxycholic Acid/Retinoic Acid Inhibit Entry and Survival of *Leishmania promastigotes* in a Time Dependent Manner

To examine the entry and intracellular survival of *L. donovani* in TACO downregulated macrophages, cells were pre-treated with maximum TACO mRNA downregulated doses of Vit.D_3/RA and CDCA/RA (treatment before parasite infection) for 24 h. Further, to investigate the parasite survival when TACO gene is downregulated, macrophages were infected with promastigotes at 1:10 ratio (**Figure 7**), and subsequently time kinetics of THP-1 cell infection by *L. donovani* were assessed at early (2 and 4 h), middle (24 and 48 h), and late (72 and 96 h) stages. The rate of entry and survival was observed at different time intervals.

Treatment with Vit.D_3/RA before *Leishmania* promastigote infection revealed that the entry and survival of parasites within these cells varied at different time intervals. At 2 h, 31% ($p = 0.506$) reduction and at 4 h, 13% ($p = 0.387$) reduction in parasite load was observed, but there was no significant difference between control and treated cells. At 24 h, we observed 47% ($p < 0.0001$) reduction, at 48 h 57% ($p < 0.002$) reduction, at 72 h 60% ($p < 0.0001$) reduction and at 96 h maximum reduction, i.e., 80% reduction in parasite load ($p < 0.001$; **Figure 8**) compared to the control.

Similarly, in cells after CDCA/RA pre-treatment, there was no significant difference in parasite load at 2 h (15% reduction; $p = 0.517$), and at 4 h it showed 5% reduced parasite load ($p = 0.553$). However, significant reduction in parasite loads at 24 (28%, $p < 0.04$), 48 (30%, $p < 0.016$), 72 (26%, $p < 0.014$), and 96 h (50%, $p < 0.004$) were observed compared to controls (**Figure 8**). The results showed that Vit.D_3/RA displayed a maximum 80% ($p < 0.001$) suppression of parasite multiplication and entry of promastigote in THP-1 macrophages, while CDCA/RA treatment showed 50% reduction ($p < 0.004$; **Figure 8**).

Discussion

Intracellular infection by the *Leishmania* parasite depends on a sequence of events including attachment, internalization, amastigote differentiation and intracellular survival. Understanding the impact of intracellular pathogens on the behavior of their host cell is the key to designing new

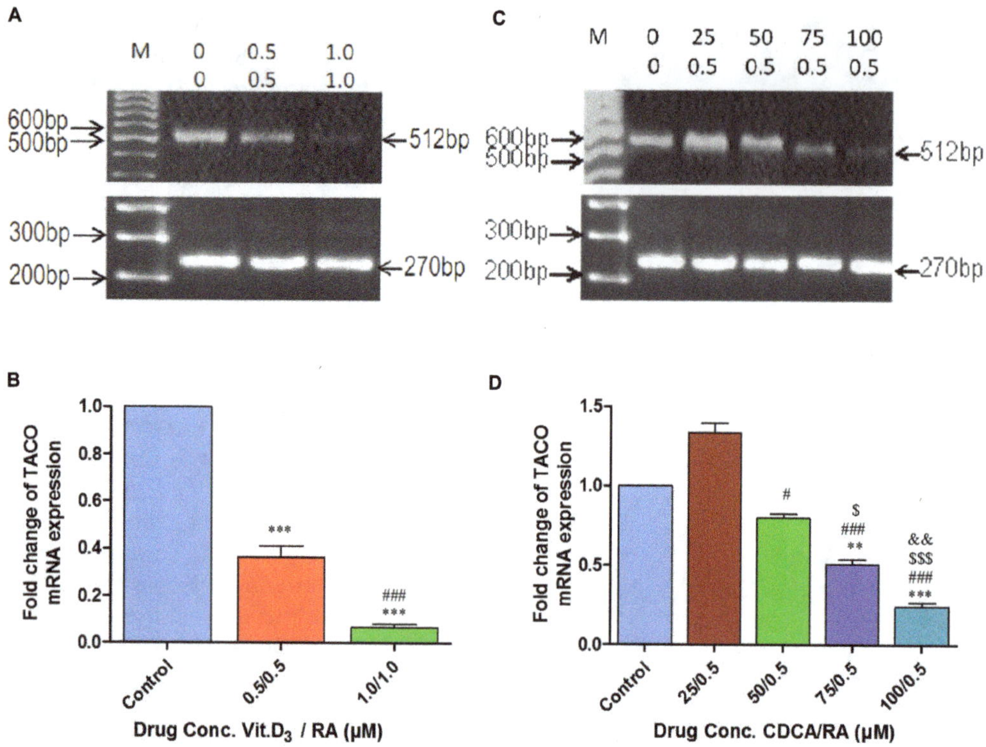

FIGURE 6 | Polymerase chain reaction (PCR) amplification showing synergistic action of Vitamin D_3/Retinoic acid (Vit.D_3/RA) and chenodeoxycholic acid/Retinoic acid (CDCA/RA) on mRNA expression of TACO gene. (A,C) Representative agarose gel photographs showing ethidium bromide stained Real Time PCR products of TACO and GAPDH genes. **(B,D)** The relative levels of TACO mRNA expression represented in fold change. Each data point in the graph represents mean ± SD of three independent experiments. ***$p < 0.001$ (Control Vs 0.5/0.5 μM; 1.0/1.0 μM), ###$p < 0.001$ (0.5/0.5 μM Vs 1.0/1.0 μM), ***$p < 0.001$ (Control Vs 75/0.5 μM; 100/0.5 μM), #$p < 0.05$, ###$p < 0.001$ (25/0.5 μM Vs 50/0.5 μM; 75/0.5 μM; 100/0.5 μM), \$$p < 0.05$, \$\$\$$p < 0.001$ (50/0.5 μM Vs 75/0.5 μM; 100/0.5 μM), &&$p < 0.05$ (75/0.5 μM Vs 100/0.5 μM).

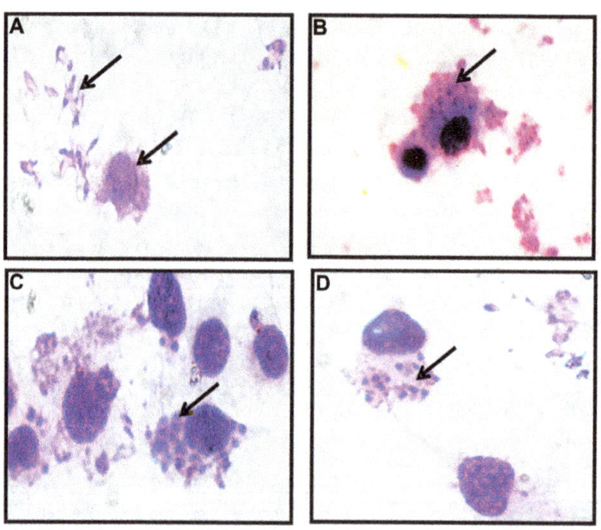

FIGURE 7 | Giemsa Stained micro-photographs of Vit.D_3/RA and CDCA/RA pre-treated THP-1 macrophage infected with promastigotes. (A) Promastigotes and Macrophages; **(B–D)** Conversion to amastigotes after internalization (indicated by arrowheads).

interventions. The present study was based on the hypothesis that the transcriptional manipulation of the TACO gene leads to phagosome (carrying parasite) maturation, which will affect the survival and replication of intracellular pathogens.

In the present study, Vit.D_3 and RA combination showed significant TACO mRNA downregulation in a dose dependent manner (**Figure 6**). Biological effects of Vit.D_3 are mediated by vitamin D receptor (VDR), a member of a superfamily of nuclear hormone receptors (Carlberg, 2003). Similarly RA modulates transcription through the ligand dependent transcription factor RXR, which binds to a particular response element in the promoter region of target genes (Giguere, 1999). The heterodimeric complex VDR/RXR then binds to a different set of response elements within effector genes. RXR ligands have been reported to synergize with Vit.D_3 to activate the 25 hydroxy-vitamin D_3-24-hydroxylase promoter (Zou et al., 1997), whereas VDR/RXR ligands that have been reported to inhibit transcriptional activity of rat osteocalcin gene (MacDonald et al., 1993; Anand and Kaul, 2003) showed similar results with these molecules. Therefore, it is reasonable to speculate that Vit.D_3 and RA act synergistically to downregulate TACO mRNA expression (Anand and Kaul, 2003).

In the present study, mevalonate-pathway derived isoprenoids, i.e., CDCA along with RA, were also used to evaluate

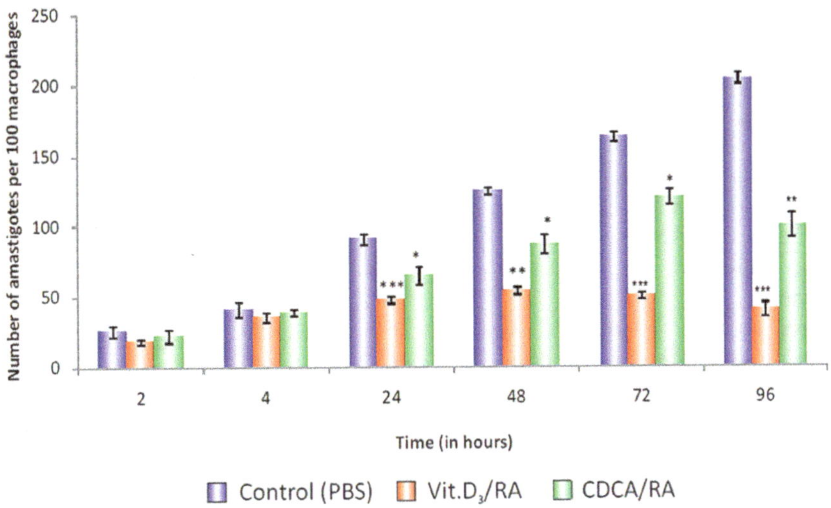

FIGURE 8 | Parasite load in Vit.D3/RA and CDCA/RA pre-treated THP-1 macrophage cells infected with promastigotes. THP-1 human macrophage cell lines were pre-treated with Vit.D3/RA, CDCA/RA for 24 h to downregulate the TACO gene, then infected with *L. donovani* promastigotes. Parasite loads were determined by calculating the total number of amastigotes per 100 macrophages at different time intervals (2, 4, 24, 48, 72, and 96 h) post-infection. The values listed are mean ± SD of three independent cultures. Significant differences are indicated by asterisks: *$p < 0.05$, **$p < 0.01$, ***$p < 0.001$.

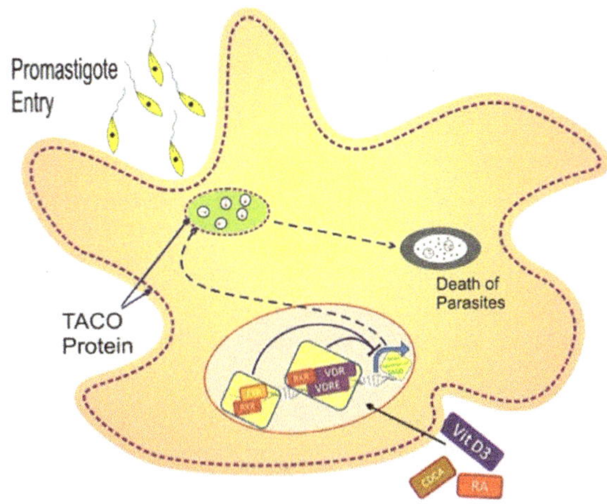

FIGURE 9 | Hypothetical model of transcriptional regulation of TACO gene with various effector molecules. *Leishmania* promastigotes enter the macrophage by phagocytosis, after which phagosomes are formed that retain tryptophan–aspartate containing coat protein (TACO). Such retention of TACO may support survival of the parasite along with late maturation and late fusion with late endosomes. Vit.D3/RA and CDCA/RA treatment leads to the downregulation of the *TACO* gene, which is possibly responsible for the detachment of TACO protein over the phagosome, and consequently, early maturation and phagolysosomal killing of the parasite.

TACO mRNA expression in a dose dependent fashion. Initially, a moderate increase in TACO mRNA expression was observed (**Figure 6**). An increased dose combination with CDCA/RA was observed to be more potent in downregulating TACO mRNA expression, initiating a pronounced downregulatory effect on TACO gene transcription (**Figure 6**). It is pertinent to note that CDCA is a potent activator of FXR, which is ligand-dependent transcription factor (Giguere, 1999). On activation, the receptor translocates into the nucleus and regulates a number of genes, either alone or in combination with its heterodimeric partner retinoid-X-receptor (RXR; Grober et al., 1999; Edwards et al., 2002). This raises the possibility that CDCA and RA, when used in combination, show a synergistic effect by activating the ligand-dependent heterodimeric complex FXR/RXR.

In support of this, Anand and Kaul (2003) demonstrated the mechanism of transcriptional repression by Vit.D3/RA and CDCA/RA through a planned bioinformatic approach coupled with reporter assay technology that was used to pinpoint the promoter region of the TACO gene. This region was evaluated for the presence and functional status of response elements corresponding to VDR/RXR and FXR/RXR. It has been noted that the three compounds that showed transcriptional repression of TACO mRNA expression are potent activators/inhibitors of these transcription factors (Anand and Kaul, 2003).

Keeping in view the positive role of TACO in *Leishmania* entry and survival, it is likely that downregulation of TACO mRNA could be accompanied by inhibition of leishmanial entry and survival within the macrophage. Consequently, investigation was carried out to discover whether or not treatment with these molecules suppress TACO mRNA, and their affects on *Leishmania* entry and survival. THP-1 macrophages were pre-treated with different effector molecules followed by *Leishmania* promastigote infection. The results of entry and survival of the parasite were analyzed by Giemsa staining at different time-periods.

Vit.D3/RA pre-treatment revealed 80% inhibition of parasite load as compared to untreated control groups (**Figure 8**). It was observed at 96 h as analyzed in *Leishmania* infected macrophages. Previously, Vit.D3 and RA had been reported to restrict the intracellular growth of *M. tuberculosis* (Wilkinson et al., 2000;

Anand and Kaul, 2003). Similarly, Sly et al. (2001) reported that Vit.D_3 treatment of *M. tuberculosis* infected THP-1 cells activated PI3K. PI3K was shown to be essential for the formation of the phagosomal cup (class-1A PI3K) and its fusion with lysosomes in normal cells (Fratti et al., 2001). In our study, we also observed that Vit.D_3/RA acts synergistically and downregulates TACO gene expression significantly (**Figure 8**). Anand and Kaul (2003) reported that the effect of Vit.D_3/RA on TACO gene expression was not evident when either was used alone, and explained that this mode of synergetic action was due to the activation of VDR/RXR transcription factors.

Similarly, CDCA/RA pre-treatment restricted *Leishmania* entry by 50% as observed at 96 h after exposure compared to control groups (**Figure 8**). Accumulating evidence suggests that bile acids modulate various signal transduction pathways including the protein kinase A, protein kinase C, c-Jun N-terminal kinase and MAP-kinase dependent cascades (Bouscarel et al., 1999; Alpini et al., 2004; De Fabiani et al., 2004). Further, no previous study has shown a direct link between CDCA and *Leishmania.* The results of the experiments in this study indicate a potential role of CDCA in killing *Leishmania.*

Altogether, the results reveal that Vit.D3/RA and CDCA/RA suppress TACO mRNA expression to significant levels. Such expression has been reported to operate through the activity of transcription factors VDR/RXR and FXR/RXR. Consequently, TACO gene suppression with these molecules led to inhibition of *Leishmania* entry and survival, thus proving Vit.D3/RA and CDCA/RA combinations, we found that Vit.D_3/RA combination showed highly effective levels of parasite suppression compared with the CDCA/RA combination. These observations suggest that TACO gene downregulation may modulate the invasion of parasite phagolysosomal maturation in macrophages following phagocytosis of *L. donovani* carrying promastigotes (**Figure 9**). The current study provides evidence that TACO gene downregulation modulates parasite entry and survival in macrophages following the phagocytosis of *L. donovani* promastigotes.

The conclusions derived from this study suggest that the effect of TACO gene downregulation can help elucidate the pathophysiology of host and parasite interactions, thereby unraveling the probable potential preventive and therapeutic alternatives against leishmaniasis. To the best of our knowledge, this study is the first to report the effect of TACO gene downregulation at the transcriptional level using vitamins and isoprenoids on *L. donovani* infection, which could prove to be a basis for the development of novel approaches in the control of leishmaniasis.

Acknowledgments

This work was supported by a grant received from the Indian Council of Medical Research (ICMR), New Delhi, India in the form of Senior Research Fellowship to Dr. VG (First author). We thank Loula Burton for proofreading assistance.

References

Alpini, G., Kanno, N., Phinizy, J. L., Glaser, S., Francis, H., Taffetani, S., et al. (2004). Tauroursodeoxycholate inhibits human cholangiocarcinoma growth via Ca2+-, PKC-, and MAPK-dependent pathways. *Am. J. Physiol. Gastrointest. Liver Physiol.* 286, G973–G982. doi: 10.1152/ajpgi.00270.2003

Anand, P. K., and Kaul, D. (2003). Vitamin D3-dependent pathway regulates TACO gene transcription. *Biochem. Biophys. Res. Commun.* 310, 876–877. doi: 10.1016/j.bbrc.2003.09.087

Anand, P. K., and Kaul, D. (2005). Downregulation of TACO gene transcription restricts mycobacterial entry/survival within human macrophages. *FEMS Microbiol. Lett.* 250, 137–144. doi: 10.1016/j.femsle.2005.06.056

Bouscarel, B., Kroll, S. D., and Fromm, H. (1999). Signal transduction and hepatocellular bile acid transport: cross talk between bile acids and second messengers. *Gastroenterology* 117, 433–452. doi: 10.1053/gast.1999.0029900433

Burrows, T. D., King, A., Smith, S. K., and Loke, Y. W. (1995). Human trophoblast adhesion to matrix proteins: inhibition and signal transduction. *Hum. Reprod.* 10, 2489–2500. doi: 10.1093/oxfordjournals.humrep.a136329

Carlberg, C. (2003). Molecular basis of the selective activity of vitamin D analogues. *J. Cell. Biochem.* 88, 274–281. doi: 10.1002/jcb.10337

Chomczynski, P., and Sacchi, N. (1987). Single-step method of RNA isolation by acid guanidinium thiocyanate-phenol-chloroform extraction. *Anal. Biochem.* 162, 156–159. doi: 10.1006/abio.1987.9999

De Fabiani E., Mitro, N., Godio, C., Gilardi, F., Caruso, D., and Crestani, M. (2004). Bile acid signaling to the nucleus: finding new connections in the transcriptional regulation of metabolic pathways. *Biochimie* 86, 771–778. doi: 10.1016/j.biochi.2004.09.027

Dermine, J. F., Scianimanico, S., Privé, C., Descoteaux, A., and Desjardins, M. (2000). Leishmania promastigotes require lipophosphoglycan to actively modulate the fusion properties of phagosomes at an early step of phagocytosis. *Cell Microbiol.* 2, 115–126. doi: 10.1046/j.1462-5822.2000.00037.x

Desjeux, P. (2004). Leishmaniasis: current situation and new perspectives. *Comp. Immunol. Microbiol. Infect. Dis.* 27, 305–318. doi: 10.1016/j.cimid.2004.03.004

Edwards, P. A., Kast, H. R., and Anisfeld, A. M. (2002). BAREing it all: the adoption of LXR and FXR and their roles in lipid homeostasis. *J. Lipid Res.* 43, 2–12.

Ferrari, G., Langen, H., Naito, M., and Pieters, J. (1999). A coat protein on phagosomes involved in the intracellular survival of mycobacteria. *Cell* 97, 435–447. doi: 10.1016/S0092-8674(00)80754-0

Fratti, R. A., Backer, J. M., Gruenberg, J., Corvera, S., and Deretic, V. (2001). Role of phosphatidylinositol 3-kinase and Rab5 effectors in phagosomal biogenesis and mycobacterial phagosome maturation arrest. *J. Cell Biol.* 154, 631–644. doi: 10.1083/jcb.200106049

Gatfield, J., Albrecht, I., Zanolari, B., Steinmetz, M. O., and Pieters, J. (2005). Association of the leukocyte plasma membrane with the actin cytoskeleton through coiled coil-mediated trimeric coronin 1 molecules. *Mol. Biol. Cell* 16, 2786–2798. doi: 10.1091/mbc.E05-01-0042

Giguere, V. (1999). Orphan nuclear receptors: from gene to function. *Endocr. Rev.* 20, 689–725. doi: 10.1210/edrv.20.5.0378

Grober, J., Zaghini, I., Fujii, H., Jones, S. A., Kliewer, S. A., Willson, T. M., et al. (1999). Identification of a bile acid-responsive element in the human ileal bile acid-binding protein gene. Involvement of the farnesoid X receptor/9-cis-retinoic acid receptor heterodimer. *J. Biol. Chem.* 274, 29749–29754. doi: 10.1074/jbc.274.42.29749

Hackstadt, T. (2000). Redirection of host vesicle trafficking pathways by intracellular parasites. *Traffic* 1, 93–99. doi: 10.1034/j.1600-0854.2000.010201.x

MacDonald, P. N., Dowd, D. R., Nakajima, S., Galligan, M. A., Reeder, M. C., Haussler, C. A., et al. (1993). Retinoid X receptors stimulate and 9-cis retinoic acid inhibits 1,25-dihydroxyvitamin D3-activated expression of the rat osteocalcin gene. *Mol. Cell Biol.* 13, 5907–5917.

Neer, E. J., Schmidt, C. J., Nambudripad, R., and Smith, T. F. (1994). The ancient regulatory-protein family of WD-repeat proteins. *Nature* 371, 297–300. doi: 10.1038/371297a0

Pryer, N. K., Salama, N. R., Schekman, R., and Kaiser, C. A. (1993). Cytosolic Sec13p complex is required for vesicle formation from the endoplasmic reticulum in vitro. *J. Cell Biol.* 120, 865–875. doi: 10.1083/jcb.120.4.865

Rybakin, V., and Clemen, C. S. (2005). Coronin proteins as multifunctional regulators of the cytoskeleton and membrane trafficking. *Bioessays* 27, 625–632. doi: 10.1002/bies.20235

Sly, L. M., Lopez, M., Nauseef, W. M., and Reiner, N. E. (2001). 1alpha,25-Dihydroxyvitamin D_3-induced monocyte antimycobacterial activity is regulated by phosphatidylinositol 3-kinase and mediated by the NADPH-dependent phagocyte oxidase. *J. Biol. Chem.* 276, 35482–35493. doi: 10.1074/jbc.M102876200

Sundar, S., Jha, T. K., Thakur, C. P., Sinha, P. K., and Bhattacharya, S. K. (2007). Injectable paromomycin for Visceral leishmaniasis in India. *N. Engl. J. Med.* 356, 2571–2581. doi: 10.1056/NEJMoa066536

Suzuki, K., Nishihata, J., Arai, Y., Honma, N., Yamamoto, K., Irimura, T., et al. (1995). Molecular cloning of a novel actin-binding protein, p57, with a WD repeat and a leucine zipper motif. *FEBS Lett.* 364, 283–288. doi: 10.1016/0014-5793(95)00393-N

Towbin, H., Staehelin, T., and Gordon, J. (1979). Electrophoretic transfer of proteins from polyacrylamide gels to nitrocellulose sheets: procedure and some applications. *Proc. Natl. Acad. Sci. U. S. A.* 76, 4350–4354. doi: 10.1073/pnas.76.9.4350

Tsuchiya, S., Kobayashi, Y., Goto, Y., Okumura, H., Nakae, S., Konno, T., et al. (1982). Induction of maturation in cultured human monocytic leukemia cells by a phorbol diester. *Cancer Res.* 42, 1530–1536.

Verstraelen, S., Wens, B., Hooyberghs, J., Nelissen, I., Witters, H., Schoeters, G., et al. (2008). Gene expression profiling of in vitro cultured macrophages after exposure to the respiratory sensitizer hexamethylene diisocyanate. *Toxicol. In Vitro* 22, 1107–1114. doi: 10.1016/j.tiv.2008.02.015

Wilkinson, R. J., Llewelyn, M., Toossi, Z., Patel, P., Pasvol, G., Lalvani, A., et al. (2000). Influence of vitamin D deficiency and vitamin D receptor polymorphisms on tuberculosis among Gujarati Asians in west London: a case-control study. *Lancet* 355, 618–621. doi: 10.1016/S0140-6736(99)02301-6

Zou, A., Elgort, M. G., and Allegretto, E. A. (1997). Retinoid X receptor (RXR) ligands activate the human 25-hydroxyvitamin D3-24-hydroxylase promoter via RXR heterodimer binding to two vitamin D-responsive elements and elicit additive effects with 1,25-dihydroxyvitamin D3. *J. Biol. Chem.* 272, 19027–19034. doi: 10.1074/jbc.272.8.4820

16

Prevention and Control of Antimicrobial Resistant Healthcare-Associated Infections: The Microbiology Laboratory Rocks!

Alexandra S. Simões[1], Isabel Couto[1], Cristina Toscano[2,3], Elsa Gonçalves[2,3], Pedro Póvoa[3,4], Miguel Viveiros[1] and Luís V. Lapão[1,5]*

[1] Global Health and Tropical Medicine, Instituto de Higiene e Medicina Tropical, Universidade Nova de Lisboa, Lisbon, Portugal, [2] Laboratório de Microbiologia Clínica e Biologia Molecular, Serviço de Patologia Clínica, Hospital de Egas Moniz, Centro Hospitalar de Lisboa Ocidental, Lisbon, Portugal, [3] Centro de Estudos de Doenças Crónicas, NOVA Medical School/Faculdade de Ciências Médicas, Universidade Nova de Lisboa, Lisbon, Portugal, [4] Unidade de Cuidados Intensivos Polivalente, Hospital de São Francisco Xavier, Centro Hospitalar de Lisboa Ocidental, Lisbon, Portugal, [5] WHO Collaborating Center for Health Workforce Policy and Planning, Instituto de Higiene e Medicina Tropical, Universidade Nova de Lisboa, Lisbon, Portugal

***Correspondence:**
Alexandra S. Simões
assimoes@ihmt.unl.pt

In Europe, each year, more than four milion patients acquire a healthcare-associated infection (HAI) and almost 40 thousand die as a direct consequence of it. Regardless of many stategies to prevent and control HAIs, they remain an important cause of morbidity and mortality worldwide with a significant economic impact: a recent estimate places it at the ten billion dollars/year. The control of HAIs requires a prompt and efficient identification of the etiological agent and a rapid communication with the clinician. The Microbiology Laboratory has a significant role in the prevention and control of these infections and is a key element of any Infection Control Program. The work of the Microbiology Laboratory covers microbial isolation and identification, determination of antimicrobial susceptibility patterns, epidemiological surveillance and outbreak detection, education, and report of quality assured results. In this paper we address the role and importance of the Microbiology Laboratory in the prevention and control of HAI and in Antibiotic Stewardship Programs and how it can be leveraged when combined with the use of information systems. Additionally, we critically review some challenges that the Microbiology Laboratory has to deal with, including the selection of analytic methods and the proper use of communication channels with other healthcare services.

Keywords: microbiology, healthcare-associated infections, antibiotics, antibiotic stewardship, information systems, prevention, control, communication

INTRODUTION

Healthcare-associated infections (HAIs) are a significant cause of morbidity and mortality leading to 37,000 deaths/year in Europe[1] and 75,000 deaths in USA in 2011 (Magill et al., 2014). The HAIs economic impact is also significant: about 9.8 billion dollars/year/USA for the five major infections (Zimlichman et al., 2013). Antibiotic resistance is one of the major

[1] http://ecdc.europa.eu/en/healthtopics/Healthcare-associated_infections

problems associated with HAIs (Cosgrove, 2006; Neidell et al., 2012): the Centers for Disease Prevention and Control (CDC) estimates that over two million people/year acquire antibiotic resistant infections, and 23,000 die as a result of it (CDC, 2013). In Europe, 25,000 people/year die with drug-resistant infections (ECDC, 2009).

Prevention through education is the most used strategy for HAIs control: the benefits from prevention can be as high as 5.5 billion dollars (Zimlichman et al., 2013). Reinforcing hand washing, staff education, environmental cleaning practices, Antibiotic Stewardship Programs (ASPs) and improved communication systems are measures implemented worldwide to control HAIs. However, to efficiently control HAIs, clinicians need to act quickly, which implies gathering all relevant information about the infection as soon as possible. That is why the Microbiology Laboratory is so important in HAIs prevention and control since it is in the front line for the early identification of infection, characterization of antibiotic resistance patterns and recognition of outbreaks (Diekema and Saubolle, 2011; Davey et al., 2013).

Traditionally, the tasks of the Microbiology Laboratory are to isolate, identify and determine antibiotic susceptibility patterns of pathogens (Wilson and Spencer, 1999). However, its scope covers other areas that are critical for Infection Control Programs as well as to ASPs, which should ideally include a member of the Microbiology Laboratory staff (Kolmos, 1999; Benbachir, 2008; CDC, 2014). The success of these kind of programs depends largely on the active involvement of the Microbiology Laboratory in activities beyond the regular microbiology exams, namely in results report, surveillance, communication, and other daily routine tasks of Infection Control Teams (Kalenić and Budimir, 2009).

In this paper, we describe the multiple chores of the Microbiology Laboratory highlighting its importance in HAIs prevention and control, and in ASPs, especially when combined with properly designed information systems. We also review some of the problems that the Microbiology Laboratory has to deal with when assisting Infection Control Teams, including the selection of the most appropriate analytic methods to provide fast and accurate results.

TASKS OF THE MICROBIOLOGY LABORATORY

Microbial Isolation and Identification

The Microbiology Laboratory main task is to isolate and identify the infection etiological agent (Benbachir, 2008), using the most appropriate, rapid and accurate diagnostic method. To ensure this, the Microbiology Laboratory needs to keep up-to-date materials, culture media, reagents, equipment, identification methods and trained personnel (CDC, 2003). The staff needs continuous on-the-job training in microbiological techniques and to be updated on the internationally endorsed methods for isolation and characterization of pathogens (Pfaller and Herwaldt, 1997; Benbachir, 2008). In addition, external and internal quality control and assurance programs must be implemented to guarantee the quality of the results (Benbachir, 2008).

Determination of Antimicrobial Susceptibility Patterns

The Microbiology Laboratory should provide frequently updated information on antimicrobial resistance patterns, essential to design appropriate hospital prescription guidelines, help clinicians to choose the most appropriate empiric therapy and to create a culture of patient safety (Pfaller and Herwaldt, 1997; Benbachir, 2008). This data can be analyzed in different perspectives, including infectious agent, specimen, ward, clinical specialty, antibiotics prescribed, or anatomic site of infection, among others (Pfaller and Herwaldt, 1997; Benbachir, 2008).

The availability of periodic reports on local antimicrobial resistance patterns is also relevant in ASPs, since it can be used to evaluate trends of antimicrobial resistance rates, to educate clinicians on optimal antimicrobial use and to assess the impact of prevention measures (Diekema and Saubolle, 2011).

Report of the Results

The laboratory work is completed only when it is effectively reported (Newton and Novak-Weekley, 2011). All laboratory results (preliminary and final) should be reported as soon as possible to clinicians and Infection Control Teams (Kalenić and Budimir, 2009). Daily reports on significant microbiology results and periodic reports with frequency of isolated pathogens and prevalence of resistant microorganisms provide clinicians and Infection Control Teams with accurate and timely information, essential to follow trends of hospital infections and control urgent situations (Pfaller and Herwaldt, 1997; Benbachir, 2008).

These reports can be delivered through meetings, phone, information systems alerts, paper, or e-mail. However, making results accessible through an information system is an advantage by ensuring that all results are available in an organized, easily accessible, and timely manner, and also permits links to other surveillance data systems (Cantón, 2005). Information systems that incorporate information about the patient, disease, infectious agent and antimicrobial susceptibility are fundamental because they promote timely exchange of information between healthcare workers (Schreckenberger and Binnicker, 2011). For instance, ARTEMIS (Teodoro et al., 2012) and HAITool[2] (Pinto et al., 2016) are good examples of this kind of systems. They analyze heterogeneous data sources and can be used to build antimicrobial resistance surveillance networks participating in the management and prevention of antibiotic resistant HAIs, and by doing so, optimizing human and economic resources[2] (Teodoro et al., 2012). Some of these systems alert the clinician (or the pharmacist) when laboratory results reveal that the antibiotic(s) in use may not be optimal or when de-escalation treatment is indicated (Schreckenberger and Binnicker, 2011; Pinto et al., 2016). The "processed information" generated by these systems are very useful for surveillance purposes and in supporting and leveraging ASPs (Davey et al., 2013).

[2]http://haitool.ihmt.unl.pt/

Surveillance and Outbreak Detection

Surveillance enables the identification of infected patients, the origin of HAIs and to understand their paths of spread. Since most of this data comes from microbiological isolates and other laboratory identification tests (Emori and Gaynes, 1993; Peterson and Brossette, 2002), the Microbiology Laboratory has a central role not only on the surveillance and early detection of outbreaks but also on monitoring and reporting unusual laboratory results (e.g., clusters of pathogens, emergence of multidrug-resistant organisms, isolation of unusual pathogens).

To detect outbreaks early enough to mitigate their impact on morbidity and mortality is one of the major challenges of an efficient surveillance program (Diekema and Saubolle, 2011). The Microbiology Laboratory, in association with the Infections Control Team, is the first to detect an outbreak because unusual clusters of pathogens or resistance patterns are easily noticed (Arias, 2010). During an outbreak, these two entities have to work side by side to: (i) provide information on the epidemiology of the etiologic agent; (ii) identify and store the isolates involved for further testing; (iii) define/select appropriate selective isolation media and drug susceptibility testing (if needed/when applicable); (iv) perform the appropriate tests for strain typing (or provide its dispatch to a reference laboratory); (v) and perform supplemental microbiological surveillance of patients, personnel, or environmental sources of infection (Emori and Gaynes, 1993; Pfaller and Herwaldt, 1997; Arias, 2010).

As described above, the use of surveillance systems can enhance surveillance programs by aggregating all the information related with patient, disease, infectious agent and antimicrobial susceptibility, making easier outbreaks detection.

Education

To maximize the efficacy of Infection Control programs, the Microbiology Laboratory should provide training and information on basic microbiology and biosafety for healthcare workers in areas such as: specimen collection, handling and transport, epidemiologically important pathogens vs. normal flora, colonization vs. infection, interpretation of microbiological results (Kalenić and Budimir, 2009). Written guidelines about sampling, handling and transport should be available in every ward, which can also include details on the tests available for proper isolation, identification, and typing of microorganisms (Grosek, 1999).

ANTIBIOTIC STEWARDSHIP PROGRAMS

Antibiotic Stewardship Programss should be included in all HAIs prevention and control programs and are essential for gathering information about epidemiological and molecular markers of resistance, and changes in resistance patterns. They not only contribute to the optimization of antimicrobial therapy, by ensuring proper use (indication, dose, route of administration, and duration) and minimizing side effects, but also promote education on it (Davey et al., 2013). The adoption of these programs leads to a reduction in the prevalence of antimicrobial resistance and costs (Malani et al., 2012). These programs have been implemented throughout the world and there are guidelines and recommendations for their use in the USA (CDC, 2014; Fridkin et al., 2014) and Europe (Pina, 2002; Department of Health Advisory Committee on Antimicrobial Resistance and Healthcare Associated Infection, 2011; Lower et al., 2013; Simões et al., 2015).

Also here, computerized surveillance and decision support systems are a good support for ASPs, since have proven to be effective in the prescription errors reduction, medical care improvement and compliance with recommendations (Evans et al., 1998; Pestotnik, 2005).

A schematic representation of the network of interactions in ASPs is shown in **Figure 1**. The laboratory imparts an important function in ASPs, generating most of the relevant information needed to characterize the biology of the pathogen (and the hosts), namely its identification, antimicrobial susceptibility patterns and epidemiological connections. Therefore, it is recommended that all ASPs include a microbiologist (CDC, 2014). A good example of the role of Microbiology Laboratory in ASPs is described by MacKenzie et al. (2007) who demonstrated that hospitals with routine reports on antimicrobial susceptibility patterns for restricted antibiotics had lower usage (and misusage) of these antibiotics.

ISSUES ON THE LABORATORY EFFICACY

Sample's Quality and Access to Clinical Data

The quality of the laboratory diagnosis is closely related with the quality of the collected samples (Benbachir, 2008). Samples should be taken on the correct time and from appropriate sites, using proper techniques and in amounts that makes possible to perform all the tests necessary for the isolation and identification (and other testing) of the pathogen (Department of Health Advisory Committee on Antimicrobial Resistance and Healthcare Associated Infection, 2011). Samples that are not properly collected and transported may lead to false results (Benbachir, 2008).

Relevant epidemiological and clinical information data are also important for accurate laboratory diagnosis. Every request for exam should include: name of the patient, name of the clinician in charge, location of the patient, date and time of specimen collection, short anamnesis including suspected diagnosis and underlying patient conditions and comorbidities (Benbachir, 2008; Kalenić and Budimir, 2009). The access to this pre-analytic data facilitates significantly the guidance toward pathogen detection and identification. These kind of information should be easily accessed throughout an information system.

Isolation in Culture or Molecular Identification Methods, Which One to Choose?

The use of laboratory culture methods for isolation of pathogens followed by identification procedures (biochemical, molecular, serologic, or other) has been the gold standard in Medical

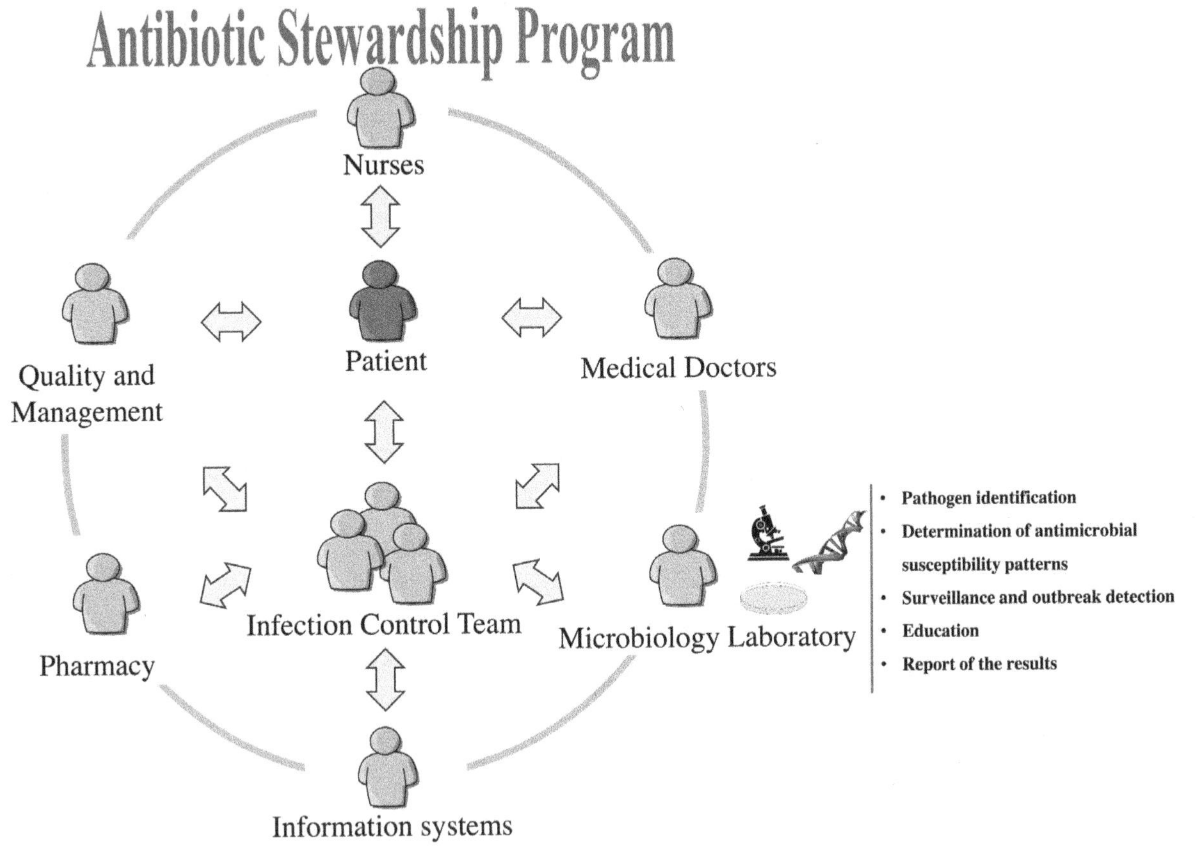

FIGURE 1 | Network of interactions in an Antibiotic Stewardship Program.

Microbiology and continues to play a vital role in the overall management of infectious diseases. As an example, blood culture is still mandatory for isolation and identification of blood pathogens and guiding therapy (Book et al., 2013). However, isolation in culture has limitations, namely being time consuming (Singh et al., 2006). Results provided 48 to 72 h after the onset of the infection often have limited impact on therapy (Tenover, 2010) and the ability of the laboratory to provide results in a timely manner is essential.

Conversely, the major benefit of direct molecular methods is related to time saving. Using Polymerase Chain Reaction (PCR) based methods, results can be obtained within 6 to 8 h, reducing greatly the time-to-result and implementation of appropriate therapy (Book et al., 2013). Molecular methods have been described as a powerful tool against the spread of microorganisms in hospital environment, in particular during outbreaks (Singh et al., 2006), and many have been used to rapidly identify microorganisms (e.g., multiplex PCR, Real-time PCR, MALDI-TOF MS), to find resistance patterns (e.g., PCR/hybridization screening of resistance determinants) and to estimate epidemiological links between bacteria (e.g., pulsed-field gel electrophoresis, multi-locus sequence typing), enabling rapid and appropriate therapeutic responses (Cantón, 2005; Simões et al., 2011; Sabat et al., 2013; Patel, 2015; Srinivasan et al., 2015). More recently whole-genome sequencing (WGS) promises to transform Infection Control. WGS provides almost all the genetic information needed for epidemiological studies (Köser et al., 2012) and has been widely used to identify and control outbreaks of antibiotic resistant HAIs (Reuter et al., 2013; Price et al., 2013). WGS can be used to quickly identify pathogenic agents from specimens and unravel many genomic single nucleotide polymorphisms and markers for drug resistance, allowing the implementation of immediate and appropriate control measures (Coll et al., 2014). However, the translation of the large amount of data generated by WGS to the clinical utility is still under development (Burke and Korngiebel, 2015).

Molecular methods have been associated with global cost reduction, due to their high specificity, sensitivity and rapid turnaround (Cantón, 2005; Tenover, 2010; Currie, 2011). Combining molecular typing with surveillance programs was shown to be cost effective and result in significant reduction of HAIs rates (Hacek et al., 1999). More recently, the integration of rapid identifications methods with stewardship interventions has been described as a way to improve time to optimal antibiotic therapy, decrease length of hospital stay and reduce mortality and healthcare costs (Huang et al., 2013; Bauer et al., 2014; Perez et al., 2014).

However, molecular methods do not solve all the problems. Several authors have described drawbacks associated with molecular methods: limited number of detectable pathogens, possibility of false positives and complex sample preparation procedures (Laxminarayan et al., 2013). In addition, molecular methods are more expensive, require specialized equipment, and training (Morshed et al., 2007) and their value in diagnosis of some infections has not been fully proven. For instance, in a recent study testing the accuracy of Septi*Fast* multi-pathogens real-time PCR, authors concluded that, despite providing faster results, this method has limited utility in bloodstream infections, when compared with conventional blood culture (Warhurst et al., 2015). Additionally, there are several microorganisms for which isolation by culture methods is the most effective and recommend procedure especially when dealing with drug-resistant inducible geno/phenotypes.

The dispute on isolation in culture followed by identification versus direct identification from specimen by molecular methods seems endless and unnecessary since both methods can be used in concert. Several authors suggested a combination of culture and molecular methods in order to increase the rate, efficacy and accuracy of pathogen detection. (Dolinger and Jacobs, 2011; Brown-Elliott and Wallace, 2012; Huttunen et al., 2013). **Table 1** summarizes some pros and cons of both strategies.

Antimicrobial Resistance Surveillance

With the emergence and spread of antimicrobial resistant pathogens, antimicrobial resistance surveillance is becoming an important task of the Microbiology Laboratory. Antimicrobial resistance surveillance is an ongoing (and organized) data collection that after being analyzed and reported provides useful information for empirical antimicrobial therapy (Cornaglia et al., 2004).

Nevertheless, a good surveillance program is time consuming and involve dedicated human resources. In addition there are several challenges on data collection, management, analysis, interpretation and reporting. For instance, promoting the use of new and low-cost technologies to improve laboratory work and to prioritize which bacteria are most important to track are issues that should be addressed (Solomon and Ijaz, 2015). Regarding interpretation, uniformization is needed: currently, different guidelines and breakpoints for evaluation of antimicrobials susceptibility patterns values are adopted in the United States of America and within several European countries (Vernet et al., 2014). Finally, the results should be presented in formats easily understandable by the clinicians (Grundmann et al., 2011).

Information systems are a good way to keep-it working smoothly (Lapão, 2007). As stated above, surveillance information systems ensure that antimicrobial resistance related data are available and organized, making easy to report it retrospectively. In addition, surveillance information systems allow better antibiotic resistance management and help to provide evidence based results that can be used for the development of control policies (Evans et al., 1998; Pestotnik, 2005).

Communication

Effective communication is critical for the Microbiology Laboratory procedures. Nevertheless, it can also be one of its major issues. Effective communication is the base of a healthy collaboration between laboratory, healthcare workers and Infection Control Teams (Kalenić and Budimir, 2009). The dialog between healthcare workers and laboratory staff must be easy and effective (Peterson et al., 2001). The existence of a dedicated laboratory staff element (privileged interlocutor) and the participation of microbiologists in regular clinician's meetings is recommended. Efficient communication between clinicians and microbiologists about the presumptive diagnosis, accelerates the diagnosis and avoids problems with inappropriate specimens (Baron et al., 2013).

In order to facilitate communication, it is recommended that the director of the Microbiology Laboratory be a clinician or a laboratory scientist with expertise in infectious diseases and

TABLE 1 | Comparison of culture and molecular identification methods.

	Culture methods	Molecular methods
Specificity	Moderate	High
Sensitivity	Low	High
Antimicrobial susceptibility	Isolates can be tested for susceptibility to relevant antibiotics	Allows the detection of some resistance markers without isolation/culturing
Amount needed to detected pathogens	High	Low
Time to obtain results	Long (especially for slow-growers organisms)	Short
Cost	Low	High (variable)
Detection of non-viable bacteria (patient in antibiotic treatment)	No	Yes
Equipment	Requires non-specialized equipment	Requires specialized equipment
Biosafety	Potential biosafety concerns	Minimizes biosafety concerns
Feasibility	Requires basic training No specialized workflow required	Requires advanced training Assays may not be commercially available
Others	Allows visual inspection of colony morphology Allows biochemical characterization of phenotype Limited potential for false positives and/or false negatives	Allows high resolution analysis Potential false positives (by cross-reaction with closely related species or contaminated amplicons) Potential false negatives (by inhibition components or target mutations)

Adapted from (Dolinger and Jacobs, 2011).

microbiology (Thomson et al., 2010) since their background on disease pathologic process facilitates the discussion of clinical cases. Additionally, information systems have an important role in communication within the hospitals by facilitating the exchange of clinical and microbiological relevant data between clinicians and laboratories (Lapão, 2007). However, it is important that information systems are defined and designed together with the healthcare workers in order to really improve communication, data quality, be useful on decision-making and be easy to use (Pinto et al., 2016).

Another reality that can affect the communication is the location of the Microbiology Laboratory. There are an increasing number of off-site laboratories providing services to hospitals and in the cases of in-house laboratories, they usually are in the basement or in an annex outside the hospital main building. It has been described that off-site laboratories delay and decrease communication, could jeopardizes infection diagnosis and treatment and weaken infection prevention and antibiotic stewardship infrastructures (Peterson et al., 2001; Dancer et al., 2015).

CONCLUSION

The Microbiology Laboratory plays a key role in HAIs prevention and control. From ensuring appropriate specimen collection and transport, to the wise selection of isolation and identification methods and finally on the antibiotic therapy guidance plus effective report and communication of the results, the laboratory covers all important aspects of infection control process. The microbiologist is a fundamental and enriching member of ASPs and Infection Control Teams. The new identifications methods (including WGS) combined with the emergence of innovative and centralized information systems that integrate the microbiology results with clinical data will revolutionize HAIs prevention and control strategies, help decision-making and resolve some of the difficulties felt by the microbiologists.

AUTHOR CONTRIBUTIONS

ASS, IC, CT, EG, PP, MV, and LVL contributed to the draft and revision of the paper and approved the final version to be published.

REFERENCES

Arias, K. M. (2010). "The role of the laboratory in outbreak detection, prevention and investigation," in *Outbreak Investigation, Prevention, and Control in Health Care Settings, Critical Issues in Patient Safety*, 2nd Edn, ed. K. M. Arias (Burlington, MA: Jones & Bartlett Learning).

Baron, E. J., Miller, J. M., Weinstein, M. P., Richter, S. S., Gilligan, P. H., Thomson, R. B., et al. (2013). A guide to utilization of the microbiology laboratory for diagnosis of infectious diseases: 2013 recommendations by the infectious diseases society of america (IDSA) and the american society for microbiology (ASM). *Clin. Infect. Dis.* 57:e22–e121. doi: 10.1093/cid/cit278

Bauer, K. A., Perez, K. K., Forrest, G. N., and Goff, D. A. (2014). Review of rapid diagnostic tests used by antimicrobial stewardship programs. *Clin. Infect. Dis.* 59(Suppl. 3), S134–S145. doi: 10.1093/cid/ciu547

Benbachir, M. (2008). "Role of the microbiology laboratory in infection control," in *Guide to Infection Control in Hospitals*, IV Edn, eds R. Wenzel, G. Bearman, T. Brewer, and J.-P. Butzler (Boston: International Society for Infectious Diseases).

Book, M., Lehmann, L. E., Zhang, X. H., and Stüber, F. (2013). Monitoring infection: from blood culture to polymerase chain reaction (PCR). Best Practice & Research. *Clin. Anaesthesiol.* 27, 279–288. doi: 10.1016/j.bpa.2013.06.010

Brown-Elliott, B. A., and Wallace, R. J. (2012). Enhancement of conventional phenotypic methods with molecular-based methods for the more definitive identification of nontuberculous *Mycobacteria*. *Clin. Microbiol. Newslett.* 34, 109–115. doi: 10.1016/j.clinmicnews.2012.06.004

Burke, W., and Korngiebel, D. M. (2015). Closing the gap between knowledge and clinical application: challenges for genomic translation. Edited by Mildred Cho. *PLoS Genet.* 11:e1004978. doi: 10.1371/journal.pgen.1004978

Cantón, R. (2005). Role of the microbiology laboratory in infectious disease surveillance, alert and response. *Clin. Microbiol. Infect.* 11(Suppl. 1), 3–8. doi: 10.1111/j.1469-0691.2005.01081.x

CDC (2003). *Manual for the Laboratory Identification and Antimicrobial Susceptibility Testing of Bacterial Pathogens of Public Health Importance in the Developing World*. Geneva: World Health Organization.

CDC (2013). *Antibiotic Resistance Threats in the United States*, 2013 Edn. Atlanta, GA: Centers for Disease Control.

CDC (2014). *Core Elements of Hospital Antibiotic Stewardship Programs*. Atlanta, GA: Centers for Disease Control. Available at: http://www.cdc.gov/getsmart/healthcare/implementation/core-elements.html

Coll, F., McNerney, R., Guerra-Assunção, J. A., Glynn, J. R., Perdigão, J., Viveiros, M., et al. (2014). A Robust SNP barcode for typing *Mycobacterium tuberculosis* complex strains. *Nat. Commun.* 5:4812. doi: 10.1038/ncomms 5812

Cornaglia, G., Hryniewicz, W., Jarlier, V., Kahlmeter, G., Mittermayer, H., Stratchounski, L., et al. (2004). European recommendations for antimicrobial resistance surveillance. *Clin. Microbiol. Infect.* 10, 349–383. doi: 10.1111/j.1198-743X.2004.00887.x

Cosgrove, S. E. (2006). The relationship between antimicrobial resistance and patient outcomes: mortality, length of hospital stay, and health care costs. *Clin. Infect. Dis.* 42(Suppl. 2), S82–S89. doi: 10.1086/499406

Currie, B. (2011). Impact of molecular diagnostics on infection control. *Infect. Dis. Special Ed.* 9, 11–15.

Dancer, S. J., Varon-Lopez, C., Moncayo, O., Elston, A., and Humphreys, H. (2015). Microbiology service centralization: a step too far. *J. Hosp. Infect.* 91, 292–298. doi: 10.1016/j.jhin.2015.08.017

Davey, P., Brown, E., Charani, E., Fenelon, L. I, Gould, M., Holmes, A., et al. (2013). Interventions to improve antibiotic prescribing practices for hospital inpatients. *Cochrane Database Syst. Rev.* 4:CD003543. doi: 10.1002/14651858.CD003543.pub3

Department of Health Advisory Committee on Antimicrobial Resistance and Healthcare Associated Infection (ARHAI) (2011). *Antimicrobial Stewardship: "Start Smart–Then Focus": Guidance for Antimicrobial Stewardship in Hospitals*. London: Public Health England.

Diekema, D. J., and Saubolle, M. A. (2011). Clinical microbiology and infection prevention. *J. Clin. Microbiol.* 49, S57–S60. doi: 10.1128/JCM. 00690-11

Dolinger, D. L., and Jacobs, A. A. (2011). "Molecular diagnostics and active screening for health care-associated infections: stepping-up the game," in *Laboratory Medicine* ed. R. L. Bertholf (Oxford: Oxford University Press).

ECDC (2009). *The Bacterial Challenge?: Time to React*. Stockholm: European Centre for Disease Prevention and Control.

Emori, T. G., and Gaynes, R. P. (1993). An overview of nosocomial infections, including the role of the microbiology laboratory. *Clin. Microbiol. Rev.* 6, 428–442. doi: 10.1128/CMR.6.4.428

Evans, R. S., Pestotnik, S. L., Classen, D. C., Clemmer, T. P., Weaver, L. K., Orme, J. F., et al. (1998). A computer-assisted management program for antibiotics and other antiinfective agents. *New Engl. J. Med.* 338, 232–238. doi: 10.1056/NEJM199801223380406

Fridkin, S., Baggs, J., Fagan, R., Magill, S., Pollack, L. A., Malpiedi, P., et al. (2014). Vital signs: improving antibiotic use among hospitalized patients. *Morb Mortal Wkly Rep.* 63, 194–200.

Grosek, S. (1999). What does a clinician expect from a microbiologist? Towards an effective joint policy. *J. Hosp. Infect.* 43. (Suppl.), S293–S296. doi: 10.1016/S0195-6701(99)90102-0

Grundmann, H., Klugman, K. P., Walsh, T., Ramon-Pardo, P., Sigauque, B., Khan, W., et al. (2011). A framework for global surveillance of antibiotic resistance. *Drug Resist. Updat.* 14, 79–87. doi: 10.1016/j.drup.2011.02.007

Hacek, D. M., Suriano, T., Noskin, G. A., Kruszynski, J., Reisberg, B., and Peterson, L. R. (1999). Medical and economic benefit of a comprehensive infection control program that includes routine determination of microbial clonality. *Am. J. Clin. Pathol.* 111, 647–654. doi: 10.1093/ajcp/111.5.647

Huang, A. M., Newton, D., Kunapuli, A., Gandhi, T. N., Washer, L. L., Isip, J., et al. (2013). Impact of rapid organism identification via matrix-assisted laser desorption/ionization time-of-flight combined with antimicrobial stewardship team intervention in adult patients with bacteremia and candidemia. *Clin. Infect. Dis.* 57, 1237–1245. doi: 10.1093/cid/cit498

Huttunen, R., Syrjänen, J., Vuento, R., and Aittoniemi, J. (2013). Current concepts in the diagnosis of blood stream infections. are novel molecular methods useful in clinical practice? *Int. J. Infect. Dis.* 17, e934–e938. doi: 10.1016/j.ijid.2013.04.018

Kalenić, S., and Budimir, A. (2009). The role of the microbiology laboratory in healthcare-associated infection prevention. *Int. J. Infect. Control* 60, (Suppl.), S57–S60. doi: 10.3396/ijic.V5i2.014.09

Kolmos, H. J. (1999). Interaction between the microbiology laboratory and clinician: what the microbiologist can provide. *J. Hosp. Infect.* 43(Suppl. 1), doi: 10.1016/S0195-6701(99)90101-9

Köser, C. U., Ellington, M. J., Cartwright, E. J., Gillespie, S. H., Brown, N. M., Farrington, M., et al. (2012). Routine use of microbial whole genome sequencing in diagnostic and public health microbiology. *PLoS Pathog.* 8:e1002824. doi: 10.1371/journal.ppat.1002824

Lapão, L. V. (2007). Survey on the status of the hospital information systems in portugal. *Methods Informat. Med.* 46, 493–499. doi: 10.1160/ME9055

Laxminarayan, R., Duse, A., Wattal, C., Zaidi, A. K. M., Wertheim, H. F. L., Sumpradit, N., et al. (2013). Antibiotic resistance—the need for global solutions. *Lancet Infect. Dis.* 13, 1057–1098. doi: 10.1016/S1473-3099(13)70318-9

Lower, H. L., Eriksen, H. M., Aavitsland, P., and Skjeldestad, F. E. (2013). Methodology of the norwegian surveillance system for healthcare-associated infections: the value of a mandatory system, automated data collection, and active postdischarge surveillance. *Am. J. Infect. Control* 41, 591–596. doi: 10.1016/j.ajic.2012.09.005

MacKenzie, F. M. I., Gould, M., Bruce, J., Mollison, J., Monnet, D. L., Krcmery, V., et al. (2007). The role of microbiology and pharmacy departments in the stewardship of antibiotic prescribing in european hospitals. *J. Hosp. Infect.* 65, 73–81. doi: 10.1016/S0195-6701(07)60019-X

Magill, S. S., Edwards, J. R., Bamberg, W., Beldavs, Z. G., Dumyati, G., Kainer, M. A., et al. (2014). Multistate point-prevalence survey of health care-associated infections. *New Engl. J. Med.* 370, 1198–1208. doi: 10.1056/NEJMoa1306801

Malani, A. N., Richards, P. G., Kapila, S., Otto, M. H., Czerwinski, J., and Singal, B. (2012). Clinical and economic outcomes from a community hospital's antimicrobial stewardship program. *Am. J. Infect. Control* 41, 145–148. doi: 10.1016/j.ajic.2012.02.021

Morshed, M. G., Lee, M., Jorgensen, D., and Isaac-Renton, J. L. (2007). Molecular methods used in clinical laboratory: prospects and pitfalls. *FEMS Immunol. Med. Microbiol.* 49, 184–191. doi: 10.1111/j.1574-695X.2006.00191.x

Neidell, M. J., Cohen, B., Furuya, Y., Hill, J., Jeon, C. Y., Glied, S., et al. (2012). Costs of healthcare- and community-associated infections with antimicrobial-resistant versus antimicrobial-susceptible organisms. *Clin. Infect. Dis.* 55, 807–815. doi: 10.1093/cid/cis552

Newton, D. W., and Novak-Weekley, S. (2011). Enhancing the function of clinical microbiology laboratories: can we navigate the road less traveled? *J. Clin. Microbiol.* 49 9(Suppl.), S72–S76. doi: 10.1128/JCM.00691-11

Patel, R. (2015). MALDI-TOF MS for the diagnosis of infectious diseases. *Clin. Chem.* 61, 100–111. doi: 10.1373/clinchem.2014.221770

Perez, K. K., Olsen, R. J., Musick, W. L., Cernoch, P. L., Davis, J. R., Peterson, L. E., et al. (2014). Integrating rapid diagnostics and antimicrobial stewardship improves outcomes in patients with antibiotic-resistant gram-negative bacteremia. *J. Infect.* 69, 216–225. doi: 10.1016/j.jinf.2014.05.005

Pestotnik, S. L. (2005). Expert clinical decision support systems to enhance antimicrobial stewardship programs: insights from the society of infectious diseases pharmacists. *Pharmacotherapy* 25, 1116–1125. doi: 10.1592/phco.2005.25.8.1116

Peterson, L. R., and Brossette, S. E. (2002). Hunting health care-associated infections from the clinical microbiology laboratory: passive, active, and virtual surveillance. *J. Clin. Microbiol.* 40, 1–4. doi: 10.1128/JCM.40.1.1-4.2002

Peterson, L. R., Hamilton, J. D., Baron, E. J., Tompkins, L. S., Miller, J. M., Wilfert, C. M., et al. (2001). Role of clinical microbiology laboratories in the management and control of infectious diseases and the delivery of Health Care. *Clin. Infect. Dis.* 32, 605–611. doi: 10.1086/318725

Pfaller, M. A., and Herwaldt, L. A. (1997). The clinical microbiology laboratory and infection control: emerging pathogens, antimicrobial resistance, and new technology. *Clin. Infect. Dis.* 25, 858–870. doi: 10.1086/515557

Pina, E. (2002). *Prevenção de Infecções Adquiridas No Hospital - Um Guia Prático*, 2ª Edição. Lisboa: Instituto Nacional de Saúde Dr. Ricardo Jorge.

Pinto, P., Gil, M., Simões, A. S., da Silva, M. M., and Lapão, L. V. (2016). "Using design science research methodology to implement a surveillance and decision-support information system to manage healthcare associated infections and antibiotic use in hospitals," in *Conference Proceedings of European, Mediterranean & Middle Eastern Conference on Information Systems*, Krakow.

Price, J., Gordon, N. C., Crook, D., Llewelyn, M., and Paul, J. (2013). The usefulness of whole genome sequencing in the management of *Staphylococcus aureus* infections. *Clin. Microbiol. Infect.* 19, 784–789. doi: 10.1111/1469-0691.12109

Reuter, S., Harrison, T. G., Koser, C. U., Ellington, M. J., Smith, G. P., Parkhill, J., et al. (2013). A pilot study of rapid whole-genome sequencing for the investigation of a legionella outbreak. *BMJ Open* 3:e002175. doi: 10.1136/bmjopen-2012-002175

Sabat, A. J., Budimir, A., Nashev, D., Sá-Leão, R., van Dijl, J. M., Laurent, F., et al. (2013). Overview of molecular typing methods for outbreak detection and epidemiological surveillance. *Euro Surveill* 18:20380.

Schreckenberger, P. C., and Binnicker, M. J. (2011). Optimizing antimicrobial susceptibility test reporting. *J. Clin. Microbiol.* 49(Suppl.), S15–S19. doi: 10.1128/JCM.00712-11

Simões, A. S., Valente, C., de Lencastre, H., and Sá-Leão, R. (2011). Rapid Identification of Noncapsulated *Streptococcus pneumoniae* in nasopharyngeal samples allowing detection of co-colonization and reevaluation of prevalence. *Diagn. Microbiol. Infect. Dis.* 71, 208–216. doi: 10.1016/j.diagmicrobio.2011.07.009

Simões, A. S., Gregório, J., Póvoa, P., and Lapão, L V. (2015). *Practical Guide for the Implementation of Antibiotic Stewardship Programs.* Lisboa: Instituto de Higiene e Medicina Tropical.

Singh, A., Goering, R. V., Simjee, S., Foley, S. L., and Zervos, M. J. (2006). Application of molecular techniques to the study of hospital infection. *Clin. Microbiol. Rev.* 19, 512–530. doi: 10.1128/CMR.00025-05

Solomon, S., and Ijaz, K. (2015). *Surveillance and Monitoring of Antimicrobial Resistance (AMR).* Geneva: World Health Organization.

Srinivasan, R., Karaoz, U., Volegova, M., MacKichan, J., Kato-Maeda, M., Miller, S., et al. (2015). Use of 16S rRNA gene for identification of a broad range of clinically relevant bacterial pathogens. *PLoS ONE* 10:e0117617. doi: 10.1371/journal.pone.0117617

Tenover, F. C. (2010). Potential impact of rapid diagnostic tests on improving antimicrobial use. *Ann. N. Y. Acad. Sci.* 1213, 70–80. doi: 10.1111/j.1749-6632.2010.05827.x

Teodoro, D., Pasche, E., Gobeill, J., Emonet, S., Ruch, P., and Lovis, C. (2012). Building a transnational biosurveillance network using semantic web technologies: requirements, design, and preliminary evaluation. *J. Med. Internet. Res.* 14:e73. doi: 10.2196/jmir.2043

Thomson, R. B., Wilson, M. L., and Weinstein, M. P. (2010). The clinical microbiology laboratory director in the united states hospital setting. *J. Clin. Microbiol.* 48, 3465–3469. doi: 10.1128/JCM.01575-10

Vernet, G., Mary, C., Altmann, D. M., Doumbo, O., Morpeth, S., Bhutta, Z. A., et al. (2014). Surveillance for antimicrobial drug resistance in under-resourced countries. *Emerg. Infect. Dis.* 20, 434–441. doi: 10.3201/EID2003.121157

Warhurst, G., Maddi, S., Dunn, G., Ghrew, M., Chadwick, P., Alexander, P., et al. (2015). Diagnostic accuracy of septifast multi-pathogen real-time pcr in the setting of suspected healthcare-associated bloodstream infection. *Intensive Care Med.* 41, 86–93. doi: 10.1007/s00134-014-3551-x

Wilson, M. P., and Spencer, R. C. (1999). Laboratory role in the management of hospital acquired infections. *J. Hosp. Infect.* 42, 1–6. doi: 10.1053/jhin.1998.0545

Zimlichman, E., Henderson, D., Tamir, O., Franz, C., Song, P., Yamin, C. K., et al. (2013). Health care–associated infections a meta-analysis of costs and financial impact on the us health care system. *JAMA Int. Med.* 173:2039. doi: 10.1001/jamainternmed.2013.9763

17

Hospital Effluents are One of Several Sources of Metal, Antibiotic Resistance Genes and Bacterial Markers Disseminated in Sub-Saharan Urban Rivers

*Amandine Laffite [1], Pitchouna I. Kilunga [2], John M. Kayembe [3], Naresh Devarajan [1], Crispin K. Mulaji [2], Gregory Giuliani [1,4,5], Vera I. Slaveykova [1] and John Poté [1,2,3]**

[1] Faculty of Science, Earth and Environmental Science Section, F.-A. Forel Institute and Institute of Environmental Sciences, University of Geneva, Geneva, Switzerland, [2] Department of Chemistry, Faculty of Science, University of Kinshasa, Kinshasa, Democratic Republic of the Congo, [3] Département de Géographie-Science de l'Environnement, Faculté des Sciences, Université Pédagogique Nationale, Kinshasa, Democratic Republic of the Congo, [4] enviroSPACE Lab., Institute for Environmental Sciences, University of Geneva, Geneva, Switzerland, [5] United Nations Environment Programme, Division of Early Warning and Assessment, Global Resource Information Database – Geneva, International Environment House, Geneva, Switzerland

***Correspondence:**
John Poté
john.pote@unige.ch

Data concerning the occurrence of emerging biological contaminants such as antibiotic resistance genes (ARGs) and fecal indicator bacteria (FIB) in aquatic environments in Sub-Saharan African countries is limited. On the other hand, antibiotic resistance remains a worldwide problem which may pose serious potential risks to human and animal health. Consequently, there is a growing number of reports concerning the prevalence and dissemination of these contaminants into various environmental compartments. Sediments provide the opportunity to reconstruct the pollution history and evaluate impacts so this study investigates the abundance and distribution of toxic metals, FIB, and ARGs released from hospital effluent wastewaters and their presence in river sediments receiving systems. ARGs (bla_{TEM}, $bla_{\mathrm{CTX\text{-}M}}$, bla_{SHV}, and *aadA*), total bacterial load, and selected bacterial species FIB [*Escherichia coli*, *Enterococcus* (ENT)] and species (Psd) were quantified by targeting species specific genes using quantitative PCR (qPCR) in total DNA extracted from the sediments recovered from 4 hospital outlet pipes (HOP) and their river receiving systems in the City of Kinshasa in the Democratic Republic of the Congo. The results highlight the great concentration of toxic metals in HOP, reaching the values (in mg kg^{-1}) of 47.9 (Cr), 213.6 (Cu), 1434.4 (Zn), 2.6 (Cd), 281.5 (Pb), and 13.6 (Hg). The results also highlight the highest ($P < 0.05$) values of 16S rRNA, FIB, and ARGs copy numbers in all sampling sites including upstream (control site), discharge point, and downstream of receiving rivers, indicating that the hospital effluent water is not an exclusive source of the biological contaminants entering the urban rivers. Significant correlation were observed between (i) all analyzed ARGs and total bacterial load (16S rRNA) 0.51 to 0.72 ($p < 0.001$, $n = 65$); (ii) ARGs (except bla_{TEM}) and FIB and Psd $0.57 < r < 0.82$ ($p < 0.001$, $n = 65$); and (iii) ARGs (except

bla_{TEM}) and toxic metals (Cd, Cr, Cu, and Zn) 0.44 to 0.72, ($p < 0.001$, $n = 65$). These findings demonstrate that several sources including hospital and urban wastewaters contribute to the spread of toxic metals and biological emerging contaminants in aquatic ecosystems.

Keywords: hospital and urban wastewater, water pollution, sediment receiving system, toxic metals, antibiotic resistance genes, fecal indicator bacteria, Sub-Saharan Africa, tropical conditions

INTRODUCTION

Contamination of freshwater resources with anthropogenic pollutants is a growing concern of interest because safe and readily available water is needed for drinking, domestic use, food production, and recreational purposes (WHO, 2015). Freshwater resource pollution by various contaminants including toxic metals, persistent organic pollutants, pathogenic organisms, antibiotic resistant bacteria (ARB), and antibiotic resistant genes (ARGs) is still a major problem in many parts of the world (Poté et al., 2008; Knapp et al., 2012; Bréchet et al., 2014; Czekalski et al., 2014; Devarajan et al., 2015b). The situation is particularly alarming in developing regions such as in Sub-Saharan Africa where most rivers, lakes, and lagoons are receiving untreated hospital and industrial effluent water, mining effluents, and urban storm water runoff affected by anthropogenic pollutants due to intensive and uncontrolled urbanization (Feng et al., 2004; Chatterjee et al., 2007; Gnandi et al., 2011; Atibu et al., 2013; Mwanamoki et al., 2014, 2015).

Hospital effluents are a particular case of anthropogenic pollutants. Indeed, hospital wastewaters are complex mixtures of chemical and biological substances which are continually discharged (Barcelo and Barceló, 2003; Boillot et al., 2008; Verlicchi et al., 2010). This mixture is the result of diagnostic laboratory and research activity waste and medicine excretion which include active principles from medicinal products and their metabolites, chemicals, disinfecting agents, specific detergents, radioactive markers, iodinated contrast media, nutrients, and bacteria and their antimicrobial resistance genes (Verlicchi et al., 2010). Particularly studied among these hospital contaminants are bacteria and their antimicrobial resistance genes because of their great ability to disseminate and their clinical and financial impact (Davies et al., 1995; Cosgrove, 2006). The remarkable effectiveness of antibiotics has reduced mortality linked to bacterial diseases in only a few decades but their over- and mis-use has rapidly lead to a dramatic exponential increase in antibiotic resistance and multidrug-resistant bacteria throughout the world (Davies and Davies, 2010; Fair and Tor, 2014). The speed with which resistance has spread is explained by acquired resistance. In contrast to chromosomal resistance which is responsible for resistance to an antibiotic or an antibiotic class, acquired resistance by genetic material acquisition may be responsible for resistance against many antibiotics or antibiotic classes (INSERM, 2013). This resistance is harbored by many human and animal, pathogenic, and potentially pathogenic bacteria and can easily be spread by either conjugation, transformation, or transduction of resistance genes which are generally located on mobile elements (plasmids, transposons, integrons; Carattoli, 2009; Cambray et al., 2010; Aminov, 2011). It is well-known that both metals and antibiotic resistance genes are located on the same mobile elements, leading to a co-selection of ARGs by metals (Baker-Austin et al., 2006; Seiler and Berendonk, 2012). Metal contaminations are widely spread in anthropogenic environment contributing on ARGs propagations (Sakan et al., 2009; Ji et al., 2012; Seiler and Berendonk, 2012).

The question of the environmental and human risks of an increasing release of bacteria carrying ARGs into the natural environment has been a subject of intense scientific and political debate in recent years. Consequently, there are a growing number of reports concerning the prevalence and dissemination of ARBs and ARGs into various environmental compartments (e.g., Kümmerer, 2004; Martínez, 2008; CDC, 2013; WHO, 2014; Devarajan et al., 2015a). Effluents from hospitals, industry, municipal organizations, and urban/agricultural runoff in many developing countries represent a significant source of emerging contaminants (metals, ARGs, ARB) in the receiving environment as the effluents are discharged into sewer systems, rivers, lakes, and seas without prior treatment which may then accumulate in sediments (Spindler et al., 2012; Mwanamoki et al., 2014; Devarajan et al., 2015a). Rivers and lakes are considered to be putative reservoirs of emerging contaminants (medicinal products, metals, ARGs) since they collect wastewaters containing various contaminants from various origins (Kümmerer, 2004; Poté et al., 2008; Allen et al., 2010). Furthermore, the sediments may accumulate 100 to 1000 times as many heavy metals, FIB and ARGs as the overlying water (e.g., Poté et al., 2008; Haller et al., 2009; Thevenon et al., 2012a,b; Mubedi et al., 2013; Mwanamoki et al., 2014, 2015; Devarajan et al., 2015a,b) and offer the opportunity for reconstructing the pollution history and evaluating the impacts.

Many studies have been performed to quantify ARB and ARGs in different environmental compartments around the world and explained the role of aquatic ecosystems as reservoirs of antibiotic resistance (e.g., Schwartz et al., 2003; Kümmerer, 2004; Levy and Marshall, 2004; Martínez, 2008; Stoll et al., 2012; Marti et al., 2014; WHO, 2014). Most of these studies formulated recommendations and hypotheses including the suggestion of further researches in different regions according to the source of drinking and recreational water, the practice of wastewater management, economic situation and sociocultural aspects of population, and climatic conditions. Nevertheless, many studies have not considered the influence of tropical conditions (e.g., in developing nations such as Sub-Saharan African countries) on the accumulation of these emerging contaminants in aquatic environment, which can vary considerably with developed countries (under temperate conditions; e.g., Czekalski et al., 2014; Devarajan et al., 2015a). Consequently, little data are available on the assessment of heavy metals and neither there is no much information found regarding quantitative and qualitative aspects of ARB as well as ARGs in the aquatic environment under tropical conditions, which have an average daily peak temperatures reaching 30°C. Measures to reduce the potential human and environmental risks caused by hazardous substances (such as toxic metals), ARB, and ARGs include their characterizations and selection of target ARB and ARG, identification of potential sources as well as risk assessment, the development of reliable surveillance and risk assessment procedures, and finally, the implementation of technological solutions that can prevent environmental contamination with ARB and ARGs (WHO, 2014; Berendonk et al., 2015; Devarajan et al., 2015a).

The aim of the research presented in this paper is to assess the role of untreated hospital effluents discharged into freshwater receiving system under tropical conditions. This assessment was based on: (i) sediment physicochemical characterization including sediment grain size, total organic matter (OM; loss on ignition), and toxic metals including Cr, Co, Ni, Cu, Zn, As, Cd, Pb, and Hg - (ii) quantitative polymerase chain reaction (qPCR) on ARGs (bla_{TEM}, $bla_{CTX\text{-}M}$, bla_{SHV}, and *aadA*), total bacterial load, and selected bacterial marker genes of fecal indicator bacteria [FIB; *E. coli* and *Enterococcus* (ENT)] and *Pseudomonas* species (Psd). To the knowledge of the authors this is first report on the accumulation of emerging microbial contaminants in the sediments of freshwater receiving systems in a central African region and specifically in the city of Kinshasa, the capital of the Democratic Republic of the Congo. Nevertheless, it should be noted that, one may argue that studies that analyze the DNA such as this study, while providing information on the presence/absence or even quantitative data but do not provide information on the expression of these ARGs (Lachmayr et al., 2009). However, the expression of genes is not the central query of this study when the purpose of this study is to address the evaluation of the tropical aquatic environment to serve as reservoirs of heavy metals and ARGs (that could be potentially transferred to other bacterial cells through horizontal gene transfer; Devarajan et al., 2016). The parameters analyzed were correlated in order to identify the potential sources of receiving system contamination.

MATERIALS AND METHODS

Study Site and Sampling

Kinshasa, the capital and largest city in the Democratic Republic of the Congo (DRC; **Figure 1**), is the 27th largest urban area in the world with 11,587,000 inhabitants and covering 9′965 km^2. The climate is classified as humid and dry with an average temperature of 21–30°C. The city has ~20 hospitals and various medical centers and polyclinics with different intrinsic characteristics (size, type of services, medical practices...). The wastewater effluents are discharged from the big hospitals into drainage systems and ejected into the urban river receiving systems without prior treatment. For small hospitals and many medical centers, wastewaters are directly rejected onto the soil, septic tanks, wells, or into rivers, and even using buckets. The selection of hospitals was done on the basis of the hospital size relatively to the practice of wastewater management as described above, and the hospital location in relation with the river receiving system. Three rivers receiving hospital effluent waters were selected for this study. They are affected by one very large hospital and three recent and innovative hospitals. No industry is located near the hospitals selected.

The sampling took place in December 2014. The surface sediments (0–4 cm layer) were collected from (i) outlet pipes (HOP) of the 4 hospitals selected, labeled H1, H2, H3, and H4. The collection points were adjacent to the hospital effluent outlet pipe before discharge into rivers. This sampling point is named E, (ii) at the HOP discharge points into the rivers (point named RP), (iii) in the rivers 50 m upstream from HOP discharge points (point named US), and (iv) in the rivers 50 m downstream from HOP discharge points (point named DS). Approximately 400–500 g of sediment were taken from each site in triplicate. All samples were stored in an icebox at 4°C until shipping (Mubedi et al., 2013; Mwanamoki et al., 2015; Devarajan et al., 2015b) and analyzed within 2 weeks.

Sediment Grain Size, Organic Matter, and Water Content

The sediment particle grain size was measured using a Laser Coulter® LS-100 diffractometer (Beckman Coulter, Fullerton, CA, USA), following 5 min ultrasonic dispersal in deionized water according to the method described by Loizeau et al. (1994). The sediment total organic matter (OM) content was estimated by loss on ignition at 550°C for 1 h in a Salvis oven (Salvis AG, Emmenbrücke, Lucerne, Switzerland). Sediment total water content was measured by drying the samples at 60°C for overnight and the weight loss was taken for the percentage of water content.

Toxic Metal Analysis

Before being analyzed, sediment samples were lyophilized at −45°C after homogenization and air-drying at ambient room temperature. Toxic metals including Cr, Cu, Zn, Cd, and Pb were determined by Inductively Coupled Plasma Mass Spectrometry (ICP-MS, Agilent model 7700 series) following the digestion of sediments in Teflon bombs heated to 150°C in analytical grade 2M HNO_3 (Loizeau et al., 1994; Pardos et al., 2004; Poté et al., 2008). Multi-element standard solutions at different concentrations (0, 0.02, 1, 5, 20, 100, and 200 μg/L) were used for calibration. Total variation coefficients of triplicate sample measurements were under 5% and chemical blanks for the procedure were less than 2% of the sample signal. The metal concentrations of sediments were expressed in ppm (mg kg^{-1} dry weight sediment).

Total Hg analysis was carried out using the Atomic Absorption Spectrophotometer (AAS) for mercury determination (Advanced Mercury Analyser; AMA 254, Altec s.r.l., Czech Rep.) following the method described by Hall and Pelchat (1997) and Roos-Barraclough et al. (2002). The method is based on sample combustion, gold amalgamation, and

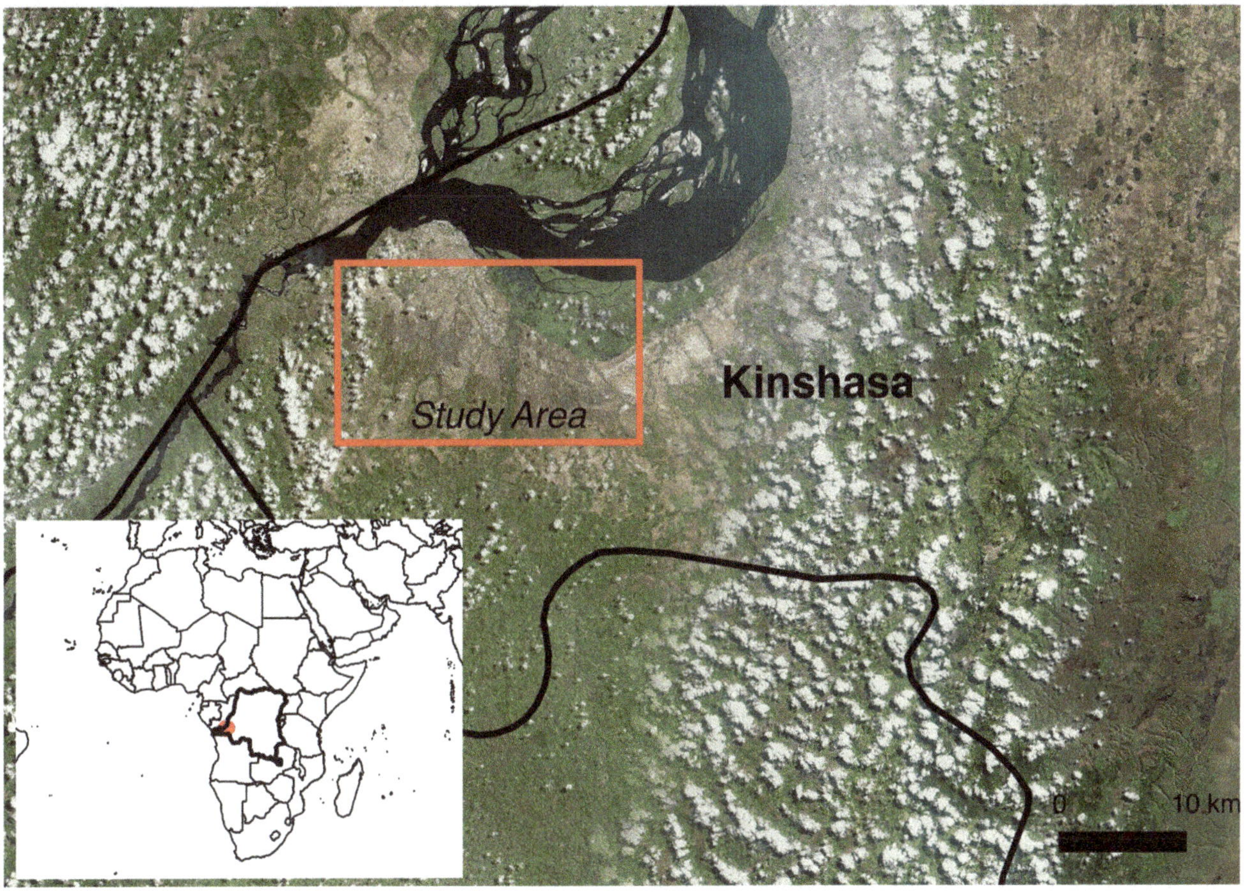

FIGURE 1 | Localization of the sampling site in the province of Kinshasa, Republic Democratic of Congo (Adapted from Google Maps).

AAS. The detection limit (3 SD blank) was 0.005 mg kg^{-1} and the reproducibility better than 2%.

Total DNA Extraction

Total DNA from sediment samples was extracted using the PowerSoil® DNA Isolation Kit (MoBio Laboratories, Carlsbad, USA) according to manufacturer's instructions. DNA extraction was performed with three replicate sample (from the same sediment sample) to compensate for heterogeneity. The concentration of extracted DNA was measured using a Qubit Fluorimeter (Life Technologies Europe B.V., Zug, Switzerland). The isolated DNA was stored at −20°C until used.

qPCR Quantification of Selected Genes in Sediments: 16S rRNA, ARGs, and FIB

Quantification of ARGs (bla_{TEM}, $bla_{CTX\text{-}M}$, bla_{SHV}, and *aadA*), bacterial gene markers for *E. coli, Enterococcus and Pseudomonas* species, and 16S rRNA genes by qPCR was performed [qPCR reactions, control plasmids, calculation for absolute gene copy numbers (gene concentration) and the gene copy numbers normalized to 16S rRNA (abundance)] as previously described by Devarajan et al. (2015a). Briefly; Genes were quantified with Eco qPCR system (Illumina, Switzerland) using KAPA SYBR® FAST qPCR Master Mix Universal Kit (KAPA Biosystems, USA). The primer sequences and reaction conditions are provided in **Table 1**. The following cycling parameters were applied: 10 min at 95°C for the polymerase activation; followed by 40 cycles of 95°C for 30 s, optimal Tm for 30 s and 72°C for 30 s. The temperature melting curve profile was obtained using the following conditions; 95°C for 30 s, optimal Tm for 30 s, followed by 95°C for 30 s.

All the reactions included negative (with no template DNA) and positive controls (10-fold serial dilutions of pGEM-T plasmid with respective target gene insert). All negative controls resulted either in no amplification or a threshold cycle (Ct) higher than the most diluted standard (pGEM-T plasmid). A sample was considered to be below the limit of detection (LOD) or negative for a target gene if ≥2 out of 3 technical replicates were negative or if sample Ct values were ≥Ct of negative controls. Samples above LOD were considered to be below the limit of quantification when the standard deviation of Ct values of methodological triplicates was 40.5 and their Ct value was higher than the Ct of the most diluted standard whose standard deviation of Ct values was ≤0.5. For each reaction the efficiency of the assay was measured using the slope of the standard curve measures ($E = 10^{[-1/slope]} - 1$). The absolute copy number of

TABLE 1 | Primers used in this study.

Target organism/gene	Primer	Oligonucleotide sequence (5′-3′)	Tm (°C)	Size (bp)	References
Bacterial 16S rRNA	338F	ACTCCTACGGGAGGCAGCAG	55	197	Ovreås et al., 1997
	518R	ATTACCGCGGCTGCTGG			
E. coli (*uidA*)	Uida405F	CAACGAACTGAACTGGCAGA	55	121	Chern et al., 2011
	Uida405R	CATTACGCTGCGATGGAT			
ENT (16S rRNA)	Ent376F	GGACGMAAGTCTGACCGA	55	221	Ram et al., 2004
	Ent578R	TTAAGAAACCGCCTGCGC			
Pseudomonas spp.	Pse435F	ACTTTAAGTTGGGAGGAAGGG	55	251	Bergmark et al., 2012
	Pse435R	ACACAGGAAATTCCACCACCC			
bla_{TEM}	TEM-RT-F	GCKGCCAACTTACTTCTGACAACG	55	247	Sidrach Cardona et al., 2014
	TEM-RT-R	CTTTATCCGCCTCCATCCAGTCTA			
bla_{CTX-M}	blaCTX-M-rt-f	ATTCCRGGCGAYCCGCGTGATACC	62	227	Fujita et al., 2011
	blaCTX-M-rt-r	ACCGCGATATCGTTGGTGGTGCCAT			
bla_{SHV}	blaSHV-rt-f	CGCTTTCCCATGATGAGCACCTTT	60	110	Xi et al., 2009
	blaSHV-rt-r	TCCTGCTGGCGATAGTGGATCTTT			
aadA	aadA-F	GCAGCGCAATGACATTCTTG	55	282	Madsen et al., 2000
	aadA-R	ATCCTTCGGCGCGATTTTG			

each reaction was quantified by referring to the corresponding standard curve obtained by plotting the copy number of the constructed pGEM-T plasmid vs. threshold cycles. The serial 10-fold dilutions of plasmid DNA containing the respective target gene copies were used for the standard curve. To emphasize the relative abundance of the resistance genes the concentrations of the gene copy numbers were presented as percentage of "copy number of a gene/copy number of 16S rRNA" for each sample.

Data Analysis

The 16S rRNA (total bacterial load), FIB and the selected marker genes and ARGs in the samples are expressed as "gene copy numbers" in per gram of dry sediment weight normalized to the DNA extraction yield. The "relative abundance" of the selected genetic marker genes (normalized to 16S rRNA) were emphasized by the ratio = (copy number of a gene) / (copy number of 16S rRNA) for each sample (Czekalski et al., 2014; Devarajan et al., 2015a). A statistical treatment of data; Correlation matrix (Pearson), Principal component analysis (PCA) and its extensions to between (BGA), and within groups (WGA) analyses (ade4 package in R) was used to analyze the grouping hospital/sampling point samples by monitoring quality variables (metal content, FIB abundance, ARGs, mean grain size and OM content). The statistical software was R version 3.2.2 (Team, 2015). Linear fixed model were fitted to the data using the functionality of the package lme4 (Bates et al., 2015). Average concentrations of gene copy numbers was modeled using the hospital and the sampling point as fixed effects and technical and biological effects as random effects. Significance of fixed effects was assessed by a t-test using a significance level of 5%. Model checking was based residual plots and normal probability checking using the raw residuals. Models were reduced using the likelihood ratio test. Pairwise comparison were evaluated based on adjusted p-values obtained using single-step method (Hothorn et al., 2008).

RESULTS AND DISCUSSION

Sediment Physicochemical Parameters and Metal Content

Sediment characteristics including particle grain-size and total organic matter (OM) are presented in **Table 2**. The sediment grain size and the OM varied substantially internally within the sampling sites ($p < 0.05$). Surface sediments of rivers in all sites studied are generally sandy-silt. The maximum value of clay observed at sites H1, H2, and H3 was less than 3%. H4 presented the maximum value of clay (11%). The same distribution was observed for sediment OM content ($p < 0.05$). The values ranged from 15.0 to 46.2% (H1), 4.7–9.4% (H2), and 0.7–8.7%. No great difference in OM was observed in the sampling sites of H4 (8.3–8.5%). Previous studies have reported that there are large variations in the distribution of sediment OM and grain size in freshwater, lakes, rivers, and reservoirs. The OM in non-contaminated freshwater sediments varies from 0.1 to 6.0% (Poté et al., 2008; Haller et al., 2009; Mubedi et al., 2013). The sediment from all sites (US: upstream; E: exit (outlet); RP: reject point (outlet discharge) and DS: downstream) of H1 and H4 are contaminated by organic matter. These results support the hypothesis that hospital effluents are one of many sources

TABLE 2 | Physico-chemical parameters of surface sediments from sampling points of each hospital site.

Hospital	Sampling point[b]	Clay (%)	Silt (%)	Sand (%)	Mean grain size (μm)	OM[c] (%)
Hospital 1	US	3.21	27.46	69.33	46.57	15.03
	E	2.61	47.96	49.43	65.69	46.15
	RP	3.36	58.44	38.20	42.70	34.78
	DS	1.31	25.45	73.24	139.10	18.10
Hospital 2	US	0.41	14.00	85.59	157.20	6.05
	E	ND[a]	ND	ND	ND	ND
	RP	0.48	13.46	86.06	229.10	9.37
	DS	1.85	63.27	34.88	48.67	4.74
Hospital 3	US	0.13	10.66	89.21	226.00	0.75
	E	0.78	9.46	89.76	205.80	3.91
	RP	0.38	7.31	92.31	234.20	1.79
	DS	0.27	27.47	72.26	135.20	8.72
Hospital 4	US	5.68	38.71	55.61	52.67	8.33
	E	0.37	58.23	41.40	58.71	8.40
	RP	10.83	57.51	31.66	24.04	8.44
	DS	0.94	26.00	73.06	82.54	8.51

[a]*ND: not determinated.*
[b]*US, upstream; E, exit; RP, reject point; DS, downstream.*
[c]*OM, organic matter.*

of contamination and that the contamination occurs at multiple points of entry along the river bank.

The results of the toxic metal analysis are reported in **Table 3**. The maximum concentration was observed in sediments at H1, reaching values (in mg kg^{-1}) of 47.9 (Cr), 213.6 (Cu), 1434.4 (Zn), 2.6 (Cd), 274.2 (Pb), and 13.6 (Hg). Sewages and rivers, which receive the majority of drained urban wastewaters of the city of Kinshasa, are used by the local population as uncontrolled landfills for domestic solid wastes. This can explain the presence of high metal concentrations in sediment (Mavakala et al., 2016). As the studied rivers flow through the City of Kinshasa, additional pollutant sources such as domestic sewages, uncontrolled landfills and artisanal activities located in the banks of rivers can probably explain the presence of contaminants accumulation in sediment. However, the presence of other non-identified sources and untreated hospital effluent water discharge cannot be excluded. In general, the concentration of toxic metals at points E, RP, and DS are higher for all sampling sites than the upstream sampling points indicating the effect of hospital effluent waters on the contamination of rivers by toxic metals.

Metals accumulation in sediments is one of a good indicators for predicting the deterioration of a contaminated environment with inorganic pollutants. The release of heavy metals into the aquatic ecosystem can lead to the pollution of water resources and may place aquatic organisms and human health at risk. The main human and environmental risk is remobilization of the contaminants and their return to the hydrosphere either by sediment re-suspension or by infiltration into groundwater (Wildi et al., 2004; Poté et al., 2008).

The evaluation of the potential deleterious effects of the metals toward benthic fauna, which is based on sediment quality guidelines (SQG; CCME, 1999; MacDonald et al., 2000; Long et al., 2006) provides an estimate of the hazard that the sediments may represent to the local biota. The authors proposed a "Threshold effect concentration" (TEC) for specific metals which is the level above which an organism is affected (or responds) and below which it does not, and a "probable effect level" (PEL), a contaminant level that is likely to have an adverse effect on biota (Mwanamoki et al., 2014). According to the SQGs and PEL (**Table 3**), the concentration of Cr, Cu, Zn, Pb, and Hg in sediment may present a potential toxic effect on indigenous fauna and flora living in these aquatic environments. Furthermore, the high PEL values observed upstream of hospital effluent discharges indicate that hospital effluents are only one of several sources of contamination. Indeed, many anthropogenic activities (i.e., industrial, sewage, agricultural land field, mining...) are known to be responsible of heavy metal release in the environment (Poté et al., 2008; Lim et al., 2013; Devarajan et al., 2015b; Niane et al., 2015) and may be responsible of the high metal values observed upstream HOP effluents discharge.

Abundance of Bacterial Population

The total bacterial load in sediment samples is presented in **Figure 2** (based on 16S rRNA gene copy numbers). In general, 16S rRNA gene copy numbers varied significantly between sampling sites ($p < 0.05$) with values of (log copy numbers g^{-1} of dry sediment). The 16S rRNA gene copy numbers in samples from H1 were several orders of magnitude higher than those observed in others hospitals. However, these results are in conformity with those found in sediment from contaminated sediments receiving WWTP effluent waters (Devarajan et al., 2015a). Furthermore, the total bacterial load after the effluent discharge (RP) for H1 and H4 were respectively 10 and 7.85 times higher than the values observed in their respective control sites (US). In contrast, the total bacterial load in the points RP for H2 and H3 was 3.7 to 6.8 times lower than their respective control site (US), indicating the possible presence of other sources of contamination.

The average copy number of FIB bacterial marker genes including *E. coli*, ENT, and Psd in the sediment samples is presented in **Figure 3**. The bacterial density varies considerably depending on the sampling point and the type of hospital. For example, the *E. coli* range at the US site (log copy numbers g^{-1} of dry sediment) was 6.44, 6.30, 6.67, and 4.21 for H1, H2, H3, and H4, respectively; ENT range (copy numbers g^{-1} of dry sediment) of 7.28, 7.59, 7.87, and 5.41 for H1, H2, H3, and H4, respectively; and Psd range (log copy numbers g^{-1} of dry sediment) was 6.96, 6.94, 7.10, and 5.49 for H1, H2, H3, and H4, respectively. The input of hospital wastewater in the receiving system lead to a 6, 1, and 288 times greater abundance of *E. coli* for H1, H2, and H4, respectively. In H3 RP sampling point, a 6.2 times decrease in *E. coli* abundance was measured after wastewater discharge showing that H3 wastewater did not contribute more than the environmental enrichment in *E. coli*.

Raw load of selected bacterial marker genes followed the 16S rRNA trend. To avoid inconstancies between qPCR assays,

TABLE 3 | Metal content of surface sediment samples from sampling point of each hospital site, analyzed by ICP-MS (expressed in mg. kg^{-1}).

Hospital	Sampling point	Cr	Co	Ni	Cu	Zn	Cd	Pb	Hg
Hospital 1	US	34.32	4.29	14.24	**107.45**	**884.61**	**1.79**	**189.62**	**1.43**
	E	**45.54**	4.55	17.42	**213.59**	**1004.47**	**1.88**	**137.08**	**13.60**
	RP	**47.87**	4.97	17.42	**204.13**	**1077.17**	**2.07**	**124.40**	**3.94**
	DS	**47.58**	7.11	21.20	**184.67**	**1434.78**	**2.65**	**274.19**	**3.25**
Hospital 2	US	13.03	1.79	6.29	**59.18**	**410.69**	0.57	**86.67**	**0.64**
	E	ND	ND	ND	ND	ND	ND	ND	ND
	RP	11.96	1.81	13.48	34.18	**304.92**	0.54	**281.52**	**0.44**
	DS	10.43	1.61	5.67	**51.91**	**352.41**	0.46	**81.15**	**0.74**
Hospital 3	US	3.20	0.37	16.73	**46.06**	87.21	0.18	**36.38**	0.15
	E	7.81	0.83	14.63	22.08	**147.29**	0.29	34.48	**0.68**
	RP	4.18	0.44	13.57	8.86	68.27	0.08	15.82	**0.31**
	DS	4.97	0.62	3.79	22.65	**153.77**	0.22	**40.75**	**0.37**
Hospital 4	US	15.36	0.99	4.85	9.38	71.99	0.10	14.96	**0.39**
	E	27.92	2.68	9.98	**47.54**	**365.75**	0.52	**75.98**	**0.56**
	RP	21.91	1.20	5.96	12.66	98.75	0.16	20.98	**0.51**
	DS	15.23	1.13	5.10	12.86	100.30	0.14	20.73	**0.44**
	SQGs[a]	37.30			35.70	123.00	0.60	35.00	0.17
	PEL[b]	90.00			197.00	315.00	3.50	91.30	0.49

[a] *Sediment quality guidelines (mg.kg^{-1}).*
[b] *Probable effect level (mg.kg^{-1}).*
In bold: values above SQGs.
Cr, chromium; Co, cobalt; Ni, nickel; Cu, copper; Zn, zinc; Cd, cadmium; Pb, lead; Hg, mercury.

including suboptimal efficiencies, selected bacterial species marker genes and ARGs were normalized using 16S rRNA (**Figures 4, 6**). The greatest abundance of bacterial populations was recorded at H1 and H4 sampling sites (except *E. coli* for H1 and Psd for H4). H2 and H3 did not show any significant increase in bacterial marker genes abundance, which was also the case for 16S rRNA abundance ($0.20 < p < 0.98$ for H3 and $0.06 < p < 0.91$ for H3). The abundance of bacterial marker genes can be either accumulated or diluted depending on the river characteristics (depth, flow rate, turbulences). No uncultivable quantitative data is available for RDC aquatic systems but the high level of total bacteria and FIB in US sampling points is consistent with data from highly contaminated sediments (Devarajan et al., 2015a,b). Compared to other hospitals, the H1 sampling site had higher values for total bacterial load which could be explained by the larger size of the hospital and the shared drainage of urban and hospital wastewater. The three other hospitals are smaller than H1 which results in smaller amounts of contaminants in their effluents. In the case of H2, no canalization of hospital wastewater was used. The cumulative effect of no drainage system and the presence of wild discharge next to the US sampling point may explain why hospital effluents discharge showed no significant increase in FIB abundance in the receiving system (Orsi et al., 2007; Graham and Polizzotto, 2013). This effluent didn't contribute more to already environmental abundance and the observed decrease in FIB abundance may be due to contaminant dilution and transport downstream by river flow (Knapp et al., 2012; Chen et al., 2013).

FIB including *E. coli* and ENT are commonly used to assess microbial safety of aquatic systems. It is well-known that many *E. coli* and ENT are also responsible for numerous health care-associated infections of the bloodstream, urinary tract, and surgical incision sites (Alm et al., 2014). To develop this high level of pathogenicity, these bacteria have acquired islands of pathogenicity including antibiotic, heavy metal resistance genes, and virulence factors. Several studies in other parts of the world have revealed the presence of pathogenic micro-organisms which are multi-resistant to antibiotics in hospital effluents (Emmanuel et al., 2009). In the absence of wastewater treatment as is the case in the hospitals in the study presented in this paper, these bacteria will be discharged directly into aquatic receiving systems. It is well-known that FIB are able to survive and proliferate in sediments as sediments provide favorable conditions for proliferation and growth. (Poté et al., 2009). Furthermore, FIB have a great ability to acquire ARG (Levy and Marshall, 2004) and are able to transfer their resistance to autochthonous bacteria by HGT (Sidrach Cardona et al., 2014). Consequently, the discharge of raw hospital wastewater could lead to an environmental reservoir of clinical resistant bacteria and their associated genes developing in the sediment (Marti et al., 2014).

Quantification of Antibiotic Resistance Genes

qPCR was performed to quantify the selected ARGs conferring resistance to ß-lactam (bla_{TEM}, bla_{CTX-M}, and bla_{SHV}) and aminoglycoside (*aadA*) in DNA extracted from the sediment

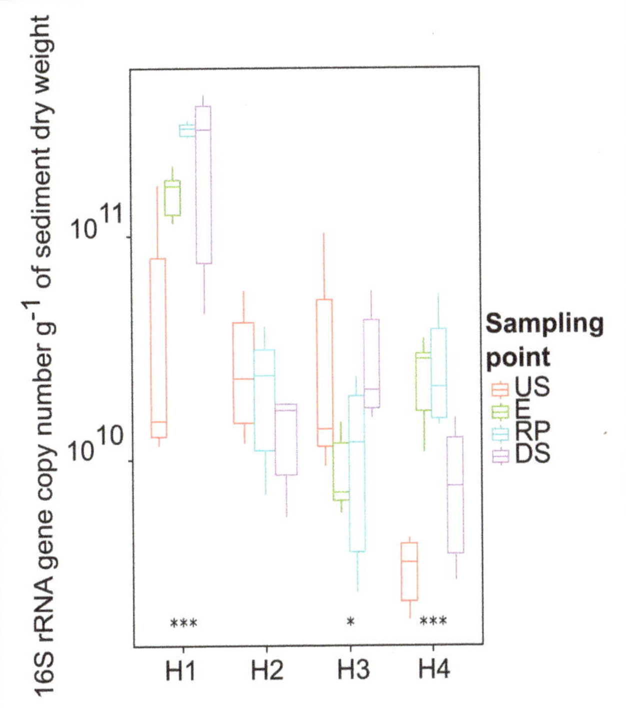

FIGURE 2 | Raw 16S rRNA copy number detected in hospital receiving systems (16S rRNA gene copy number / g of DS) at each sampling point. Significant stars represent significant variation between US and RP point, ***-$p < 0.01$; and * $0.1 > p > 0.05$. For the pairs not marked the statistical difference between US and RP was statistically insignificant. The line in each box marks the media and boxes: 25th and 75th percentiles; whiskers: 5th and 95th percentiles and outliers ± 1.5*IQ. US, upstream; E, hospital outlet effluent; RP, reject point; DS, downstream.

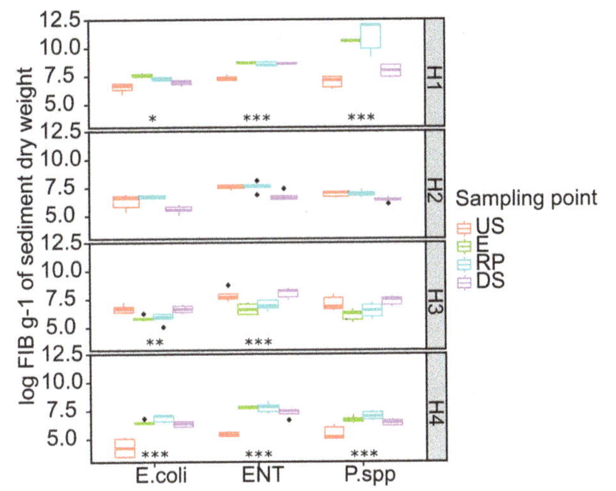

FIGURE 3 | Raw FIB copy number detected in hospital receiving systems at each sampling point. Significant stars represent significant variation between US and RP point, ***-$p < 0.01$, ** $0.01 > p > 0.01$ and * $0.1 > p > 0.05$. For the pairs not marked the statistical difference between US and RP was statistically insignificant. The line in each box marks the media and boxes: 25th and 75th percentiles; whiskers: 5th and 95th percentiles and outliers ± 1.5*IQR. US, upstream; E, hospital outlet effluent; RP, reject point; DS, downstream; ENT, Enterococcus; Psd, Pseudomonas species.

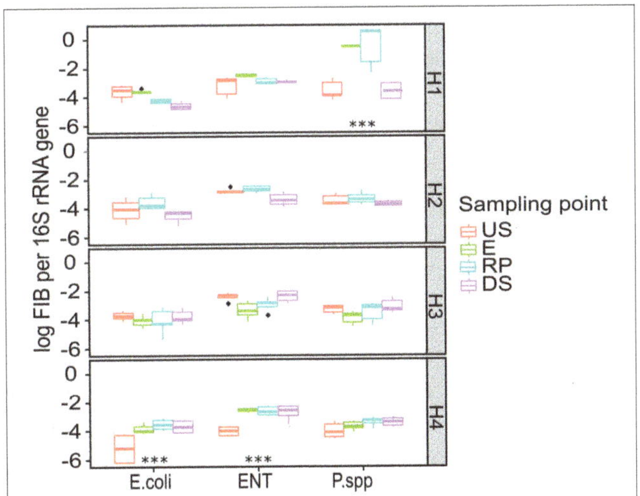

FIGURE 4 | Normalized FIB copy number detected in hospital receiving systems at each sampling point. Significant stars represent significant variation between US and RP point, ***-$p < 0.01$. For the pairs not marked the statistical difference between US and RP was statistically insignificant. The line in each box marks the media and boxes: 25th and 75th percentiles; whiskers: 5th and 95th percentiles and outliers ± 1.5*IQR. US, upstream; E, hospital outlet effluent; RP, reject point; DS, downstream; ENT, Enterococcus; Psd, Pseudomonas species.

samples. ARG selection was based on various criteria including (Devarajan et al., 2016): (i) clinically relevant genes (human risk); (ii) genes conferring resistance to frequently used antibiotics; (iii) ARGs previously reported in mobile genetic elements; and (iv) the antibiotics used in 6 pilot hospitals in Kinshasa (Nzolo et al., 2013). The raw gene copy number (ARGs g^{-1} of dry sediment) was used to estimate the general changes in ARGs level in receiving systems. The results are presented in **Figure 5**. The ARGs copy number (ARGs g^{-1} of dry sediment) for *aadA*, bla_{CTX-M}, bla_{SHV}, and bla_{TEM} varied, respectively from 4.64 to 7.83, 4.67 to 5.01, 3.92 to 4.66, and 4.23 to 4.86 at US sites, and from 5.33 to 9.24, 4.55 to 5.61, 3.76 to 6.17, and 4.36 to 5.46 at RP/DS sampling sites. The great abundance of bla_{TEM} and *aadA* genes at all sampling sites (US, E, RP, and DS) could be explained by their ubiquitous presence as housekeeping genes, which has previously been shown to occur frequently among soil bacteria as well as by their presence in sewage and effluent receiving systems (Demanèche et al., 2008; Thevenon et al., 2012a; Suzuki et al., 2015). A relevant increase in ARG level after wastewater discharge is only observed in H1 sediments ($p < 0.05$) with a 25.6, 45.0, and 148 times increase observed between US and RP sampling points for bla_{CTX-M}, bla_{SHV}, and *aadA*, respectively. For the others hospitals, the general trend of ARGs increased after wastewater discharge was no longer observed. The abundance of ARGs and associated bacteria in a receiving system may vary depending on the size of the hospital and type of services.

The normalized/relative abundances of 16S rRNA were found in order to quantify relative change in ARGs abundances, that is, whether or not more or fewer ARGs appear per microbial genome (Laht et al., 2014). The relative abundance of ARGs in

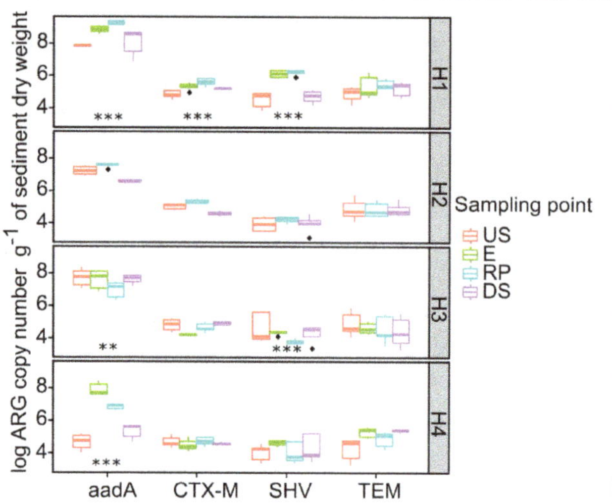

FIGURE 5 | Raw ARGs copy number detected in hospital receiving systems at each sampling point. Significant stars represent significant variation between US and RP point, ***-$p < 0.01$; and ** $0.01 > p > 0.01$. For the pairs not marked the statistical difference between US and RP was statistically insignificant. The line in each box marks the media and boxes: 25th and 75th percentiles; whiskers: 5th and 95th percentiles and outliers ± 1.5*IQR. US, upstream; E, hospital outlet effluent; RP, reject point; DS, downstream.

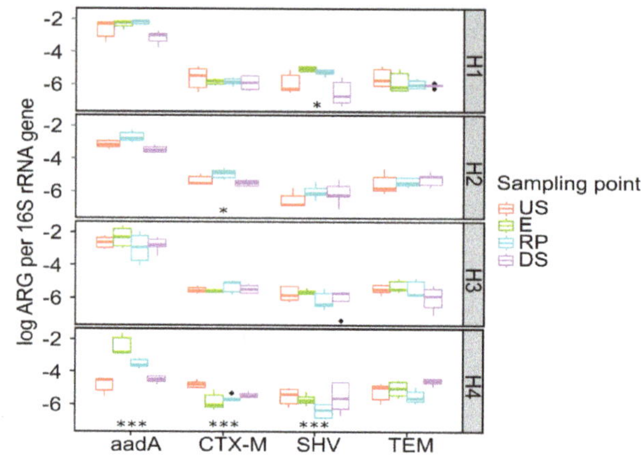

FIGURE 6 | Normalized ARGs copy number detected in hospital receiving systems at each sampling point. Significant stars represent significant variation between US and RP point, ***-$p < 0.01$; and * $0.1 > p > 0.05$. For the pairs not marked the statistical difference between US and RP was statistically insignificant. The line in each box marks the media and boxes: 25th and 75th percentiles; whiskers: 5th and 95th percentiles and outliers ± 1.5*IQR. US, upstream; E, hospital outlet effluent; RP, reject point; DS, downstream.

the sediment samples is presented in **Figure 6**. In general, the influence of hospital effluents was not observed in the relative abundance of ARGs copy numbers in receiving systems. Some specific cases such as *aadA* in H4, bla_{SHV} in H1, and $bla_{CTX\text{-}M}$ in H2 increased significantly after hospital effluent discharge ($p < 0.01$). These data suggest that increases in ARGs abundances are directly related to wastewater discharge depending on hospital type and disposal practices, although unknown sources and/or causes also exist (Graham et al., 2011; Marti et al., 2014). The prevalence of microbial contaminants in the control sites (upstream) could be explained by, for example, input from major activities such as agricultural runoff, open defecation, urban discharge, and other anthropogenic activities along the river banks, which receives considerable amounts of wastewaters (Dekov et al., 1998; Tshibanda et al., 2014). The abundance of total bacterial load, ARGs, and FIB showed a relevant increase after wastewater discharge but the results highlight that hospital wastewater effluents are not the only source of micropollutant accumulation.

Interestingly, the relative abundances of ARGs observed in this study were greater than in other studies performed in a similar environment under tropical conditions (Graham et al., 2011; Devarajan et al., 2016) and can be compared to data obtained in industrialized countries (Devarajan et al., 2015a). However, the lack of background information and the knowledge gap in our pristine study site does not help in understanding the trends observed. ESBLs are mostly TEM, SHV, and CTX-M derivatives. The great abundance of clinically relevant ARGs such as $bla_{CTX\text{-}M}$ and bla_{SHV} in the sediments studied may indicate the possible presence of ESBL in these systems (Poirel et al., 2012). The presence of ESBL in rivers (such as the sites studied) is highly alarming because the majority of ESBL are resistant to first line antibiotics but are also resistant to a large number of relevant antibiotics (Tacao et al., 2014). Furthermore, such a large abundance of ARGs represents a serious threat from resistance propagation because gene exchange can take place in sediment between both dead and living bacteria (Mao et al., 2014). It has been determined that approximately 90 bacterial species have natural transformability competences. Among them are many human pathogens, including the genera *Campylobacter, Haemophilus, Helicobacter, Nesseiria, Pseudomomas, Staphylococcus*, and *Streptococcus* (Mao et al., 2014). So the reservoir of ARGs in river sediments can be easily used by other bacteria to become ever more resistant.

The abundance of ARGs in the receiving systems reported in this study can be considered as alarming. Results indicate clearly that sediment receiving system under tropical condition can act as reservoirs of ARGs including bla_{TEM}, $bla_{CTX\text{-}M}$, bla_{SHV}, and *aadA*. It has been demonstrated that the intensive use of antibiotics for humans, animals, and agricultural purpose has led to the release (e.g., through the disposal of human and animal wastes) of ARB and ARGs into soil and aquatic environment (Martínez, 2008; Sommer et al., 2009). In the study region as well as in many Sub-Saharan African countries, there is no regulation for the use of antibiotics in humans, animals as well as for agricultural purpose, and data concerning the occurrence of ARGs and ARBs in aquatic environments is limited (WHO, 2014; Devarajan et al., 2016). Additionally, there is no policies and management tools to facilitate the urban wastewater treatment in study region. Thus, according to the results of this study, we strongly recommend the prudence and regulation for the use of antibiotics in humans and animals consumption, to limit spread

TABLE 4 | Spearman's Rank-Order Correlation of selected parameters analyzed in sediment samples [*n* = 65, statistically significant coefficients ($p < 0.05$) are in bold].

	Cd	Cr	Cu	Grain size	Hg	16S rRNA	aadA	CTX-M	*E. coli*	ENT	Psd	SHV	TEM	OM	Pb	Zn
Cd		**0.90**	**0.95**	**−0.24**	**0.64**	**0.59**	**0.66**	**0.54**	−0.10	**0.47**	**0.64**	**0.60**	**0.25**	**0.76**	**0.63**	**0.99**
Cr			**0.89**	**−0.52**	**0.66**	**0.61**	**0.59**	**0.44**	−0.05	**0.51**	**0.67**	**0.67**	**0.35**	**0.83**	**0.43**	**0.89**
Cu				**−0.29**	**0.78**	**0.67**	**0.71**	**0.57**	−0.11	**0.54**	**0.78**	**0.72**	**0.25**	**0.87**	**0.49**	**0.95**
Grain size					−0.26	−0.33	−0.01	0.03	−0.05	−0.20	**−0.29**	**−0.32**	**−0.33**	**−0.41**	0.23	**−0.26**
Hg						**0.51**	**0.52**	**0.37**	−0.05	**0.46**	**0.70**	**0.63**	0.08	**0.89**	**0.25**	**0.63**
16S							**0.72**	**0.67**	−0.19	**0.83**	**0.80**	**0.63**	**0.51**	**0.72**	0.24	**0.57**
aadA								**0.58**	**−0.36**	**0.74**	**0.73**	**0.66**	0.18	**0.63**	**0.43**	**0.65**
CTX-M									−0.11	**0.57**	**0.62**	**0.56**	**0.24**	**0.59**	**0.52**	**0.51**
E. coli										**−0.34**	−0.17	−0.13	−0.04	−0.04	−0.12	−0.11
ENT											**0.73**	**0.59**	**0.47**	**0.59**	**0.27**	**0.45**
Psd												**0.82**	**0.26**	**0.86**	0.21	**0.61**
SHV													0.15	**0.79**	0.19	**0.57**
TEM														0.23	0.12	**0.25**
OM															**0.32**	**0.74**
Pb																**0.63**
Zn																

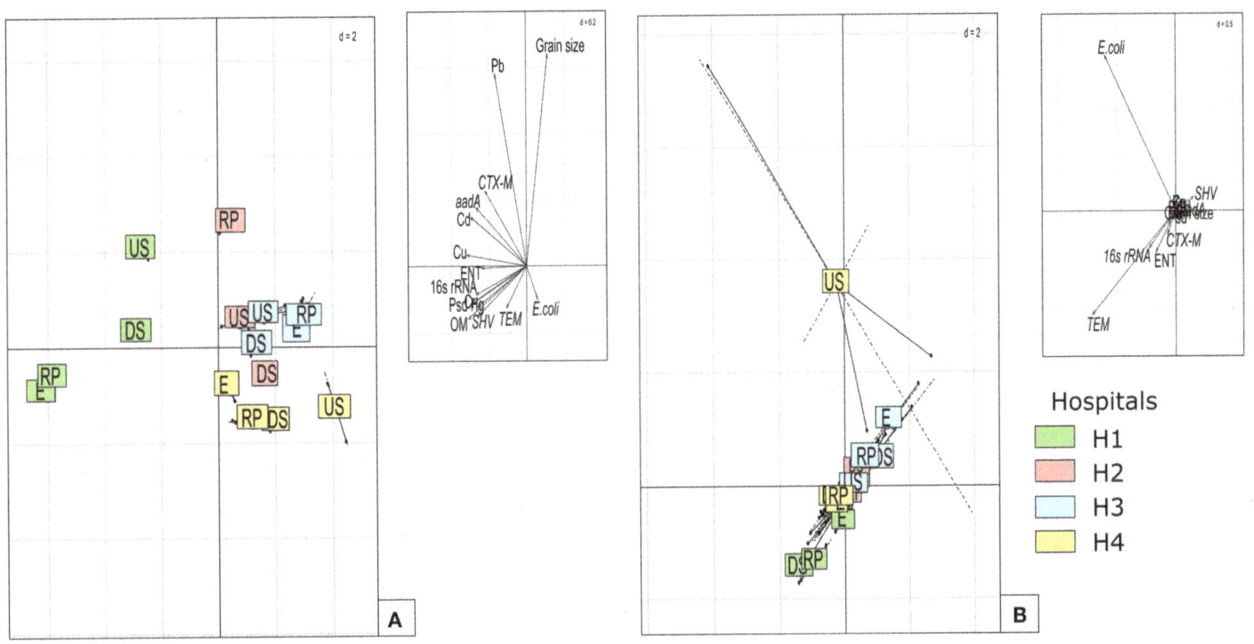

FIGURE 7 | Grouping of each sampling point according to ARGs, FIB, toxic metals, grain size, and OM. (A) plot using between group analyses to discriminate each points in various hospital receiving system. **(B)** same samples plotted after decomposing differences in each sampling point by within group analysis. Right upper panels show correlation with variables (PCA variable scores).

of ARGs and ARB into the environment. Furthermore, the need of a strategy for hospital and urban wastewater treatment.

Statistical Correlation

Correlation analysis between total bacterial load, FIB, ARGs, toxic metals, total organic matter, and sediment grain size was carried out to determine potential links between both parameters analyzed and possible origins of contaminants with the results being presented in **Table 4**. Total organic matter content, metal concentrations, bacterial indicator genetic markers (except *E. coli*), and ARGs were mostly significantly, positively, and mutually correlated. Nevertheless, all ARGs studied at hospital and sampling points are significantly correlated with total bacterial load (16S rRNA): 0.51 to 0.72 ($p < 0.001$, $n = 65$). ARGs (except for bla_{TEM}) have a positive correlation with *E. coli*, ENT, and Psd ($0.57 < r < 0.82$, $p < 0.05$, $n = 65$) and the metals (Cd, Cr, Cu, Hg, and Zn): ($0.37 < r < 0.71$, $p < 0.001$, $n = 65$). Strong positive and mutual correlation was observed between 16S rRNA, *E. coli*, ENT, and Psd with ARGs (except bla_{TEM}). These results indicate that these biological contaminants could originate from common sources and they are carried to the receiving system by common transporters (Thevenon et al., 2012b; Devarajan et al., 2015a). In addition, there was a positive correlation between total organic content and the metals in sediments. This observation is also supported by the fact that the contaminants are attached to both large organic and small inorganic particles such as clay and they could behave in a similar way in transporting contaminants to the receiving system (Poté et al., 2008; Zhao et al., 2015).

BGA on PCA analysis (**Figure 7**) showed that sampling points varied greatly between hospital sites revealing the impact of (i) initial background level in ARGs, heavy metals, and FIB and (ii) the hospital type (**Figure 7**-left). To analyze effluent effect independently of the hospital, sampling points were decomposed before fitting (WGA on PCA using hospital as "within group" factor) (**Figure 7**-right). The results show a large increase in ARGs, FIB, toxic metals, and OM for hospital H1 and H4 linked to wastewater discharge. Lastly, these results indicate that river receiving systems could depend on hospital practices but also that river sediments are already significantly contaminated by unknown sources. As the rivers flow through the City of Kinshasa, additional pollutant sources such as domestic sewage, uncontrolled landfill and artisanal activities located in the banks of rivers can probably explain the presence of contaminants accumulation in sediment (Mubedi et al., 2013; Ngelinkoto et al., 2014; Mwanamoki et al., 2015).

CONCLUSION

The research presented in this paper investigates the abundance and dissemination of metal, FIB and ARGs released from hospital effluents into the urban river receiving systems. It's important to note that one of the main concerns of this research consists on the evaluation of the degree to which river receiving system under tropical conditions can act as reservoir of metals, FIB and ARGs. Results demonstrate accumulation of toxic metals, *E. coli*, *Enterococcus*, and *Pseudomonas* species as well as ARGs in sediment, indicating that river receiving systems under tropical conditions (developing countries such as our study region) can act as a reservoir for metals and emerging microbial contaminants such as FIB and ARGs which can be transferred to human pathogens. Thus, the river receiving systems under tropical conditions which has average daily peak temperatures reaching 30°C, could potentially favor the transfer of mobile genetic elements carrying ARGs to susceptible bacterial pathogens. On the other hand, the presence of higher values of FIB and ARGs in sediment samples located upstream of the hospital outlet discharges (control sites) indicates that the hospital effluent wastewaters are not the only source of deterioration of bacteriological quality of studied rivers. The pollution in the cases studied in this paper may be explained by probable multiple diffuse pollution sources including open defecation, uncontrolled landfills, unregulated effluent discharges, and inadequate sewage collection near the sites studied.

Rivers in most developing nations (such as our study region) serve as a basic network for human and animal consumption as well as irrigation for fresh urban produces. High values of metals, FIB and ARGs observed in river receiving systems indicate the human and environmental potential risks. However, further studies are required to find the pathways used by ARGs to spread, exploring their potential transfer into clinically relevant bacteria and human commensal as well as assessing the human exposure and environment potential risks. To our knowledge, this is the first study to be performed in the region regarding the quantification of ARGs in receiving systems. The quantification of FIB and ARGs as performed in this study can therefore facilitate improved risk assessments for the prudent use of antibiotics in human, animal and agriculture, and provide baseline information for developing strategies (such as hospital and urban wastewater treatment) to limit the spread of these emerging contaminants under tropical conditions.

AUTHOR CONTRIBUTIONS

AL, CM, GG, VS, and JP conceived and designed research; AL, ND, PK, JK, and CM performed research: sampling and laboratory analysis; AL, GG, ND, and JP analyzed data; and AL, CM, VS, and JP wrote the paper. All authors have read, reviewed and approved the manuscript before submission.

REFERENCES

Allen, H. K. H., Donato, J. J., Wang, H. H. H., Cloud Hansen, K. A. K., Davies, J. J., and Handelsman, J. J. (2010). Call of the wild: antibiotic resistance genes in natural environments. *Nat. Rev. Microbiol.* 8, 251–259. doi: 10.1038/nrmicro2312

Alm, E. W., Zimbler, D., Callahan, E., and Plomaritis, E. (2014). Patterns and persistence of antibiotic resistance in faecal indicator bacteria from freshwater recreational beaches. *J. Appl. Microbiol.* 117, 273–285. doi: 10.1111/jam.12512

Aminov, R. I. R. (2011). Horizontal gene exchange in environmental microbiota. *Front. Microbiol.* 2:158. doi: 10.3389/fmicb.2011.00158

Atibu, E. K., Devarajan, N., Thevenon, F., Mwanamoki, P. M., Tshibanda, J. B., Mpiana, P. T., et al. (2013). Concentration of metals in surface water and sediment of Luilu and Musonoie Rivers, Kolwezi-Katanga, Democratic Republic of Congo. *Appl. Geochem.* 39, 26–32. doi: 10.1016/j.apgeochem.2013.09.021

Baker-Austin, C., Wright, M. S., Stepanauskas, R., and McArthur, J. V. (2006). Co-selection of antibiotic and metal resistance. *Trends Microbiol.* 14, 176–182. doi: 10.1016/j.tim.2006.02.006

Barcelo, D., and Barceló, D. (2003). Emerging pollutants in water analysis. TrAC. *Trends Analytical Chem.* 22, xiv–xvi. doi: 10.1016/s0165-9936(03)01106-3

Bates, D., Mächler, M., Bolker, B., and Walker, S. (2015). Fitting linear mixed-effects models using lme4. *J. Statist. Softw.* 67, 1–48. doi: 10.18637/jss.v067.i01

Berendonk, T. U., Manaia, C. M., Merlin, C., Fatta-Kassinos, D., Cytryn, E., Walsh, F., et al. (2015). Tackling antibiotic resistance: the environmental framework. *Nat. Rev. Microbiol.* 13, 310–317. doi: 10.1038/nrmicro3439

Bergmark, L. L., Poulsen, P. H., Al-Soud, W. A., Norman, A. A., Hansen, L. H., and Sørensen, S. J. S. (2012). Assessment of the specificity of Burkholderia and Pseudomonas qPCR assays for detection of these genera in soil using 454 pyrosequencing. *FEMS Microbiol. Lett.* 333, 77–84. doi: 10.1111/j.1574-6968.2012.02601.x

Boillot, C., Bazin, C., Tissot-Guerraz, F., Droguet, J., Perraud, M., Cetre, J. C., et al. (2008). Daily physicochemical, microbiological and ecotoxicological fluctuations of a hospital effluent according to technical and care activities. *Sci. Total Environ.* 403, 113–129. doi: 10.1016/j.scitotenv.2008.04.037

Bréchet, C., Plantin, J., Sauget, M., Thouverez, M., Talon, D., Cholley, P., et al. (2014). Wastewater treatment plants release large amounts of extended-spectrum beta-lactamase-producing *Escherichia coli* into the environment. *Clin. Infect. Dis.* 58, 1658–1665. doi: 10.1093/cid/ciu190

Cambray, G. G., Guerout, A. A.-M., and Mazel, D. D. (2010). Integrons. *Annu. Rev. Genet.* 44, 141–166. doi: 10.1146/annurev-genet-102209-163504

Carattoli, A. (2009). Resistance plasmid families in enterobacteriaceae. *Antimicrobial Agents Chemother.* 53, 2227–2238. doi: 10.1128/AAC.01707-08

CCME (1999). *Canadian Sediment Quality Guidelines for the Protection of Aquatic Life*. EPC 98-E, Canadian Environmental Quality Guidelines, Canadian Council of Ministers of the Environment. Available online at: http://www.ccme.ca/

CDC (2013). *Antibiotic Resistance and Threats in the United States.* Centers for Disease Control and Prevention. Available online at: http://www.cdc.gov/drugresistance/threat-report-2013

Chatterjee, M., Silva Filho, E. V., Sarkar, S. K., Sella, S. M., Bhattacharya, A., Satpathy, K. K., et al. (2007). Distribution and possible source of trace elements in the sediment cores of a tropical macrotidal estuary and their ecotoxicological significance. *Environ. Int.* 33, 346–356. doi: 10.1016/j.envint.2006.11.013

Chen, B., Liang, X., Huang, X., Zhang, T., and Li, X. (2013). Differentiating anthropogenic impacts on ARGs in the Pearl River Estuary by using suitable gene indicators. *Water Res.* 47, 2811–2820. doi: 10.1016/j.watres.2013.02.042

Chern, E. C., Siefring, S., Paar, J., Doolittle, M., and Haugland, R. A. (2011). Comparison of quantitative PCR assays for *Escherichia coli* targeting ribosomal RNA and single copy genes. *Lett. Appl. Microbiol.* 52, 298–306. doi: 10.1111/j.1472-765X.2010.03001.x

Cosgrove, S. E. S. (2006). The relationship between antimicrobial resistance and patient outcomes: mortality, length of hospital stay, and health care costs. *Clin. Infect. Dis.* 42(Suppl. 2), S82–S89. doi: 10.1086/499406

Czekalski, N., Gascón Díez, E., and Bürgmann, H. (2014). Wastewater as a point source of antibiotic-resistance genes in the sediment of a freshwater lake. *ISME J.* 8, 1381–1390. doi: 10.1038/ismej.2014.8

Davies, C. M., Long, J. A. H., Donald, M., and Ashbolt, N. J. (1995). Survival of fecal microorganisms in marine and fresh-water sediments. *Appl. Environ. Microbiol.* 61, 1888–1896.

Davies, J. J., and Davies, D. D. (2010). Origins and evolution of antibiotic resistance. *Microbiol. Mol. Biol. Rev.* 74, 417–433. doi: 10.1128/MMBR.00016-10

Dekov, V. M., Araujo, F., Van Grieken, R., Subramanian, V., and Vangrieken, R. (1998). Chemical composition of sediments and suspended matter from the Cauvery and Brahmaputra rivers (India). *Sci. Total Environ.* 212, 89–105. doi: 10.1016/S0048-9697(97)00132-0

Demanèche, S., Sanguin, H., Poté, J., Navarro, E., Bernillon, D., Mavingui, P., et al. (2008). Antibiotic-resistant soil bacteria in transgenic plant fields. *Proc. Natl. Acad. Sci. U.S.A.* 105, 3957–3962. doi: 10.1073/pnas.0800072105

Devarajan, N., Laffite, A., Graham, N. D., Meijer, M., Prabakar, K., Mubedi, J. I., et al. (2015a). Accumulation of clinically relevant antibiotic-resistance genes, bacterial load, and metals in freshwater lake sediments in Central Europe. *Environ. Sci. Technol.* 49, 6528–6537. doi: 10.1021/acs.est.5b01031

Devarajan, N., Laffite, A., Mulaji, C. K., Otamonga, J.-P., and Mpiana, P. T., Mubedi, J.I., et al. (2016). Occurrence of antibiotic resistance genes and bacterial markers in a tropical river receiving hospital and urban wastewaters. *PLoS ONE* 11:e0149211. doi: 10.1371/journal.pone.0149211

Devarajan, N., Laffite, A., Ngelikoto, P., Elongo, V., Prabakar, K., Mubedi, J., et al. (2015b). Hospital and urban effluent waters as a source of accumulation of toxic metals in the sediment receiving system of the Cauvery River, Tiruchirappalli, Tamil Nadu, India. *Environ. Sci. Poll. Res.* 22, 12941–12950. doi: 10.1007/s11356-015-4457-z,

Emmanuel, E. E., Perrodin, Y. Y., and Pierre, M. G. M. (2009). Groundwater contamination by microbiological and chemical substances released from hospital wastewater: health risk assessment for drinking water consumers. *Environ. Int.* 35, 718–726. doi: 10.1016/j.envint.2009.01.011

Fair, R. J., and Tor, Y. (2014). Antibiotics and bacterial resistance in the 21st century. *Perspect. Medicin. Chem.* 6, 25–64. doi: 10.4137/PMC.S14459

Feng, H., Han, X., Zhang, W., and Yu, L. (2004). A preliminary study of heavy metal contamination in Yangtze River intertidal zone due to urbanization. *Mar. Pollut. Bull.* 49, 910–915. doi: 10.1016/j.marpolbul.2004.06.014

Fujita, S. S.-I., Yosizaki, K. K., Ogushi, T. T., Uechi, K. K., Takemori, Y. Y., Senda, Y. Y., et al. (2011). Rapid identification of gram-negative bacteria with and without CTX-M extended-spectrum -lactamase from positive blood culture bottles by PCR followed by microchip gel electrophoresis. *J. Clin. Microbiol.* 49, 1483–1488. doi: 10.1128/JCM.01976-10

Gnandi, K., Han, S., Rezaie-Boroon, M. H., Porrachia, M., and Deheyn, D. (2011). Increased bioavailability of mercury in the Lagoons of Lomé, Togo: the possible role of dredging. *Ambio* 40, 26–42. doi: 10.1007/s13280-010-0094-4

Graham, D. W., Olivares-Rieumont, S., Knapp, C. W., Lima, L., Werner, D., and Bowen, E. (2011). Antibiotic resistance gene abundances associated with waste discharges to the Almendares River near Havana, Cuba. *Environ. Sci. Technol.* 45, 418–424. doi: 10.1021/es102473z

Graham, J. P., and Polizzotto, M. L. (2013). Pit latrines and their impacts on groundwater quality: a systematic review. *Environ. Health Perspect.* 121, 521–530. doi: 10.1289/ehp.1206028

Hall, G. E. M., and Pelchat, P. (1997). Evaluation of a direct solid sampling atomic absorption spectrometer for the trace determination of mercury in geological samples. *Analyst* 122, 921–924. doi: 10.1039/a700194k

Haller, L. L., Pote, J. J., Loizeau, J. J.-L., and Wildi, W. W. (2009). Distribution and survival of faecal indicator bacteria in the sediments of the Bay of Vidy, Lake Geneva, Switzerland. *Ecol. Indic.* 9, 540–547. doi: 10.1016/j.ecolind.2008.08.001

Hothorn, T. T., Bretz, F. F., and Westfall, P. P. (2008). Simultaneous inference in general parametric models. *Biometrical J.* 50, 346–363. doi: 10.1002/bimj.200810425

INSERM (2013). *Résistance Aux Antibiotiques [Online]*. Available online at: http://www.inserm.fr/thematiques/immunologie-inflammation-infectiologie-et-microbiologie/dossiers-d-information/resistance-aux-antibiotiques (Accessed October10, 2015).

Ji, X. X., Shen, Q. Q., Liu, F. F., Ma, J. J., Xu, G. G., Wang, Y. Y., et al. (2012). Antibiotic resistance gene abundances associated with antibiotics and heavy metals in animal manures and agricultural soils adjacent to feedlots in

Shanghai; China. *J. Hazard. Mater.* 235–236, 178–185. doi: 10.1016/j.jhazmat.2012.07.040

Knapp, C. W., Lima, L., Olivares-Rieumont, S., Bowen, E., Werner, D., and Graham, D. W. (2012). Seasonal variations in antibiotic resistance gene transport in the Almendares River, Havana, Cuba. *Front. Microbiol.* 3:396. doi: 10.3389/fmicb.2012.00396

Kümmerer, K. (2004). Resistance in the environment. *J. Antimicrobial Chemother.* 54, 311–320. doi: 10.1093/jac/dkh325

Lachmayr, K. L., Kerkhof, L. J., Dirienzo, A. G., Cavanaugh, C. M., and Ford, T. E. (2009). Quantifying nonspecific TEM betalactamase (blaTEM) genes in a wastewater stream. *Appl. Environ. Microbiol.* 75, 203–211. doi: 10.1128/AEM.01254-08

Laht, M., Karkman, A., Voolaid, V., Ritz, C., Tenson, T., Virta, M., et al. (2014). Abundances of tetracycline, sulphonamide and beta-lactam antibiotic resistance genes in conventional Wastewater Treatment Plants (WWTPs) with different waste load. *PLoS ONE* 9:e103705. doi: 10.1371/journal.pone.0103705

Levy, S. B. S., and Marshall, B. B. (2004). Antibacterial resistance worldwide: causes, challenges and responses. *Nat. Med.* 10, S122–S129. doi: 10.1038/nm1145

Lim, W. Y., Aris, A. Z., and Tengku, H. T. H. (2013). Spatial geochemical distribution and sources of heavy metals in the sediment of Langat River, Western Peninsular Malaysia. *Environ. Forensics* 14, 133–145. doi: 10.1080/15275922.2013.781078

Loizeau, J. L., Arbouille, D., Santiago, S., and Vernet, J. P. (1994). Evaluation of a wide range laser diffraction grain size analyser for use with sediments. *Sedimentology* 41, 353–361. doi: 10.1111/j.1365-3091.1994.tb01410.x

Long, E. R., Ingersoll, C. G., and MacDonald, D. D. (2006). Calculation and uses of mean sediment quality guideline quotients: a critical review. *Environ. Sci. Technol.* 40, 1726–1736. doi: 10.1021/es058012d

MacDonald, D. D., Ingersoll, C. G., and Berger, T. A. (2000). Development and evaluation of consensus-based sediment quality guidelines for freshwater ecosystems. *Arch. Environ. Contam. Toxicol.* 39, 20–31. doi: 10.1007/s002440010075

Madsen, L., Aarestrup, F. M., and Olsen, J. E. (2000). Characterisation of streptomycin resistance determinants in Danish isolates of Salmonella Typhimurium. *Vet. Microbiol.* 75, 73–82. doi: 10.1016/S0378-1135(00)00207-8

Mao, D., Luo, Y., Mathieu, J., Wang, Q., Feng, L., Mu, Q., et al. (2014). Persistence of extracellular DNA in river sediment facilitates antibiotic resistance gene propagation. *Environ. Sci. Technol.* 48, 71–78. doi: 10.1021/es404280v

Marti, E., Variatza, E., Luis Balcazar, J., and Balcazar, J. L. (2014). The role of aquatic ecosystems as reservoirs of antibiotic resistance. *Trends Microbiol.* 22, 36–41. doi: 10.1016/j.tim.2013.11.001

Martínez, J. L. (2008). Antibiotics and antibiotic resistance genes in natural environments. *Science* 321, 365–367. doi: 10.1126/science.1159483

Mavakala, B. K., Le Faucheur, S., Mulaji, C. K., Laffite, A., Devarajan, N., Biey, E. M., et al. (2016). Leachates draining from controlled municipal solid waste landfill: Detailed geochemical characterization and toxicity tests. *Waste Manag.* doi: 10.1016/j.wasman.2016.04.028. [Epub ahead of print].

Mubedi, J. I., Devarajan, N., Le Faucheur, S., Mputu, J. K., Atibu, E. K., Sivalingam, P., et al. (2013). Effects of untreated hospital effluents on the accumulation of toxic metals in sediments of receiving system under tropical conditions: case of South India and Democratic Republic of Congo. *Chemosphere* 93, 1070–1076. doi: 10.1016/j.chemosphere.2013.05.080

Mwanamoki, P. M., Devarajan, N., Thevenon, F., Atibu, E. K., Tshibanda, J. B., Ngelinkoto, P., et al. (2014). Assessment of pathogenic bacteria in water and sediment from a water reservoir under tropical conditions (Lake Ma Vall,e), Kinshasa Democratic Republic of Congo. *Environ. Monit. Assess.* 186, 6821–6830. doi: 10.1007/s10661-014-3891-6

Mwanamoki, P. M., Devarajan, N., Niane, B., Ngelinkoto, P., Thevenon, F., Nlandu, J. W., et al. (2015). Trace metal distributions in the sediments from river-reservoir systems: case of the Congo River and Lake Ma Vallée, Kinshasa (Democratic Republic of Congo). *Environ. Sci. Pollut. Res. Int.* 22, 586–597. doi: 10.1007/s11356-014-3381-y

Ngelinkoto, P., Thevenon, F., Devarajan, N., Birane, N., Maliani, J., Buluku, A., et al. (2014). Trace metal pollution in aquatic sediments and some fish species from the Kwilu-Ngongo River, Democratic Republic of Congo (Bas-Congo). *Toxicol. Environ. Chem.* 96, 48–57. doi: 10.1080/02772248.2014.910211

Niane, B., Guedron, S., Moritz, R., Cosio, C., Ngom, P. M., Deverajan N., et al. (2015). Human exposure to mercury in artisanal small-scale gold mining areas of Kedougou region, Senegal, as a function of occupational activity and fish consumption. *Environ. Sci. Pollut. Res.* 22, 7101–7111. doi: 10.1007/s11356-014-3913-5

Nzolo, D. D., Mulungo, P. R., and avec le soutien du Programme SIAPS (2013). *Évaluation de l'utilisation des Médicaments dans Six Hôpitaux Pilotes où les CPT Sont Fonctionnels en République Démocratique du Congo*. Arlington, VA: Management Sciences for Health.

Orsi, R. H., Stoppe, N. C., Sato, M. I. Z., Gomes, T. A. T., Prado, P. I., Manfio, G. P., et al. (2007). Genetic variability and pathogenicity potential of *Escherichia coli* isolated from recreational water reservoirs. *Res. Microbiol.* 158, 420–427. doi: 10.1016/j.resmic.2007.02.009

Ovreås, L., Forney, L., Daae, F. L. and Torsvik, V. (1997). Distribution of bacterioplankton in meromictic Lake Saelenvannet, as determined by denaturing gradient gel electrophoresis of PCR-amplified gene fragments coding for 16S rRNA. *Appl. Environ. Microbiol.* 63, 3367–3373.

Pardos, M., Benninghoff, C., De Alencastro, L. F., and Wildi, W. (2004). The impact of a sewage treatment plant's effluent on sediment quality in a small bay in Lake Geneva (Switzerland–France). Part 1: Spatial distribution of contaminants and the potential for biological impacts. *Lakes Reservoirs Res. Manage.* 9, 41–52. doi: 10.1111/j.1440-1770.2004.00233.x

Poirel, L. L., Nordmann, P. P., and Bonnin, R. A. R. (2012). Genetic support and diversity of acquired extended spectrum b-lactamases in Gram-negative rods. *Infect. Genet. Evol.* 12, 883–893. doi: 10.1016/j.meegid.2012.02.008

Poté, J., Haller, L., Kottelat, R., Sastre, V., Arpagaus, P., and Wildi, W. (2009). Persistence and growth of faecal culturable bacterial indicators in water column and sediments of Vidy Bay, Lake Geneva, Switzerland. *J. Environ. Sci.* 21, 62–69. doi: 10.1016/S1001-0742(09)60012-7

Poté, J., Haller, L., Loizeau, J.-L., Garcia Bravo, A., Sastre, V., and Wildi, W. (2008). Effects of a sewage treatment plant outlet pipe extension on the distribution of contaminants in the sediments of the Bay of Vidy, Lake Geneva, Switzerland. *Bioresour. Technol.* 99, 7122–7131. doi: 10.1016/j.biortech.2007.12.075

Ram, J. L. J., Ritchie, R. P. R., Fang, J. J., Gonzales, F. S. F., and Selegean, J. P. J. (2004). Sequence-based source tracking of *Escherichia coli* based on genetic diversity of beta-glucuronidase. *J. Environ. Qual.* 33, 1024–1032. doi: 10.2134/jeq2004.1024

Roos-Barraclough, F., Givelet, N., Martinez-Cortizas, A., Goodsite, M. E., Biester, H., and Shotyk, W. (2002). An analytical protocol for the determination of total mercury concentrations in solid peat samples. *Sci. Total Environ.* 292, 129–139. doi: 10.1016/S0048-9697(02)00035-9

Sakan, S. M., Dordevic, D. S., Manojlovic, D., Dragana, D. S., Dragan, D., Predrag, P. S., et al. (2009). Assessment of heavy metal pollutants accumulation in the Tisza river sediments. *J. Environ. Manage.* 90, 3382–3390. doi: 10.1016/j.jenvman.2009.05.013

Schwartz, T., Kohnen, W., Hansen, B., and Obst, U. (2003). Detection of antibiotic-resistant bacteria and their resistance genes in wastewater, surface water, and drinking water biofilms. *FEMS Microbiol. Ecol.* 43, 325–335. doi: 10.1111/j.1574-6941.2003.tb01073.x

Seiler, C., and Berendonk, T. U. (2012). Heavy metal driven co-selection of antibiotic resistance in soil and water bodies impacted by agriculture and aquaculture. *Front. Microbiol.* 3:399. doi: 10.3389/fmicb.2012.00399

Sidrach Cardona, R., Marti, E., Balcazar, J. L., Becares, E., Hijosa Valsero, M., and Balcázar, J. L. (2014). Prevalence of antibiotic-resistant fecal bacteria in a river impacted by both an antibiotic production plant and urban treated discharges. *Sci. Total Environ.* 488–489, 220–227. doi: 10.1016/j.scitotenv.2014.04.100

Sommer, M. O., Dantas, G., and Church, G. M. (2009). Functional characterization of the antibiotic resistance reservoir in the human microflora. *Science*, 325, 1128–1131. doi: 10.1126/science.1176950

Spindler, A. A., Fuentefria, D. B. D., Corcao, G. G., Otton, L. M. L., and Corção, G. G. (2012). Beta-lactams resistance and presence of class 1 integron in *Pseudomonas* spp. isolated from untreated hospital effluents in Brazil. *Anton. van Leeuwenhoek* 102, 73–81. doi: 10.1007/s10482-012-9714-2

Stoll, C., Sidhu, J. P. S., Tiehm, A., and Toze, S. (2012). Prevalence of clinically relevant antibiotic resistance genes in surface water samples collected from Germany and Australia. *Environ. Sci. Technol.* 46, 9716–9726. doi: 10.1021/es302020s

Suzuki, S., Ogo, M., Koike, T., Takada, H., and Newman, B. (2015). Sulfonamide and tetracycline resistance genes in total- and culturable-bacterial assemblages in South African aquatic environments. *Front. Microbiol.* 6:796. doi: 10.3389/fmicb.2015.00796

Tacao, M. M., Moura, A. A., Henriques, I. I., Tacão, M. M., and Correia, A. A. (2014). Co-resistance to different classes of antibiotics among ESBL-producers from aquatic systems. *Water Res.* 48, 100–107. doi: 10.1016/j.watres.2013.09.021

Team, R. C. (2015). *R: A Language and Environment for Statistical Computing.* Vienne: R Foundation for Statistical Computing.

Thevenon, F., Adatte, T., Wildi, W., and Pote, J. (2012a). Antibiotic resistant bacteria/genes dissemination in lacustrine sediments highly increased following cultural eutrophication of Lake Geneva (Switzerland). *Chemosphere* 86, 468–476. doi: 10.1016/j.chemosphere.2011.09.048

Thevenon, F., Regier, N., Benagli, C., Tonolla, M., Adatte, T., Wildi, W., et al. (2012b). Characterization of fecal indicator bacteria in sediments cores from the largest freshwater lake of Western Europe (Lake Geneva, Switzerland). *Ecotoxicol. Environ. Saf.* 78, 50–56. doi: 10.1016/j.ecoenv.2011.11.005

Tshibanda, J. B., Devarajan, N., Birane, N., Mwanamoki, P. M., Atibu, E. K., Mpiana, P. T., et al. (2014). Microbiological and physicochemical characterization of water and sediment of an urban river: N'Djili River, Kinshasa, Democratic Republic of the Congo. *Sustainability Water Qual. Ecol.* 3–4, 47–54. doi: 10.1016/j.swaqe.2014.07.001

Verlicchi, P., Galletti, A., Petrovic, M., and Barceló, D. (2010). Hospital effluents as a source of emerging pollutants: an overview of micropollutants and sustainable treatment options. *J. Hydrol.* 389, 416–428. doi: 10.1016/j.jhydrol.2010.06.005

WHO (2014). *Antimicrobial Resistance. Global Report on Surveillance.* Geneva: World Health Organization.

WHO (2015). *Drinking-water Quality.* Geneva: World Health Organization.

Wildi, W., Dominik, J., Loizeau, J. L., Thomas, R. L., Favarger, P.-Y., Haller, L., et al. (2004). River, reservoir and lake sediment contamination by heavy metals downstream from urban areas of Switzerland. *Lakes Reservoir. Res. Manag.* 9, 75–87. doi: 10.1111/j.1440-1770.2004.00236.x

Xi, C. C., Zhang, Y. Y., Marrs, C. F. C., Ye, W. W., Simon, C. C., Foxman, B. B., et al. (2009). Prevalence of antibiotic resistance in drinking water treatment and distribution systems. *Appl. Environ. Microbiol.* 75, 5714–5718. doi: 10.1128/AEM.00382-09

Zhao, L., Mi, D., Chen, Y., Wang, L., and Sun, Y. (2015). Ecological risk assessment and sources of heavy metals in sediment from Daling River basin. *Environ. Sci. Pollut. Res.* 22, 5975–5984. doi: 10.1007/s11356-014-3770-2

18

Effect of Tulathromycin on Colonization Resistance, Antimicrobial Resistance and Virulence of Human Gut Microbiota in Chemostats

Haihong Hao[1,2†], *Shengxi Zhou*[2†], *Guyue Cheng*[2], *Menghong Dai*[2], *Xu Wang*[1], *Zhenli Liu*[1], *Yulian Wang*[1,2*] *and Zonghui Yuan*[1,2*]

[1] *National Reference Laboratory of Veterinary Drug Residues and MAO Key Laboratory for Detection of Veterinary Drug Residues, Huazhong Agricultural University, Wuhan, China,* [2] *MOA Laboratory for Risk Assessment of Quality and Safety of Livestock and Poultry Products, Huazhong Agricultural University, Wuhan, China*

***Correspondence:**
Yulian Wang
wangyulian@mail.hzau.edu.cn;
Zonghui Yuan
yuan5802@mail.hzau.edu.cn

†These authors have contributed equally to this work.

To evaluate microbiological safety of tulathromycin on human intestinal bacteria, tulathromycin (0, 0.1, 1, 10, and 100 μg/mL) was added into Chemostats. Before and after drug exposure, we monitored (1) population, SCFA products, antimicrobial resistance, and colonization resistance of gut microbiota, and (2) the antimicrobial resistance genes, transferability, virulent genes, pathogenicity of *Enterococus faecalis*. Results showed that low level of tulathromycin did not exhibit microbiological hazard on resistance selection and colonization resistance. However, high level of tulathromycin (10 and 100 μg/mL) may disturb colonization resistance of human gut microbiota and select antimicrobial resistant *E. faecalis*. Most of the selected resistant *E. faecalis* carried resistant gene of *ermB*, transferable element of Tn*1545* and three virulence genes (*esp*, *cylA*, and *ace*). One of them (*E. faecalis* 143) was confirmed to have higher horizontal transfer risk and higher pathogenicity. The calculated no observable adverse effect concentration (NOAEC) and microbiological acceptable daily intake (mADI) in our study was 1 μg/mL and 14.66 μg/kg.bw/day, respectively.

Keywords: tulathromycin, gut microbiota, colonization resistance, antimicrobial resistance, chemostat

INTRODUCTION

Tulathromycin is the first and only member of the triamilide sub-class of macrolide. Tulathromycin is used therapeutically in treatment of respiratory disease in swine and cattle at a single dose of 2.5 mg/kg.bw. It has been registered in more than 30 countries across America, Europe, Oceania, and Asia and played important role in veterinary medicine (FDA, 2004). This agent is characterized by rapid absorption from the injection site, extensive distribution to tissue, and slow elimination. The withdrawal period for cattle and swine is 22 and 5 days, respectively. This drug is excreted primarily unchanged (90%) in feces (2/3) and in urine (1/3), suggesting that it may reach to human colon and remain its antimicrobial activity (Benchaoui et al., 2004; EMEA, 2004; Nowakowski et al., 2004).

The residue of tulathromycin in animal food may have unintended microbiological effects on human gut microbiota. The possible harmful effects may be: (1) shifts in bacterial counts and biochemistry, (2) destruction of colonization resistance, (3) emergence of antimicrobial resistant bacteria (Cerniglia and Kotarski, 1999; Nutsch et al., 2005). Additionally, antibiotic resistant bacteria may have enhanced fitness or high virulence (Mundy et al., 2000). Human intestinal strains may also serve as reservoirs for antimicrobial resistant determinations and mediates the gene transfer (Salyers et al., 2004).

Based on *in vitro* antibiotic susceptibility tests, microbiological ADIs recommended by Food and Drug Administration (FDA), European Medicine Agency (EMA), and Australian Pesticides and Veterinary Medicines Authority (APVMA) were 50, 10.99, and 5 μg/kg.bw/d, respectively. The large difference in these mADI may due to the disadvantage and limitation of short-term *in vitro* antibiotic susceptibility tests in evaluation of long-term effects of tulathromycin residues posed on human intestinal bacteria and in analyze of impact of tulathromycin on colonization resistance and emergence of antimicrobial resistance of human colonic microbiota (Cerniglia and Kotarski, 2005). Therefore, microbiological safety assessment measures of tulathromycin residues is largely inadequate. It is largely unknown that what is the effect of long-term exposure to tulathromycin on colonization resistance of human intestinal microbiota and on antimicrobial resistance development, virulence change, and gene transfer in some specific intestinal bacteria.

In the present article, the chemostat model of human colonic gut, which is an approach recommended by VICH (VICH GL-36) and some previous studies (Carman and Woodburn, 2001; Carman et al., 2004, 2005), is used to evaluate microbiological safety of tulathromycin on human intestinal microbiota.

MATERIALS AND METHODS

Chemicals

The tulathromycin (TUL), erythromycin (ERY), and lincomycin (LIN) were dissolved in methanol and then diluted with deionized water. The ciprofloxacin (CIP), tetracycline (TET), and rifampicin (RIF) were dissolved in deionized water. Tulathromycin was purchased from Liu He animal Pharmaceutical Co., Ltd. (Qingdao, China). The erythromycin, lincomycin, ciprofloxacin, tetracycline, and rifampicin were purchased from SIGMA.

Bacteria Strains

The *E. coli* ATCC 25922, *Enterococcus faecalis* ATCC29212, and *Micrococcus luteus* ATCC 9341 were purchased from American Type Culture Collection (ATCC). The *E. coli* ATCC 25922 and *E. faecalis* ATCC29212 were used as quality controls for species identification and minimum inhibitory concentration (MIC) determination. The *M. luteus* ATCC 9341 were used as an indicator for determination of the concentration of tulathromycin. *E. faecalis* JH2-2 (Rifampicin MIC > 50 μg/mL) and *E. coli* NK5449 (Rifampicin MIC > 100 μg/mL), purchased from Belgian coordinated collections of microorganisms and Institute of microbiology in Chinese academy of sciences, respectively, were used as receptors for conjugation test. The *Salmonella* Typhimurium SI3 was a ciprofloxacin resistant strain which was selected in our previous study (Sun et al., 2011). This strain was used as the challenge strain for evaluating the colonization resistance of chemostat.

Preparation of Fresh Fecal Samples and Strain Isolation

Fresh fecal samples from six adult volunteers who had no history of antibiotic usage and gastrointestinal disturbance within the preceding 3 months were prepared following previous method (Carman and Woodburn, 2001; Hao et al., 2013). The use of human fecal samples was approved by the ethical Committee of Huazhong Agricultural University (approval number hzauch 2013-002).

Strain Isolation and MIC Determination from Fresh Fecal Samples

The four predominant intestinal bacteria (*E. coli*, *Enterococcus*, *Bifidobacterium*, and Bacteroides *fragilis*) were isolated from the fresh fecal samples of six adult volunteers by selective agars (Eosin methylene blue agar, bile esculin azide agar, BBL media, and bacteroides bile esculin agar). Ten isolates of each species were obtained from fresh fecal sample of each volunteer. After species identification by classic biochemical tests and ABI 3130 system (Applied Biosystem, USA), 32 isolated strains of each species were subjected to MIC determination by agar dilution method provide by CLSI (document M7-A5 for aerobic bacterial and document M11-A5 for anaerobic bacterial). The *E. coli* ATCC25922 and *E. faecalis* ATCC 29212 were used as quality control for MIC determination. The minimum concentration to inhibit 50% of isolates (MIC_{50}) and the minimum concentration to inhibit 90% of isolates (MIC_{90}) was calculated based on the MIC distribution and estimated by probability analysis using SPSS statistical package (Kays and Graff, 2002; Xu et al., 2013).

Designation of Tulathromycin Dosage in Preliminary Test

The preliminary test for selection of tulathromycin concentration was carried out following the method in previous study (Hao et al., 2013). Briefly, different concentrations of tulathromycin (0, 0.5, 10, 20, 40, 60, 80, 100 μg/mL) were mixed with 50 mL prepared fecal samples at the final concentration of 20% (w/v). The activity of tulathromycin on populations of four different bacteria (*E. coli*, *Enterococcus*, *Bifidobacterium*, and *B. fragilis*) were determined by bacterial colony count using selective agars. The highest concentration of tulathromycin was selected for further experiments as it was able to significantly change the population of four predominant intestinal bacteria.

The low to intermediate concentration of tulathromycin (0.1, 1, and 10 μg/mL) were designed based on the acceptable daily intake (ADI) recommended by FDA (50 μg/kg.bw/d), EMA (10.99 μg/kg.bw/d), and APVMA (5 μg/kg.bw/d). In those designed concentration, 1 μg/mL tulathromycin was the mean MIC_{50}-value to the most sensitive *Bifidobacterium* strains. One group was drug free methanol control (0 μg/mL tulathromycin).

Establishment of Chemostats and the Time Schedule

The establishment of chemostat models and the time schedule were carried out following the method in previous studies (Carman and Woodburn, 2001; Hao et al., 2013). Briefly, 50 mL prepared fecal suspension at the final concentration of 20% (w/v) was inoculated into each culture vessel. After 7 h incubation, culture medium was pumped into and out of the culture vessel at a uniform rate of 35 mL/h to maintain 500 mL of culture medium.

After 7 days running, the chemostats reached to a steady state. From 7th to 13th day, the chemostats were kept on running on steady state without administration of tulathromycin(Chen et al., 2011, 2014). From 14th to 20th day, five designed concentrations of tulathromycin (0, 0.1, 1, 10, and 100 μg/mL) were, respectively, infused into the culture medium. During 20th–22nd day, the tulathromycin was withdrawn from chemostat models and 1 mL of 6×10^8 CFU/mL (2X McFarland) *Salmonella* Typhimurium SI3 were daily inoculated into each chemostat. Then the chemostats continued to run for another 7 days (to 29th day) without challenge of *Salmonella* Typhimurium (Moffatt, 2007).

Monitoring Bacterial Counts in the Chemostats

During day 7–20, samples were daily taken from each chemostat. The changes of four predominant bacteria (*E. coli*, *Enterococcus*, *B. fragilis*, and *Bifidobacterium*) were measured by viable cell counting (Hao et al., 2013, 2015).

Monitoring Short Chain Fatty Acids (SCFAs) in the Chemostats

During day 7–20, samples were daily taken from each chemostat. The concentration of three primary SCFAs (acetic acid, butryric acid, and propionic acid) were monitored using a developed gas chromatographic (GC) method (Hao et al., 2013, 2015).

Evaluation of Colonization Resistance in the Chemostats

From day 20th to 29th, samples were taken from each chemostat to monitor the population of *Salmonella* Typhimurium SI3 using bismuth sulfite (BS) agar containing 4 μg/mL ciprofloxacin(Sun et al., 2011; Hao et al., 2013, 2015). The colonization resistance was disrupted if *Salmonella* Typhimurium SI3 was successfully colonized into chemostat models.

Monitoring Resistance Rate in the Chemostats

During day 8–20, samples were daily taken from each chemostat. The change of resistance rate was also monitored following the method in previous study (Hao et al., 2013, 2015). The resistance rates of *E. coli* and *Enterococcus* were equal to the number of resistant colonies on the selective agars containing 4-fold MIC_{90} of tulathromycin divided by the number of total colonies on the selective agars without tulathromycin. The 4-fold MIC_{90} was used for selection of tulathromycin resistance on basis of VICH GL-36 document and some previous reports of resistance selection (Allen and Bierman, 2009; Kadlec et al., 2011).

Determination of Resistance Pheno- and Geno-type in the Selected *E. faecalis*

During day 8–20, a total of 70 Enterococcus isolates were random selected from samples in the chemostat containing 100 μg/mL tulathromycin. After species identification by biochemical tests and PCR amplification, 64 isolates were identified as *E. faecalis*. Among these *E. faecalis*, 34 isolates were obtained before the administration of tulathromycin, while 30 isolates were selected after the treatment with tulathromycin. The susceptibility of the 64 *E. faecalis* to macrolide, lincosamides, and tetracycline were determined by agar dilution method.

The genes involved in macrolide-lincosamides-streptogramins (MLS) resistance with a methylation mechanism were determined by PCR amplification of known *erm* genes using specific primers for *ermA*, *ermB*, and *ermC* (see **Table 1**). The genes involved in antibiotic efflux systems were determined using specific primers for the *mefA/E* gene (see **Table 1**). The PCR procedure was followed the method in previous published paper (Portillo et al., 2000).

Detect Transfer Risk of the Selected Macrolide Resistant *E. faecalis*

The macrolide-resistant isolates containing *ermB* gene were selected to determine the presence of transposons Tn*1545* and

TABLE 1 | PCR primers and products for detection of macrolides resistance gene and transposons and virulence determinants in *E. faecalis*.

Primers	5′–3′	Target fragment (bp)	GeneBank no.
ermA	F: GTTCAAGAACAATCAATACAGAG R: GGATCAGGAAAAGGACATTTTAC	421	FN668375
ermB	F: GAAAAGGTACTCAACCAAATA R: AGTAACGGTACTTAAATTGTTTAC	639	NC_014498
ermC	F: AATCGGCTCAGGAAAAGG R: ATCGTCAATTCCTGCATG	534	NC_014498
mef (A/E)	F: AGTATCATTAATCACTAGTGC R: TTCTTCTGGTACTAAAAGTGG	346	NC_018641
Tn *1545*	F: CTTAGAAGCAAACTTAAGAGTGTGT R: GGTTGAGTA CCTTTTCATTCGTTAA	382	NC_013644
Tn *917*	F: ATCTGACGGTGACATCTCTC R: GGTTGAGTACCTTTTCATTCGTTAA	652	NC_017312
oop	F: TTGCTAATGCTAGTCCACGACC R: GCGTCAACACTTGCATTGCCGA	032	AF034770
gelE	F: ACCCCGTATCATTGGTTT R: ACGCATTGCTTTTCCATC	405	M37185
cylA	F: GACTCGGGGATTGATAGGC R: GCTGCTAAAGCTGCGCTTAC	688	AD1CLYL
ace	F: GGAATGACCGAGAACGATGGC R: GCTTGATGTTGGCCTGCTTCCG	616	AF159247
asal	F: CCAGCCAACTATGGCGGAATC R: CCTGTCGCAAGATCGACTGTA	529	SFPASA1

Tn*917* using the primers (see **Table 1**) and method established in previous study (Okitsu et al., 2005). Filter mating method was used to investigate the conjugative transfer of the selected macrolide resistant *E. faecalis*. A representative macrolide-resistant isolate containing *ermB* and composite transposon was selected as donor strain. The recipients were two rifampicin-resistant strains, *E. faecalis* JH2-2 (Rif MIC > 50 μg/mL) and *E. coli* NK5449 (Rif MIC > 100 μg/mL). The donor and recipient strains were mixed into the conjugation system at the ratio of 1:9 and incubated on the serum agar for 48 h at 37°C. The number of donor, recipient and transconjugants were counted by agar plate containing rifampicin and/or erythromycin.

Determination of Virulence in the Selected *E. faecalis*

The presence of virulence factors, including the surface protein (*esp*), haemolysin activator (*cylA*), gelatinase (*gelE*), collagen binding protein (*ace*), and aggregation substances (*asal*), were determined by PCR in the 64 *E. faecalis* isolates obtained in the pre- and post-treatment of tulathromycin in the chemostat. PCR primers used in this study were listed in **Table 1**. The annealing temperatures of five virulence factors were 65°C for *esp*, 51°C for *gelE*, 61°C for *CylA*, 61°C for *ace* and 63°C for *asal* gene, respectively.

In order to compare the changes of pathogenicity of *E. faecalis*, two representative *E. faecalis* isolates (*E. faecalis* 143 and *E. faecalis* 174) were subjected to determine the median lethal dose (LD_{50}). Briefly, the 72 SPF Kunming mice with body weight of 25–28 g were randomly divided into nine groups with half males and half females. The groups were, respectively, challenged with *E. faecalis* isolate by intraperitoneal injection of 0.5 mL diluted concentration of bacteria suspension (10^7–10^{10} CFU/mouse). The dead mice were carefully dissected in a bacteria-free operating environment. The LD_{50} was calculated by improved Karber method. All experimental procedures were performed according to the guidelines of the committee on the use and care of the laboratory animals in Hubei province China. The study was approved by the Animal Care Center, Hubei Science and Technology Agency in China. All the animals were monitored throughout the study for any sign of adverse effect.

Statistical Analysis

All experiments were performed in triplicate. The statistical analysis was performed following the previous study (Hao et al., 2013, 2015). Briefly, a "mean pre-treatment" level and 95% prediction interval (PI95) for each parameter was set up based on the data obtained from each culture vessel during steady state (day 7–13) and used as reference boundaries for assessing the effect of tulathromycin on each parameter in the drug exposure period (day 14–20).

NOAEC and mADI Calculation

The NOAEC was the no observable adverse effect concentration in this study. The microbiological acceptable daily intake (mADI) for tulathromycin was calculated following the guideline of VICH GL-36. The formula used for mADI calculation was that mADI = NOAEC × daily fecal bolus/(fraction of oral dose available for micro-organisms × weight of human).

RESULTS

MIC_{90} of the Strains Isolated from Fresh Fecal Samples

The 32 strains of each species (*E. coli*, *Enterococcus*, *Bifidobacterium*, and *B. fragilis*) were isolated from fresh fecal samples of six volunteers. The MIC for 90% of isolates (MIC_{90}) of tulathromycin for *E. coli*, *Enterococcus*, *Bifidobacterium*, and *B. fragilis* were 5.53, 7.87, 1.35, and 2.30 μg/mL, respectively. After dilution, the methanol used for dissolving tulathromycin did not exert some antimicrobial effect.

The Designed Four Tulathromycin Concentration

From the preliminary test, 100 μg/mL was the highest concentration of tulathromycin which could significantly change the population of four predominant intestinal bacteria. Based on the ADI-values recommended by FDA, EMA, and APVMA, the lower concentration of tulathromycin were designed as 0.1, 1, and 10 μg/mL.

Effect of Tulathromycin on Bacterial Counts

The population of *E. coli* was kept between 3.667 × 10^6 and 5.482 × 10^6 CFU/mL in steady state based on statistical data among five chemostats (**Figure 1A**). Three days after administration of 100 μg/mL tulathromycin, the population of *E. coli* was decreased to 6.556 × 10^5 CFU/mL which was ~6-fold lower than 95% lower confidence limit. However, the three low concentration of tulathromycin (0.1, 1, and 10 μg/mL) did not significantly change the number of *E. coli*.

Pre-treatment of tulathromycin (day 8–13), the *Enterococcus* counts was in the range of 9.526 × 10^4–8.674 × 10^5 CFU/mL (**Figure 1B**). Under exposure to 10 μg/mL tulathromycin, *Enterococcus* count was decreased ~1.6-fold in the 5th day of post-treatment. On the contrary, the total number of *Enterococcus* was increased almost 3-fold from 18th day after administration of 100 μg/mL tulathromycin.

The number of *Bifidobacterium* varied from 1.105 × 10^7 to 2.70 × 10^8 CFU/mL (**Figure 1C**) during day 8–13. The administration of 100 μg/mL tulathromycin significantly decreased the number of *Bifidobacterium* in the chemostat. It was shown that *Bifidobacterium* count was decreased ~10-fold lower than 95% lower confidence limit.

Significant and dose-dependent effects of tulathromycin on *B. fragilis* counts were observed in all tested concentration of tulathromycin. After treatment by 10 and 100 μg/mL tulathromycin, *B. fragilis* count was decreased 6- and 90-fold lower than 95% lower confidence limit, respectively (**Figure 1D**).

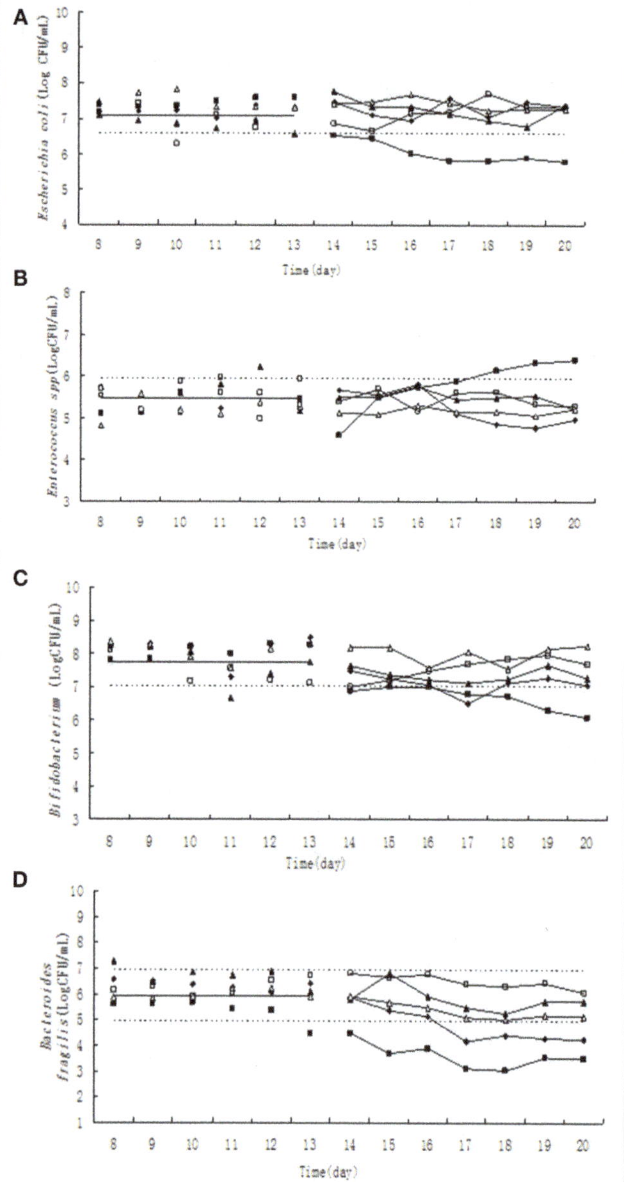

FIGURE 1 | Effect of tulathromycin on *Escherichia coli* (A), *Enterococcus* (B), *Bifidobacterium* (C), *Bacteroides fragilis* (D) in chemostat model. □, 0 μg/ mL; Δ, 0.1 μg/ mL; ▲, 1 μg/mL; ♦, 10 μg/mL; ■, 100 μg/mL; ———, pre-treatment mean; --------, 95% predicated interval.

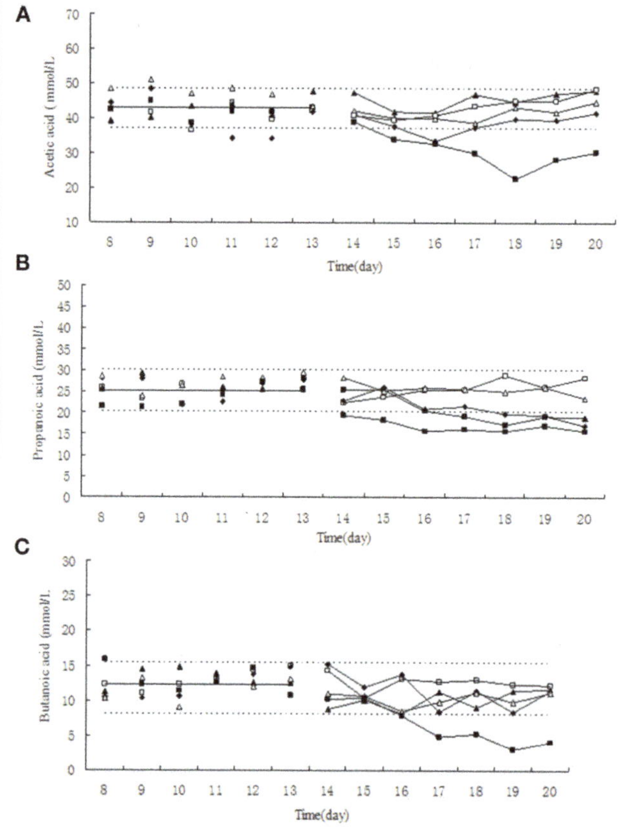

FIGURE 2 | Effect of tulathromycin on acetic acid (A), propionic acid (B), butyric acid (C) in chemotat models. □, 0 μg/mL; Δ, 0.1 μg/mL; ▲, 1 μg/mL; ♦, 10 μg/mL; ■, 100 μg/mL; ———, pre-treatment mean; --------, 95% predicated interval.

Effect of Tulathromycin on Short Chain Fatty Acid (SCFA)

The relative low concentration of tulathromycin (0, 0.1, and 1 μg/mL) did not significantly change the molar concentration of acetic acid, propionc acid and butyric acid (**Figure 2**). Under exposure to 10 μg/mL tulathromycin, the concentration of acetic acid and propionc acid was slightly decreased. Upon the administration of 100 μg/mL tulathromycin, the concentration of acetic acid, propionc acid, and butyric acid were decreased ~1.3, 1.3, and 2.68-fold lower than 95% lower confidence limit, respectively. Among the three dominant SCFAs, the concentration of propionc acid was changed remarkably under exposure of tulathromycin and present significant dose-dependent effect of tulathromycin.

Effect of Tulathromycin on Colonization Resistance

In the single growth control group, the growth of *Salmonella* Typhimurium was stable at the level of 3.75×10^7–1.54×10^8 CFU/mL, indicating that *Salmonella* Typhimurium grew well in the chemostat model containing no drug and gut microbiome (**Figure 3**). However, the colony number of *Salmonella* Typhimurium tapered to 10^2 CFU/mL on day 31 in the chemostat containing stable gut microbiome, suggesting that the gut microbiome may establish colonization resistance to exogenous pathogens. After treatment of lower concentration of tulathromycin (10, 1, and 0.1 μg/mL), the number of *Salmonella* Typhimurium was also decreased to the level of 10^2 CFU/mL. In contrast, the colonization number of *Salmonella* Typhimurium was in the range of 2.08×10^5–7.15×10^6 CFU/mL in the chemostat administrated by highest concentration of tulathromycin (100 μg/mL), suggesting that the high concentration of drug may disturb the colonization resistance of gut microbiome and induce the proliferation of pathogen (**Figure 3**).

Effect of Tulathromycin on Resistant Rate

Before the treatment of tulathromycin, 10–30% of tulathromycin resistance was observed in *Escherichia coli* and in *Enterococcus* strains (**Figures 4A,B**). Under exposure to 10 μg/mL tulathromycin, the percentage of resistant *Enterococcus* was slight increased (**Figure 4B**). After treatment with 100 μg/mL tulathromycin, the resistant rates in *E. coli* and *Enterococcus* were obviously higher than control group, especially in *Enterococcus*, it reach up to 80% (**Figures 4A,B**). After administration of different concentration of tulathromycin, regular changes were not observed in *Bifidobacterium* and *Bacteroides fragilis* (**Figures 4C,D**).

Resistant Phenotype and Genotype of the Selected *E. faecalis*

After species confirmation, 34 and 30 *E. faecalis* isolates were selected from chemostats pre- and post-treatment, respectively. The MIC_{50} and MIC_{90} of these 64 *E. faecalis* strains to erythromycin, tulathromycin, lincomycin, and tetracycline were showed in **Table 2**. The 34 *E. faecalis* strains isolated from chemostats before administration of tulathromycin exhibited high susceptibility to erythromycin, tulathromycin and tetracycline (MIC $\leq$ 4 μg/mL), and low resistance to lincomycin (MIC = 16, 32 μg/mL). However, after treatment with tulathromycin, 30 *E. faecalis* isolates (except for the strains of 141, 142, 144, and 164) showed high-level resistance to the four tested antibiotics (MIC $\geq$ 4 μg/mL). The MIC_{50} of erythromycin, tulathromycin, lincomycin, and tetracycline to *E. faecalis* were considerably increased for 88.9, 49.8, 5.1, and 45.4-fold, respectively.

About 88.46% of the tulathromycin resistant *E. faecalis* isolated from chemostats harbored macrolide resistance associated gene of *ermB* (**Table 3**). However, the tested macrolide resistance associated genes (*ermABC* and *mefA/E*) were free in the tulathromycin resistant *E. faecalis* strains (**Table 3**).

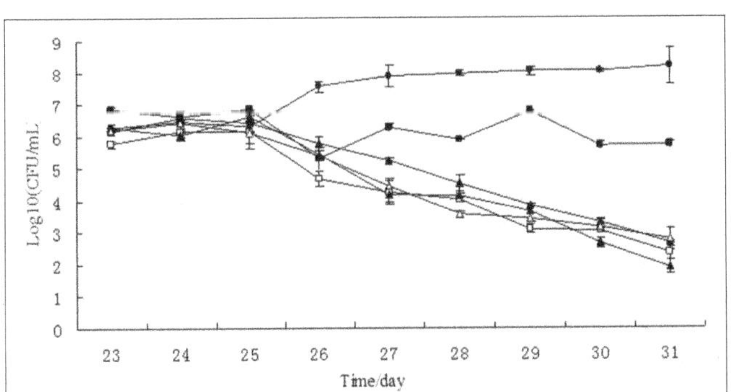

FIGURE 3 | Growth curves of *Salmonella* Typhimurium in chemostat models. □, 0 μg/mL; Δ, 0.1 μg/mL; ▲, 1 μg/mL; ♦, 10 μg/mL; ■, 100 μg/mL; •, growth control.

Transfer Risk of Macrolide Resistant *E. faecalis*

All of *ermB* containing *E. faecalis* strains also harbored composite transposon of Tn*1545* (**Table 3**). When the *E. faecalis* 143 strain containing both *ermB* and Tn*1545* was selected as donor strain and subjected to conjugation transfer test, the result showed that macrolide resistant determinants could transfer to *E. faecalis* JH2-2 and *E. coli* NK5449 at the frequencies of 10^{-6}–10^{-7} (**Table 4**).

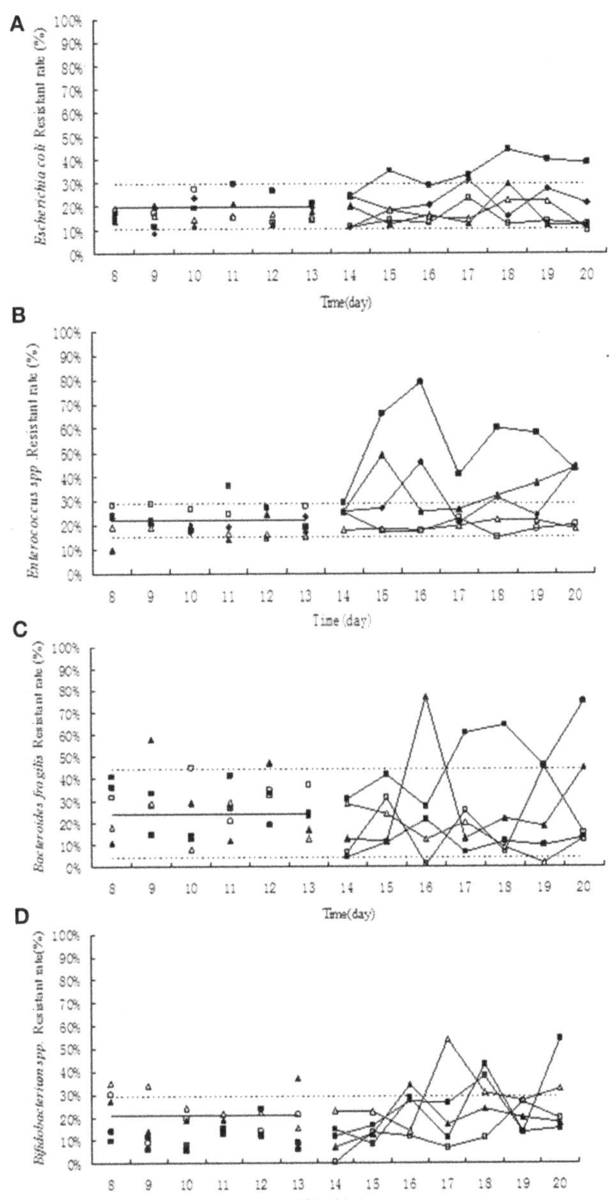

FIGURE 4 | Effect of tulathromycin on resistance in *Escherichia coli* (A), *Enterococcus* (B), Bifidobacterium (C), *Bacteroides fragilis* (D) in chemostat model. □, 0 μg/mL; Δ, 0.1 μg/mL; ▲, 1 μg/mL; ♦, 10 μg/ mL; ■, 100 μg/ mL; ———, pre-treatment mean; - - - - - - - -, 95%predicated interval.

TABLE 2 | Comparison of MICs of separated *E. faecalis* strains, before and after treated with four drugs.

Drug	Pre- or post-treatment	Strains (*N*)	MICs (μg/mL)											MIC_{50} (μg/mL)	MIC_{90} (μg/mL)
			256	128	64	32	16	8	4	2	1	0.5	0.25		
ERY	Pre-	34						1	2	26	4		1	2.610	5.211
ERY	Post-	30	17	9						3	1			231.698	–
TLU	Pre-	34							31	2			1	4.904	10.995
TLU	Post-	30	21	4					3	2				244.149	–
LIN	Pre-	34				27	6						1	41.706	221.77
LIN	Post-	30	21	1	2	6								213.721	669.13
TET	Pre-	34								33			1	2.552	4.437
TET	Post-	30		22	2					5		1		115.681	–

MIC_{50} = minimum concentration to inhibit 50% of isolates; MIC_{90} = minimum concentration to inhibit 90% of isolates. MIC_{90}- and MIC_{50}-values are estimated values by probability analysis by SPSS (Kays and Graff, 2002; Xu et al., 2013); "–" datas not given; white areas was pre-treatment group; gray areas was post-treatment group; ERY, erythromycin; TLU, tulathromycin; LIN, lincomycin tetracycline.

TABLE 3 | The relationship of MIC, resistant gene and virulence gene in *E. faecalis* isolated during drug administration.

Isolates no.	MICs				Resistant gene		Virulence determinants			
	ERY	TLU	LIN	TET	*ermB*	Tn1545	*esp*	*cylA*	*gelE*	*ace*
141	2	4	32	2	–	–	–	–	+	+
142	2	4	32	2	–	–	–	–	+	+
143	128	256	256	128	+	+	+	+	–	+
144	2	4	32	2	–	–	–	–	+	+
145	256	256	32	2	–	+	–	–	+	+
151	128	256	256	128	+	–	+	+	–	+
152	128	128	256	128	+	+	+	+	–	+
154	1	2	32	2	–	–	–	–	+	+
155	128	128	32	0.5	–	–	–	–	+	+
161	256	256	256	128	+	+	+	+	–	+
162	256	256	256	128	+	+	+	+	–	+
164	256	256	256	128	+	+	+	+	–	+
165	256	256	256	128	+	+	+	+	–	+
171	256	256	256	128	+	+	+	+	–	+
172	128	256	64	64	+	–	–	–	–	–
174	256	256	64	64	–	+	–	–	–	–
181	128	256	256	128	+	+	+	+	–	+
182	256	256	256	128	+	+	+	+	–	+
183	256	256	256	128	+	+	+	+	–	+
185	256	256	256	128	+	+	–	–	–	–
191	128	256	256	128	+	+	+	+	–	+
192	128	128	256	128	+	+	+	+	–	+
193	256	256	256	128	+	+	+	+	–	+
194	256	256	256	128	+	+	+	+	–	+
195	256	256	256	128	+	+	+	+	–	+
201	128	128	128	128	+	+	+	+	–	+
202	256	256	256	128	+	+	+	+	–	+
203	256	256	256	128	+	+	+	+	–	–
204	256	256	256	128	+	+	+	+	–	+
205	256	256	256	128	+	+	+	+	–	+

The isolate was numbered by isolated day and strain number. For example, isolate 143 was the third isolate obtained in 14th day. Gray shades used to distinct the positive and negative of special virulence factor.

TABLE 4 | The frequencies of conjugation transfer between donor and host strains.

Receptor strains	Times	Donor strain (CFU/mL)	Host strain (CFU/mL)	Transconjugant (CFU/mL)	Transfer frequency
E. faecalis JH2-2	1	1.21×10^9	2.62×10^8	2.04×10^3	7.79×10^{-6}
	2	4.30×10^9	6.75×10^8	9.40×10^2	1.39×10^{-6}
	3	3.72×10^9	4.35×10^8	2.60×10^3	5.98×10^{-6}
E. coli NK5449	1	8.42×10^8	6.82×10^8	1.90×10^2	2.79×10^{-7}
	2	1.25×10^9	3.71×10^8	2.20×10^2	5.93×10^{-7}
	3	1.13×10^9	1.65×10^8	6.60×10^2	4.00×10^{-6}

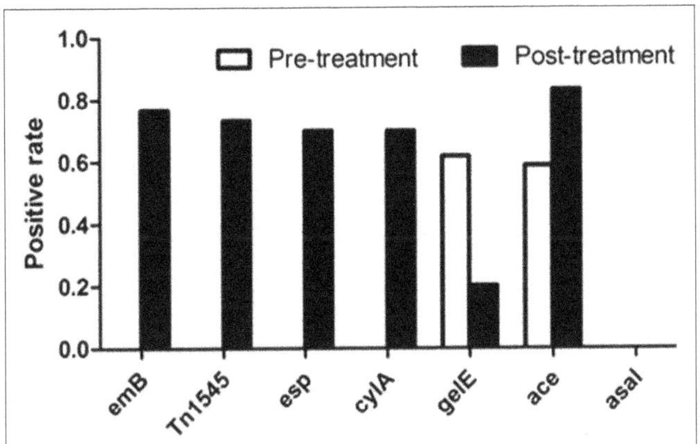

FIGURE 5 | Comparison of positive rate of resistant determinants and virulence genes of *E. faecalis* before and after experiment with drug.

Virulence of the Selected *E. faecalis*

In the 34 *E. faecalis* stains selected in the pre-treatment, positive ratios of *esp*, *gelE*, *clyA*, *ace*, and *asal* were 0, 61.76, 0, 58.8% and 0, respectively. However, these changed into 70, 20, 70, 83.3% and 0, respectively, in the 30 *E. faecalis* stains selected in the post-treatment (**Figure 5**). The positive rates of surface protein (*esp*) and hemolysin activator (*cylA*) were significantly increased (0–70%). To the contrary, the carriage ratios of gelatinase (*gelE*) had a downside (61.76–20%). Aggregation substances (*asal*) were not found in all of the 64 strains *E. faecalis*. As shown in **Table 3**, most of the antimicrobial resistance in *E. faecalis* selected after treating with tulathromycin carried resistance gene of *ermB*, transferable element of Tn*1545* and three virulence gens (*esp*, *cylA*, and *ace*).

After infection with *E. faecalis* 143 (harboring *ermB*, Tn*1545*, *esp*, *cylA*, and *ace*), mice died within 8 h which was earlier than the death of mice infected with *E. faecalis* 174 (free of *ermB*, *esp*, *cylA*, and *ace*). The LD_{50} of the two *E. faecalis* strains was calculated by improved Karber method. The detailed results were shown in **Table 5**. The LD_{50} *E. faecalis* 143 (5.970×10^9 μg/mL) was three-times higher than that of *E. faecalis* 174(1.603×10^9 μg/mL), suggesting that *E. faecalis* 143 strain harboring virulence factors (*esp*, *cylA*, and *ace*) was more virulent than the strain without these two virulence genes.

NOAEC and mADI Calculation

Based on our results, the NOAEC was set up as 1 μg/mL. The daily fecal bolus was known as 220 mL. The fraction of oral dose available for microorganisms in the intestinal tract was 0.25 which can be split into two factors of 0.5 each. One factor of 0.5 was based on results for reduced availability of the substance due to interaction with fecal matter (EMEA, 2004) and the other factor of 0.5 was based on the impact of acidic colonic pH on tulathromycin availability for gut bacteria(USFDA, 2004). The weight of human was 60 kg/person. Therefore, our established mADI was 14.66 μg/kg.bw/d.

DISCUSSION

This study is the first of its kind to assess the effect of tulathromycin on human microbiota using the chemostat model. In addition, this study concentrated on the antimicrobial resistance development and virulence change of *E. faecalis* isolates in chemostats under long term exposure to a range of tulathromycin concentrations.

The present study showed that the intermediate concentration (10 μg/mL) slightly change the population of *Enterococci* and *Bacteroides fragilis*, while the highest concentration (100 μg/mL) inhibited the growth of three type of bacteria except for *Enterococcus*. This result was similar with our previous results that the numbers of some intestinal bacteria (e.g., *B. fragilis*) underwent significant changes during exposure to tilmicosin (Hao et al., 2015). As one of the most predominant bacteria in the intestinal microbiota, *B. fragilis* may be a most sensitive indicator of gut microbiome under exposure to macrolide drugs including erythromycin, tilmicosin, and tulathromycin (Carman et al., 2005; Merck sharp and D. Corp., 2011; Hao et al., 2015).

The present study and our previous investigation suggested that in the chemostat model high concentration of macrolide drugs (tilmicosin and tulathromycin) could significantly reduce the population of *B. fragilis* and subsequently resulted into the decline of the three main SCFAs especially propionic acid (Hao et al., 2015). The related change of propionic acid with *B. fragilis* population that we found was also observed in human flora associated (HFA) mice model (MacNeil, 2005).

Similar to previous studies, the colonization resistance of human intestinal microbiota in the chemostat was disrupted

TABLE 5 | Comparing the LD_{50} of *E. faecalis* 143 and 174 in the mice experiment.

E. faecalis no.	Inoculated dose (CFU/mouse)	Total mice number	Dead mice number during experiment				$lgLD_{50}$	LD_{50} (CFU/mL)
			0–8 h	8–24 h	24–48 h	>48 h		
14-3	1.60×10^{10}	8	7	0	0	0	9.205	1.603×10^{9}
	1.60×10^{9}	8	3	1	1	0		
	1.60×10^{8}	8	0	0	0	0		
	1.60×10^{7}	8	0	0	0	0		
	0	8	0	0	0	0		
17-4	1.06×10^{10}	8	2	1	1	0	9.776	5.970×10^{9}
	1.06×10^{9}	8	0	0	1	0		
	1.06×10^{8}	8	0	0	0	0		
	1.06×10^{7}	8	0	0	0	0		
	0	8	0	0	0	0		

under 7 days exposure to high concentration of antibiotics (Carman et al., 2004; Hao et al., 2013). Coincidently, in our chemostat model, there were significant alterations in the populations of *E. coli, B. fragilis, Enterococcus,* and *Bifidobacterium* which appeared to be indicator of intestinal microbiota and contributed a lot to the colonization resistance (Corpet, 1993; Nuding et al., 2013). As previously reported, 10^5 CFU/mL of *E. coli* had a complete inhibitory effect on the growth of *Salmonella* (Carman et al., 2004). However, in our previous result, the treatment of tilmicosin did change the colonization resistance (Hao et al., 2015). This difference suggested that disruption of colonization resistance was largely depended on antimicrobial agents and their concentrations (Carman et al., 2004; Ferreira et al., 2011).

Similar to previous results, resistance rate in *E. coli* did not change in the chemostat and HFA rodent models treated by tilmicosin (EMEA, 1997; Cerniglia and Kotarski, 2005; Hao et al., 2015). This may be due to the inherent resistance to macrolide drugs in *E. coli* (Phuc Nguyen et al., 2009). However, the resistance rate of *Enterococcus, Bifidobacterium,* and *B. fragilis* was significantly increased under the selective pressure of 100 and 10 μg/mL tulathromycin in our study. Consistently, the subtherapeutic and therapeutic administration of tulathromycin also significantly increased the proportion of erythromycin resistant enterococci in beef cattle (Zaheer et al., 2013).

Our study showed that most of the isolated tulathromycin resistant enterococcicontained *ermB*. The *ermB* gene in different gram-positive bacteria has been well-documented (Schmitz et al., 2000; Perreten et al., 2005; Littauer et al., 2006; Tremblay et al., 2011; Zmantar et al., 2011). The occurrence of macrolide resistance mediated by *ermB* was also found in enterococci originating from swine and cattle due to the subtherapeutic use of tylosin and tulathromycin (Jackson et al., 2004; Chen et al., 2008; Zaheer et al., 2013).

Tn*1545* was found in almost of the high-level macrolides resistant *Enterococcus* harboring *ermB* gene. Our conjugation test also showed that the *Enterococcus* isolate containing Tn*1545* and *ermB* can transfer its resistance to *E. faecalis* JH2-2 and *E. coli* NK5449. The transferability of *ermB* located in transposon may play an important role on the increase of resistance rate in *Enterococcus, Bifidobacterium,* and *B. fragilis* (Okitsu et al., 2005; Ciric et al., 2013).

Both the previous study and our study found that *gelE* gene was one of the predominant virulence genes in *E. faecalis* (Di Rosa et al., 2006). A positive correlation between macrolide resistance and *gelE* virulence gene was observed in an epidemiological investigation (Zou et al., 2011; Lins et al., 2013). High level expression of *gelE* has also been observed in multi-drug resistant Enterococci and in macrolide resistant *E. feacalis* containing *ermB* gene (Arciola et al., 2008; Hao et al., 2015). However, the *E. feacalis* containing both *ermB* gene and gelatinase (*gelE*) did not occur in our study.

Most of *E. faecalis* harboring both virulence factors (*esp* and *cylA*) and resistance gene of *ermB* were selected after treatment with tulathromycin, however, no *E. faecalis* isolates containing these two virulence genes was found before tulathromycin treatment. Coincidently, recent studies also found the existence of a large pool of potentially virulent and multidrug resistant *E. faecalis* in diseased farm animals (Seputiene et al., 2012). The presence and expression of some virulence determinants (e.g., *esp* and *cylA*) may enhance the colonization and invasion of *E. faecalis* to the epithelial cell of host (Trieu-Cuot et al., 1990; Littauer et al., 2006; Heikens et al., 2009; Johanson et al., 2012; Cafini et al., 2015; Kafil and Mobarez, 2015). The acute toxicity test with SPF mice indicated that *E. faecalis* harboring the macrolide resistant gene of *ermB* and two virulence genes (*esp* and *cylA*) had higher toxicity and pathogenicity.

Our established mADI (14.6 μg/kg.bw/d) was slightly higher than the mADI (10.97 μg/kg.bw/d) recommended by EMA-CVMP and the mADI (5 μg/kg.bw/d) recommended APVMA. Recently, EMA-CVMP revised the mADI of tulathromycin to 55 μg/kg.bw/d (EMA/CVMP, 2015). As a new approved drug, more work of safety assessment needs to be done to establish the final mADI of tulathromycin.

EXECUTIVE SUMMARY

Dose dependent effect on colonization resistance

10 μg/mL tulathromycin would significantly decrease the population but increase the resistance rate of *Enterococcus* and *Bacteroides fragilis*.
100 μg/mL tulathromycin significantly decreased population of *Escherichia coli*, *Bifidobacterium* and *B. fragilis* and SCFAs.
The colonization resistance was disturbed by higher concentration of tulathromycin.

Antimicrobial resistance inducement and risk of resistant factors

10 μg/mL tulathromycin would significantly increase the resistance rate of *Enterococcus* and *Bacteroides fragilis*.
100 μg/mL tulathromycin largely increased resistant rate of *Enterococcus* and selected multidrug resistant *E. faecalis*.
The selected resistant *E. faecalis* always carried *ermB* gene. It was located in transposons Tn*1545* and had ability of horizontal gene transfer (HGT).

The virulence change under drug exposure

The *E. faecalis* harboring resistance gene of *ermB* gene and virulence gene of *esp* and *cylA* was only selected after administration of high concentration of tulathromycin.
The *E. faecalis* harboring *esp* and *cylA* had higher pathogenicity.

Microbiological acceptable daily intake (mADI) of tulathromycin

The mADI was calculated as 14.66 μg/kg bw/day based on our study.

CONCLUSIONS

In conclusion, the established NOAEC and mADI in our study was 1 μg/mL and 14.66 μg/kg.bw/day, respectively. The low concentration of tulathromycin had no significant microbiological hazard with regard to colonization resistance and antimicrobial resistance. However, the long-term exposure to high concentration of tulathromycin (100 μg/mL) may damage the colonization resistance of human gut microbiota and induce the development of antimicrobial resistance in *Enterococcus*. The *E. feacalis* containing both transferable resistance determinant (*ermB* in Tn*1545*) and virulence genes (*esp* and *cylA*) were selected after administration of high level tulathromycin. More work need to be done to systematically assessment the safety of tulathromycin on human public health.

AUTHOR CONTRIBUTIONS

Experiment designation: HH, SZ, YW, and ZY; Experiment implement: SZ, HH, and ZL; Data analysis: SZ, HH, XW, YW, and ZY; Manuscript writing: SZ and HH; Manuscript modification: HH, GC, MD, YW, and ZY.

FUNDING

This work was supported by Grants from National Basic Research program of China (2013CB127200), project supported by the morning program of Wuhan in China (2015070404010191), Fundamental Research Funds for the Central Universities (2662015PY035), National Natural Science Foundation of China (31101856 and 31272614), and National Program for Risk Assessment of Quality and Safety of Livestock and Poultry Products (GJFP2016008).

ACKNOWLEDGMENTS

We give our sincere appreciation to Carl E. Cerniglia and Sangeeta Khare from National Center of Toxicological Research, USFDA due to their help on modification of this manuscript.

REFERENCES

Allen, G. P., and Bierman, B. C. (2009). *In vitro* analysis of resistance selection by linezolid in vancomycin-susceptible and -resistant *Enterococcus faecalis and Enterococcus faecium*. *Int. J. Antimicrob. Agents* 34, 21–24. doi: 10.1016/j.ijantimicag.2008.12.011

Arciola, C. R., Baldassarri, L., Campoccia, D., Creti, R., Pirini, V., Huebner, J., et al. (2008). Strong biofilm production, antibiotic multi-resistance and high gelE expression in epidemic clones of *Enterococcus faecalis* from orthopaedic implant infections. *Biomaterials* 29, 580–586. doi: 10.1016/j.biomaterials.2007.10.008

Benchaoui, H. A., Nowakowski, M., Sherington, J., Rowan, T. G., and Sunderland, S. J. (2004). Pharmacokinetics and lung tissue concentrations of tulathromycin in swine. *J. Vet. Pharmacol. Ther.* 27, 203–210. doi: 10.1111/j.1365-2885.2004.00586.x

Cafini, F., Gómez-Aguado, F., Corcuera, M. T., Ramos, C., Bas, P., Collado, L., et al. (2015). Genotypic and phenotypic diversity in *Enterococcus faecalis:* is agar invasion a pathogenicity score? *Rev. Esp. Quimioter.* 28, 101–108. doi: 10.1016/j.micpath.2015.11.017

Carman, R. J., Simon, M. A., Fernandez, H., Miller, M. A., and Bartholomew, M. J. (2004). Ciprofloxacin at low levels disrupts colonization resistance of human fecal microflora growing in chemostats. *Regul. Toxicol. Pharmacol.* 40, 319–326. doi: 10.1016/j.yrtph.2004.08.005

Carman, R. J., Simon, M. A., Petzold, H. E. III, Wimmer, R. F., Batra, M. R., Fernandez, A. H., et al. (2005). Antibiotics in the human food chain: establishing no effect levels of tetracycline, neomycin, and erythromycin using a chemostat model of the human colonic microflora. *Regul. Toxicol. Pharmacol.* 43, 168–180. doi: 10.1016/j.yrtph.2005.06.005

Carman, R. J., and Woodburn, M. A. (2001). Effects of low levels of ciprofloxacin on a chemostat model of the human colonic microflora. *Regul. Toxicol. Pharmacol.* 33, 276–284. doi: 10.1006/rtph.2001.1473

Cerniglia, C. E., and Kotarski, S. (1999). Evaluation of veterinary drug residues in food for their potential to affect human intestinal microflora. *Regul. Toxicol. Pharmacol.* 29, 238–261. doi: 10.1006/rtph.1999.1300

Cerniglia, C. E., and Kotarski, S. (2005). Approaches in the safety evaluations of veterinary antimicrobial agents in food to determine the effects on the human intestinal microflora. *J. Vet. Pharmacol. Ther.* 28, 3–20. doi: 10.1111/j.1365-2885.2004.00595.x

Chen, J., Fluharty, F. L., St-Pierre, N., Morrison, M., and Yu, Z. (2008). Technical note: occurrence in fecal microbiota of genes conferring resistance to both macrolide-lincosamide-streptogramin B and tetracyclines concomitant with feeding of beef cattle with tylosin. *J. Anim. Sci.* 86, 2385–2391. doi: 10.2527/jas.2007-0705

Chen, T., Li, S., and Wei, H. (2014). Antibiotic resistance capability of cultured human colonic microbiota growing in a chemostat model. *Appl. Biochem. Biotechnol.* 173, 765–774. doi: 10.1007/s12010-014-0882-6

Chen, T., Yuan, J., Feng, X., Wei, H., and Hua, W. (2011). Effects of enrofloxacin on the human intestinal microbiota *in vitro*. *Int. J. Antimicrob. Agents* 37, 567–571. doi: 10.1016/j.ijantimicag.2011.01.013

Ciric, L., Jasni, A., de Vries, L. E., Agersø, Y., Mullany, P., and Roberts, A. P. (2013). "Landes bioscience," in *Madame Curie Bioscience Database [Internet], Bacterial Integrative Mobile Genetic Elements*, eds A. P. Roberts and P. Mullany (Austin, TX: Landes Bioscience), 2000–2013.

Corpet, D. E. (1993). An evaluation of methods to assess the effect of antimicrobial residues on the human gut flora. *Vet. Microbiol.* 35, 199–212. doi: 10.1016/0378-1135(93)90145-W

Di Rosa, R., Creti, R., Venditti, M., D'Amelio, R., Arciola, C. R., Montanaro, L., et al. (2006). Relationship between biofilm formation, the enterococcal surface protein (Esp) and gelatinase in clinical isolates of *Enterococcus faecalis* and *Enterococcus faecium*. *FEMS Microbiol. Lett.* 256, 145–150. doi: 10.1111/j.1574-6968.2006.00112.x

EMA/CVMP (2015). *Tulathromycin (Modification of the Microbiological ADI and MRLs in Bovine and Porcine Species)*. EMA/CVMP. Available online at: http://www.ema.europa.eu/docs/en_GB/document_library/Maximum_Residue_Limits_-_Report/2015/02/WC500182166.pdf

EMEA (1997). *Committee for Veterinary Medicinal Products, Tilmicosin, Summary Report (1)*. E. CVMP. EMEA/MRL/318/97-FINAL.

EMEA (2004). *Committee for Veterinary Medicinal Products, Tulathromycin, Summary Report (2)*. EMEA-CVMP. EMEA/MRL/894/04-Final.

FDA (2004) *Tulathromycin Microbiological Effects on Bacteria of Humanhealth Concern, A Qualitative Risk Estimation*, Vol. 9, 1–58.

Ferreira, R. B., Gill, N., Willing, B. P., Antunes, L. C., Russell, S. L., Croxen, M. A., et al. (2011). The intestinal microbiota plays a role in Salmonella-induced colitis independent of pathogen colonization. *PLoS ONE* 6:e20338. doi: 10.1371/journal.pone.0020338

Hao, H., Guo, W., Iqbal, Z., Cheng, G., Wang, X., Dai, M., et al. (2013). Impact of cyadox on human colonic microflora in chemostat models. *Regul. Toxicol. Pharmacol.* 67, 335–343. doi: 10.1016/j.yrtph.2013.08.011

Hao, H., Yao, J., Wu, Q., Wei, Y., Dai, M., Iqbal, Z., et al. (2015). Microbiological toxicity of tilmicosin on human colonic microflora in chemostats. *Regul. Toxicol. Pharmacol.* 73, 201–208. doi: 10.1016/j.yrtph.2015.07.008

Heikens, E., Leendertse, M., Wijnands, L. M., van Luit-Asbroek, M., Bonten, M. J., van der Poll, T., et al. (2009). Enterococcal surface protein Esp is not essential for cell adhesion and intestinal colonization of *Enterococcus faecium* in mice. *BMC Microbiol.* 9:19. doi: 10.1186/1471-2180-9-19

Jackson, C. R., Fedorka-Cray, P. J., Barrett, J. B., and Ladely, S. R. (2004). Effects of tylosin use on erythromycin resistance in enterococci isolated from swine. *Appl. Environ. Microbiol.* 70, 4205–4210. doi: 10.1128/AEM.70.7.4205-4210.2004

Johanson, J. J., Feriancikova, L., and Xu, S. (2012). Influence of enterococcal surface protein (esp) on the transport of *Enterococcus faecium* within saturated quartz sands. *Environ. Sci. Technol.* 46, 1511–1518. doi: 10.1021/es203265m

Kadlec, K., Brenner Michael, G., Sweeney, M. T., Brzuszkiewicz, E., Liesegang, H., Daniel, R., et al. (2011). Molecular basis of macrolide, triamilide, and lincosamide resistance in *Pasteurella multocida* from bovine respiratory disease. *Antimicrob. Agents Chemother.* 55, 2475–2477. doi: 10.1128/AAC.00092-11

Kafil, H. S., and Mobarez, A. M. (2015). Spread of enterococcal surface protein in antibiotic resistant *Enterococcus faecium* and *Enterococcus faecalis* isolates from urinary tract infections. *Open Microbiol. J.* 26, 14–17. doi: 10.2174/1874285801509010014

Kays, M. B., and Graff, M. A. (2002). Broth microdilution and E-test for determining fluoroquinolone activity against *Streptococcus pneumoniae*. *Ann. Pharmacother.* 36, 416–422. doi: 10.1345/aph.1A119

Lins, R. X., de Oliveira Andrade, A., Hirata, R. Jr., Wilson, M. J., Lewis, M. A., Williams, D. W., et al. (2013). Antimicrobial resistance and virulence traits of *Enterococcus faecalis* from primary endodontic infections. *J. Dent.* 41, 779–786. doi: 10.1016/j.jdent.2013.07.004

Littauer, P., Caugant, D., Sangvik, M., Høiby, E., Sundsfjord, A., and Simonsen, G. (2006). Macrolide-resistant *Streptococcus pyogenes* in Norway: population structure and resistance determinants. *Antimicrob. Agents Chemother.* 50, 1896–1899. doi: 10.1128/AAC.50.5.1896-1899.2006

MacNeil, J. D. (2005). The joint food and agriculture organization of the United Nations/World Health Organization Expert Committee on Food Additives and its role in the evaluation of the safety of veterinary drug residues in foods. *AAPS J.* 7, E274–E280. doi: 10.1208/aapsj070228

Merck sharp and D. Corp. (2011). *Antimicrobial Activity-Merck Veterianry Manual.* London: Merck sharp and D. Corp.

Moffatt, L. (2007). *Draxxin Injectable Solution-APVMA Product Number 5930. Australian Pesticides and Veterinary Medicines Authority.* Kingston, ACT. Available online at: http://apvma.gov.au/sites/default/files/publication/14156-prs-draxxin.pdf

Mundy, L., Sahm, D., and Gilmore, M. (2000). Relationships between enterococcal virulence and antimicrobial resistance. *Clin. Microbiol. Rev.* 13, 513–522. doi: 10.1128/CMR.13.4.513-522.2000

Nowakowski, M. A., Inskeep, P. B., Risk, J. E., Skogerboe, T. L., Benchaoui, H. A., Meinert, T. R., et al. (2004). Pharmacokinetics and lung tissue concentrations of tulathromycin, a new triamilide antibiotic, in cattle. *Vet. Ther.* 5, 60–74.

Nuding, S., Antoni, L., and Stange, E. F. (2013). The host and the flora. *Dig. Dis.* 31, 286–292. doi: 10.1159/000354680

Nutsch, R. G., Hart, F. J., Rooney, K. A., Weigel, D. J., Kilgore, W. R., and Skogerboe, T. L. (2005). Efficacy of tulathromycin injectable solution for the treatment of naturally occurring swine respiratory disease. *Vet. Ther.* 6, 214.

Okitsu, N., Kaieda, S., Yano, H., Nakano, R., Hosaka, Y., Okamoto, R., et al. (2005). Characterization of ermB gene transposition by Tn1545 and Tn917 in macrolide-resistant *Streptococcus pneumoniae* isolates. *J. Clin. Microbiol.* 43, 168–173. doi: 10.1128/JCM.43.1.168-173.2005

Perreten, V., Vorlet-Fawer, L., Slickers, P., Ehricht, R., Kuhnert, P., and Frey, J. (2005). Microarray-based detection of 90 antibiotic resistance genes of gram-positive bacteria. *J. Clin. Microbiol.* 43, 2291–2302. doi: 10.1128/JCM.43.5.2291-2302.2005

Phuc Nguyen, M. C., Woerther, P. L., Bouvet, M., Andremont, A., Leclercq, R., and Canu, A. (2009). *Escherichia coli* as reservoir for macrolide resistance genes. *Emerging Infect. Dis.* 15, 1648–1650. doi: 10.3201/eid1510.090696

Portillo, A., Ruiz-Larrea, F., Zarazaga, M., Alonso, A., Martinez, J. L., and Torres, C. (2000). Macrolide resistance genes in *Enterococcus* spp. *Antimicrob. Agents Chemother.* 44, 967–971. doi: 10.1128/AAC.44.4.967-971.2000

Salyers, A. A., Gupta, A., and Wang, Y. (2004). Human intestinal bacteria as reservoirs for antibiotic resistance genes. *Trends Microbiol.* 12, 412–416. doi: 10.1016/j.tim.2004.07.004

Schmitz, F.-J., Sadurski, R., Kray, A., Boos, M., Geisel, R., Köhrer, K., et al. (2000). Prevalence of macrolide-resistance genes in *Staphylococcus aureus* and *Enterococcus faecium* isolates from 24 European university hospitals. *J. Antimicrob. Chemother.* 45, 891–894. doi: 10.1093/jac/45.6.891

Seputiene, V., Bogdaite, A., Ruzauskas, M., and Suziedeliene, E. (2012). Antibiotic resistance genes and virulence factors in *Enterococcus faecium* and *Enterococcus faecalis* from diseased farm animals: pigs, cattle and poultry. *Pol. J. Vet. Sci.* 15, 431–438.

Sun, Y., Dai, M., Hao, H., Wang, Y., Huang, L., Almofti, Y. A., et al. (2011). The role of RamA on the development of ciprofloxacin resistance in *Salmonella enterica* serovar Typhimurium. *PLoS ONE* 6:e23471. doi: 10.1371/journal.pone.0023471

Tremblay, C.-L., Letellier, A., Quessy, S., Boulianne, M., Daignault, D., and Archambault, M. (2011). Multiple-antibiotic resistance of *Enterococcus faecalis* and *Enterococcus faecium* from cecal contents in broiler chicken and turkey flocks slaughtered in Canada and plasmid colocalization of tetO and ermB genes. *J. Food Prot.* 74, 1639–1648. doi: 10.4315/0362-028X.JFP-10-451

Trieu-Cuot, P., Poyart-Salmeron, C., Carlier, C., and Courvalin, P. (1990). Nucleotide sequence of the erythromycin resistance gene of the conjugative transposon Tn1545. *Nucleic Acids Res.* 18, 3660–3660. doi: 10.1093/nar/18.12.3660

USFDA (2004). *Tulathromycin Microbiological Effect*. USFDA. Available online at: http://www.fda.gov/downloads/AdvisoryCommittees/CommitteesMeetingMaterials/VeterinaryMedicineAdvisoryCommittee/UCM127196.pdf

Xu, Y., Gao, C., Li, X., He, Y., Zhou, L., Pang, G., et al. (2013). *In vitro* antifungal activity of silver nanoparticles against ocular pathogenic filamentous fungi. *J. Ocul. Pharmacol. Ther.*, 29, 270–274. doi: 10.1089/jop.2012.0155

Zaheer, R., Cook, S. R., Klima, C. L., Stanford, K., Alexander, T., Topp, E., et al. (2013). Effect of subtherapeutic vs. therapeutic administration of macrolides on antimicrobial resistance in Mannheimia haemolytica and Enterococci isolated from beef cattle. *Front. Microbiol.* 4:133. doi: 10.3389/fmicb.2013.00133

Zmantar, T., Kouidhi, B., Miladi, H., and Bakhrouf, A. (2011). Detection of macrolide and disinfectant resistance genes in clinical *Staphylococcus aureus* and coagulase-negative *Staphylococci*. *BMC Res. Notes* 4:453. doi: 10.1186/1756-0500-4-453

Zou, L. K., Wang, H. N., Zeng, B., Li, J. N., Li, X. T., Zhang, A. Y., et al. (2011). Erythromycin resistance and virulence genes in *Enterococcus faecalis* from swine in China. *New Microbiol.* 34, 73–80.

19

Fecal Carriage of *Staphylococcus aureus* in the Hospital and Community Setting

Shantelle Claassen-Weitz[1], *Adebayo O. Shittu*[2], *Michelle R. Ngwarai*[1], *Lehana Thabane*[3], *Mark P. Nicol*[1,4,5] *and Mamadou Kaba*[1,4*]

[1] Division of Medical Microbiology, Department of Pathology, Faculty of Health Sciences, University of Cape Town, Cape Town, South Africa, [2] Department of Microbiology, Obafemi Awolowo University, Ile-Ife, Nigeria, [3] Department of Clinical Epidemiology and Biostatistics, McMaster University, Hamilton, ON, Canada, [4] Institute of Infectious Disease and Molecular Medicine, Faculty of Health Sciences, University of Cape Town, Cape Town, South Africa, [5] National Health Laboratory Service of South Africa, Groote Schuur Hospital, Cape Town, South Africa

***Correspondence:**
Mamadou Kaba
mamadou.kaba@hotmail.com;
mamadou.kaba@uct.ac.za

Background and rationale: *Staphylococcus aureus* fecal carriage has been identified as a potential source for nosocomial transmission and a risk factor for disease development. This systematic review determined the overall *S. aureus* [including methicillin susceptible and resistant *S. aureus* (MSSA and MRSA)] fecal carriage rates within the community and healthcare settings.

Methodology: Peer-reviewed articles indexed in Medline, Scopus, Academic Search Premier, Africa-Wide Information, CINAHL, and Web of Science were identified using applicable and controlled vocabulary through to 11 November 2015. Eligible studies were ascertained by three independent reviewers. Random-effects meta-analyses of proportions were performed to determine *S. aureus,* MSSA and MRSA fecal carriage rates reported by eligible studies.

Results: Twenty six studies were included in this review. The pooled estimates for *S. aureus*, MSSA and MRSA fecal carriage were 26% (95% confidence interval (CI): 16.8–36.3%), 86% (95% confidence interval (CI): 65.9–97.9%) and 10% (95% CI: 0.7–27.0%), respectively. Fecal *S. aureus* carriage rates increased on average from 10 to 65% during the first 8 weeks of life, followed by an average carriage rate of 64% at 6 months and 46% at 1 year of life. Genotyping techniques were employed mainly in studies conducted in developed countries and comprised largely of gel-based techniques. Six studies reported on the role of *S. aureus* fecal strains in diarrhea ($n = 2$) and the risk for acquiring infections ($n = 4$). Eight of the 26 studies included in this review performed antibiotic susceptibility testing of *S. aureus* fecal isolates.

Conclusion: This study provides evidence that screening for *S. aureus* fecal carriage, at least in populations at high risk, could be an effective measure for the prevention of *S. aureus* transmission and infection in the healthcare and community setting. More well-structured studies need to be conducted and sequence-based genotyping techniques should be employed for the comparison of isolates on a global scale in both developing and developed countries.

Keywords: carriage, community, fecal, *Staphylococcus aureus*, systematic review

INTRODUCTION

Staphylococcus aureus is a commensal Gram-positive bacterium, which under certain circumstances may be responsible for pyogenic or toxigenic infections, such as skin and soft tissue infections, toxic shock syndrome and pneumonia (Tong et al., 2015). Its carriage is considered as an important risk factor for subsequent development of hospital and community-acquired infections (Ellis et al., 2004; Wertheim et al., 2004; Maier et al., 2005; Dukic et al., 2013; Levy et al., 2013). The anterior nares is recognized as the primary site for *S. aureus* colonization (Kluytmans et al., 1997; van Belkum et al., 2009; Sollid et al., 2014). Other anatomical niches for *S. aureus* include the skin (Popov et al., 2014), oropharynx (Mertz et al., 2007; Petersen et al., 2013), intestinal tract (Acton et al., 2009), and the vagina (Bourgeois-Nicolaos et al., 2010).

The importance of fecal carriage of *S. aureus* has been recognized more than five decades ago in a study which demonstrated that rectal *S. aureus* carriage preceded those from the nose and throat in new-borns (Hurst, 1960). Thereafter, several studies have provided evidence on the clinical importance of fecal carriage of *S. aureus* [in particular methicillin-resistant *S. aureus* (MRSA)] in the hospital setting (Acton et al., 2009). For example, it has been shown that hospitalized patients with both *S. aureus* fecal and nasal colonization are significantly more likely to have positive skin cultures compared to patients with nasal carriage only (Bhalla et al., 2007). In addition, *S. aureus* fecal carriage may serve as an important source for environmental contamination, which can potentially facilitate nosocomial transmission within the healthcare setting (Bhalla et al., 2007). Furthermore, antibiotic-associated diarrhea attributed to MRSA has also been reported (Lo and Borchardt, 2009; Sizemore et al., 2012; Avery et al., 2015); and patients with MRSA colonized diarrheal stools impact significantly on environmental contamination (Boyce et al., 2007).

Despite the potential role and significance of the sole fecal carriage of *S. aureus* (Lee et al., 1997; Squier et al., 2002; Bhalla et al., 2007) and the transmission dynamics of *S. aureus* in infection, a limited number of studies have focused on fecal *S. aureus* carriage in the hospital and community setting (Acton et al., 2009). This systematic literature review is therefore aimed to determine the overall rate of *S. aureus* [including methicillin susceptible and resistant *S. aureus* (MSSA and MRSA)] fecal carriage amongst individuals in the community and healthcare settings.

METHODOLOGY

This review followed the preferred reporting items for systematic reviews and meta-analyses (PRISMA) guidelines (Moher et al., 2009). The PRISMA check-list for this review is provided in a Supplementary Table (Table S1).

Literature Search Strategy

Peer-reviewed articles (written in English and French) published through to 11 November 2015 on *S. aureus* fecal carriage within the community and healthcare settings were evaluated using four electronic databases and a combination of keywords (**Table 1**). We also explored for additional articles by checking the references cited in the primary eligible studies included in this systematic review.

Study Selection and Data Extraction

Potentially relevant articles (selected based on their titles and abstracts) were assessed for eligibility (**Table 2**) by three independent authors. All potentially eligible articles were screened for "predatory journals" using "Beall's list" (Beall, 2015; Shen and Björk, 2015; Siebert et al., 2015). The corresponding authors of potentially relevant articles were contacted to determine the healthcare exposure status of participants so as to assess their eligibility for inclusion in this systematic review (**Table 2**). Data extraction was performed independently by two authors using a standardized data extraction form. Disagreements and inconsistencies were resolved by consensus. The following information was extracted from each eligible study: study population, number of participants screened for fecal carriage, participant characteristics (age, health status, exposure to health care settings), sample collection details (sample type, age at which samples were collected, collection site), laboratory techniques (*S. aureus* and MRSA screening methods, genotyping techniques, virulence profile assessment), as well as *S. aureus* and MRSA detection rates.

Operational Definitions of Terms Used in this Systematic Review

Community Setting

Healthy participants

- Participants reported to be healthy at the time of screening for *S. aureus* or MRSA fecal carriage without any exposure to healthcare settings during the year preceding screening (McKinnell et al., 2013);

TABLE 1 | Search strategy performed in four databases.

Database	Search mode	Keywords
Medline via Pubmed	All fields	("staphylococcus aureus") AND ("gut" OR "gastrointestinal" OR "anal" OR "anus" OR "intestinal" OR "rectum" OR "rectal" OR "stool" OR "feces" OR "faeces" OR "fecal" OR "faecal") AND ("epidemiology" OR "incidence" OR "prevalence" OR "carriage" OR "carriage rate" OR carrier*) AND ("humans" OR "human")
Scopus via SciVerse	Article title, abstract, keywords	
Academic Search Premier, Africa-Wide Information and CINAHL via EBSCOHost	Boolean/Phrase	
Web of Science via Web of Knowledge	Topic	

TABLE 2 | Eligibility criteria.

Inclusion criteria for systematic review	Exclusion criteria for systematic review
• Studies published from 1920 to 11 November 2015 were included in the search. • Studies reporting on *S. aureus* or MRSA carriage from fecal/rectal/anal specimens from humans. • Studies providing information on the prevalence of *S. aureus* or MRSA fecal carriage. • Healthcare exposure data should include information on whether or not participants were: 1. Hospitalized in the 12 months prior to screening nursing home residents, health care workers, or patients transferred from other hospitals or wards (McKinnell et al., 2013). 2. Screened for *S. aureus* or MRSA fecal carriage within > or ≤ 48 hours of healthcare contact (Folden et al., 2005; Millar et al., 2007; Otter and French, 2011). • Studies published in either English or French.	• Studies screening for *S. aureus* or MRSA from samples other than feces/rectal swabs/anal swabs. • Fecal samples studied for parasites or bacteria other than *S. aureus*. • Articles reporting on the number of *S. aureus* or MRSA isolates detected from fecal specimens or on the number of fecal specimens positive for *S. aureus* or MRSA, but not providing information on the number of participants testing positive for *S. aureus* or MRSA fecal carriage. • Studies not providing the necessary healthcare exposure data for participants (via the published article or via correspondence with the authors), in order to categorize participants into Healthy participants, Out-patients, In-patients and Healthcare personnel. • Articles published in predatory journals (Beall, 2015). • Articles not obtainable from the electronic databases, the University of Cape Town (UCT) library or the UCT inter-library loans.
Inclusion criteria for meta-analysis of proportions	**Exclusion criteria for meta-analysis of proportions**
• Overall fecal carriage prevalence for *S. aureus* and/or MRSA must be available.	• Studies providing fecal carriage rates for participants for which fecal carriage rates have previously been reported. • Studies not providing information on the age at which participants were screened. • Studies screening a pre-selected group of participants based on microbiological assessments. • Studies for which MRSA was not confirmed using molecular methods.

- Pregnant women visiting obstetric clinics;
- New-borns and mothers at maternity wards during the time of delivery;
- Mothers and infants reported as healthy at the time of screening for *S. aureus* or MRSA fecal carriage, but exposed to the delivery unit or maternity ward during the year preceding screening.

Out-patients

Patients screened for *S. aureus* or MRSA fecal carriage with ≤48 h of healthcare contact (Folden et al., 2005; Millar et al., 2007; Otter and French, 2011). Patients should not have had contact with healthcare settings in the year preceding the study.

Healthcare Setting

In-patients

Patients screened for *S. aureus* or MRSA fecal carriage with >48 h of healthcare contact. Patients screened within ≤48 h after admission should be those transferred from another hospital/ward which will allow for >48 h of hospital contact.

Healthcare personnel

Participants screened for *S. aureus* or MRSA fecal carriage working at a healthcare setting with or without any illness.

Developed and Developing Countries

Countries were categorized as developed or developing countries based on data from the International Monetary Fund (http://www.imf.org/external/pubs/ft/weo/2015/01/weodata/groups.htm).

Antibiotic Susceptibility Results

The percentage of isolates (obtained from participants with *S. aureus* or MRSA fecal carriage) resistant to each of the antibiotics assayed was calculated from studies that provided adequate data on antibiotic susceptibility test results. Our review noted susceptibility tests results whether or not the respective studies incorporated published guidelines [such as Clinical Laboratory Standards Institute (CLSI), National Committee on Clinical Laboratory Standards (NCCLS), European Committee on Antimicrobial Susceptibility Testing (EUCAST), Antibiogram Committee of the French Society of Microbiology (CA-SFM), or the Swedish Reference Group for Antibiotics (SRGA) guidelines] in assessing the antibiotic resistance profiles.

Statistical Analysis and Data Visualization

The *S. aureus,* MRSA and MSSA fecal carriage rates for studies included in this systematic review were calculated as follows:

$$\textit{S. aureus}\text{ fecal carriage rate (\%)} = \frac{\text{Participants positive for }\textit{S. aureus}\text{ fecal carriage}}{\text{Participants screened for }\textit{S. aureus}\text{ fecal carriage}}$$

$$\text{MRSA fecal carriage rate (\%)} = \frac{\text{Participants positive for MRSA fecal carriage}}{\text{Participants screened for }\textit{S. aureus}\text{ or MRSA fecal carriage}}$$

$$\text{MSSA fecal carriage rate (\%)} = \frac{(\text{Participants positive for }\textit{S. aureus}\text{ fecal carriage} - \text{Participants positive for MRSA fecal carriage})}{\text{Participants screened for }\textit{S. aureus}\text{ fecal carriage}}$$

Individual reports assessing the same participants for *S. aureus*, MSSA or MRSA fecal carriage were considered as a single report. Calculated fecal *S. aureus* carriage rates were used to derive longitudinal data of individual studies, as well as the average carriage rate amongst these studies, at each time-point. Meta-analyses of proportions were performed to determine the overall *S. aureus*, MSSA and MRSA fecal carriage rates (pooled estimates) among individuals in the community and healthcare settings. Meta-analyses of proportions for MRSA and MSSA did not include studies for which MRSA was not confirmed using molecular methods. For all meta-analyses of proportions, studies screening for MRSA amongst pre-selected vancomycin resistant enterococci (VRE) fecal carriers were excluded. Similarly, meta-analyses of proportions did not include studies that screened for MRSA fecal carriage solely from pre-selected MRSA carriers (MRSA identified from other body sites). Meta-analyses were performed using StatsDirect statistical software version 3.0.165 [England: StatsDirect Ltd. 2016] for studies adhering to the inclusion criteria summarized in **Table 2**. The StatsDirect statistical software version 3.0.165 [England: StatsDirect Ltd. 2016] was also applied to assess the heterogeneity between the studies included in the meta-analyses (Cochran Q-test) (Cochran, 1954) and to determine the inconsistency across the studies included (I^2 statistic) (Higgins et al., 2003). The criterion for statistical significance for the test for heterogeneity was set at alpha = 0.05. The risk of publication bias was assessed and visualized by a Funnel plot (Egger et al., 1997; Sterne et al., 2011).

RESULTS

Study Selection and Characteristics

S. aureus Study Selection

Figure 1 outlines the study selection process and the broad reasons for exclusion. The search strategy identified 2522 records. An additional record was identified from the reference list of one of the eligible articles included in the review. A total of 124 potentially eligible reports were identified, of which 69 fulfilled the primary inclusion criteria (**Figure 1**). The vast majority (80%; 55/69) of these potentially eligible articles did not provide information on healthcare exposure during the year preceding screening and/or did not indicate the duration for which patients were admitted prior to the time of screening. Following correspondence with authors, seven articles were excluded as these reports did not fulfill our inclusion criteria. Moreover, 36 articles were excluded due to lack of required information from corresponding authors or as a result of unavailable author contact information. Consequently, only 26 (11 and 15 reports based on their full texts and information obtained from the authors, respectively) of the 69 studies could be included in our systematic review. The main findings reported by each of the 26 eligible studies are summarized in detail in **Tables 3, 4**. Select studies that screened for *S. aureus* fecal carriage from both community and healthcare settings are also reported accordingly in **Tables 3, 4**.

Characteristics of Reports from Community and Healthcare Settings

Reports on S. aureus fecal carriage

A total of 19 reports investigated fecal *S. aureus* carriage within the community setting, of which five and 14 studies reported on fecal carriage rates from outpatients and healthy participants, respectively (**Table 3**). Moreover, the majority (64%; 9/14) of reports on fecal *S. aureus* carriage rates from healthy participants were of longitudinal design and investigated infants up until one year of age (**Table 3**). Of the five reports on fecal carriage rates from outpatients, a single study performed a longitudinal analysis of *S. aureus* fecal carriage (Efuntoye and Adetosoye, 2003) and another investigated infants during the first year of life (Shehabi et al., 2013). Study sizes for the community setting ranged between 21 and 1761 participants (**Table 3**).

Fecal *S. aureus* carriage within the healthcare setting was noted in 12 reports (**Table 4**). Of these, 10 were from inpatients and two from healthcare personnel. All reports on inpatients were of cross-sectional design and the majority (60%; 6/10) did not provide information on the age of the participants. In addition, the two studies on healthcare personnel were cross-sectional in design and carried out in the United States of America (USA) (Carmeli et al., 1998; Andrews et al., 2009). Study sizes for healthcare-based reports ranged between 37 and 2727 participants (**Table 4**).

Reports on methicillin susceptible and resistant S. aureus fecal carriage

Six of the 19 reports on *S. aureus* fecal carriage from the community setting provided MRSA fecal carriage rates confirmed by molecular methods (**Table 3**). Five of these studies (conducted in developed countries) reported both *S. aureus* and MRSA fecal carriage rates which allowed for the calculation of MSSA fecal carriage rates. Only one study within the healthcare setting (conducted in the USA) confirmed fecal MRSA carriage by screening specimens using a molecular approach (Andrews et al., 2009).

Pooled Estimates of *S. aureus* Fecal Carriage Rates Assessed by Meta-Analyses

Studies included in all of the proportional meta-analyses were heterogeneous, as determined by the Cochrane Q test and I^2 statistic (**Figures 2–4**). We could not determine pooled MSSA or MRSA fecal carriage rates within the healthcare setting as only a single study was considered eligible for this analysis.

The pooled random-effects estimate for *S. aureus* fecal carriage within the community and healthcare settings was 26% (95% *CI* = 16.8–36.3; **Figure 5**). Sub-analyses of *S. aureus* fecal carriage within the community and healthcare settings resulted in pooled random-effects estimates of 31% (95% *CI* = 17.8–46.3) and 5% (95% CI = 1.7–8.9), respectively.

MSSA fecal carriage was estimated at 86% (95% *CI* = 65.9–97.9) using the random-effects model (**Figure 6**). Within the community setting, the random effects estimate for MSSA fecal

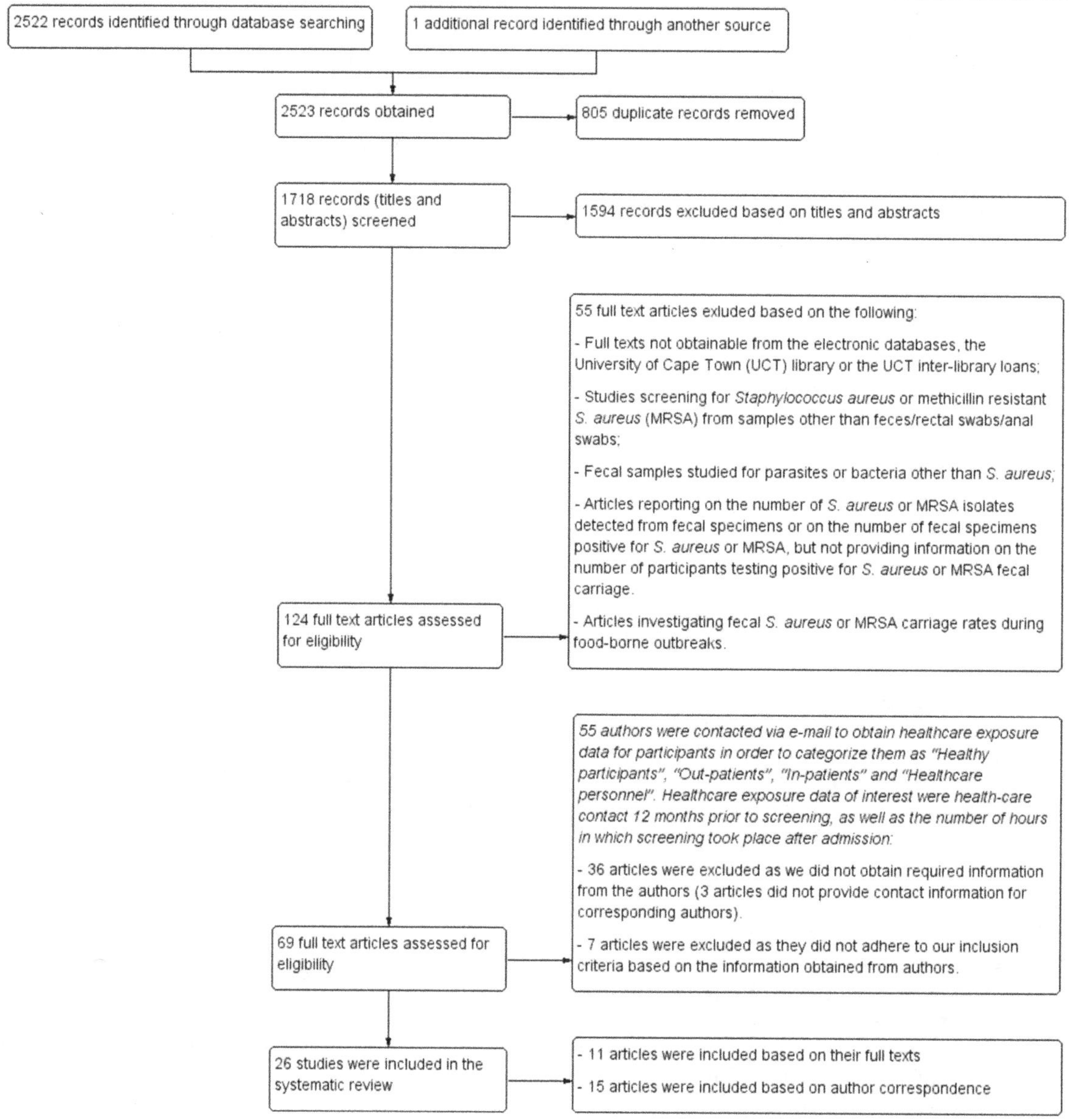

FIGURE 1 | Study selection. Flow diagram of identification and selection process for studies included in the systematic review.

carriage was 86% (95% *CI* = 62.3–98.5). The pooled random-effects estimates for MRSA fecal carriage were 10% (95% *CI* = 0.7–27.0; **Figure 7**); and 10% (95% *CI* = 0.4–28.9) within the community setting.

S. aureus Fecal Carriage Rates According to the Age of Participants

The report on this section is not based on meta-analysis. *S. aureus* fecal carriage rates within the community setting were higher during the first year of life (**Figure 8**). On average, reports from longitudinal studies revealed an increase in *S. aureus* fecal carriage rates from approximately 10–65% during the first 8 weeks of life (**Figure 8**). At 6 months of age, the average fecal carriage rate was 64%, thereafter it decreased to approximately 46% at 1 year of life. A longitudinal investigation of fecal MRSA carriage rates from healthy participants from the USA showed an increase in fecal MRSA carriage from 0 to 9% during the first 2 weeks of life (Gries et al., 2009). The highest MRSA fecal carriage rate (23%) reported was from Spanish infants screened at $\leq$1 year of life (Benito et al., 2015).

Assessment of Antibiotic Susceptibility of Fecal *S. aureus* Isolates

Eight of the 26 eligible studies (31%) included in this review assayed for antibiotic susceptibility of fecal *S. aureus* or MRSA isolates (**Table 5**). Overall, *S. aureus* or MRSA isolates were

TABLE 3 | Characteristics of eligible studies analysing fecal carriage of *Staphylococcus aureus* or MRSA from the community.

Study population setting	Participants screened for fecal[Ψ] carriage (n)	Participant characteristics			Sample collection			Laboratory technique(s)				*S. aureus* detection	MRSA detection	References
		Age range	Health status	Exposure to healthcare setting 12 months prior to screening[†]	Sample type	Age at which samples were collected	Site at which samples were collected	*S. aureus* detection	MRSA detection	Genotyping	Virulence profile analysis	% (n/N)	& (n/N)	
CATEGORY: HEALTHY PARTICIPANTS														
Italy	100	Birth to 12 months	Healthy	At time of delivery	Rectal swabs	3 days	Delivery unit	Phenotypic	NP	RAPD	SE TSST	5 (5/100)[φ]	NA	Lindberg et al., 2010
					Feces	1 week	Home					15 (15/100)[φ]		
						2 weeks						24 (24/100)[φ]		
						4 weeks						34 (34/100)[φ]		
						8 weeks						45 (45/100)[φ]		
						6 months						52 (52/100)[φ]		
						1 year						31 (27/86)[φ]		
						Overall prevalence						66 (66/100)[φ]		
Mozambique	121	≤14 days to 1 year	Apparently healthy	NR	Feces	≤14 days to 1 year	Home	Molecular	NP	NP	NP	77 (92/120)	NA	González et al., 2013
Nigeria	120	15–35 years	Healthy	No	Feces	15 to 35 years	Provided by participants	Phenotypic	Phenotypic	NP	NP	32 (38/120)	34 (13/38)[¶]	Onanuga and Temedie, 2011
Spain	21	7–35 days	Healthy	At time of delivery[φ]	Feces	1 week	Home	Phenotypic and Molecular	Phenotypic and Molecular	*spa* typing	SE	10 (2/21)		Benito et al., 2015
						2 weeks				*agr* typing	PVL	14 (3/21)		
						5 weeks				MLST	ET	48 (10/21)		
						Overall prevalence				PFGE	TSST AUR BAP CNA	57 (12/21)	42 (5/12)	

(Continued)

TABLE 3 | Continued

Study population setting	Participants screened for fecal$^{\Psi}$ carriage (n)	Participant characteristics			Sample collection			Laboratory technique(s)				*S. aureus* detection	MRSA detection	References
		Age range	Health status	Exposure to healthcare setting 12 months prior to screening†	Sample type	Age at which samples were collected	Site at which samples were collected	*S. aureus* detection	MRSA detection	Genotyping	Virulence profile analysis	% (n/N)	& (n/N)	
Spain	100	2–89 years	Healthy	No$^{\varphi}$	Feces	2–89 years	NR	Phenotypic and Molecular	Phenotypic and Molecular	*spa* typing *agr* typing MLST	SE PVL ET TSST AUR BAP CNA	15 (15/100)	0 (0/15)	Benito et al., 2013
Spain	50	7–23 months	Healthy	At time of delivery$^{\varphi}$	Feces	7–23 months	Nurseries	Phenotypic and Molecular	Phenotypic and Molecular	NP	NP	6 (3/50)	0 (0/3)	Domínguez et al., 2002
Sweden	100	Birth to 12 months	Healthy	At time of delivery	Rectal swabs	3 days	Delivery unit	Phenotypic	NP	RAPD	SE TSST	16 (16/100)$^{\varphi}$	NA	Lindberg et al., 2010
					Feces	1 week	Home					48 (48/100)$^{\varphi}$		
						2 weeks						56 (56/100)$^{\varphi}$		
						4 weeks						64 (64/100)$^{\varphi}$		
						8 weeks						72 (72/100)$^{\varphi}$		
						6 months						68 (68/100)$^{\varphi}$		
						1 year						55 (55/100)$^{\varphi}$		
						Overall prevalence						78 (78/100)$^{\varphi}$		
Sweden	64	Birth to 8 weeks	Healthy	At time of delivery	Rectal swabs	3 days$^{\varphi}$	Delivery unit$^{\varphi}$	Phenotypic	NP	NP	SE TSST	13 (8/64)$^{\varphi}$	NA	Lundell et al., 2009
					Feces	1 week	Home$^{\varphi}$					39 (25/64)$^{\varphi}$		
						2 weeks						53 (33/62)$^{\varphi}$		
						4 weeks						59 (37/63)$^{\varphi}$		
						8 weeks						71 (44/62)$^{\varphi}$		
						Overall prevalence						73 (47/64)$^{\varphi}$		

(Continued)

TABLE 3 | Continued

Study population setting	Participants screened for fecal[Ψ] carriage (n)	Participant characteristics			Sample collection			Laboratory technique(s)				*S. aureus* detection	MRSA detection	References
		Age range	Health status	Exposure to healthcare setting 12 months prior to screening[†]	Sample type	Age at which samples were collected	Site at which samples were collected	*S. aureus* detection	MRSA detection	Genotyping	Virulence profile analysis	% (n/N)	& (n/N)	
Sweden	50	Birth to 12 months	Healthy	At time of delivery	Rectal swabs	3 days 1 week 2 weeks 4 weeks 8 weeks Overall prevalence	Delivery unit Home	Phenotypic	NP	RAPD PFGE	ET TSST	20 (10/50) 40 (20/50) 52 (26/50) 60 (30/50) 64 (32/50) 68 (34/50)	NA	Lindberg et al., 2004a
	37	Apparently healthy[φ]	Allergic and non-allergic mothers	At time of delivery	Feces	1 week after delivery or at a later stage	Home					24 (9/37)	NA	
Sweden	81	Birth to 12 months	Healthy	At time of delivery	Rectal swabs	3 days 1 week 2 weeks 4 weeks 8 weeks 6 months 1 year	Delivery unit at 3 days and home at 1 week to 1 year	Phenotypic	Phenotypic	RAPD	ET TSST	NR	0 (0/81)[φ]	Lindberg et al., 2004b
Sweden	49	Birth to 12 months	Healthy	At time of delivery	Rectal swabs Feces	3 days 1 week 2 weeks 4 weeks 8 weeks 6 months 1 year Overall prevalence	Delivery unit Home	Phenotypic	NP	RAPD	ET TSST	16 (8/49) 57 (28/49) 65 (32/49) 65 (32/49) 73 (36/49) 73 (36/49) 53 (26/49) 86 (42/49)[φ]	NA	Lindberg et al., 2000

(Continued)

TABLE 3 | Continued

Study population setting	Participants screened for fecal$^{\Psi}$ carriage (n)	Participant characteristics			Sample collection			Laboratory technique(s)				S. aureus detection	MRSA detection	References
		Age range	**Health status**	**Exposure to healthcare setting 12 months prior to screening†**	**Sample type**	**Age at which samples were collected**	**Site at which samples were collected**	***S. aureus* detection**	**MRSA detection**	**Genotyping**	**Virulence profile analysis**	**% (n/N)**	**& (n/N)**	
United Kingdom	30	2–7 months	Healthy	NR	Feces	2 weeks 10 weeks 7 months Overall prevalence	Home	Phenotypic	NP	NP	SE TSST	37 (11/30) 40 (12/30) 40 (12/30) 40 (12/30)	NA	Harrison et al., 2009
United States of America	147	>18 years	Healthy pregnant women at 35-37 weeks of pregnancy	No$^{\varphi}$	Rectal swabs	>18 years	Obstetric clinics	Phenotypic	Phenotypic and Molecular	SCC*mec* typing PFGE	PVL	4 (6/147)$^{\varphi}$	0 (0/6)$^{\varphi}$	Andrews et al., 2009
United States of America	38	1 day to 2 weeks	Healthy	At time of delivery	Feces	1–2 days 2 weeks Overall prevalence	New-born unit	Phenotypic	Phenotypic and Molecular	PFGE	PVL	0 (0/38) 26 (6/23) 26 (6/23)	0 (0/38) 33 (2/6) 33 (2/6)	Gries et al., 2009
CATEGORY: OUTPATIENTS														
India	100	16–88 years	Patients at admission	No long hospital stay or admission to other hospitals	Feces	16–88 years	Hospital	Phenotypic	NP	NP	NP	0 (0/100)	NA	Deepa et al., 2014
Jordan	216	≤28 days to 1 year	NR	No	Feces	≤28 days to 1 year	Clinic	Phenotypic	Phenotypic	SCC*mec* typing	ET PVL SE TSST	17 (37/216)	59 (22/37)	Shehabi et al., 2013

(Continued)

TABLE 3 | Continued

Study population setting	Participants screened for fecal[Ψ] carriage (n)	Participant characteristics			Sample collection			Laboratory technique(s)				*S. aureus* detection	MRSA detection	References
		Age range	Health status	Exposure to healthcare setting 12 months prior to screening[†]	Sample type	Age at which samples were collected	Site at which samples were collected	*S. aureus* detection	MRSA detection	Genotyping	Virulence profile analysis	% (n/N)	& (n/N)	
Nigeria	1761	≤5 years	Diarrhoeic children	No[φ]	Feces	<1 year	Hospital	Phenotypic	Phenotypic	NP	ET	3 (11/416)	NR	Efuntoye and Adetosoye, 2003
						1.1–2.0 years						4 (13/323)	NR	
						2.1–3.0 years						4 (12/309)	NR	
						3.1–4.0 years						5 (15/292)	NR	
						4.1–5.0 years						5 (21/421)	NR	
						Overall prevalence						4 (72/1761)	NR	
Saudi Arabia	58	NR	Patients at admission (<48 h)[φ] with diarrhea or abdominal pain	No[φ]	Feces	NR	Hospital	Phenotypic	Phenotypic	NP	NP	NA	9 (5/58)	Babay and Somily, 2009
United States of America	150	Birth to 18 years	Children requiring abscess drainage (n = 60)	No[φ]	Rectal swabs	Birth to 18 years	Hospital	Phenotypic and Molecular	Molecular	MLVA SCC*mec* typing	PVL	47 (28/60)	NR	Faden et al., 2010
			Children requiring general surgery (n=90)									1 (1/90)	NR	

[Ψ]Fecal samples, rectal swabs, anal swabs, peri-rectal or peri-anal swabs.

[†]Hospital, long-term care facility, nursing homes, maternity wards.

[¶]Resistant to cefoxitin.

[φ]Information obtained from the author.

Phenotypic identification: culture characteristics on mannitol salt agar, Baird-Parker agar, Tripticase soy agar, Chapman agar, Staphylococcus medium 110, positive results for Gram stain, catalase, coagulase and DNase Tests.

agr, Accessory gene regulator; AUR, Aureolysin; BAP, biofilm-associated protein; CAN, collagen-binding protein; ET, Exfoliative toxins; MLVA, Multiple-locus variable-number tandem repeat analysis; MRSA, methicillin resistant Staphylococcus aureus; NR, Not reported; NP, Not performed; NA, Not applicable; PFGE, pulsed-field gel electrophoresis; PVL, Panton-Valentine Leukocidin; RAPD, random amplified polymorphic DNA; SCCmec, staphylococcal cassette chromosome mec; SE, Staphylococcal enterotoxins; spa, Staphylococcus aureus protein A; TSST, Toxic shock syndrome toxin.

TABLE 4 | Characteristics of eligible studies analysing fecal carriage of *Staphylococcus aureus* or MRSA from the healthcare setting.

Study population setting	Participants screened for fecal[φ] carriage (n)	Participant characteristics			Sample collection			Laboratory technique(s)				*S. aureus* detection	MRSA detection	Reference
		Age range	Health status	Exposure to healthcare setting 12 months prior to screening[†]	Sample type	Age at which samples were collected	Site at which samples were collected	*S. aureus* detection	MRSA detection	Genotyping	Virulence profile analysis	% (n/N)	& (n/N)	
CATEGORY: IN-PATIENTS														
France	748	Mean age: 55 years±12	Liver cirrhosis	Hospitalized for minimum of 2 weeks	Feces	Mean age: 55 years±12	Hospital	Phenotypic	Phenotypic	NP	NP	NR	12 (93/748)	Campillo et al., 2001
France	327	NR	Chronic liver disease, post-surgical patients, patients with alcohol withdrawal and digestive tract diseases	Patients transferred from other hospitals	Feces	NR	Hospital	Phenotypic and Molecular	Phenotypic	PFGE	NP	NR	11 (36/327)	Dupeyron et al., 2002
Germany	2727	NR	Nosocomial diarrhea	≥72 h at the time of study	Feces	NR	Hospital	Phenotypic	Phenotypic	NP	SE	7 (198/2727)	15 (29/198)	Flemming and Ackermann, 2007
Germany	131	NR	NR	Inpatients positive for MRSA	Rectal swabs	NR	Hospital	Phenotypic and Molecular	Phenotypic and Molecular	PFGE	SE	NR	47 (61/131)	Klotz et al., 2005
Jordan	214	≤28 days to 1 year	NR	NR	Feces	≤28 days to 1 year	NICU	Phenotypic	Phenotypic	SCC*mec* typing	ET PVL SE TSST	2 (5/214)	20 (1/5)	Shehabi et al., 2013
Saudi Arabia	122	NR	NR	≥72 h at the time of study	Feces	NR	Hospital	Phenotypic	Phenotypic	NP	NP	NA	7 (9/122)	Babay and Somily, 2009
United States of America	810 (2000-01) 925 (2006-07)	NR	Cancer	Inpatients[φ]	Rectal swabs	NR	Hospital	Phenotypic and Molecular	Phenotypic	*spa* typing MLST PFGE	PVL	NR	0.6 (5/810)[φ] 2.9 (27/925)[φ]	Srinivasan et al., 2010

(Continued)

TABLE 4 | Continued

Study population setting	Participants screened for fecal[Ψ] carriage (n)	Participant characteristics			Sample collection			Laboratory technique(s)				*S. aureus* detection	MRSA detection	Reference
		Age range	Health status	Exposure to healthcare setting 12 months prior to screening[†]	Sample type	Age at which samples were collected	Site at which samples were collected	*S. aureus* detection	MRSA detection	Genotyping	Virulence profile analysis	% (n/N)	& (n/N)	
United States of America	161	57–103 years	Fecal and urinary in-continence, pressure ulcers, diabetes, COPD, heart failure	Long-term care facility residents	Rectal swabs	57-103 years	Long-term care wards	NP	Phenotypic	PFGE	NP	NA	3 (4/161)	O'Fallon et al., 2009
United States of America	37	48–91 years	Chronic renal failure, diabetes, chronic dermato-logic infections	Inpatients positive for VRE	Feces	48 to 91 years	Hospital	Phenotypic	Phenotypic	PFGE	NP	62 (23/37)	87 (20/23)	Ray et al., 2003
United States of America	114	NR	NR	Skilled-care patients admitted for long-term care	Rectal swabs		Hospital	Phenotypic	Phenotypic	PFGE	NP	NR	5 (6/114)	Trick et al., 2001
CATEGORY: HEALTHCARE PERSONNEL														
United States of America	62	>18 years	Healthy pregnant women at 35–37 weeks of pregnancy	No[φ]	Rectal swabs	> 18 years	Obstetric clinics	Phenotypic	Phenotypic and Molecular	SCC*mec* typing PFGE	PVL	3 (2/62)[φ]	0 (0/2)[φ]	Andrews et al., 2009
United States of America	55	36 years±11	NR	Nurses (n = 29), Physicians (n = 15), Others (n = 9), Unknown (n = 2) (mean patient contact years: 13 years±9)	Fecal	36 years±11	NR	NP	Phenotypic	NP	NP	NA	0 (0/55)	Carmeli et al., 1998

[Ψ]*Fecal samples, rectal swabs, anal swabs, peri-rectal or peri-anal swabs.*

[†]*Hospital, long-term care facility, nursing homes, maternity wards.*

[φ]*Information obtained from the author.*

Phenotypic identification: culture characteristics on mannitol salt agar, Baird-Parker agar, Tripticase soy agar, Chapman agar, Staphylococcus medium 110, positive results for Gram stain, catalase, coagulase and DNase Tests.

agr, Accessory gene regulator; AUR, Aureolysin; BAP, biofilm-associated protein; CNA, collagen-binding protein; COPD, chronic obstructive pulmonary disorder; ET, Exfoliative toxins; MLVA, Multiple-locus variable-number tandem repeat analysis; MRSA, methicillin resistant Staphylococcus aureus; NICU, Neonatal intensive care unit; NR, Not reported; NP, Not performed; NA, Not applicable; PFGE: pulsed-field gel electrophoresis; PVL, Panton-Valentine Leukocidin; SCCmec, staphylococcal cassette chromosome mec; SE, Staphylococcal enterotoxins; spa, Staphylococcus aureus protein A; TSST, Toxic shock syndrome toxin; VRE, Vancomycin-resistance enterococci.

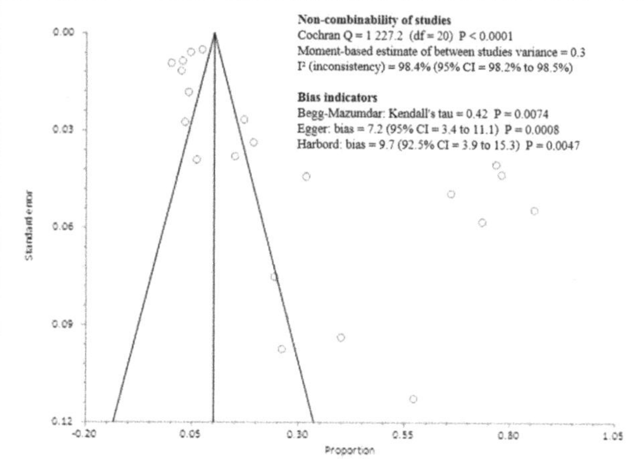

FIGURE 2 | Bias assessment (Funnel) plot for studies assessing *Staphylococcus aureus* fecal carriage rates.

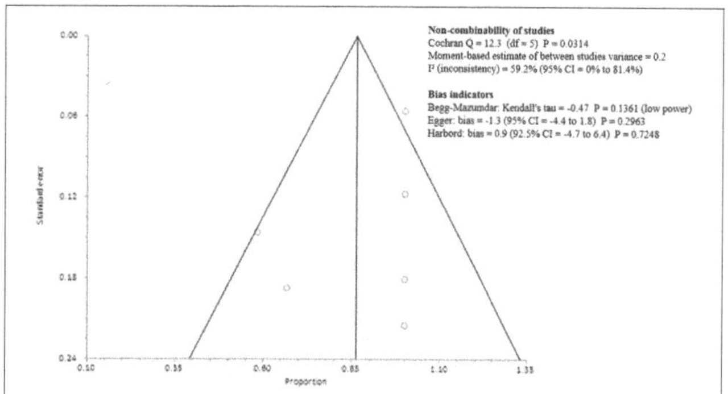

FIGURE 3 | Bias assessment (Funnel) plot for studies assessing Methicillin susceptible *Staphylococcus aureus* fecal carriage rates.

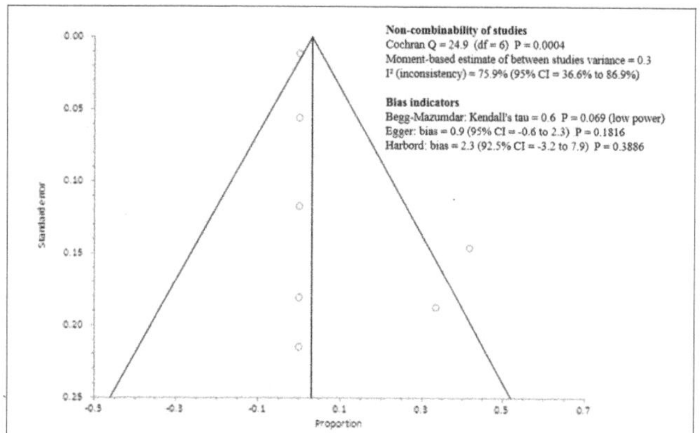

FIGURE 4 | Bias assessment (Funnel) plot for studies assessing Methicillin resistant *Staphylococcus aureus* fecal carriage rates.

screened with 32 different antibiotics across the respective studies using disk diffusion, agar dilution, or the Vitek Legacy System. The use of published guidelines for susceptibility testing were reported by six of the eight studies (**Table 5**). Susceptibility testing to erythromycin was performed most frequently (88%; 7/8), followed by chloramphenicol, clindamycin, ciprofloxacin, gentamicin, penicillin and vancomycin (75%; 6/8) (**Table 5**). Vancomycin intermediate or resistant *S. aureus* (VISA/VRSA) were not identified in five of the six studies that screened for vancomycin resistance (**Table 5**). Only the study by Onanuga and Temedie (2011) reported fecal VRSA carriage of 37% (14/38).

Genotyping of *S. aureus* Isolated from Fecal Specimens

Techniques used to genotype *S. aureus* isolated from fecal specimens included multiple-locus variable-number tandem repeat analysis (MLVA), pulsed-field gel electrophoresis (PFGE), random amplified polymorphic DNA (RAPD) analysis, staphylococcal cassette chromosome *mec* (SCC*mec*), accessory gene regulator (*agr*) and *Staphylococcus aureus* protein A (*spa*) typing (**Tables 3, 4**). Genotyping was performed in slightly more reports from the healthcare setting (67%; 8/12) compared to the community (58%; 11/19). Gel-based methods (PFGE, RAPD and MLVA) were employed in 58% (7/12) and 42% (8/19) of studies in the healthcare and community settings, respectively. In addition, similar rates (26% vs. 25%) in the use of sequence-based methods (*spa* typing, SCC*mec* typing and MLST) for genotyping of *S. aureus* strains were reported from community and healthcare settings. Only a single study conducted in a developing country (Jordan) performed genotyping of the *S. aureus* strains (Shehabi et al., 2013).

Assessment of the Detection of *S. aureus* Virulence Genes

Virulence genes screened included the aureolysin enzyme, biofilm-associated protein, collagen-binding protein, exfoliative toxins (ETs), staphylococcal enterotoxins (SEs), toxic shock syndrome toxin (TSST), and Panton-Valentine leukocidin (PVL) (**Tables 3, 4**). More community-based investigations screened for *S. aureus* virulence genes compared to reports from the healthcare setting. Thus, 53% (10/19), 37% (7/19), and 37% (7/19) of studies conducted in the community setting reported on TSSTs, SEs, ETs, respectively, using PCR, reverse passive latex agglutination tests or enzyme-linked immunosorbent assays. Approximately one third of the studies conducted in the community setting (6/19) reported on PCR detection of the PVL genes. In studies conducted in the healthcare setting; 8% (1/12), 25% (3/12.), 8% (1/12), and 25% (3/12) reported on TSSTs, SEs, ETs, and PVL, respectively.

S. aureus and MRSA Fecal Carriage as Risk Factors for Disease Development

Two studies included in this review identified enterotoxin producing *S. aureus* strains from fecal specimens of patients with diarrhea (Efuntoye and Adetosoye, 2003; Flemming and Ackermann, 2007). Another study reported that all patients colonized with MRSA in both the nares and rectum (8/8) developed an infection (Srinivasan et al., 2010). In addition, two of the nine patients, colonized with MRSA in the rectum only, were concurrently or subsequently infected. *Spa* typing on a

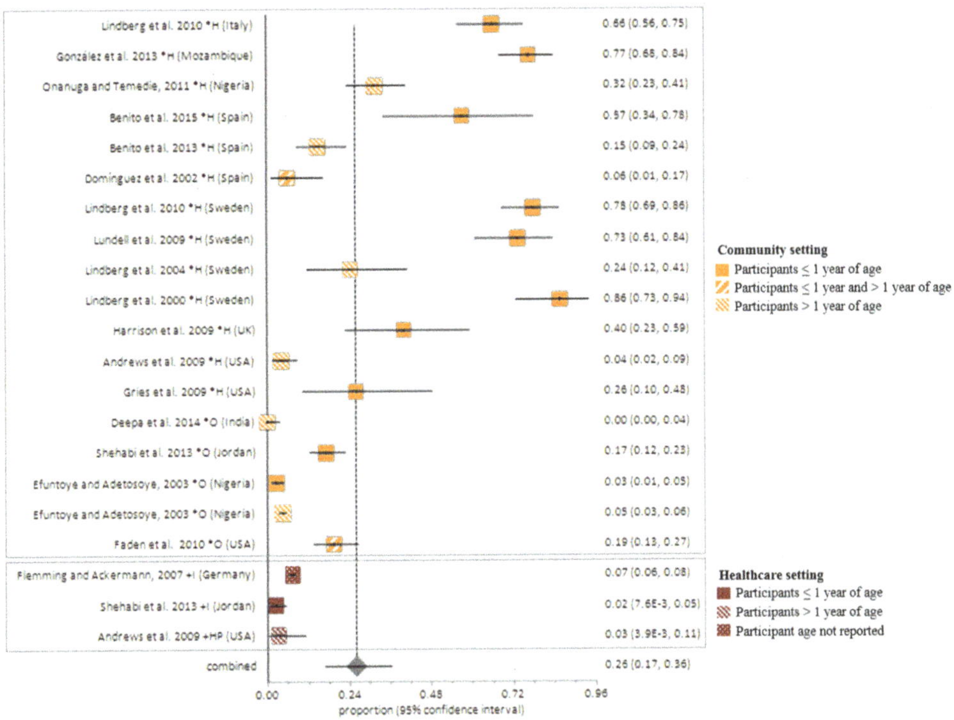

FIGURE 5 | Meta-analysis of proportions on *S. aureus* fecal carriage rates. *, Community setting; +, Healthcare setting; H, Healthy participants; O, Outpatients; I, Inpatients; HP, Healthcare personnel.

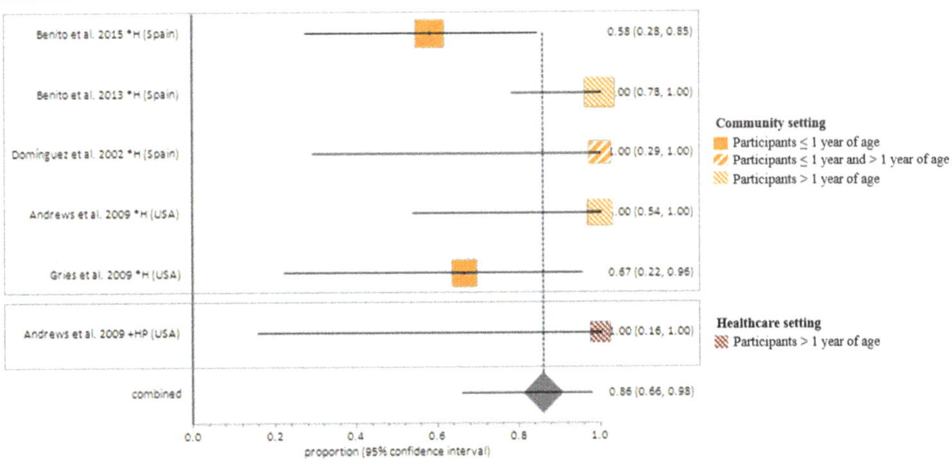

FIGURE 6 | Meta-analyses of proportions on Methicillin susceptible *Staphylococcus aureus* fecal carriage rates. Pooled random-effects estimate of MSSA fecal carriage within the community and healthcare setting. *, Community setting; +, Healthcare setting; H, Healthy participants; HP, Healthcare personnel.

subset of colonizing isolates from the nares and rectum noted that the majority (69%; 9/13) were clonally related to infecting isolates (Srinivasan et al., 2010). In support of the potential of fecal carriage for infection, it has also been shown that *S. aureus* detection occurs more frequently from rectal specimens of children with skin and soft tissue abscesses (47%; 28/60) compared with the control group (1%; 1/90) ($P = 0.0001$) (Faden et al., 2010).

DISCUSSION

Our results clearly showed that fecal *S. aureus* carriage from healthy infants is high during the first year of life. Specifically, *S. aureus* fecal carriage rates increased during the first 8 weeks of life followed by a gradual decrease towards 1 year of life. The reasons for this abrupt increase in fecal carriage very early in life (especially from healthy infants) is not yet clear,

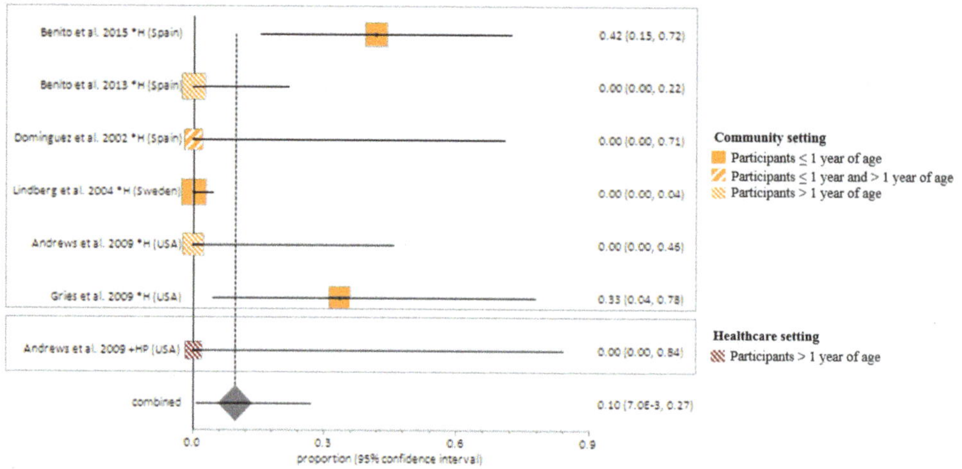

FIGURE 7 | Meta-analyses of proportions on Methicillin resistant *Staphylococcus aureus* fecal carriage rates. Pooled random effects estimate of MRSA fecal carriage within community and healthcare settings. *, Community setting; +, Healthcare setting; H, Healthy participants; HP, Healthcare personnel.

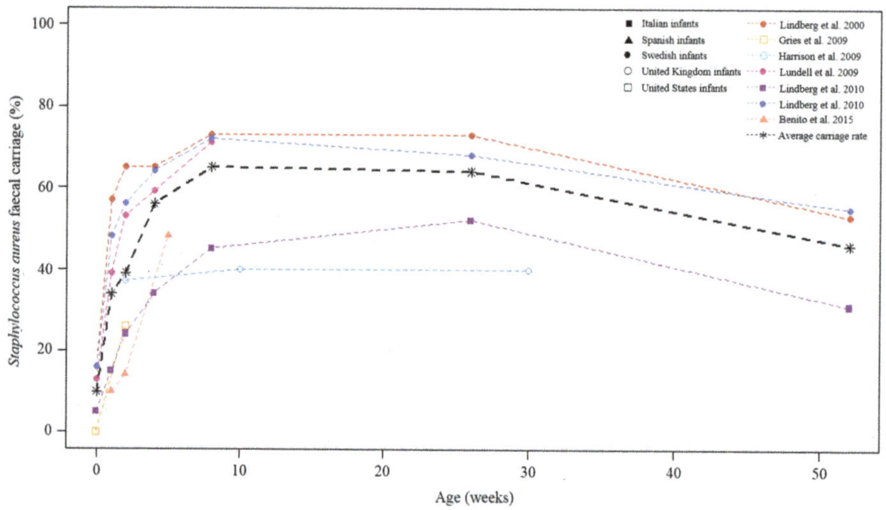

FIGURE 8 | Longitudinal *S. aureus* fecal carriage rates during the first year of life. The lines in color indicated fecal carriage rates (%) at each of the time-points measured by the respective studies. The different cohorts are shown by different symbols at each of the time-points studied. The black broken line is the average fecal *S. aureus* carriage rate calculated from all longitudinal studies at the respective time-points under study.

however a potential explanation may be early life care-giving practices, particularly breastfeeding. For example, colostrum contains the highest levels of human milk oligosaccharides (HMOs) (Bode, 2012), which have been suggested to stimulate *S. aureus* growth (Hunt et al., 2012). Moreover, *S. aureus* strains may be transmitted from parents via skin contact (Lindberg et al., 2004a) or from the mother via breastfeeding (Kawada et al., 2003; Lindberg et al., 2004a; Benito et al., 2015). Furthermore, staphylococci from the maternal GIT or skin surrounding the areola may be transferred to breast milk during lactation (Thum et al., 2012; Fernández et al., 2013). Higher *S. aureus* fecal carriage rates have also been noted from breast-fed in comparison to formula-fed or mixed-fed infants (González et al., 2013; Salminen et al., 2015). The observed change in the dynamics of *S. aureus* fecal carriage after 8 weeks of life may be explained by the increase in anaerobic bacteria from around 1 week of life (Bezirtzoglou, 1997; Adlerberth et al., 2006; Adlerberth and Wold, 2009; Jost et al., 2012), as well as the introduction of formula feeding (González et al., 2013) and solid foods (Bergström et al., 2014; Voreades et al., 2014). Infant fecal bacterial profiles have also been shown to change during the course of the lactation period (Cabrera-Rubio et al., 2012; González et al., 2013).

This systematic review does not only provide insight into the dynamics of fecal *S. aureus* carriage rates during the first year of life; but also highlights that *S. aureus* and MRSA fecal carriage is a potential risk factor for subsequent infections. Vancomycin is

TABLE 5 | Antibiotic resistance profiles across participants screened for fecal *S. aureus* or MRSA.

Study	Guide-lines applied	Techniques applied	Total number of *S. aureus* or MRSA isolates screened for resistance	Antibiotic resistance profiles of fecal S. aureus or MRSA isolates (%)																															
				Aminoglycosides					β-lactam/β-lactamase inhibitors	Cephalosporin			Fluoroquinolones			Glycopeptides		Lincosamides	Lipopeptides		Macrolides		Oxazolidinones	Penicillins				Phenicols	Pseudomonic acid	Pyrimidines	Pyrimidines/Sulfonamides	Streptogramin	Steroidal	Tetracyclines	
				Amikacin	Gentamicin	Kanamycin	Streptomycin	Tobramycin	Amoxicillin-clavulanic acid	Cefoxitin	Cefuroxime	Cephalothin	Ciprofloxacin	Levofloxacin	Ofloxacin	Teicoplanin	Vancomycin	Clindamycin	Colistin	Polymyxin B	Erythromycin	Spiramycin	Linezolid	Ampicillin	Methicillin	Penicillin	Oxacillin	Chloramphenicol	Mupirocin	Trimethoprim	Co-trimoxazole	Virginiamycin	Fusidic acid	Doxycycline	Tetracycline
Domínguez et al., 2002	NR	Agar dilution method	3		0	0	0	0					0			0	0	0			67					100	0	0							0
Efuntoye and Adetosoye, 2003	NCCLS	Disk diffusion method	72			22						0						9	99	99	67			79	7	100		0							
Lindberg et al., 2004b	SRGA	Disk diffusion method	116		0			0					0			0	0	1			3					78	0	0		0			1		2
Flemming and Ackermann, 2007	NR	Disk diffusion method	198																								15								
Srinivasan et al., 2010	CLSI	Vitek Legacy System	31*		3					100			0	32			0	32			81					100			0		3				
Onanuga and Temedie, 2011	CLSI	Disk diffusion and agar dilution method	38	0	5				18	34	24		8		8		37				34	0		68				34			37	0		61	
Benito et al., 2013	CLSI CA-SFM	Disk diffusion method	15		0	0	0	7		0			0				0	20			20		0			60	0	0	7		0		0		0
Benito et al., 2015	CLSI EUCAST	Disk diffusion method	25		36	0	16	36		40			4				0	32			36		0			40	40	0	0		0		4		0

(CA-SFM), Antibiogram Committee of the French Society of Microbiology; (CLSI), Clinical Laboratory Standards Institute; (EUCAST), European Committee on Antimicrobial Susceptibility; (NCCLS), National Committee on Clinical Laboratory Standards; (SRGA), Swedish Reference Group for Antibiotics; NR, Not reported.

**Number of MRSA isolates (detected using oxacillin screening agar) screened for antibiotic resistance*

Antibiotic resistance rates (%): 0; > 0–10; > 10–20; > 20–30; > 30–40; > 40–50; > 50–60; > 60–70; > 70–80; > 80–90; > 90–100.

regarded as one of the drugs of choice for MRSA infections (Tarai et al., 2013); however the emergence of vancomycin resistant *S. aureus* (VRSA) poses yet another threat to infection control (Hiramatsu, 1998; Spagnolo et al., 2014). The intestinal tract, in particular, may be a key potential reservoir for the emergence and transmission of VRSA isolates due to the intestinal coexistence (Ray et al., 2003), and potential transfer of the *vanA* gene from VRE to MRSA (Courvalin, 2006). Although, 23% of the studies included in this review screened for fecal carriage of VRSA within community and healthcare settings (Domínguez et al., 2002; Lindberg et al., 2004b; Srinivasan et al., 2010; Onanuga and Temedie, 2011; Benito et al., 2013, 2015); only a single study, performed in Nigeria, reported VRSA fecal carriage (Onanuga and Temedie, 2011). It is noteworthy, however, that this finding should be interpreted with caution as the disk diffusion method was used to screen for vancomycin resistance at 30 μg/ml, which is not recommended by the CLSI guidelines (Clinical Laboratory Standards Institute, 2012).

Healthcare associated fecal screening for *S. aureus* and MRSA is of key importance in infection control (Campillo et al., 2001; Ray et al., 2003; Bhalla et al., 2007). For example, it has been shown that select staphylococcal enterotoxins (SEs) may contribute to the colonizing success of *S. aureus* strains in the GIT (Nowrouzian et al., 2011), which could potentially facilitate in its transmission. Moreover, *S. aureus* and MRSA fecal carriage may complicate de-colonization, with a potential to contribute to infections within the healthcare setting (Campillo et al., 2001; Dupeyron et al., 2002; Ray et al., 2003; Srinivasan et al., 2010). To prevent nosocomial transmission and infection, two recent studies (Roth et al., 2016; Senn et al., 2016) have also highlighted the importance of screening for *S. aureus* fecal carriage on admission in the following risk groups: patients admitted to surgery or intensive care units with a history of MRSA colonization or infection; hospitalization during the past year; or direct transfer from another healthcare facility. Only a single study was considered eligible for inclusion in our meta-analyses of the proportions on MSSA and MRSA fecal carriage within the healthcare setting. Therefore we could not determine the fecal carriage rate for MSSA or MRSA within this setting.

A major limitation in this systematic review is the poor study design and limited data available from studies assessing the fecal carriage rates of *S. aureus* and MRSA. For example, a large proportion of potentially eligible articles were excluded due to the lack of information regarding participants' contact with healthcare facilities as well as the duration of hospital admission prior to *S. aureus* and MRSA screening. This information is essential in comparing fecal carriage rates from community and healthcare settings. Furthermore, a number of studies could not be included in calculating the pooled estimates for MSSA and MRSA fecal carriage (from both community and healthcare settings) due to the lack of molecular techniques incorporated to confirm MRSA carriage. On the other hand, the extent in which our observations could have changed if unavailable articles were included is unclear. However, based on the rigorous appraisal of various studies in this systematic review, we conclude that the excluded articles are not likely to impact significantly on observations presented in the manuscript. In addition, more studies from both developed and developing countries are needed in order to determine *S. aureus* and MRSA fecal carriage and transmission within and between the community and healthcare settings. In support of this, rural areas and low socioeconomic status have been shown to contribute to higher fecal transmission rates of *S. aureus* and MRSA (Vale and Vítor, 2010). Finally, there is the need for more sequence-based genotyping data on *S. aureus* and MRSA fecal carriage as the majority of studies from developed countries made use of gel-based methods which are not ideal when comparing isolates on a global level.

CONCLUSION

S. aureus, MSSA and MRSA fecal carriage rates within both the community and healthcare setting are not negligible and estimated at 26, 86, and 10%, respectively. Therefore, preventative strategies which include fecal *S. aureus* screening of high risk patients are necessary for infection control within these settings. More studies are needed to determine the role of fecal *S. aureus* carriage as a risk factor for disease development; as well as fecal carriage rates of MSSA, MRSA, and VRSA from both community and healthcare settings. Furthermore, well-structured research should be conducted and sequence-based genotyping techniques should be employed. The latter will allow for comparison of isolates on a global level in both developing and developed countries.

AUTHOR CONTRIBUTIONS

MK and SC initiated the project. SC, MRN, and MK searched the databases for potentially eligible articles based on their titles and abstracts. SC extracted the data and contacted authors of potentially eligible publications to obtain healthcare information on participants when this information was unclear or not provided by the articles. SC, MK, and AS reviewed the articles. SC, LT, and MK performed the statistical analysis and interpreted the results. SC, LT, AS, MPN, and MK wrote the manuscript. All the authors reviewed the final version of the manuscript prior to submission for publication.

FUNDING

This work was supported by the Bill and Melinda Gates Foundation Global Health Grant (OPP1017641), the National Research Foundation (South Africa), the Carnegie Corporation of New York (United States of America), the US National Institutes of Health (1U01AI110466-01A1), and the Wellcome Trust, United Kingdom (102429/Z/13/Z).

ROLE OF FUNDING SOURCE

Any opinions, findings and conclusions, or recommendations expressed in this review are those of the authors, and therefore do not represent the official position of the funders. The funders had no role in the study design, data collection and analysis, decision to publish, or preparation of the manuscript. The first and the corresponding author had full access to the study data.

All authors had final responsibility for the decision to submit the article for publication.

ACKNOWLEDGMENTS

SC is supported by the National Research Foundation and the Drakenstein Child Health Study, University of Cape Town (South Africa), a birth cohort study funded by Bill and Melinda Gates Foundation (OPP1017641). MK was a recipient of Carnegie Corporation of New York (USA) fellowship, and he is currently supported by Wellcome Trust, United Kingdom (102429/Z/13/Z).

REFERENCES

Acton, D. S., Plat-Sinnige, M. J. T., Van Wamel, W., de Groot, N., and van Belkum, A. (2009). Intestinal carriage of *Staphylococcus aureus*: how does its frequency compare with that of nasal carriage and what is its clinical impact? *Eur. J. Clin. Microbiol. Infect. Dis.* 28, 115–127. doi: 10.1007/s10096-008-0602-7

Adlerberth, I., Lindberg, E., Åberg, N., Hesselmar, B., Saalman, R., Strannegård, I.-L., et al. (2006). Reduced enterobacterial and increased staphylococcal colonization of the infantile bowel: an effect of hygienic lifestyle? *Pediatr. Res.* 59, 96–101. doi: 10.1203/01.pdr.0000191137.12774.b2

Adlerberth, I., and Wold, A. E. (2009). Establishment of the gut microbiota in Western infants. *Acta Paediatr.* 98, 229–238. doi: 10.1111/j.1651-2227.2008.01060.x

Andrews, J. I., Fleener, D. K., Messer, S. A., Kroeger, J. S., and Diekema, D. J. (2009). Screening for *Staphylococcus aureus* carriage in pregnancy: usefulness of novel sampling and culture strategies. *Am. J. Obstet. Gynecol.* 201, 396.e1–e5. doi: 10.1016/j.ajog.2009.06.062

Avery, L. M., Zempel, M., and Weiss, E. (2015). Case of antibiotic-associated diarrhea caused by *Staphylococcus aureus* enterocolitis. *Am. J. Health Syst. Pharm.* 72, 943–951. doi: 10.2146/ajhp140672

Babay, H. A. H., and Somily, A. M. (2009). Intestinal carriage of methicillin resistant *Staphylococcus aureus* and extended -spectrum beta-lactamase-producing Enterobacteriacae in hospitalized and nonhospitalized patients and their clinical implications. *Asian Pac. J. Trop. Med.* 2, 41–45.

Beall, J. (2015). *Beall's List: Potential, Possible, or Probable Predatory Scholarly Open-Access Publishers.* Available online at: http://scholarlyoa.com/publishers/

Benito, D., Lozano, C., Gómez-Sanz, E., Zarazaga, M., and Torres, C. (2013). Detection of Methicillin-susceptible *Staphylococcus aureus* ST398 and ST133 strains in gut microbiota of healthy humans in Spain. *Microb. Ecol.* 66, 105–111. doi: 10.1007/s00248-013-0240-1

Benito, D., Lozano, C., Jiménez, E., Albújar, M., Gómez, A., Rodríguez, J. M., et al. (2015). Characterization of *Staphylococcus aureus* strains isolated from faeces of healthy neonates and potential mother-to-infant microbial transmission through breastfeeding. *FEMS Microbiol. Ecol.* 91:fiv007. doi: 10.1093/femsec/fiv007

Bergström, A., Skov, T. H., Bahl, M. I., Roager, H. M., Christensen, L. B., Ejlerskov, K. T., et al. (2014). Establishment of intestinal microbiota during early life: a longitudinal, explorative study of a large cohort of Danish infants. *Appl. Environ. Microbiol.* 80, 2889–2900. doi: 10.1128/AEM.00342-14

Bezirtzoglou, E. (1997). The intestinal microflora during the first weeks of life. *Anaerobe* 3, 173–177. doi: 10.1006/anae.1997.0102

Bhalla, A., Aron, D. C., and Donskey, C. J. (2007). *Staphylococcus aureus* intestinal colonization is associated with increased frequency of *S. aureus* on skin of hospitalized patients. *BMC Infect. Dis.* 7:105. doi: 10.1186/1471-2334-7-105

Bode, L. (2012). Human milk oligosaccharides: every baby needs a sugar mama. *Glycobiology* 22, 1147–1162. doi: 10.1093/glycob/cws074

Bourgeois-Nicolaos, N., Lucet, J. C., Daubié, C., Benchaba, F., Rajguru, M., Ruimy, R., et al. (2010). Maternal vaginal colonisation by *Staphylococcus aureus* and newborn acquisition at delivery. *Paediatr. Perinat. Epidemiol.* 24, 488–491. doi: 10.1111/j.1365-3016.2010.01139.x

Boyce, J. M., Havill, N. L., Otter, J. A., and Adams, N. M. T. (2007). Widespread environmental contamination associated with patients with diarrhea and methicillin-resistant *Staphylococcus aureus* colonization of the gastrointestinal tract. *Infect. Control Hosp. Epidemiol.* 28, 1142–1147. doi: 10.1086/520737

Cabrera-Rubio, R., Collado, M. C., Laitinen, K., Salminen, S., Isolauri, E., and Mira, A. (2012). The human milk microbiome changes over lactation and is shaped by maternal weight and mode of delivery. *Am. J. Clin. Nut.* 96, 544–551. doi: 10.3945/ajcn.112.037382

Campillo, B., Dupeyron, C., and Richardet, J. P. (2001). Epidemiology of hospital-acquired infections in cirrhotic patients: effect of carriage of methicillin-resistant *Staphylococcus aureus* and influence of previous antibiotic therapy and norfloxacin prophylaxis. *Epidemiol. Infect.* 127, 443–450. doi: 10.1017/S0950268801006288

Carmeli, Y., Venkataraman, L., DeGirolami, P. C., Lichtenberg, D. A., Karchmer, A. W., and Samore, M. H. (1998). Stool colonization of healthcare workers with selected resistant bacteria. *Infect. Control Hosp. Epidemiol.* 19, 38–40.

Cochran, W. G. (1954). The combination of estimates from different experiments. *Biometrics* 10, 101–129.

Courvalin, P. (2006). Vancomycin resistance in gram-positive cocci. *Clin. Infect. Dis.*, 42, S25–S34. doi: 10.1086/491711

Deepa, S., Vandana, S., and Venkatesha, D. (2014). Screening at admission for carrier prevalence of multidrug resistant organisms: a hospital based observational study. *Biosci. Biotechnol. Res. Asia* 11, 309–316. doi: 10.13005/bbra/1273

Domínguez, E., Zarazaga, M., and Torres, C. (2002). Antibiotic resistance in *Staphylococcus* isolates obtained from fecal samples of healthy children. *J. Clin. Microbiol.* 40, 2638–2641. doi: 10.1128/JCM.40.7.2638

Dukic, V. M., Lauderdale, D. S., Wilder, J., Daum, R. S., and David, M. Z. (2013). Epidemics of community-associated methicillin-resistant *Staphylococcus aureus* in the United States: a meta-analysis. *PLoS ONE* 8:e52722. doi: 10.1371/journal.pone.0052722

Dupeyron, C., Campillo, B., Bordes, M., Faubert, E., Richardet, J.-P, and Mangeney, N. (2002). A clinical trial of mupirocin in the eradication of methicillin-resistant *Staphylococcus aureus* nasal carriage in a digestive disease unit. *J. Hosp. Infect.* 52, 281–287. doi: 10.1053/jhin.2002.1287

Efuntoye, M. O., and Adetosoye, A. I. (2003). Enterotoxigenicity and drug sensitivity of staphylococci from children aged five years and below with sporadic diarrhoea. *East Afr. Med. J.* 80, 656–659. doi: 10.4314/eamj.v80i12.8784

Egger, M., Davey Smith, G., Schneider, M., and Minder, C. (1997). Bias in meta-analysis detected by a simple, graphical test. *BMJ* 315, 629–634.

Ellis, M. W., Hospenthal, D. R., Dooley, D. P., Gray, P. J., and Murray, C. K. (2004). Natural history of community-acquired methicillin-resistant *Staphylococcus aureus* colonization and infection in soldiers. *Clin. Infect. Dis.* 39, 971–979. doi: 10.1086/423965

Faden, H., Lesse, A. J., Trask, J., Hill, J. A., Hess, D. J., Dryja, D., et al. (2010). Importance of colonization site in the current epidemic of staphylococcal skin abscesses. *Pediatrics* 125, e618–e624. doi: 10.1542/peds.2009-1523

Fernández, L., Langa, S., Martín, V., Maldonado, A., Jiménez, E., Martín, R., et al. (2013). The human milk microbiota: origin and potential roles in health and disease. *Pharmacol. Res.* 69, 1–10. doi: 10.1016/j.phrs.2012.09.001

Flemming, K., and Ackermann, G. (2007). Prevalence of enterotoxin producing *Staphylococcus aureus* in stools of patients with nosocomial diarrhea. *Infection* 35, 356–358. doi: 10.1007/s15010-007-6268-8

Folden, D. V., Machayya, J. A., Sahmoun, A. E., Beal, J. R., Holzman, G. S., Helgerson, S. D., et al. (2005). Estimating the proportion of community-associated methicillin-resistant *Staphylococcus aureus*: two definitions used in the USA yield dramatically different estimates. *J. Hosp. Infect.* 60, 329–332. doi: 10.1016/j.jhin.2004.12.025

González, R., Mandomando, I., Fumadó, V., Sacoor, C., Macete, E., Alonso, P. L., et al. (2013). Breast milk and gut microbiota in African mothers and infants from an area of high HIV prevalence. *PLoS ONE* 8:e80299. doi: 10.1371/journal.pone.0080299

Gries, D. M., Zemzars, T. F., Gibson, K. A., O'Hern, E., Iyer, M., Myers, M., et al. (2009). A pilot study to assess frequency of carriage and routes of acquisition of *Staphylococcus aureus* by healthy infants. *Am. J. Infect. Control* 37, 598–600. doi: 10.1016/j.ajic.2008.12.003

Harrison, L. M., Morris, J. A., Lauder, R. M., and Telford, D. R. (2009). Staphylococcal pyrogenic toxins in infant urine samples: a possible marker of transient bacteraemia. *J. Clin. Pathol.* 62, 718–735. doi: 10.1136/jcp.2008.057232

Higgins, J. P. T., Thompson, S. G., Deeks, J. J., and Altman, D. G. (2003). Measuring inconsistency in meta-analyses. *BMJ* 327, 557–560. doi: 10.1136/bmj.327.7414.557

Hiramatsu, K. (1998). Vancomycin resistance in staphylococci. *Drug Resist. Updat.* 1, 135–150. doi: 10.1016/S1368-7646(98)80029-0

Hunt, K. M., Preuss, J., Nissan, C., Davlin, C. A., Williams, J. E., Shafii, B., et al. (2012). Human milk oligosaccharides promote the growth of staphylococci. *Appl. Environ. Microbiol.* 78, 4763–4770. doi: 10.1128/AEM.00477-12

Hurst, V. (1960). Transmission of hospital staphylococci among newborn infants: II. Colonization of the skin and mucous membranes of the infants. *Pediatrics* 25, 204–214.

Jost, T., Lacroix, C., Braegger, C. P., and Chassard, C. (2012). New insights in gut microbiota establishment in healthy breast fed neonates. *PLoS ONE* 7:e44595. doi: 10.1371/journal.pone.0044595

Kawada, M., Okuzumi, K., Hitomi, S., and Sugishita, C. (2003). Transmission of *Staphylococcus aureus* between healthy, lactating mothers and their infants by breastfeeding. *J. Hum. Lact.* 19, 411–417. doi: 10.1177/0890334403257799

Klotz, M., Zimmermann, S., Opper, S., Heeg, K., and Mutters, R. (2005). Possible risk for re-colonization with methicillin-resistant *Staphylococcus aureus* (MRSA) by faecal transmission. *Int. J. Hyg. Environ. Health* 208, 401–405. doi: 10.1016/j.ijheh.2005.05.004

Kluytmans, J., van Belkum, A., and Verbrugh, H. (1997). Nasal carriage of *Staphylococcus aureus*: epidemiology, underlying mechanisms, and associated risks. *Clin. Microbiol. Rev.* 10, 505–520.

Lee, Y. L., Cesario, T., Gupta, G., Flionis, L., Tran, C., Decker, M., et al. (1997). Surveillance of colonization and infection with *Staphylococcus aureus* susceptible or resistant to methicillin in a community skilled-nursing facility. *Am. J. Infect. Control* 25, 312–321. doi: 10.1016/S0196-6553(97)90023-7

Levy, P. Y., Ollivier, M., Drancourt, M., Raoult, D., and Argenson, J. N. (2013). Relation between nasal carriage of *Staphylococcus aureus* and surgical site infection in orthopedic surgery: the role of nasal contamination. A systematic literature review and meta-analysis. *Orthop. Traumatol. Surg. Res.* 99, 645–651. doi: 10.1016/j.otsr.2013.03.030

Lindberg, E., Adlerberth, I., Hesselmar, B., Saalman, R., Strannegård, I.-L., Åberg, N., et al. (2004a). High rate of transfer of *Staphylococcus aureus* from parental skin to infant gut flora. *J. Clin. Microbiol.* 42, 530–534. doi: 10.1128/JCM.42.2.530-534.2004

Lindberg, E., Adlerberth, I., Matricardi, P., Bonanno, C., Tripodi, S., Panetta, V., et al. (2010). Effect of lifestyle factors on *Staphylococcus aureus* gut colonization in Swedish and Italian infants. *Clin. Microbiol. Infect.* 17, 1209–1215. doi: 10.1111/j.1469-0691.2010.03426.x

Lindberg, E., Adlerberth, I., and Wold, A. E. (2004b). Antibiotic resistance in *Staphylococcus aureus* colonising the intestines of Swedish infants. *Clin. Microbiol. Infect.* 10, 890–894. doi: 10.1111/j.1469-0691.2004.01002.x

Lindberg, E., Nowrouzian, F., Adlerberth, I., and Wold, A. E. (2000). Long-time persistence of superantigen-producing *Staphylococcus aureus* strains in the intestinal microflora of healthy infants. *Pediatr. Res.* 48, 741–747. doi: 10.1203/00006450-200012000-00007

Lo, T. S., and Borchardt, S. M. (2009). Antibiotic-associated diarrhea due to methicillin-resistant *Staphylococcus aureus*. *Diagn. Microbiol. Infect. Dis.* 63, 388–389. doi: 10.1016/j.diagmicrobio.2008.12.007

Lundell, A. C., Hesselmar, B., Nordström, I., Saalman, R., Karlsson, H., Lindberg, E., et al. (2009). High circulating immunoglobulin A levels in infants are associated with intestinal toxigenic *Staphylococcus aureus* and a lower frequency of eczema. *Clin. Exp. Allergy* 39, 662–670. doi: 10.1111/j.1365-2222.2008.03176.x

Maier, J., Melzl, H., Reischl, U., Drubel, I., Witte, W., Lehn, N., et al. (2005). Panton-Valentine leukocidin-positive methicillin-resistant *Staphylococcus aureus* in Germany associated with travel or foreign family origin. *Eur. J. Clin. Microbiol. Infect. Dis.* 24, 637–639. doi: 10.1007/s10096-005-0008-8

McKinnell, J. A., Miller, L. G., Eells, S. J., Cui, E., and Huang, S. S. (2013). A systematic literature review and meta-analysis of factors associated with methicillin-resistant *Staphylococcus aureus* colonization at time of hospital or intensive care unit admission. *Infect. Control Hosp. Epidemiol.* 34, 1077–1086. doi: 10.1086/673157

Mertz, D., Frei, R., Jaussi, B., Tietz, A., Stebler, C., Flückiger, U., et al. (2007). Throat swabs are necessary to reliably detect carriers of *Staphylococcus aureus*. *Clin. Infect. Dis.* 45, 475–477. doi: 10.1086/520016

Millar, B. C., Loughrey, A., Elborn, J. S., and Moore, J. E. (2007). Proposed definitions of community-associated meticillin-resistant *Staphylococcus aureus* (CA-MRSA). *J. Hosp. Infect.* 67, 109–113. doi: 10.1016/j.jhin.2007.06.003

Moher, D., Liberati, A., Tetzlaff, J., and Altman, D. G. (2009). Preferred reporting items for systematic reviews and meta-analyses: the PRISMA statement. *PLoS Med.* 6:1000097, DOI: 10.1371/journal.pmed.1000097

Nowrouzian, F. L., Dauwalder, O., Meugnier, H., Bes, M., Etienne, J., Vandenesch, F., et al. (2011). Adhesin and superantigen genes and the capacity of *Staphylococcus aureus* to colonize the infantile gut. *J. Infect. Dis.* 204, 714–721. doi: 10.1093/infdis/jir388

O'Fallon, E., Schreiber, R., Kandel, R., and D'Agata, E. M. C. (2009). Multidrug-Resistant gram-negative bacteria at a long-term care facility: assessment of residents, healthcare workers, and inanimate surfaces. *Infect. Control Hosp. Epidemiol.* 30, 1172–1179. doi: 10.1086/648453

Onanuga, A., and Temedie, T. C. (2011). Multidrug-resistant intestinal *Staphylococcus aureus* among self-medicated healthy adults in Amassoma, South-South, Nigeria. *J. Health Popul. Nutr.* 29, 446–453. doi: 10.3329/jhpn.v29i5.8898

Otter, J. A., and French, G. L. (2011). Community-associated meticillin-resistant *Staphylococcus aureus* strains as a cause of healthcare-associated infection. *J. Hosp. Infect.* 79, 189–193. doi: 10.1016/j.jhin.2011.04.028

Petersen, I. S., Larsen, P. L., Brandelev, B. L., Hald, J., Prætorius, C., Welinder, R., et al. (2013). Close association between oropharyngeal and rhinopharyngeal colonization with *Staphylococcus aureus* - clues to new insight of MRSA colonization of the oropharynx. *J. Hosp. Infect.* 84, 259–262. doi: 10.1016/j.jhin.2013.04.007

Popov, L., Kovalski, J., Grandi, G., Bagnoli, F., and Amieva, M. R. (2014). Three-dimensional human skin models to understand *Staphylococcus aureus* skin colonization and infection. *Front. Immunol.* 5:41. doi: 10.3389/fimmu.2014.00041

Ray, A. J., Pultz, N. J., Bhalla, A., Aron, D. C., and Donskey, C. J. (2003). Coexistence of vancomycin-resistant enterococci and *Staphylococcus aureus* in the intestinal tracts of hospitalized patients. *Clin. Infect. Dis.* 37, 875–881. doi: 10.1086/377451

Roth, V. R., Longpre, T., Taljaard, M., Coyle, D., Suh, K. N., Muldoon, K. A., et al. (2016). Universal vs risk factor screening for Methicillin-Resistant *Staphylococcus aureus* in a Large Multicenter Tertiary Care Facility in Canada. *Infect. Control Hosp. Epidemiol.* 37, 41–48. doi: 10.1017/ice.2015.230

Salminen, S., Endo, A., Isolauri, E., and Scalabrin, D. (2015). Early gut colonization with Lactobacilli and *Staphylococcus* in infants: the Hygiene Hypotphesis extended. *J. Pediatr. Gastroenterol. Nutr.* 62, 80–86. doi: 10.1097/MPG.0000000000000925

Senn, L., Clerc, O.,Zanetti, G., Basset, P., Prod'hom, G., Gordon, N. C., et al. (2016). The Stealthy Superbug: the role of asymptomatic enteric carriage inmaintaining a long-term hospital outbreak of ST228 methicillin-resistant *Staphylococcus aureus*. *MBio* 7, e02039–e02015. doi: 10.1128/mBio.02039-15

Shehabi, A. A., Abu-Yousef, R., Badran, E., Al-Bakri, A. G., Abu-Qatouseh, L. F., and Becker, K. (2013). Major characteristics of *Staphylococcus aureus* colonizing Jordanian infants. *Pediatr. Int.* 55, 300–304. doi: 10.1111/ped.12060

Shen, C., and Björk, B. C. (2015). "Predatory" open access: a longitudinal study of article volumes and market characteristics. *BMC Med.* 13:230. doi: 10.1186/s12916-015-0469-2

Siebert, S., Machesky, L. M., and Insall, R. H. (2015). Overflow in science and its implications for trust. *Elife* 4:e10825. doi: 10.7554/eLife.10825

Sizemore, E. N., Rivas, K. M., Valdes, J., and Caballero, J. (2012). Enteral vancomycin and probiotic use for methicillin-resistant *Staphylococcus aureus* antibiotic-associated diarrhoea. *BMJ Case Rep.* 2012, 1–5. doi: 10.1136/bcr-2012-006366

Sollid, J. U. E., Furberg, A. S., Hanssen, A. M., and Johannessen, M. (2014). *Staphylococcus aureus*: determinants of human carriage. *Infect. Genet. Evol.* 21, 531–541. doi: 10.1016/j.meegid.2013.03.020

Spagnolo, A. M., Orlando, P., Panatto, D., Amicizia, D., Perdelli, F., and Cristina, M. L. (2014). *Staphylococcus aureus* with reduced susceptibility to vancomycin in healthcare settings. *J. Prev. Med. Hyg.* 55, 137–144. doi: 10.15167/2421-4248/jpmh2014.55.4.454

Squier, C., Rihs, J. D., Risa, K. J., Sagnimeni, A., Wagener, M. M., Stout, J., et al. (2002). *Staphylococcus aureus* rectal carriage and its association with infections in patients in a surgical intensive care unit and a liver transplant unit. *Infect. Control Hosp. Epidemiol.* 23, 495–501. doi: 10.1086/500651

Srinivasan, A., Seifried, S. E., Zhu, L., Srivastava, D. K., Perkins, R., Shenep, J. L., et al. (2010). Increasing prevalence of nasal and rectal colonization with methicillin-resistant *Staphylococcus aureus* in children with cancer. *Pediatr. Blood Cancer* 55, 1317–1322. doi: 10.1002/pbc.22815

Clinical and Laboratory Standards Institute (2012). *Performance Standards for Antimicrobial Disk Susceptibility Tests; Approved Standard - Eleventh Edition. M02-A11, Vol.* 32. Wayne, PA: Clinical and Laboratory Standards Institute.

Sterne, J. A. C., Sutton, A. J., Ioannidis, J. P. A., Terrin, N., Jones, D. R., Lau, J., et al. (2011). Recommendations for examining and interpreting funnel plot asymmetry in meta-analyses of randomised. *BMJ* 342, 1–8. doi: 10.1136/bmj.d4002

Tarai, B., Das, P., and Kumar, D. (2013). Recurrent Challenges for Clinicians: emergence of Methicillin-Resistant *Staphylococcus aureus*, vancomycin resistance, and current treatment options. *J. Lab. Physicians* 5, 71–78. doi: 10.4103/0974-2727.119843

Thum, C., Cookson, A. L., Otter, D. E., Mcnabb, W. C., Hodgkinson, A. J., Dyer, J., et al. (2012). Can nutritional modulation of maternal intestinal microbiota influence the development of the infant gastrointestinal tract? *J. Nutr.* 142, 1921–1928. doi: 10.3945/jn.112.166231.1921

Tong, S. Y. C., Davis, J. S., Eichenberger, E., Holland, T. L., and Fowler, V. G. Jr. (2015). *Staphylococcus aureus* infections: epidemiology, pathophysiology, clinical manifestations, and management. *Clin. Microbiol. Rev.* 28, 603–661. doi: 10.1128/CMR.00134-14

Trick, W. E., Weinstein, R. A., DeMarais, P. L., Kuehnert, M. J., Tomaska, W., Nathan, C., et al. (2001). Colonization of skilled-care facility residents with antimicrobial-resistant pathogens. *Am. Geriatr. Soc.* 49, 270–276. doi: 10.1046/j.1532-5415.2001.4930270.x

Vale, F. F., and Vítor, J. M. B. (2010). Transmission pathway of *Helicobacter pylori*: does food play a role in rural and urban areas? *Int. J. Food Microbiol.* 138, 1–12. doi: 10.1016/j.ijfoodmicro.2010.01.016

van Belkum, A., Melles, D. C., Nouwen, J., van Leeuwen, W. B., van Wamel, W., Vos, M. C., et al. (2009). Co-evolutionary aspects of human colonisation and infection by *Staphylococcus aureus*. *Infect. Genet. Evol.* 9, 32–47. doi: 10.1016/j.meegid.2008.09.012

Voreades, N., Kozil, A., and Weir, T. L. (2014). Diet and the development of the human intestinal microbiome. *Front. Microbiol.* 5:494. doi: 10.3389/fmicb.2014.00494

Wertheim, H. F. L., Vos, M. C., Ott, A., van Belkum, A., Voss, A., Kluytmans, J. A. J. W., et al. (2004). Risk and outcome of nosocomial *Staphylococcus aureus* bacteraemia in nasal carriers versus non-carriers. *Lancet* 364, 703–705. doi: 10.1016/S0140-6736(04)16897-9

20

The IncP-6 Plasmid p10265-KPC from *Pseudomonas aeruginosa* Carries a Novel ΔIS*Ec33*-Associated *bla*$_{KPC-2}$ Gene Cluster

Xiaotian Dai[1], Dongsheng Zhou[2], Wei Xiong[1], Jiao Feng[2], Wenbo Luo[2,3], Guangming Luo[1], Haijing Wang[1], Fengjun Sun[3]* and Xiangdong Zhou[1]*

[1] Department of Pulmonology, Southwest Hospital, Third Military Medical University, Chongqing, China, [2] State Key Laboratory of Pathogen and Biosecurity, Beijing Institute of Microbiology and Epidemiology, Beijing, China, [3] Department of Pharmacy, Southwest Hospital, Third Military Medical University, Chongqing, China

***Correspondence:**
Xiangdong Zhou
xiangdongzhou@126.com;
Fengjun Sun
fengj_sun@163.com

Pseudomonas aeruginosa strain 10265 was recovered from a patient with pneumonia in a Chinese public hospital, and it displays the carbapenem resistance phenotype due to the acquisition of a non-conjugative but mobilizable IncP-6-type plasmid p10265-KPC. p10265-KPC carries a Tn*5563*-borne defective *mer* locus, and a novel ΔIS*Ec33*-associated *bla*$_{KPC-2}$ gene cluster without paired inverted repeats and paired direct repeats at both ends. Mobilization of this ΔIS*Ec33*-associated element in p10265-KPC would be attributed to homologous recombination-based insertion of a foreign structure Tn*3*-IS*Apu1*-*orf7*-IS*Apu2*- IS*Kpn27*-Δ*bla*$_{TEM-1}$-*bla*$_{KPC-2}$-ΔIS*Kpn6*-*korC*-*orf6*-*klcA*-Δ*repB* into a pre-existent intact IS*Ec33*, making IS*Ec33* truncated at the 3′ end. The previously reported pCOL-1 represents the first sequenced KPC-producing IncP-6 plasmid, while p10265-KPC is the second one. These two plasmids carry two distinct *bla*$_{KPC-2}$ gene clusters, which are inserted into the different sites of the IncP-6 backbone and have different evolutionary histories of assembly and mobilization. This is the first report of identification of the IncP-6-type resistance plasmid in China.

Keywords: *Pseudomonas aeruginosa*, KPC-2, p10265-KPC, IncP-6

INTRODUCTION

Klebsiella pneumoniae carbapenamases (KPCs) were initially discovered in USA in 1996, and they have disseminated worldwide among Enterobacteriaceae, *Pseudomonas* and *Acinetobacter* with *K. pneumoniae* being the most predominate species (Munoz-Price et al., 2013; Chen et al., 2014b). At least 23 KPC protein variants (KPC-2 to KPC-24, KPC-1 is essentially identical to KPC-2) have been identified[1]. The *bla*$_{KPC}$ genes are typically present on plasmids, varying in size, genetic structure and incompatibility group (e.g., IncFII, FIA, I2, A/C, N, X, R, P, U, W, L/M, and ColE; Munoz-Price et al., 2013; Chen et al., 2014b). Chromosomal location of *bla*$_{KPC}$ has also been evidenced in *Pseudomonas aeruginosa*, indicating that the *bla*$_{KPC}$ genes can be integrated into host genome (Villegas et al., 2007; Cuzon et al., 2011). KPC-producing bacteria are resistant to almost all β-lactams and often to other classes of antibiotics (such as aminoglycosides, quinolones, and tetracyclines), resulting from the co-selection of additional resistance determinants encoded by

[1]http://www.lahey.org/studies/

insertion sequence-, integron- and transposon-associated mobile gene clusters and, thereby, leaves few or no antimicrobial treatment options (Munoz-Price et al., 2013; Chen et al., 2014b).

At least thirteen incompatibility groups, IncP-1 to IncP-7 and IncP-9 to IncP-14, have been recognized for the plasmids found in the natural isolates of *Pseudomonas*, and about one third of these plasmids characterized belong to the IncP-2 group which typically have a size > 300 kb (Sagai et al., 1976; Boronin, 1992). Plasmids belonging to IncP-2, IncP-5, IncP-7, IncP-10, IncP-12, and IncP-13 incompatibility groups have a narrow host range and cannot be transferred from *Pseudomonas* to *Escherichia coli*, while the other IncP types especially including IncP-1, IncP-4, and IncP-6 seem to have a broad host range (Sagai et al., 1976; Boronin, 1992; Xiong et al., 2013). IncP-1 corresponds to IncP in the *E. coli* plasmid classification system, and plasmids of this group can transfer and replicate virtually in all Gram-negative bacteria, contributing to the spread of antibiotic and heavy metal resistance (Popowska and Krawczyk-Balska, 2013).

The IncP-6 plasmids are capable of replicating in both *E. coli* (where there are assigned into the IncG group) and *Pseudomonas*. Only a few IncP-6 plasmids, such as Rms149 from *P. aeruginosa* (Haines et al., 2005), pCOL-1 from *P. aeruginosa* (Naas et al., 2013) and pRIO-5 from *Serratia marcescens* (Bonnin et al., 2012), have been fully sequenced, and all these plasmid have acquired various mobile genetic structures harboring resistance markers. In addition, pRSB105 from an uncultured eubacterium represents a mosaic plasmid that carries the IncP-6 backbone as well as the Rep1 replicon module, most likely contributing to the extension of plasmid's host range (Schluter et al., 2007).

Data presented here reveal that *P. aeruginosa* strain 10265 harbors a novel IncP-6 resistance plasmid p10265-KPC. The complete sequence of p10265-KPC was determined and compared with other sequenced IncP-6 plasmids. p10265-KPC carries a novel Δ*ISEc33*-associated bla_{KPC-2} gene cluster as well as a Tn*5563*-borne defective mercury resistance (*mer*) gene locus, providing further insights into drug resistance mechanism of the KPC-encoding IncP-6 plasmids.

MATERIALS AND METHODS

Bacterial species was identified using Bruker MALDI Biotyper (Bruker Daltonics, Bremen, Germany) and 16S rRNA gene sequencing (Frank et al., 2008). The major acquired carbapenemase and extended-spectrum β-lactamase genes were detected by PCR, followed by amplicon sequencing on ABI 3730 Sequencer (Applied Biosystems, Foster City, CA, USA; Chen et al., 2015). The experimental protocols were approved by the Ethics Committee of the Third Military Medical University.

Plasmid electroporation or conjugal transfer was performed with *E. coli* TOP10 ($LacZ^-$, resistant to streptomycin and tetracycline) and EC600 ($LacZ^-$, resistant to nalidixic acid and rifampicin) being used as recipient for selection of bla_{KPC}-positive electroporants or transconjugants, respectively (Chen et al., 2015). Transfer of the bla_{KPC} gene on the plasmid was determined by S1-PFGE and Southern blot hybridization (Lee et al., 2012; Chen et al., 2015).

Activity of Ambler class A/B/D carbapenemases in bacterial cell extracts was determined by CarbaNP test (Dortet et al., 2012) with modifications (Chen et al., 2015). Bacterial antimicrobial susceptibility was tested by VITEK 2 (BioMérieux Vitek, Hazelwood, MO, USA) and interpreted as per Clinical and Laboratory Standards Institute guidelines (Twenty-Fourth Informational Supplement M10-S24, 2014).

Plasmid DNA was isolated from *E. coli* electroporant using Qiagen large construct kit (Qiagen, Hilden, Germany), and sequenced by whole-genome shotgun strategy in combination with Illumina HiSeq 2500 (Illumina, San Diego, CA, USA) sequencing technology. The contigs were assembled with Velvet, and the gaps were filled through combinatorial PCR and Sanger sequencing on ABI 3730 Sequencer. The genes were predicted with GeneMarkS^{TM} and further annotated by BLASTP and BLASTN against UniProt and NR databases. Gene organization diagrams were drawn with Inkscape[2]. The complete sequence of p10265-KPC was submitted to GenBank under accession number KU578314.

RESULTS AND DISCUSSION

Case Report

In September 2010, an 81-year-old male with hemafecia visited a public hospital in Beijing of China, and the progressive symptoms of fever, couch, and pulmonary infection were observed after hospitalization. The patient had the underlying diseases hypertension, diabetes, multiple cerebral infarction, and chronic renal insufficiency. The patient received long-term hospital care under the hospital and was bed-ridden with indwelling catheter. His symptoms of hemafecia were generally well controlled during hospitalization, but he started to suffer from the recurrent urinary tract infections since August 2013. About 2 weeks later, bacterial colonies were observed after cultivation of the urine specimens on the Mueller-Hinton agar, and the bacterial isolate designated 10265 was identified as *P. aeruginosa*. Based on the antimicrobial susceptibility test results, the patient received the intravenous administration with amikacin, and his symptoms associated with urinary tract infections progressively disappeared.

Overview of Plasmid p10265-KPC

Screening for the bla_{GES}, bla_{KPC}, bla_{SME}, bla_{IMI}, bla_{BIC}, bla_{IMP}, bla_{VIM}, bla_{NDM}, bla_{TMB}, bla_{FIM}, bla_{SPM}, bla_{DIM}, bla_{GIM}, bla_{SIM}, bla_{AIM}, bla_{SMB}, bla_{OXA}, bla_{CTX-M}, bla_{TEM}, bla_{SHV}, bla_{GES}, bla_{PER}, bla_{VEB}, and bla_{OXA} genes by PCR (Chen et al., 2015) indicated the presence of only bla_{KPC-2} (but not any of the other *bla* genes tested) in strain 10265. Electroporation of the plasmid DNA of strain 10265 into *E. coli* TOP10 generated a bla_{KPC}-positive electroporant 10265-KPC-TOP10, but repeated attempts of plasmid conjugal transfer with *E. coli* EC600 being used as recipient and strain 10265 as donor failed to obtain a bla_{KPC}-positive *E. coli* transconjugant. S1-PFGE followed by Southern hybridization (Chen et al., 2015) indicated the presence

[2]https://inkscape.org/

of a ~40 kb plasmid, being able to hybridize with a bla_{KPC}-specific probe (Lee et al., 2012), in both 10265 and 10265-KPC-TOP10 (data not shown)·10265 and 10265-KPC-TOP10 but not TOP10 have the class A carbapenemase activity (data not shown). Strain 10265 is resistant to all the β-lactam, β-lactamase inhibitor, fluoroquinolone, and sulfonamide drugs tested but remains susceptible to aminoglycosides, while 10265-KPC-TOP10 is resistant to β-lactams and β-lactamase inhibitors but remains susceptible to all the other drugs (**Table 1**). Taken together, strain 10265 harbors a non-conjugative plasmid p10265-KPC, which carries the bla_{KPC-2} gene to mediate the resistance to β-lactams including monobactam and carbapenems.

The complete sequence of p10265-KPC, recovered from the 10265-KPC-TOP10 strain, was determined with a mean coverage of 124, resulting in a circular plasmid sequence of 38,939 bp with an average G + C content of 58.2% (**Figure 1**). Sequence annotation generated a total of 41 predicted open reading frames. The modular structure of p10265-KPC is divided into the backbone [especially including the regions for plasmid replication (*repA*) and stability (*parABC* and *mob*)], and three separate accessory modules (a novel bla_{KPC-2} gene cluster, Tn*5563*, and IS*Pa19*) inserted at the different sites of the backbone.

Accessory Modules of p10265-KPC

The rapid spread of bla_{KPC} genes in European and American countries is linked to their location in a Tn*3*-family unit transposon Tn*4401* with at least eight designated isoforms *a* to *g* and a separate *d* (Chen et al., 2012; Bryant et al., 2013; Chmelnitsky et al., 2014). Tn*4401b* is the prototype one and has a modular structure *tnpRA* (transposition core module)-IS*Kpn7*-bla_{KPC}-IS*Kpn6*, which is delimited by two 39 bp inverted repeats (IRs), and the other isoforms result from distinct deletion or insertion events occurring at the different sites of Tn*4401b* (Chen et al., 2012; Bryant et al., 2013; Chmelnitsky et al., 2014).

In China, Tn*4401* is rarely found (Ho et al., 2013) and, instead, a core module Tn*3*-IS*Kpn27*-bla_{KPC}-ΔIS*Kpn6* is frequently identified as the bla_{KPC} platform (Shen et al., 2009; Chen et al., 2014a,c; Li et al., 2015). For generation of the above core module, an intact IS*Kpn27* is inserted into the 3′-end of Tn*3*, and then the resulting Tn*3*-IS*Kpn27* is connected with bla_{KPC-2} and ΔIS*Kpn6* (**Figure 2**). This core module is imbedded in two major classes of transposons (Wang et al., 2015), the Tn*1722*-based unit transposons [e.g., pKP048 (Shen et al., 2009)] and the IS*26*-based composite transposons [e.g., pKPC-LKEc (Chen et al., 2014c)].

The Tn*1722*-based transposon in pKP048 (Shen et al., 2009) looks like a prototype one, and it is generated from the

TABLE 1 | Antimicrobial resistance phenotypes of *Pseudomonas aeruginosa* and *Escherichia coli* with plasmid p10265-KPC.

Antibiotics	MIC (mg/L)/antimicrobial susceptibility		
	P. aeruginosa 10265	*E. coli* 10265-KPC-TOP10	*E. coli* TOP10
Penicillins			
Ampicillin	≥32/R	≥32/R	4/S
Ampicillin/sulbactam	≥32/R	≥32/R	4/S
Piperacillin	≥128/R	≥128/R	≤4/S
Piperacillin/tazobactam	≥128/R	≥128/R	≤4/S
Cephalosporins			
Cefazolin	≥64/R	≥64/R	≤4/S
Cefuroxime sodium	≥64/R	≥64/R	4/S
Cefuroxime axetil	≥64/R	≥64/R	4/S
Cefotetan	≥64/R	32/R	≤4/S
Ceftriaxone	≥64/R	≥64/R	≤1/S
Ceftazidime	≥64/R	≥64/R	≤1/S
Carbapenems			
Imipenem	≥16/R	≥16/R	≤1/S
Meropenem	≥16/R	8/R	≤0.25/S
Monobactam			
Aztreonam	≥64/R	≥64/R	≤1/S
Fluoroquinolones			
Ciprofloxacin	≥4/R	≤0.25/S	≤0.25/S
Levofloxacin	≥8/R	≤0.25/S	≤0.25/S
Sulfonamide			
Trimethoprim/sulfamethoxazole	≥320/R	≤20/S	≤20/S
Aminoglycosides			
Amikacin	≤2/S	≤2/S	≤2/S
Gentamicin	≤1/S	≤1/S	≤1/S
Tobramycin	2/S	≤1/S	≤1/S

S, susceptible; R, resistant.

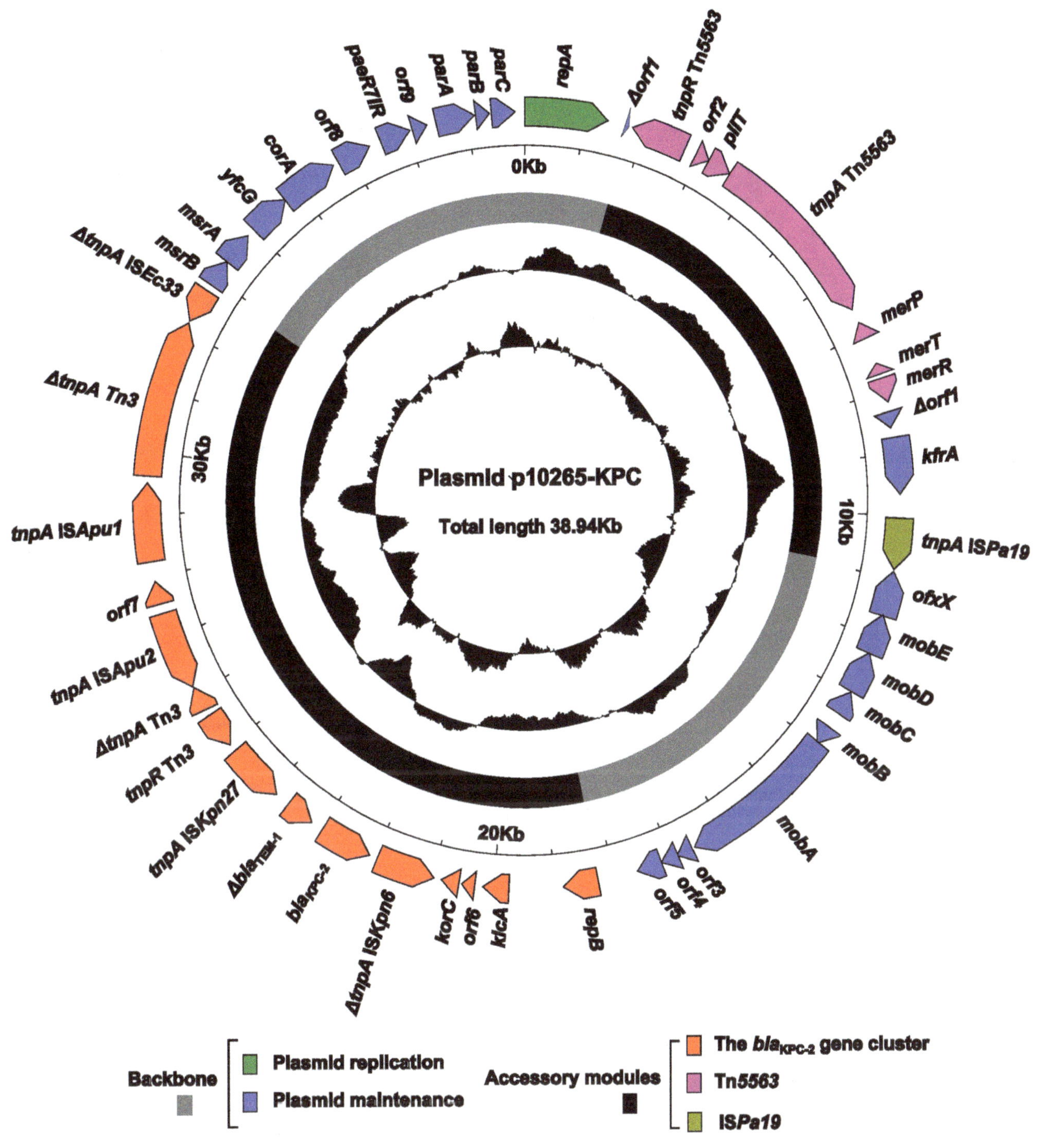

FIGURE 1 | Schematic maps of p10265-KPC. Genes are denoted by arrows and colored based on gene function classification. The innermost two circles indicate the GC-Skew [(G-C)/(G + C)] and the GC content.

insertion of IS*Kpn27*-*bla*$_{KPC-2}$-ΔIS*Kpn6*-*korC*-*orf6*- *klcA*-Δ*repB* into the *mcp* gene of the cryptic transposon Tn*1722*, making *mcp* to be truncated; moreover, it is bounded by 39 bp IRs and further flanked by 5 bp direct repeats (DRs: target site duplications which are usually the signature of a transposition event) at both ends (**Figure 2**). Before being captured by Tn*1722*, the above mentioned core module IS*Kpn27*-*bla*$_{KPC-2}$-ΔIS*Kpn6* is connected with a gene cluster *korC*-*orf6*-*klcA*-Δ*repB*.

In p10265-KPC, the primary genetic content Tn3-IS*Kpn27*-*bla*$_{KPC-2}$-ΔIS*Kpn6* -*korC*-*orf6*-*klcA*-Δ*repB* is also found but it has undergone two major evolutionary events: (i) the

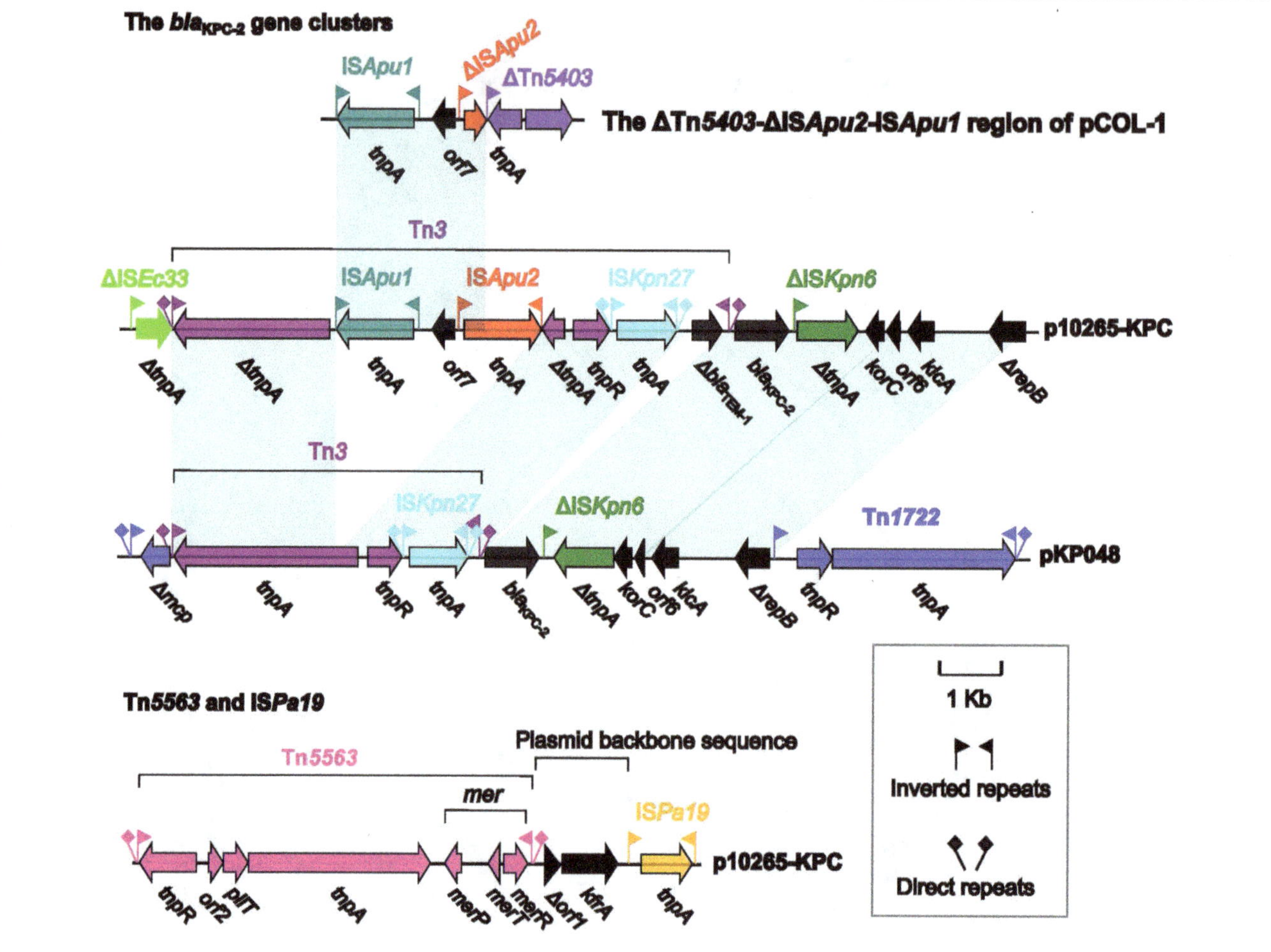

FIGURE 2 | Accessory modules of p10265-KPC and comparison with related genetic contents. Genes are denoted by arrows and colored based on gene function classification. Shading regions denote shared regions of homology (>95% nucleotide similarity).

insertion of a Δbla_{TEM-1} gene between IS*Kpn27* and the Tn*3* IRR (IR right), and (ii) the insertion of IS*Apu1*-*orf7*-IS*Apu2* into the Tn*3* *tnpA* gene, disrupting it into two separate parts (**Figure 2**). The resulting structure is then connected with ΔIS*Ec33* to finally constitute a 15.1 kb ΔIS*Ec33*-associated element ΔIS*Ec33*-Tn*3*-IS*Apu1*-*orf7*-IS*Apu2*-IS*Kpn27*-Δbla_{TEM-1}-bla_{KPC-2}-ΔIS*Kpn6*-*korC*- *orf6*-*klcA*-Δ*repB* (**Figure 2**). In contrast to the Tn*1722*-based unit transposons, the ΔIS*Ec33*-associated element is not bracketed by IRs and DRs. In addition, the Tn*3* in this ΔIS*Ec33*-associated element is heavily fragmented due to insertion of various elements and most likely defective in the activity of transposition. The mobilization of this ΔIS*Ec33*-associated element in p10265-KPC would attribute to homologous recombination-based insertion of a foreign element Tn*3*-IS*Apu1*-*orf7*-IS*Apu2*-IS*Kpn27*-Δbla_{TEM-1}-bla_{KPC-2}-ΔIS*Kpn6*-*korC*-*orf6*-*klcA*-Δ*repB* into a pre-existent intact IS*Ec33* element (making it truncated at 3′ end), rather than resulting from a transposition event of the whole ΔIS*Ec33*-associated element followed by the deletion of its adjacent extremities removing IR and DR sequences.

In p10265-KPC, the 6.5 kb transposon Tn*5563* is located upstream of IS*Pa19*, with two consecutive backbone genes *orf6* and *kfrA* as the interval between Tn*5563* and IS*Pa19*. IS*Pa19* contains the single transposase gene *tnpA*, and this insertion sequence is bordered by 18 bp IRs; this insertion sequence was initially described in plasmid Rms149 (Haines et al., 2005). Tn*5563*, belonging to the Tn*3* subgroup of the Tn*3* family transposons, was initially identified in plasmid pRA2 from *P. alcaligenes* and organized sequentially as *tnpR* (resolvase), *orf2* (hypothetical protein), *pliT* (PilT domain-containing protein), *tnpA*, *merP* (mercuric transport protein periplasmic componen), *merT* (mercuric transport protein), and *merR* (mercuric resistance operon regulatory protein); this gene cluster is bounded by 39 bp IRs and further flanked by 5 bp (this study) or 7 bp DRs at both ends (Yeo et al., 1998). Various truncated versions of Tn*5563* are also found in pOZ176 (Xiong et al., 2013) and pUM505 (Ramirez-Diaz et al., 2011) from *P. aeruginosa*. The Tn*5563* element of p10265-KPC differs from the prototype Tn*5563* of pRA2 with a 286 bp insertion (nucleotide position 7270 to 7555) between *merP* and *merT*. The above observations indicate the frequent inter-plasmid transmission of Tn*5563* among *Pseudomonas* species.

Replication and Maintenance Determinants of p10265-KPC

Plasmid p10265-KPC belongs to the IncP-6 incompatibility group because it carries three partition genes *parABC* and a downstream replicase gene *repA*, which constitute an IncP6-type consecutive *par-rep* gene cluster. The *parA* gene encodes an ATPase, whereas *parB* and *parC* encode auxiliary partition proteins. The *repA* gene and the *parABC* locus of p10265-KPC show >97% and >99%, respectively, nucleotide sequence identity with the three IncP-6 plasmids Rms149, pRIO-5, and pCOL-1. The Rms149 RepA has been shown to confer the plasmid's replication ability in *E. coli*, *P. aeruginosa*, and *P. putida* (Haines et al., 2005), while the pRIO-5 RepA is able to replicate in *S. marcescens* and *Acinetobacter baumannii* but not in *P. aeruginosa* (Bonnin et al., 2012). The *parABC* locus of Rms149 is known to promote the plasmid mobilization in *E. coli* (Haines et al., 2005).

All of p10265-KPC, Rms149, pRIO-5, and pCOL-1 contain a 5.6 kb MOB_P family mobilization module (Francia et al., 2004), which is composed of six genes *mobA* (relaxase/primase fusion protein), *mobB* (*oriT* recognition-like protein), *mobC* (relaxosome protein), and *mobD* and *mobE* (auxiliary proteins). The study with Rms149 denotes that the *mob* gene cluster is functional for the plasmid mobilization in *E. coli* (Haines et al., 2005). In addition, the above *mob* gene clusters are similar to those of the IncQ plasmids pTF-FC2 and pTC-F14; as shown by the genetic analysis using these two plasmids, the minimal region essential for mobilization are *mobA*, *mobB*, and *mobC*, while *mobD* and *mobE* are non-essential but together they greatly enhance the mobilization frequency (van Zyl et al., 2003).

Genomic Comparison of p10265-KPC with pCOL-1

pCOL-1 represents the first sequenced KPC-producing IncP-6 plasmid (Naas et al., 2013), while p10265-KPC is the second one. The *par-rep* regions for partition-replication and the *mob* gene modules for mobilization are conserved in the p10265-KPC and pCOL-1 backbones (**Figure 3**), allowing these two plasmids to transfer if a conjugative plasmid is also present in the cell. The p10265-KPC and pCOL-1 backbones lack the conjugal transfer gene regions, which is in accordance with the fact that these two plasmids are unable to self-transfer their drug resistance markers via conjugation. An inversion of the backbone gene cluster *msrB-msrA-yfcG-corA-orf8* in p10265-KPC turns it into Δ*orf8-corA'-yfcG-msrA-msrB* in pCOL-1 with a truncation of *orf8* and, moreover, *corA* becomes a pseudo gene with the accumulation of multiple indels.

A 206 bp fragment comprising 12 copies of tandem repeat of GCGCCTGCCTTTGAGTA is inserted into the *repA-orf1* intergenic region of pCOL-1 relative to p10265-KPC (**Figures 3** and **4**). The open reading frame *orf1* is disrupted at two distinct sites, respectively, by the insertion of two different accessory elements, namely a 10 kb bla_{KPC-2}-carrying Tn*4401b* in pCOL-1 and a *mer* locus-carrying *Tn5563* in p10265-KPC (**Figures 3** and **4**).

pCOL-1 and p10265-KPC share the accessory element IS*Pa19*, which is inserted between the backbone genes *kfrA* and *ofxX* (**Figure 3**). Downstream of the backbone gene *orf5* of p10265-KPC and pCOL-1 are two distinct inserted accessory regions, namely the ΔIS*Ec33*-associated bla_{KPC-2} gene cluster and a 4.3 kb ΔTn*5403*-ΔIS*Apu2*-IS*Apu1* region (showing sequence similarity to the ΔIS*Ec33*-associated element), respectively (**Figures 2** and **3**).

Remarkably, pCOL-1 and p10265-KPC carry two distinct bla_{KPC-2} gene clusters, Tn*4401b* and the ΔIS*Ec33*-associated

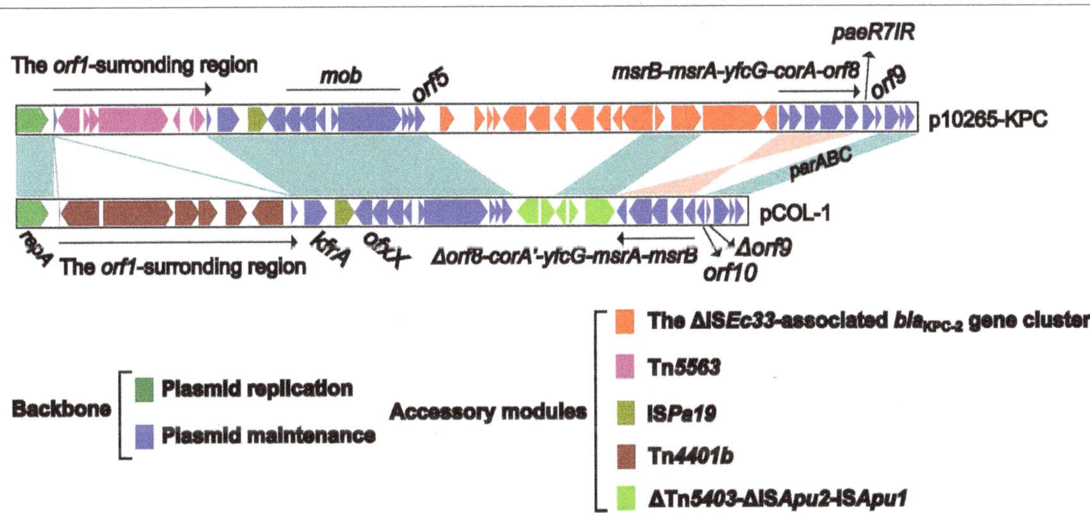

FIGURE 3 | Linear comparison of sequenced plasmids p10265-KPC and pCOL-1. Genes are denoted by arrows and colored based on gene function classification. Shading regions denote shared regions of homology (>95% nucleotide similarity).

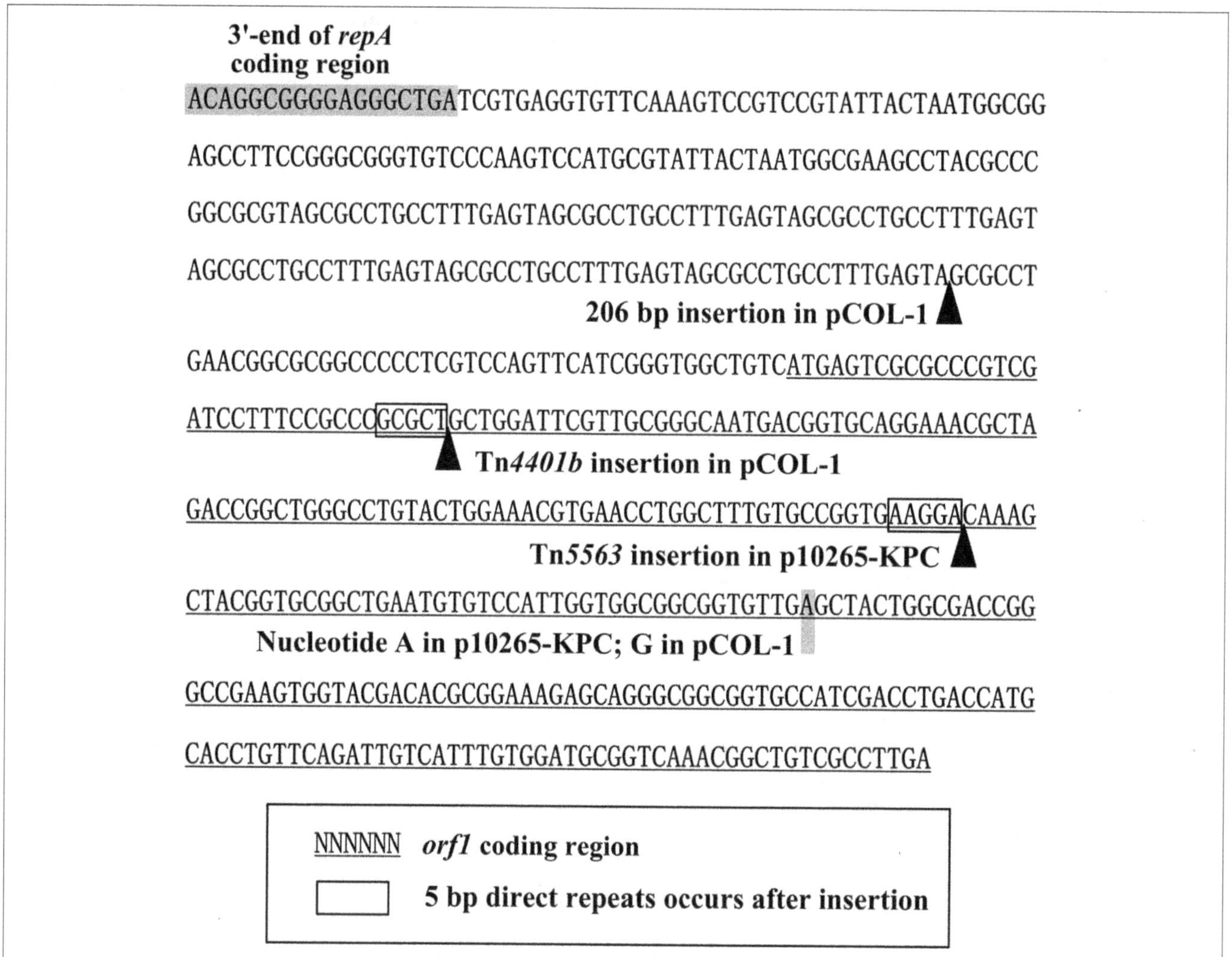

FIGURE 4 | *orf1*-surrounding regions. Shown are the *orf1*-surrounding DNA regions of p10265-KPC and pCOL-1 with inserted genetic contents.

element, respectively; these two gene clusters are inserted at two different sites of the IncP-6 backbone and seem to have completely different evolutionary histories of genetic assembly and transposition.

CONCLUSION

Plasmid p10265-KPC is a novel IncP-6 resistance plasmid from *P. aeruginosa*, and it carries the IncP-6-type replication, partition and mobilization systems and a novel ΔIS*Ec33*-associated bla_{KPC-2} gene cluster accounting for carbapenem resistance. The ΔIS*Ec33*-associated element has a complex mosaic structure, which is genetically related to the previously characterized Tn*1722*-based bla_{KPC-2}-carrring unit transposons (Wang et al., 2015). Besides bla_{KPC-2}, p10265-KPC still carries a truncated bla_{TEM-1} gene in the bla_{KPC-2} gene cluster and an incomplete *mer* locus in Tn*5563*, both of which are thought defective to mediate the corresponding resistance phenotypes. KPC-2 appears to be the sole determinant of antimicrobial resistance for p10265-KPC. Epidemiological study and routine surveillance of p10265-KPC-like plasmids in China is needed.

The IncP-6 resistance plasmids are not commonly found in the natural isolates of *P. aeruginosa*. The accumulating complete sequences of the IncP-6 plasmids would make it possible to chart their evolutionary history and to draw the inferences about the processes that lead to these complex plasmid genomes. As seen from p10265-KPC, Rms149, pRIO-5, and pCOL-1, the IncP-6 plasmid backbones are able to integrate a wide variety of foreign genetic contents through transposition or homologous recombination mediated by the transposable elements such as insertion sequences, transposons and integrons. The IncP-6 plasmids are quite unusual in having a relatively small backbone but carrying a large amount of accessory modules which are mainly composed of mobile genetic elements and resistance determinants. It is worth elucidating whether there are specific mechanisms associated with the IncP-6 plasmids to promote the involvement of themselves in the complex processes of acquisition of foreign genetic contents.

AUTHOR CONTRIBUTIONS

DZ, FS, and XZ designed the study. XD, WX, JF, WL, GL, HW, and FS performed experiments. DZ, XD, and FS analyzed data. XD, WX, JF, WL, GL, HW, and FS contributed reagents, materials and analysis tools. DZ, XD, FS, and XZ wrote this manuscript.

ACKNOWLEDGMENTS

This work was funded by the Chongqing Application and Development Program (cstc2014yykfA110021), the National Basic Research Program of China (2015CB554202), and the National High-Tech Research and Development Program of China (2014AA021402).

REFERENCES

Bonnin, R. A., Poirel, L., Sampaio, J. L., and Nordmann, P. (2012). Complete sequence of broad-host-range plasmid pRIO-5 harboring the extended-spectrum-β-lactamase gene blaBES-1. *Antimicrob. Agents Chemother.* 56, 1116–1119. doi: 10.1128/AAC.00480-11

Boronin, A. M. (1992). Diversity of *Pseudomonas* plasmids: to what extent? *FEMS Microbiol. Lett.* 100, 461–467. doi: 10.1111/j.1574-6968.1992.tb05740.x

Bryant, K. A., Van Schooneveld, T. C., Thapa, I., Bastola, D., Williams, L. O., Safranek, T. J., et al. (2013). KPC-4 Is encoded within a truncated Tn4401 in an IncL/M plasmid, pNE1280, isolated from *Enterobacter cloacae* and *Serratia marcescens*. *Antimicrob. Agents Chemother.* 57, 37–41. doi: 10.1128/AAC.01062-12

Chen, L., Chavda, K. D., Mediavilla, J. R., Jacobs, M. R., Levi, M. H., Bonomo, R. A., et al. (2012). Partial excision of blaKPC from Tn4401 in carbapenem-resistant *Klebsiella pneumoniae*. *Antimicrob. Agents Chemother.* 56, 1635–1638. doi: 10.1128/AAC.06182-11

Chen, L., Hu, H., Chavda, K. D., Zhao, S., Liu, R., Liang, H., et al. (2014a). Complete sequence of a KPC-producing IncN multidrug-resistant plasmid from an epidemic *Escherichia coli* sequence type 131 strain in China. *Antimicrob. Agents Chemother.* 58, 2422–2425. doi: 10.1128/AAC.02587-13

Chen, L., Mathema, B., Chavda, K. D., Deleo, F. R., Bonomo, R. A., and Kreiswirth, B. N. (2014b). Carbapenemase-producing *Klebsiella pneumoniae*: molecular and genetic decoding. *Trends Microbiol.* 22, 686–696. doi: 10.1016/j.tim.2014.09.003

Chen, Y. T., Lin, J. C., Fung, C. P., Lu, P. L., Chuang, Y. C., Wu, T. L., et al. (2014c). KPC-2-encoding plasmids from *Escherichia coli* and *Klebsiella pneumoniae* in Taiwan. *J. Antimicrob. Chemother.* 69, 628–631. doi: 10.1093/jac/dkt409

Chen, Z., Li, H., Feng, J., Li, Y., Chen, X., Guo, X., et al. (2015). NDM-1 encoded by a pNDM-BJ01-like plasmid p3SP-NDM in clinical *Enterobacter* aerogenes. *Front. Microbiol.* 6:294. doi: 10.3389/fmicb.2015.00294

Chmelnitsky, I., Shklyar, M., Leavitt, A., Sadovsky, E., Navon-Venezia, S., Ben Dalak, M., et al. (2014). Mix and match of KPC-2 encoding plasmids in *Enterobacteriaceae*-comparative genomics. *Diagn. Microbiol. Infect. Dis.* 79, 255–260. doi: 10.1016/j.diagmicrobio.2014.03.008

Cuzon, G., Naas, T., Villegas, M. V., Correa, A., Quinn, J. P., and Nordmann, P. (2011). Wide dissemination of *Pseudomonas aeruginosa* producing β-lactamase blaKPC-2 gene in Colombia. *Antimicrob. Agents Chemother.* 55, 5350–5353. doi: 10.1128/AAC.00297-11

Dortet, L., Poirel, L., and Nordmann, P. (2012). Rapid identification of carbapenemase types in *Enterobacteriaceae* and *Pseudomonas* spp. by using a biochemical test. *Antimicrob. Agents Chemother.* 56, 6437–6440. doi: 10.1128/AAC.01395 12

Francia, M. V., Varsaki, A., Garcillan-Barcia, M. P., Latorre, A., Drainas, C., and De La Cruz, F. (2004). A classification scheme for mobilization regions of bacterial plasmids. *FEMS Microbiol. Rev.* 28, 79–100. doi: 10.1016/j.femsre.2003.09.001

Frank, J. A., Reich, C. I., Sharma, S., Weisbaum, J. S., Wilson, B. A., and Olsen, G. J. (2008). Critical evaluation of two primers commonly used for amplification of bacterial 16S rRNA genes. *Appl. Environ. Microbiol.* 74, 2461–2470. doi: 10.1128/AEM.02272-07

Haines, A. S., Jones, K., Cheung, M., and Thomas, C. M. (2005). The IncP-6 plasmid Rms149 consists of a small mobilizable backbone with multiple large insertions. *J. Bacteriol.* 187, 4728–4738. doi: 10.1128/JB.187.14.4728-4738.2005

Ho, P. L., Cheung, Y. Y., Lo, W. U., Li, Z., Chow, K. H., Lin, C. H., et al. (2013). Molecular characterization of an atypical IncX3 plasmid pKPC-NY79 carrying blaKPC-2 in a *Klebsiella pneumoniae*. *Curr. Microbiol.* 67, 493–498. doi: 10.1007/s00284-013-0398-2

Lee, C. M., Liao, C. H., Lee, W. S., Liu, Y. C., Mu, J. J., Lee, M. C., et al. (2012). Outbreak of *Klebsiella pneumoniae* carbapenemase-2-producing *K. pneumoniae* sequence type 11 in Taiwan in 2011. *Antimicrob. Agents Chemother.* 56, 5016–5022. doi: 10.1128/AAC.00878-12

Li, G., Zhang, Y., Bi, D., Shen, P., Ai, F., Liu, H., et al. (2015). First report of a clinical, multidrug-resistant *Enterobacteriaceae* isolate coharboring fosfomycin resistance gene fosA3 and carbapenemase gene blaKPC-2 on the same transposon, Tn1721. *Antimicrob. Agents Chemother.* 59, 338–343. doi: 10.1128/AAC.03061-14

Munoz-Price, L. S., Poirel, L., Bonomo, R. A., Schwaber, M. J., Daikos, G. L., Cormican, M., et al. (2013). Clinical epidemiology of the global expansion of *Klebsiella pneumoniae* carbapenemases. *Lancet Infect. Dis.* 13, 785–796. doi: 10.1016/S1473-3099(13)70190-7

Naas, T., Bonnin, R. A., Cuzon, G., Villegas, M. V., and Nordmann, P. (2013). Complete sequence of two KPC-harbouring plasmids from *Pseudomonas aeruginosa*. *J. Antimicrob. Chemother.* 68, 1757–1762. doi: 10.1093/jac/dkt094

Popowska, M., and Krawczyk-Balska, A. (2013). Broad-host-range IncP-1 plasmids and their resistance potential. *Front. Microbiol.* 4:44. doi: 10.3389/fmicb.2013.00044

Ramirez-Diaz, M. I., Diaz-Magana, A., Meza-Carmen, V., Johnstone, L., Cervantes, C., and Rensing, C. (2011). Nucleotide sequence of *Pseudomonas aeruginosa* conjugative plasmid pUM505 containing virulence and heavy-metal resistance genes. *Plasmid* 66, 7–18. doi: 10.1016/j.plasmid.2011.03.002

Sagai, H., Hasuda, K., Iyobe, S., Bryan, L. E., Holloway, B. W., and Mitsuhashi, S. (1976). Classification of R plasmids by incompatibility in *Pseudomonas aeruginosa*. *Antimicrob. Agents Chemother.* 10, 573–578. doi: 10.1128/AAC.10.4.573

Schluter, A., Szczepanowski, R., Kurz, N., Schneiker, S., Krahn, I., and Puhler, A. (2007). Erythromycin resistance-conferring plasmid pRSB105, isolated from a sewage treatment plant, harbors a new macrolide resistance determinant, an integron-containing Tn402-like element, and a large region of unknown function. *Appl. Environ. Microbiol.* 73, 1952–1960. doi: 10.1128/AEM.02159-06

Shen, P., Wei, Z., Jiang, Y., Du, X., Ji, S., Yu, Y., et al. (2009). Novel genetic environment of the carbapenem-hydrolyzing β-lactamase KPC-2 among *Enterobacteriaceae* in China. *Antimicrob. Agents Chemother.* 53, 4333–4338. doi: 10.1128/AAC.00260-09

van Zyl, L. J., Deane, S. M., and Rawlings, D. E. (2003). Analysis of the mobilization region of the broad-host-range IncQ-like plasmid pTC-F14 and its ability to interact with a related plasmid, pTF-FC2. *J. Bacteriol.* 185, 6104–6111. doi: 10.1128/JB.185.20.6104-6111.2003

Villegas, M. V., Lolans, K., Correa, A., Kattan, J. N., Lopez, J. A., and Quinn, J. P. (2007). First identification of *Pseudomonas aeruginosa* isolates producing a KPC-type carbapenem-hydrolyzing β-lactamase. *Antimicrob. Agents Chemother.* 51, 1553–1555. doi: 10.1128/AAC.01405-06

Wang, L., Fang, H., Feng, J., Yin, Z., Xie, X., Zhu, X., et al. (2015). Complete sequences of KPC-2-encoding plasmid p628-KPC and CTX-M-55-encoding p628-CTXM coexisted in *Klebsiella pneumoniae*. *Front. Microbiol.* 6:838. doi: 10.3389/fmicb.2015.00838

Xiong, J., Alexander, D. C., Ma, J. H., Deraspe, M., Low, D. E., Jamieson, F. B., et al. (2013). Complete sequence of pOZ176, a 500-kilobase IncP-2 plasmid encoding IMP-9-mediated carbapenem resistance, from outbreak isolate *Pseudomonas aeruginosa* 96. *Antimicrob. Agents Chemother.* 57, 3775–3782. doi: 10.1128/AAC.00423-13

21

Monitoring the Microevolution of *Salmonella enterica* in Healthy Dairy Cattle Populations at the Individual Farm Level Using Whole-Genome Sequencing

Laura M. Carroll[1†], Ariel J. Buehler[1], Ahmed Gaballa[1], Julie D. Siler[2], Kevin J. Cummings[2], Rachel A. Cheng[1] and Martin Wiedmann[1]*

[1] Department of Food Science, Cornell University, Ithaca, NY, United States, [2] Department of Population Medicine and Diagnostic Sciences, Cornell University, Ithaca, NY, United States

***Correspondence:**
Laura M. Carroll
lmc297@cornell.edu

†Present address:
Laura M. Carroll,
Structural and Computational Biology Unit, EMBL, Heidelberg, Germany

Livestock represent a possible reservoir for facilitating the transmission of the zoonotic foodborne pathogen *Salmonella enterica* to humans; there is also concern that strains can acquire resistance to antimicrobials in the farm environment. Here, whole-genome sequencing (WGS) was used to characterize *Salmonella* strains (n = 128) isolated from healthy dairy cattle and their associated environments on 13 New York State farms to assess the diversity and microevolution of this important pathogen at the level of the individual herd. Additionally, the accuracy and concordance of multiple *in silico* tools are assessed, including: (i) two *in silico* serotyping tools, (ii) combinations of five antimicrobial resistance (AMR) determinant detection tools and one to five AMR determinant databases, and (iii) one antimicrobial minimum inhibitory concentration (MIC) prediction tool. For the isolates sequenced here, *in silico* serotyping methods outperformed traditional serotyping and resolved all un-typable and/or ambiguous serotype assignments. Serotypes assigned *in silico* showed greater congruency with the *Salmonella* whole-genome phylogeny than traditional serotype assignments, and *in silico* methods showed high concordance (99% agreement). *In silico* AMR determinant detection methods additionally showed a high degree of concordance, regardless of the pipeline or database used (≥98% agreement among susceptible/resistant assignments for all pipeline/database combinations). For AMR detection methods that relied exclusively on nucleotide BLAST, accuracy could be maximized by using a range of minimum nucleotide identity and coverage thresholds, with thresholds of 75% nucleotide identity and 50–60% coverage adequate for most pipeline/database combinations. *In silico* characterization of the microevolution and AMR dynamics of each of six serotype groups (*S.* Anatum, Cerro, Kentucky, Meleagridis, Newport, Typhimurium/Typhimurium variant Copenhagen) revealed that some lineages were strongly associated with individual farms, while others were distributed across multiple farms. Numerous AMR determinant acquisition and loss events were identified, including the recent acquisition of cephalosporin resistance-conferring *bla*$_{CMY}$- and *bla*$_{CTX-M}$-type beta-lactamases. The results presented here provide high-resolution insight into the temporal dynamics of AMR *Salmonella* at the scale of the individual farm and highlight both the strengths and limitations of WGS in tracking zoonotic pathogens and their associated AMR determinants at the livestock-human interface.

Keywords: *Salmonella*, antimicrobial resistance, serotyping, dairy cattle, whole-genome sequencing, evolution, livestock

INTRODUCTION

The foodborne pathogen *Salmonella enterica* is estimated to be responsible for 1.35 million infections, 26,500 hospitalizations, and 420 deaths each year in the United States alone (Centers for Disease Control and Prevention, 2021). Despite the fact that over 2,600 *Salmonella* serotypes have been described (Issenhuth-Jeanjean et al., 2014), fewer than 100 of these serotypes are responsible for the majority of human infections (Centers for Disease Control and Prevention, 2020). In line with this, some *Salmonella* serotypes may share strong associations with a specific host, an extreme example of which can be seen in the human-restricted nature of *Salmonella* Typhi (Uzzau et al., 2000; Boore et al., 2015). Other serotypes, while not confined exclusively to infection of a single host, may be adapted to a given reservoir; for example, *Salmonella* Choleraesuis, while largely adapted to swine, occasionally infects humans (Uzzau et al., 2000; Chiu et al., 2004).

Cattle are a potential reservoir from which humans can acquire salmonellosis, and infected animals can shed *Salmonella* at irregular intervals for varying periods of time, regardless of whether they express clinical signs of bovine salmonellosis or not (Cummings et al., 2010b; Davidson et al., 2018; Holschbach and Peek, 2018). The bovine reservoir boasts its own repertoire of serotypes that can infect humans, with bovine-associated *Salmonella* serotype Dublin, known for its rare but frequently invasive infections in humans, being arguably the most noteworthy (Taylor et al., 1982; Uzzau et al., 2000; Rodriguez-Rivera et al., 2014; Harvey et al., 2017; Mohammed et al., 2017). However, a range of *Salmonella* serotypes can persist and thrive in cattle, potentially infecting humans via either direct contact with infected animals or through food (Gutema et al., 2019). In a previous survey of 46 dairy cattle herds in New York State, *Salmonella* strains isolated from subclinically infected dairy cattle and associated farm environments spanned 26 serotypes, the most common being Cerro, Kentucky, Typhimurium, Newport, and Anatum (Rodriguez-Rivera et al., 2014). Additionally, antimicrobial resistant (AMR) isolates were observed on several farms, on numerous occasions, suggesting subclinically infected dairy cattle as a potential source of AMR *Salmonella* (Rodriguez-Rivera et al., 2014).

Numerous studies have employed whole-genome sequencing (WGS) to characterize *Salmonella* from bovine sources (Mather et al., 2013; Agren et al., 2016; Carroll et al., 2017b; Delgado-Suarez et al., 2018; Liao et al., 2019); however, little is known regarding the evolution and AMR acquisition and loss dynamics of *Salmonella* at the single herd/farm level. Furthermore, the bulk of bovine-associated *Salmonella* WGS efforts have focused on clinical veterinary samples and/or epidemic lineages (e.g., *S.* Typhimurium DT104). In this study, 128 non-typhoidal *S. enterica* strains isolated from repeated sampling on 13 New York State dairy cattle farms between 2007 and 2009 were characterized using WGS. All strains were isolated from apparently healthy, subclinically infected bovine hosts, as well as the associated farm environment (Rodriguez-Rivera et al., 2014). Using WGS, the microevolution of these persistent lineages within each herd is characterized, as well as the temporal acquisition and loss of AMR determinants among them. In addition to offering insight into the genomics of *Salmonella* isolated from healthy bovine populations at the individual herd/farm level, the accuracy and concordance of multiple *in silico* serotyping and AMR prediction tools are evaluated. Finally, an in-depth, critical analysis of the strengths and limitations of the methods used here is provided, which includes guidance to researchers who wish to employ WGS for herd-level pathogen monitoring.

MATERIALS AND METHODS

Isolate Selection

Salmonella enterica isolates (n = 128) obtained from one of 13 dairy farms in New York State were selected to undergo WGS for this study (**Supplementary Table 1**). All strains were isolated from farms that had undergone surveillance for *Salmonella* for a period of at least 12 months as described previously (Cummings et al., 2010a; Rodriguez-Rivera et al., 2014). Strains were isolated from repeated sampling on each farm between October 2007 and August 2009, from either (i) fecal samples from healthy, subclinically infected dairy cows (referred to hereafter as "bovine" isolates), or (ii) farm environmental swabs (referred to hereafter as "farm environmental" isolates) (Cummings et al., 2010a). All isolates underwent serotyping, phenotypic antimicrobial susceptibility testing, and pulsed-field gel electrophoresis (PFGE) as described previously (Rodriguez-Rivera et al., 2014).

Whole-Genome Sequencing and Data Pre-processing

Genomic DNA extraction and sequencing library preparation were performed as described previously (Carroll et al., 2017b), and the genomes of all 128 *Salmonella* isolates were sequenced using an Illumina HiSeq platform and 2 × 250 bp paired-end reads. Illumina sequencing adapters and low-quality bases were trimmed using Trimmomatic version 0.33 (using default parameters for Nextera paired-end reads) (Bolger et al., 2014), and FastQC version 0.11.9 (Andrews, 2019) was used to confirm adapter removal and assess read quality. SPAdes version 3.8.0

(Bankevich et al., 2012) was used to assemble genomes *de novo* (using the "careful" option and *k*-mer sizes of 21, 33, 55, 77, 99, and 127), and QUAST version 4.5 (Gurevich et al., 2013) and the "lineage_wf" workflow implemented in CheckM version 1.1.3 (Parks et al., 2015) were used to assess the quality of the resulting assemblies. MultiQC version 1.8 (Ewels et al., 2016) was used to aggregate genome quality metrics. Genome quality statistics are available for all isolates (**Supplementary Table 1**).

In silico Serotyping

In addition to undergoing traditional serotyping in a laboratory setting (i.e., serological detection of expressed O and H antigens using the White-Kauffmann-Le Minor scheme) as described previously (Rodriguez-Rivera et al., 2014), all 128 assembled *Salmonella* genomes (see section "Whole-Genome Sequencing and Data Pre-processing" above) underwent *in silico* serotyping using the command line implementations of (i) the *Salmonella in silico* Typing Resource (SISTR) version 1.0.2 (Yoshida et al., 2016) and (ii) SeqSero2 version 1.1.1 (Zhang et al., 2019) (using SeqSero2's *k*-mer based workflow). Serotypes assigned using all three methods are available for all 128 isolates (**Supplementary Table 1**). In cases where a discrepancy existed among the traditional serotype designation and one or more of the *in silico* methods, the serotype assigned using two out of the three methods was selected as the final serotype to be reported (e.g., when assigning strain names to isolates in the manuscript, for phylogeny annotation). To confirm that all serotype assignments were reasonable, a phylogeny was constructed using core single nucleotide polymorphisms (SNPs) detected in all *Salmonella* genomes in this study (see section "Reference-Free Single Nucleotide Polymorphism Identification and Phylogeny Construction" below).

In silico Antimicrobial Resistance Determinant Detection

Antimicrobial resistance determinants were detected in each of the 128 *Salmonella* genomes using five separate approaches: (i) ABRicate[1] version 0.8 (Seemann, 2018), (ii) AMRFinderPlus version 3.2.3 (Feldgarden et al., 2019), (iii) ARIBA version 2.14.1 (Hunt et al., 2017), (iv) BTyper version 2.3.3 (Carroll et al., 2017a), and (v) SRST2 version 0.2.0 (Inouye et al., 2014). Assembled genomes were used as input for the ABRicate and BTyper approaches, while trimmed Illumina reads were used as input for the SRST2 and ARIBA approaches. Prokka version 1.12 (Seemann, 2014) was used to annotate each assembled genome, and the resulting GFF (.gff) and FASTA (.faa and .ffn) files were used as input for the AMRFinderPlus approach. For the ABRicate approach, the following AMR gene databases were tested (each accessed June 11, 2018 via ABRicate's abricate-get_db command): (i) the Antibiotic Resistance Gene-ANNOTation database (ARG-ANNOT) (Gupta et al., 2014), (ii) the Comprehensive Antibiotic Resistance Database (CARD) (Jia et al., 2017), (iii) the National Center for Biotechnology Information's (NCBI's) Bacterial AMR Reference Gene Database (NCBI) (Feldgarden et al., 2019), and (iv) the ResFinder database (ResFinder) (Zankari et al., 2012). For each genome and database combination, minimum AMR gene identity and coverage thresholds ranging from 50 to 100% (5% increments) and 0–100% (10% increments) were tested, respectively. For the BTyper approach, the (i) ARG-ANNOT v3 and (ii) MEGARes version 1.0.1 (Lakin et al., 2017) databases available with BTyper version 2.3.3 were used, with the minimum AMR gene identity and coverage thresholds varied in a manner identical to the ABRicate approach. For the SRST2 approach, the (i) ARG-ANNOT and (ii) ResFinder databases available with SRST2 version 0.2.0 were tested, using default thresholds. For the ARIBA approach, the following databases were tested (each accessed June 13, 2019 using ARIBA's getref command): (i) the version of ARG-ANNOT available with SRST2, (ii) CARD, (iii) MEGARes, (iv) NCBI, and (v) ResFinder, with all default thresholds used. For the AMRFinder approach, the latest version of the AMRFinder database was used (accessed December 6, 2019), along with the organism-specific database for *Salmonella*.

[1]https://github.com/tseemann/abricate

In silico Prediction of Antimicrobial Minimum Inhibitory Concentration Values

The PATRIC3 antimicrobial minimum inhibitory concentration (MIC) prediction model for *Salmonella* (Nguyen et al., 2019) (accessed June 13, 2019) was used to predict MIC values for each of the 128 *Salmonella* isolates in this study, using the assembled genome of each as input (**Supplementary Text**).

Prediction of Phenotypic Susceptible-Intermediate-Resistant Classifications Using *in silico* Methods

All 128 *Salmonella* isolates underwent phenotypic antimicrobial susceptibility testing with a panel of 15 antimicrobials (i.e., amikacin, amoxicillin-clavulanic acid, ampicillin, cefoxitin, ceftiofur, ceftriaxone, chloramphenicol, ciprofloxacin, gentamicin, kanamycin, nalidixic acid, streptomycin, sulfamethoxazole-trimethoprim, sulfisoxazole, and tetracycline) using the Sensititre system (Trek Diagnostic Systems Ltd., Cleveland, OH, United States) available at Cornell University's Animal Health Diagnostic Center as described previously (Rodriguez-Rivera et al., 2014). A "true" (i.e., phenotypic) susceptible-intermediate-resistant (SIR) classification for each of the 15 antimicrobials was obtained for 126 *Salmonella* isolates by comparing raw MIC values to NARMS breakpoints for *Salmonella* (accessed March 23, 2020; **Supplementary Table 1**). For streptomycin, the 1996–2013 NARMS breakpoints were used, as this was compatible with the concentrations used at the time of phenotypic testing (Rodriguez-Rivera et al., 2014). For sulfisoxazole, isolates with MIC > 256 were classified as resistant, as a concentration of 512 μg/mL was not tested. While raw MIC values were unavailable for two isolates (BOV_KENT_16_04-03-08_R8-0967 and ENV_MELA_01_01-10-08_R8-0165; **Supplementary Table 1**), both isolates had previously been categorized as pan-susceptible to all 15 antimicrobials (a classification that was maintained here, as all *in silico* methods correctly classified these isolates as pan-susceptible).

Known AMR determinant/phenotype associations for AMR determinants detected by each of the AMR determinant detection pipeline/database combinations described above (see section "*In silico* Antimicrobial Resistance Determinant Detection") were obtained from (i) Supplementary Table 4 of the AMRFinder validation paper (Feldgarden et al., 2019) and (ii) CARD (**Supplementary Table 2** and **Supplementary Text**). An isolate was predicted to be resistant to a particular antimicrobial if it possessed one or more AMR determinants known to confer resistance to that antimicrobial; if it did not possess any AMR determinants known to confer resistance to that antimicrobial, the isolate was predicted to be susceptible to that antimicrobial (**Supplementary Table 2**). For each AMR determinant detection pipeline/database combination, the caret package (Kuhn, 2008) in R version 3.6.1 (R Core Team, 2019) was used to construct a confusion matrix and calculate accuracy scores, Cohen's kappa coefficients, and other statistics (**Supplementary Table 3**) by treating "true" susceptible/resistant classifications obtained using phenotypic susceptibility testing as a reference. Cases of intermediate phenotypic resistance were treated as susceptible, as it resulted in slightly higher accuracy scores for all pipeline/database combinations for this particular data set. Because *in silico* prediction of susceptibility/resistance was highly dependent on prior knowledge of AMR determinants and the antimicrobials to which they conferred resistance, the concordance of all pipeline/database combinations was assessed by comparing each pipeline/database combination to results obtained using the SRST2 pipeline/ARG-ANNOT database combination.

To assess the ability of the MIC prediction method implemented in PATRIC3 to predict *Salmonella* SIR classification (see section "*In silico* Prediction of Antimicrobial Minimum Inhibitory Concentration Values" above), predicted MIC values for 14 antimicrobials produced using PATRIC3 were used to predict the SIR status of each of the 128 *Salmonella* isolates using the same NARMS breakpoints used for phenotypic testing. Azithromycin MICs produced by PATRIC3 were excluded, as azithromycin was not among the 15 antimicrobials used here for phenotypic testing. The ability of PATRIC3 to predict amikacin resistance was also not evaluated, as amikacin is not among the antimicrobials queried by PATRIC3. A confusion matrix was constructed as described above, using predicted SIR classifications derived from predicted MIC values produced by PATRIC3 and NARMS breakpoints. Additionally, the deviation of raw MIC predictions produced by PATRIC3 ($MIC_{PATRIC3}$) from "true" raw MIC predictions produced using phenotypic testing ($MIC_{Phenotypic}$) in number of dilution factors ($N_{dilution\ factors}$) was assessed using the following equation:

$$N_{dilution\ factors} = \frac{\ln(\frac{MIC_{PATRIC3}}{MIC_{Phenotypic}})}{\ln(2)}$$

where ln corresponds to the natural logarithm. For example: if PATRIC3 predicted an MIC value of 8 and the "true" MIC value obtained with phenotypic testing was 2, then $\ln(8/2)/\ln(2) = 2$; this means that the PATRIC3 prediction of 8 is +2 dilution factors away from the "true" MIC of 2 (as dilution used for MIC are 2 fold serial dilutions, e.g., 2, 4, and 8 μg/mL).

Re-testing of Isolates With Highly Incongruent Antimicrobial Resistance Phenotypes

Several (n = 21) isolates possessed a phenotypic AMR SIR profile which was deemed to be highly incongruent with its predicted *in silico* AMR profile, regardless of the *in silico* pipeline/database used (**Supplementary Table 4**). For example, *S.* Cerro isolate BOV_CERO_35_10−02−08_R8−2685 was resistant to nine antimicrobials but did not harbor any known acquired AMR genes (**Supplementary Table 4**). Similarly, *S.* Newport isolate ENV_NEWP_62_03−05−09_R8−3442 itself was pan-susceptible, but harbored multiple acquired AMR genes (e.g., bla_{CMY-2}, *floR*, *sul2*, and *tetA*), which conferred multidrug resistance in closely related *S.* Newport isolates (**Supplementary Table 4**). To address these incongruencies, 21 selected *Salmonella* isolates underwent phenotypic antimicrobial susceptibility re-testing (conducted September 16, 2020) as described above (see section "Prediction of Phenotypic Susceptible-Intermediate-Resistant Classifications Using *in silico* Methods"), with the exception of amikacin and kanamycin, as the contemporary panel did not include these antimicrobials (**Supplementary Table 4**).

Kanamycin testing was conducted separately using a gradient diffusion assay (Jorgensen and Ferraro, 2009) according to the manufacturer's instructions (BioMérieux Kanamycin Strip KM 256, product number 412381). Briefly, bacterial isolates were streaked for single colonies onto Brain Heart Infusion [BHI, Becton Dickinson (BD), Franklin Lakes, NJ, United States] agar plates from frozen glycerol stocks. Pre-cultures were prepared by inoculating a single colony in 3 mL Mueller-Hinton (MH) broth (BD Difco), followed by incubating at 37°C with shaking at 200 rpm for 12–14 h. The pre-cultures were used to inoculate tubes with 5 mL MH broth at 1:200 dilution, and the tubes were incubated at 37°C with shaking at 200 rpm for 5 h. Four mL of melted MH soft agar medium (0.7% agar) were mixed with 100 μL of culture and poured onto Petri plates containing 15 mL of MH agar medium (0.7% agar), and the plates were dried for 5 min. Kanamycin gradient strips were laid on top of the soft agar, and the plates were incubated at 35°C for 18 h. MIC values were determined by evaluating the inhibition zone using a magnifying lens according to the manufacturer's instructions.

Minimum inhibitory concentration values obtained from re-testing these isolates were interpreted within NARMS breakpoints as described above (see section "Prediction of Phenotypic Susceptible-Intermediate-Resistant Classifications Using *in silico* Methods") and are reported in the main manuscript (with the exception of amikacin; due to its exclusion from the contemporary panel, original MIC values are reported). Original and updated MIC and SIR values for all 21 isolates are available in **Supplementary Table 4.**

In silico Plasmid Replicon Detection

Plasmid replicons were detected in all *Salmonella* genome assemblies using ABRicate and the PlasmidFinder database (accessed June 11, 2018 via ABRicate's abricate-get_db command). For a plasmid replicon to be considered present in a genome, minimum nucleotide BLAST (BLASTN) (Camacho et al., 2009) identity and coverage values of 80 and 60%, respectively, were used (Carattoli et al., 2014).

Reference-Free Single Nucleotide Polymorphism Identification and Phylogeny Construction

A reference-free approach was used to compare the 128 *Salmonella* genomes sequenced in this study to 442 of the 445 *Salmonella* genomes described by Worley et al. (2018); three genomes were omitted because their Sequence Read Archive (SRA) data was not publicly available at the time of access (February 20, 2019). Raw reads for each of the 442 publicly available genomes were downloaded from SRA (Leinonen et al., 2011; Kodama et al., 2012) and processed and assembled as described above (see section "Whole-Genome Sequencing and Data Pre-processing" described above). kSNP3 version 3.1 (Gardner and Hall, 2013; Gardner et al., 2015) was used to identify core SNPs among all 570 assembled *Salmonella* genomes, using the optimal *k*-mer size determined by Kchooser (k = 19). IQ-TREE version 1.6.10 (Nguyen et al., 2015) was used to construct a maximum likelihood (ML) phylogeny using the resulting core SNPs and the optimal nucleotide substitution model identified using ModelFinder [determined using model Bayesian Information Criteria (BIC) values; **Supplementary Text**]. Bootstrapping was performed using 1,000 replicates of the Ultrafast Bootstrap method (Minh et al., 2013; Hoang et al., 2018). The resulting ML phylogeny was annotated in R using the bactaxR package (Carroll et al., 2020b; **Supplementary Text**).

Pan-Genome Characterization

GFF files produced by Prokka (see section "*In silico* Antimicrobial Resistance Determinant Detection" above) were used as input for Roary version 3.12.0 (Page et al., 2015), which was used to identify orthologous gene clusters at a 70% protein BLAST (BLASTP) identity threshold. The resulting gene presence/absence matrix produced by Roary was used as input for besPLOT[2] (Carroll et al., 2020a), which was used to perform non-metric multidimensional scaling (NMDS) (Kruskal, 1964) and construct plots in two dimensions using a Jaccard distance metric (**Supplementary Text**).

Clustering based on gene presence/absence was assessed for each of the following grouping factors: (i) serotype, (ii) farm, and (iii) isolation source (i.e., bovine or farm environmental). For each of the three grouping factors, the following three statistical tests were performed, using the gene presence/absence matrix produced by Roary, a Jaccard distance metric, and 10,000 permutations: (i) the permutest and betadisper functions in R's vegan package (Oksanen et al., 2019) were used to conduct an ANOVA-like permutation test (Anderson, 2006) to test if group dispersions were homogenous (referred to hereafter as the PERMDISP2 test); (ii) analysis of similarity (ANOSIM) (Clarke, 1993) using the ANOSIM function in the vegan package in R was used to determine if the average of the ranks of within-group distances was greater than or equal to the average of the ranks of between-group distances (Anderson and Walsh, 2013); (iii) permutational analysis of variance (PERMANOVA) (Anderson, 2001) using the adonis2 function in the vegan package in R was used to determine if group centroids were equivalent. For all tests, a Bonferroni correction was applied to correct for multiple comparisons.

Potential clustering based on AMR gene presence/absence was additionally assessed for the same three grouping factors (serotype, farm, and isolation source), using the presence and absence of AMR determinants detected by AMRFinderPlus as input (i.e., AMR and stress response determinants identified using the "plus" option in AMRFinderPlus). All steps were performed as described above, and a Bonferroni correction was used to correct for multiple comparisons.

Reference-Based Core Single Nucleotide Polymorphism Identification Within Serotypes

For each individual serotype, core SNPs were identified among genomes assigned to that serotype using a reference-based approach. For each serotype, Snippy version 4.3.6[3] (Seemann, 2019) was used to identify core SNPs among all representatives assigned to the serotype, using the trimmed Illumina paired-end reads of each genome as input (see section "Whole-Genome Sequencing and Data Pre-processing" above) and one of six high-quality assembled genomes from isolates in this study as a reference genome (**Supplementary Table 1** and **Supplementary Text**). Gubbins version 2.3.4 (Croucher et al., 2015) was used to identify and remove recombination within the full alignment that resulted, and the filtered alignment produced by Gubbins was queried using snp-sites version 2.4.0 (Page et al., 2016) to produce an alignment of core SNPs for each serotype.

Construction of Within-Serotype Phylogenies

For each serotype, IQ-TREE version 1.6.10 was used to construct a ML phylogeny, using core SNPs detected among all isolates assigned to the serotype as input (see "Reference-Based Core Single Nucleotide Polymorphism Identification Within Serotypes" section above), the optimal ascertainment bias-aware nucleotide substitution model selected using ModelFinder, and 1,000 replicates of the UltraFast bootstrap approximation. The temporal structure of each resulting ML phylogeny was assessed using the R^2 value produced by the best-fitting root in TempEst version 1.5.1 (**Supplementary Table 5**; Rambaut et al., 2016).

A tip-dated phylogeny was then constructed for each serotype using BEAST version 2.5.0 (Bouckaert et al., 2014, 2019), using the serotype's corresponding core SNP alignment as input (**Supplementary Text**, **Supplementary Table 5**, and **Supplementary Figure 1**). For a detailed

[2]https://github.com/lmc297/besPLOT

[3]https://github.com/tseemann/snippy

description of all temporal phylogeny construction steps, see the **Supplementary Text**.

Data Availability

Illumina reads are available for all isolates sequenced in this study under NCBI Bioproject Accession PRJNA756552. NCBI BioSample accession numbers for each individual isolate, as well as all associated metadata and genome quality statistics, are available in **Supplementary Table 1**. All BEAST 2 XML files used for temporal phylogeny construction are available at https://github.com/lmc297/zru_farms.

RESULTS

In silico Serotyping of Bovine-Associated *Salmonella* Resolves Incongruencies Between Traditional Serotyping and Whole-Genome Phylogeny

A total of 128 *Salmonella* strains isolated from healthy (i.e., subclinically infected) dairy cattle (n = 39) and their associated farm environments (n = 89) on 13 different New York State farms underwent WGS (**Supplementary Table 1**). In addition to undergoing traditional serotyping in a laboratory setting, all isolates were assigned serotypes *in silico* using both (i) SISTR and (ii) SeqSero2 (**Supplementary Table 1**). Importantly, serotypes assigned *in silico* using SISTR and/or SeqSero2 were able to resolve all un-typable and/or ambiguous serotypes assigned using traditional serotyping (**Supplementary Table 1**). Furthermore, *in silico* serotypes assigned using (i) SISTR's core-genome multi-locus sequence typing (cgMLST) approach and (ii) SeqSero2 were both highly congruent with the *Salmonella* whole-genome phylogeny (**Figure 1**) and highly concordant with each other: 127 of 128 (99.2%) *Salmonella* isolates sequenced in this study were assigned to identical *in silico* serotypes using both SISTR cgMLST and SeqSero2 (**Supplementary Table 1**), with 100% concordance observed for six of seven observed *in silico* serotype groups (i.e., S. Anatum, S. Cerro, S. Meleagridis, S. Minnesota, S. Newport, and S. Typhimurium and its variants, assigned to n = 15, 13, 20, 1, 16, and 27 isolates, respectively). Among S. Kentucky (n = 36), a single incongruent isolate was observed (ENV_KENT_16_12-04-07_R8-0061), as SeqSero2 could not detect an O-antigen within the genome and was thus unable to assign this isolate to any serotype. This isolate was assigned a serotype of 8,20:-:z6 using traditional serotyping (S. Kentucky has antigenic formula 8,20:i:z6); SISTR classified the isolate as S. Kentucky, and the isolate clustered among the S. Kentucky isolates sequenced in this study within the *Salmonella* whole-genome phylogeny (**Figure 1** and **Supplementary Table 1**).

When variants of the S. Typhimurium serotype (n = 27) were considered, discrepancies were observed among traditional serotype assignments and both *in silico* methods (**Supplementary Table 1**). While SeqSero2 could differentiate between S. Typhimurium and the O5- variant of S. Typhimurium (also known as S. Typhimurium variant Copenhagen; "S. Typhimurium Copenhagen" is used hereafter), SISTR was unable to differentiate the two (**Supplementary Table 1**), as noted previously (Ibrahim and Morin, 2018; Zhang et al., 2019). However, S. Typhimurium and S. Typhimurium Copenhagen serotype assignments obtained using SeqSero2 and traditional serotyping did not always agree, as five of 27 S. Typhimurium/S. Typhimurium Copenhagen assignments (18.5%) differed between the two methods (**Supplementary Table 1**). For four of the five incongruent isolates, SeqSero2 assigned an isolate to S. Typhimurium Copenhagen, while traditional serotyping assigned a serotype of S. Typhimurium; for one isolate, the opposite scenario applied (**Supplementary Table 1**). Furthermore, the lineages formed by isolates classified here as S. Typhimurium Copenhagen using either traditional serotyping or SeqSero2, as well as two S. Typhimurium Copenhagen genomes from a previous study (Worley et al., 2018), were polyphyletic (**Figure 1**); consequently, the whole-genome phylogeny could not be used to reliably differentiate these two variants.

For the remainder of this study, a serotype assigned consistently with at least two out of the three methods (i.e., traditional serotyping, SeqSero2, and SISTR cgMLST) was selected as the final serotype to be reported for each isolate. Nine of the 13 farms surveyed here harbored *Salmonella* isolates that belonged to a single serotype, while two farms harbored two serotypes or serotype variants (Farms 25 and 35 harbored Typhimurium/Typhimurium Copenhagen and Cerro/Newport, respectively; **Supplementary Table 1**). The remaining two farms harbored three *Salmonella* serotypes (Farms 17 and 62 harbored Kentucky/Newport/Typhimurium and Cerro/Minnesota/Newport, respectively; **Supplementary Table 1**).

In silico Methods Predict Antimicrobial Susceptibility and Resistance Among Bovine-Associated *Salmonella* With High Accuracy and Concordance

Using a 15-antimicrobial panel and NARMS breakpoints for *Salmonella*, more than half of all isolates in this study (81 of 128; 63.3%) were classified as susceptible to all 15 antimicrobials tested, while 38 isolates (29.7%) were classified as resistant to two or more antimicrobials (obtained after the 15-antimicrobial panel was re-run for 22 isolates to resolve discrepancies between *in silico* predictions and phenotypic AMR data; **Supplementary Tables 1, 4**).

Regardless of choice of AMR determinant detection pipeline and AMR determinant database, all pipeline/database combinations performed nearly identically when given the task of predicting phenotypic AMR susceptibility/resistance to 15 antimicrobials using known AMR determinant-phenotype associations (**Figure 2**, **Table 1**, and **Supplementary Tables 2, 3**). Furthermore, all pipeline/database combinations showed an extremely high degree of concordance (98.0% or greater for all pipeline/database combinations; **Supplementary Figure 2**). The overall accuracy of all *in silico* AMR determinant detection pipeline/database combinations ranged from 95.8 to 97.4%, with the SRST2 AMR detection tool/ARG-ANNOT AMR

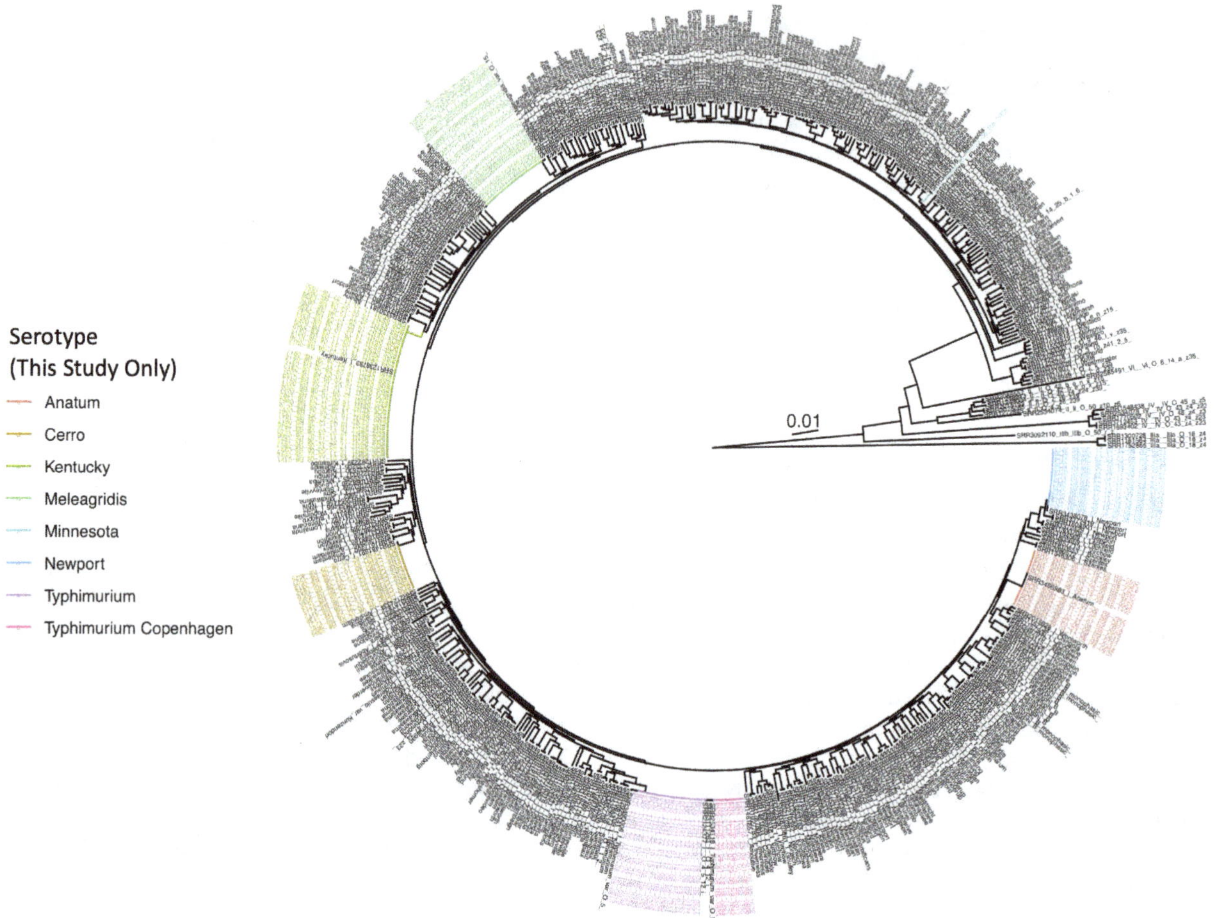

FIGURE 1 | Maximum likelihood phylogeny constructed using core SNPs identified among 570 *Salmonella* isolate genomes. Publicly available genomes are denoted by black tip labels (n = 442), while genomes of bovine- and bovine farm-associated strains isolated in conjunction with this study are denoted by colored tip labels (n = 128). In cases where a discrepancy existed between the traditional serotype designation of an isolate and one or more *in silico* methods (i.e., SISTR and SeqSero2), the serotype assigned using two out of the three methods was selected as the final serotype to be used for phylogeny annotation. The phylogeny is rooted at the midpoint with branch lengths reported in substitutions per site. Core SNPs were identified among all genomes using kSNP3, while the phylogeny was constructed and annotated using IQ-TREE and bactaxR/ggtree, respectively.

determinant database combination achieving the highest accuracy for this data set (**Figure 2**, **Table 1**, and **Supplementary Table 3**). The ARIBA/CARD pipeline/database combination achieved the highest specificity, although all pipeline/database combinations were able to predict phenotypic AMR with high specificity (>99.0%; **Figure 2**, **Table 1**, and **Supplementary Table 3**). Sensitivity ranged from 71.8 to 84.4%, with SRST2 achieving the highest sensitivities (84.4 and 84.0% for the ARG-ANNOT and ResFinder databases, respectively; **Table 1** and **Supplementary Table 3**).

For the AMR determinant detection pipelines that relied on nucleotide BLAST (i.e., ABRicate and BTyper), a range of minimum percent nucleotide identity and coverage thresholds were additionally tested (i.e., all combinations of 50–100% nucleotide identity in increments of 5% and 0–100% coverage in increments of 10%; **Supplementary Figure 3**) so that the optimal combination(s) could be established for the isolate genomes sequenced here. For ABRicate/ARG-ANNOT, ABRicate/NCBI, and ABRicate/ResFinder, maximum accuracy was achieved using minimum coverage thresholds of 60, 50, and 50–60%, respectively, and 75–95% nucleotide identity thresholds (**Supplementary Figure 3**). For ABRicate/CARD, minimum thresholds of 60% coverage and 75% nucleotide identity were optimal (**Supplementary Figure 3**). For BTyper/ARG-ANNOT, maximum accuracy was achieved using 60% coverage and 50–95% nucleotide identity; for BTyper/MEGARes, 50–60% coverage and 95% nucleotide identity were the optimal thresholds (**Supplementary Figure 3**).

The performance of the PATRIC3 *in silico* MIC prediction method was additionally evaluated (**Figure 3** and **Supplementary Figure 4**). PATRIC3 was able to correctly classify *Salmonella* isolates as SIR based on NARMS breakpoints with an overall accuracy of 92.9% [95% confidence interval 91.6–94.1%, accuracy P-value (accuracy > no information rate) < 1.25E-26; **Figure 3**]. At the individual antimicrobial level, PATRIC3 achieved >90% SIR prediction accuracy for 12 of 14 antimicrobials; only

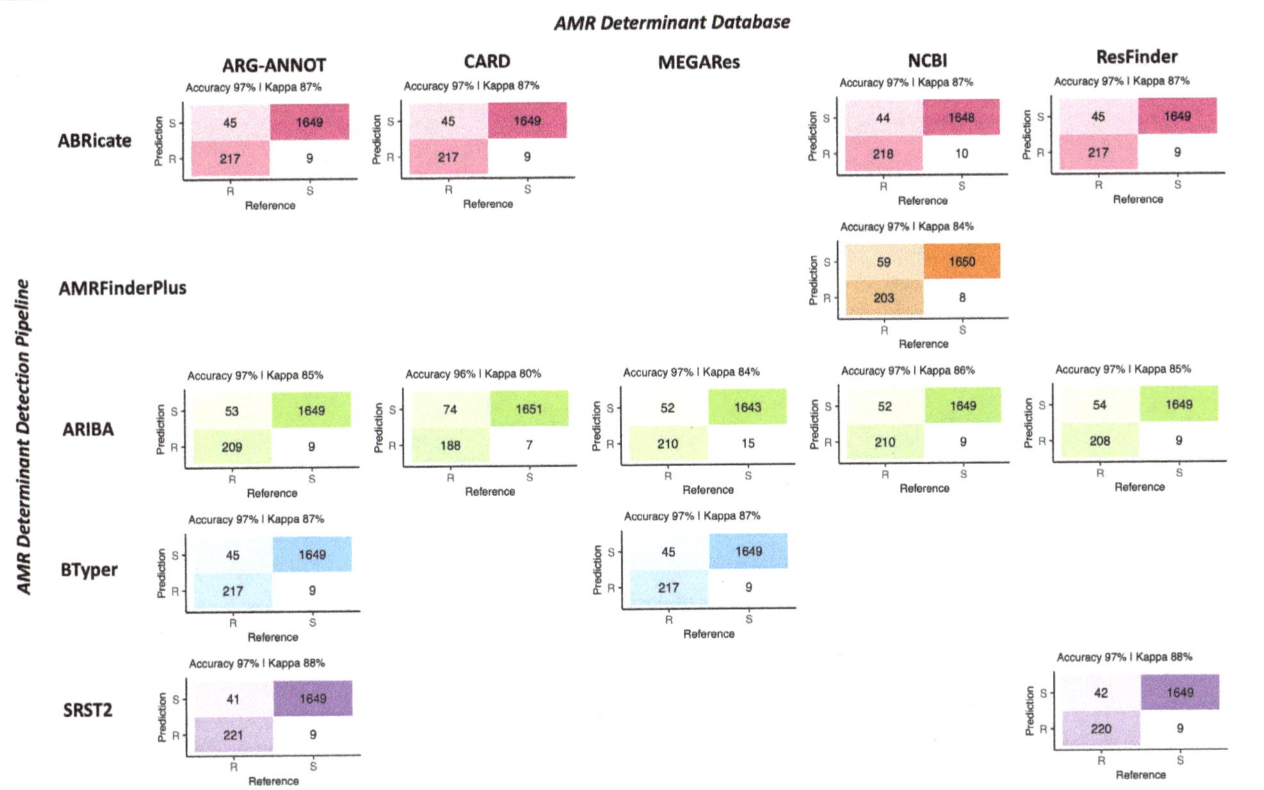

FIGURE 2 | Confusion matrices showcasing agreement between susceptible-intermediate-resistant (SIR) classification of 128 *Salmonella* isolates obtained using phenotypic resistance testing (denoted as the matrix "Reference") and five *in silico* methods (denoted as the matrix "Prediction") for 15 antimicrobials. Accuracy values above each matrix denote the percentage of correctly classified instances out of all instances. Kappa values above each matrix denote Cohen's kappa coefficient for the matrix, reported as a percent. For the phenotypic method, SIR classification was determined using NARMS breakpoints for *Salmonella* (accessed March 23, 2020). For the *in silico* antimicrobial resistance (AMR) determinant detection approaches, combinations of five pipelines and one to five AMR determinant databases were tested; isolate genomes that harbored one or more AMR determinants previously known to confer resistance to a particular antimicrobial were categorized as resistant to that antimicrobial ("R"), while those which did not were categorized as susceptible ("S"; see **Supplementary Table 2** for all detected AMR determinants and their associated resistance classifications). For all AMR determinant detection methods, isolates that showed intermediate phenotypic resistance to an antimicrobial were categorized as susceptible ("S") rather than resistant, as this classification produced slightly better accuracy scores for all pipeline/database combinations. For AMR determinant detection methods that relied on nucleotide BLAST (i.e., ABRicate and BTyper), the confusion matrix obtained using the nucleotide identity and coverage threshold combination that produced the highest accuracy are shown (**Supplementary Figure 3**); for all other methods, confusion matrices obtained using default detection parameters are shown.

sulfisoxazole and tetracycline resistance prediction accuracies were <90% (83.6 and 68.0%, respectively; **Figure 3** and **Supplementary Figure 4**).

Genomic Antimicrobial Resistance Determinants of Bovine-Associated *Salmonella* Are Serotype-Associated

Based on the presence and absence of pan-genome elements among all 128 *Salmonella* isolates sequenced here, the *Salmonella* pan-genome was more similar within serotype and within farm than between serotype and between farm, respectively (PERMANOVA and ANOSIM $P < 0.05$ after a Bonferroni correction; **Figure 4** and **Table 2**), with serotypes showing a higher degree of pan-genome dissimilarity (ANOSIM $R = 0.99$) and accounting for a larger proportion of the variance (PERMANOVA $R^2 = 0.93$) than farms (**Figure 4** and **Table 2**); however, dispersion among both serotypes and farms differed (PERMDISP2 $P < 0.05$ after a Bonferroni correction; **Table 2**), indicating that the ANOSIM and/or PERMANOVA tests could potentially be confounding dispersion with serotype/farm. Additionally, subclinical bovine *Salmonella* isolates did not significantly differ from strains isolated from the associated farm environment based on pan-genome element presence/absence (PERMANOVA, ANOSIM, and PERMDISP2 $P > 0.05$ after a Bonferroni correction; **Figure 4** and **Table 2**).

Based on the presence and absence of AMR and stress response determinants detected among all 128 *Salmonella* genomes, isolates were more similar within serotype than between serotypes (PERMANOVA and ANOSIM $P < 0.05$ and PERMDISP2 $P > 0.05$ after a Bonferroni correction; **Figure 4** and **Table 2**). Additionally, isolates were more similar within farm than between farm based on their AMR and stress response gene presence/absence profiles (PERMANOVA and ANOSIM $P < 0.05$; **Figure 4** and **Table 2**), although significant, potentially confounding dispersion differences among farms were present

TABLE 1 | Statistics for the 15-antimicrobial phenotypic susceptibility/resistance prediction task for all antimicrobial resistance (AMR) determinant pipeline/database combinations[a].

AMR Pipeline	AMR Database	% Accuracy (95% Confidence Interval)	Cohen's Kappa (%)	Corrected Accuracy *P*-Value[b]	Corrected McNemar's Test *P*-Value[b]	Sensitivity (%)	Specificity (%)
ABRicate	ARG-ANNOT	97.2 (96.3–97.9)	87.3	1.72E-59	2.67E-05	82.8	99.5
ABRicate	CARD	97.2 (96.3–97.9)	87.3	1.72E-59	2.67E-05	82.8	99.5
ABRicate	NCBI	97.2 (96.3–97.9)	87.4	1.72E-59	9.94E-05	83.2	99.4
ABRicate	ResFinder	97.2 (96.3–97.9)	87.3	1.72E-59	2.67E-05	82.8	99.5
AMRFinderPlus	NCBI	96.5 (95.6–97.3)	83.9	1.41E-50	1.41E-08	77.5	99.5
ARIBA	ARG-ANNOT	96.8 (95.9–97.5)	85.3	7.37E-54	6.63E-07	79.8	99.5
ARIBA	CARD	95.8 (94.8–96.6)	79.9	3.08E-42	3.14E-12	71.8	99.6
ARIBA	MEGARes	96.5 (95.6–97.3)	84.3	1.41E-50	1.53E-04	80.2	99.1
ARIBA	NCBI	96.8 (95.9–97.6)	85.5	1.55E-54	1.06E-06	80.2	99.5
ARIBA	ResFinder	96.7 (95.8–97.5)	85.0	3.45E-53	4.15E-07	79.4	99.5
BTyper	ARG-ANNOT	97.2 (96.3–97.9)	87.3	1.72E-59	2.67E-05	82.8	99.5
BTyper	MEGARes	97.2 (96.3–97.9)	87.3	1.72E-59	2.67E-05	82.8	99.5
SRST2	ARG-ANNOT	97.4 (96.6–98.1)	88.4	1.69E-62	1.63E-04	84.4	99.5
SRST2	ResFinder	97.3 (96.5–98.0)	88.1	9.85E-62	1.04E-04	84.0	99.5

[a]*Statistics were calculated using the confusionMatrix function in the caret package in R, with resistant ("R") phenotypes/genotypes treated as the "positive" result and susceptible ("S") phenotypes/genotypes treated as the "negative" result; See* ***Supplementary Table 3*** *for an extended version of this table.*
[b]*Adjusted using a Bonferroni correction.*

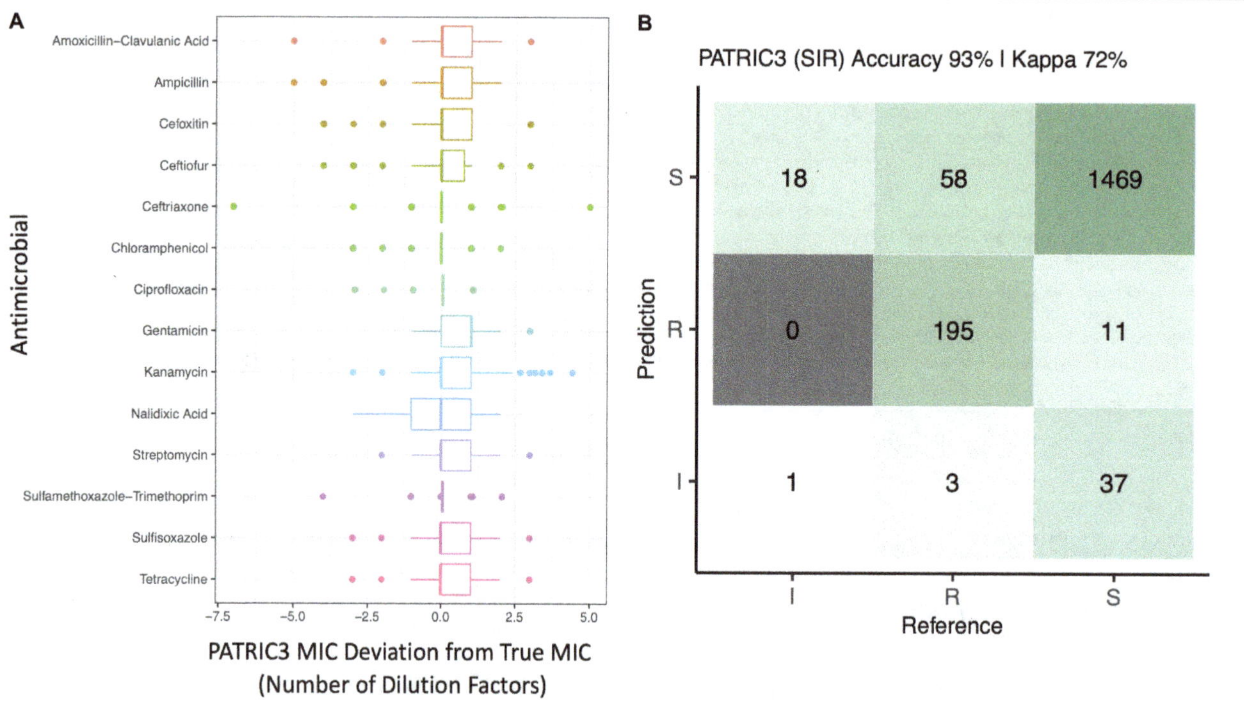

FIGURE 3 | (A) Deviation of PATRIC3 predicted minimum inhibitory concentration (MIC) values from "true" MIC values obtained using phenotypic resistance testing for 14 antimicrobials (*Y*-axis), reported in number of dilution factors (*X*-axis). For each box plot, lower and upper box hinges correspond to the first and third quartiles, respectively. Lower and upper whiskers extend from the hinge to the smallest and largest values no more distant than 1.5 times the interquartile range from the hinge, respectively. Points represent pairwise distances that fall beyond the ends of the whiskers. Only isolates with raw MIC values available are included (126 of 128 isolates). **(B)** Confusion matrix showcasing agreement between susceptible-intermediate-resistant (SIR) classification of all 128 *Salmonella* isolates obtained using phenotypic resistance testing (denoted as the matrix "Reference") and PATRIC3 (denoted as the matrix "Prediction") for 14 antimicrobials. The accuracy value above the matrix denotes the percentage of correctly classified instances out of all instances. The Kappa value above the matrix denotes Cohen's kappa coefficient for the matrix, reported as a percent. For both the phenotypic and PATRIC3 methods, SIR classification was determined using NARMS breakpoints for *Salmonella* (accessed March 23, 2020).

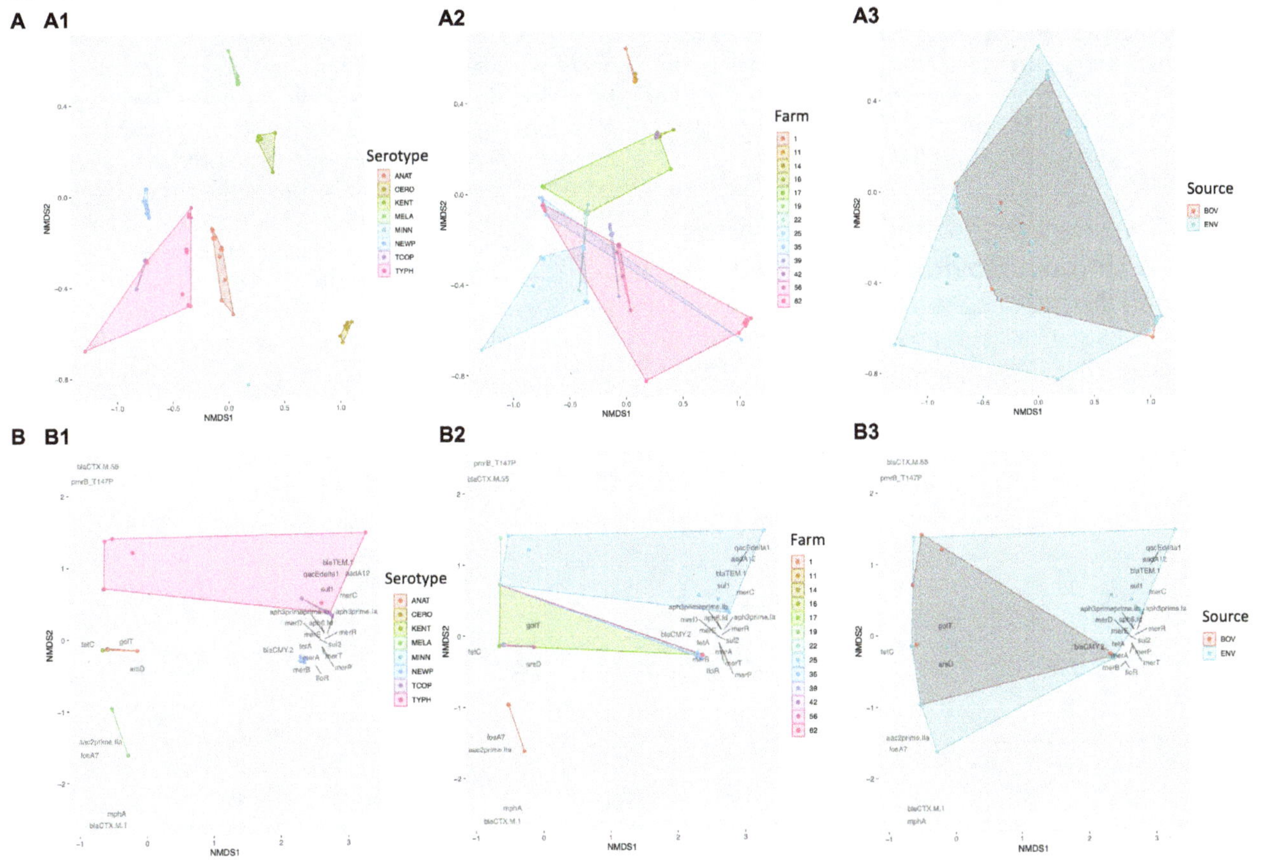

FIGURE 4 | Results of non-metric multidimensional scaling (NMDS) performed using the presence and absence of **(A)** pan-genome elements (n = 4,102; identified using Roary), and **(B)** antimicrobial resistance (AMR) and stress response genes (n = 28; detected using AMRFinderPlus) among 128 bovine-associated *Salmonella* isolates, plotted in two dimensions. Points represent isolates, while shaded regions and convex hulls correspond to isolate (1) serotypes (ANAT, Anatum; CERO, Cerro; KENT, Kentucky; MELA, Meleagridis; NEWP, Newport; TCOP, Typhimurium Copenhagen; TYPH, Typhimurium), (2) farm, and (3) source (BOV, bovine; ENV, bovine farm environment). For all plots, a Jaccard distance metric was used. For AMR/stress response genes **(B)**, gene names/scores are plotted in dark gray text.

TABLE 2 | Results of PERMDISP2, ANOSIM, and PERMANOVA tests[a].

Group	PERMDISP2 Raw *P*-Value (*F*)[b]	ANOSIM Raw *P*-Value (*R*)[c]	PERMANOVA Raw *P*-Value (R^2)[d]
Pan-genome element presence/absence (n = 4,102)[e]			
Serotype	2.0E-4 (14.3)*	<1.0E-4 (0.99)*	<1.0E-4 (0.93)*
Farm	<1.0E-4 (4.43)*	<1.0E-4 (0.54)*	<1.0E-4 (0.73)*
Source	0.071 (3.40)	0.99 (−0.07)	0.32 (0.01)
Antimicrobial resistance and stress response gene presence/absence (n = 28)[f]			
Serotype	0.013 (4.46)	<1.0E-4 (0.79)*	<1.0E-4 (0.85)*
Farm	<1.0E-4 (5.52)*	<1.0E-4 (0.30)*	<1.0E-4 (0.54)*
Source	0.74 (0.01)	0.79 (−0.03)	0.31 (0.01)

[a] *All tests were performed using a Jaccard dissimilarity metric and 10,000 permutations; raw P-values are reported for all tests, with significant P-values (P < 0.05 after a Bonferroni correction was applied to all values) denoted with an asterisk (*).*

[b] *ANOVA-like permutation test applied to results obtained using the PERMDISP2 procedure for the analysis of multivariate homogeneity of group dispersions (i.e., variances), obtained using the betadisper and permutest functions in the vegan package in R; betadisper is a multivariate analog of Levene's test for homogeneity of variances.*

[c] *Analysis of similarities (ANOSIM) test results obtained using the ANOSIM function in the vegan package in R.*

[d] *Permutational analysis of variance (PERMANOVA) test results obtained using the adonis2 function in the vegan package in R.*

[e] *Identified using Roary and a 70% protein BLAST (BLASTP) identity threshold.*

[f] *Detected using AMRFinderPlus.*

(PERMDISP2 $P < 0.05$; **Table 2**). As was the case with the pan-genome in its entirety, subclinical bovine *Salmonella* isolates did not significantly differ from farm environmental isolates based on AMR and stress response gene presence/absence (PERMANOVA, ANOSIM, and PERMDISP2 $P > 0.05$ after a Bonferroni correction; **Figure 4** and **Table 2**).

Each of Two New York State Dairy Farms Harbors a Unique, Bovine-Associated *Salmonella* Anatum Lineage

Fifteen *S.* Anatum strains encompassing four PFGE types (**Supplementary Table 1**) were isolated from subclinical bovine sources and their associated farm environments on two different New York State dairy farms (i.e., Farms 39 and 56; **Figure 5** and **Table 3**). Notably, the *S.* Anatum lineages circulating on each farm were distinct at a genomic level, with isolates from each farm forming a separate clade [posterior probability (PP) = 1 for each; **Figure 5**]. The two farm-associated lineages were predicted to share a common ancestor circa 1836 (node age 1836.28 using median node heights; **Figure 5**), although the age of the common ancestor could not be dated reliably [node height 95% highest posterior density (HPD) interval 540.85–1978.42; **Supplementary Figure 5**].

Salmonella Anatum isolates from Farm 39 shared a common ancestor circa 2005 (node age 2004.69, node height 95% HPD

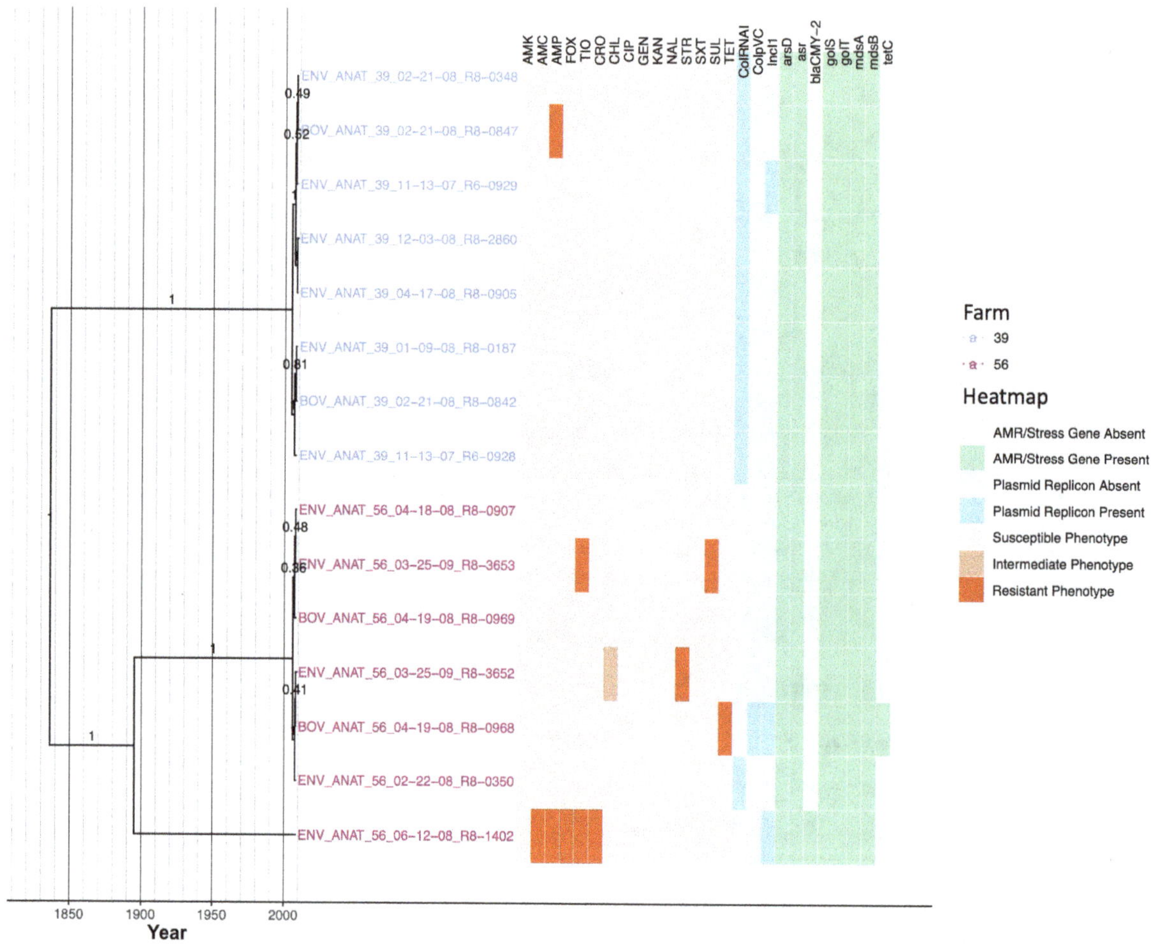

FIGURE 5 | Rooted, time-scaled maximum clade credibility (MCC) phylogeny constructed using core SNPs identified among 15 *Salmonella* Anatum genomes isolated from subclinical bovine sources and the surrounding bovine farm environment. Tip label colors denote the ID of the farm from which each strain was isolated. Branch labels denote posterior probabilities of branch support. Time in years is plotted along the *X*-axis, and branch lengths are reported in years. The heatmap to the right of the phylogeny denotes (i) the susceptible-intermediate-resistant (SIR) classification of each isolate for each of 15 antimicrobials (obtained using phenotypic testing and NARMS breakpoints; orange); (ii) presence and absence of plasmid replicons (detected using ABRicate/PlasmidFinder and minimum nucleotide identity and coverage thresholds of 80 and 60%, respectively; blue); (iii) presence and absence of antimicrobial resistance (AMR) and stress response genes (identified using AMRFinderPlus and default parameters; green). Core SNPs were identified using Snippy. The phylogeny was constructed using the results of ten independent runs using a strict clock model, the Standard_TVMef nucleotide substitution model, and the Coalescent Bayesian Skyline population model implemented in BEAST version 2.5.1, with 10% burn-in applied to each run. LogCombiner-2 was used to combine BEAST 2 log files, and TreeAnnotator-2 was used to construct the phylogeny using median node heights. Abbreviations for the 15 antimicrobials are: AMK, amikacin; AMC, amoxicillin-clavulanic acid; AMP, ampicillin; FOX, cefoxitin; TIO, ceftiofur; CRO, ceftriaxone; CHL, chloramphenicol; CIP, ciprofloxacin; GEN, gentamicin; KAN, kanamycin; NAL, nalidixic acid; STR, streptomycin; SXT, sulfamethoxazole-trimethoprim; SUL, sulfisoxazole; TET, tetracycline.

1978.46–2007.69; **Figure 5** and **Supplementary Figure 5**). All Farm 39 *S.* Anatum isolates possessed identical AMR/stress response gene profiles, and all isolates were pan-susceptible except for a single isolate that was resistant to ampicillin (**Figure 5**). All Farm 39 *S.* Anatum isolates additionally harbored ColRNAI plasmids; a single isolate additionally harbored an IncI1 plasmid that appeared to harbor no AMR genes (**Figure 5**).

Salmonella Anatum isolates from Farm 56, however, were considerably more diverse than their Farm 39 counterparts; while a clade containing six of seven strains shared a very recent common ancestor (node age 2006.16, node height 95% HPD 1985.37–2008.11; **Figure 5** and **Supplementary Figure 5**), a unique lineage represented by a single environmental isolate (ENV_ANAT_56_06-12-08_R8-1402) was present among *S.* Anatum from Farm 56 (**Figure 5**). All *S.* Anatum isolates from Farm 56 were predicted to have evolved from a common ancestor that existed circa 1895 (node age 1895.03), although this node could not be reliably dated (node height 95% HPD 1036.89–1989.944; **Supplementary Figure 5**). Additionally, *S.* Anatum isolated from Farm 56 showcased a greater degree of AMR heterogeneity than those from Farm 39 (**Figure 5**). Notably, the isolate comprising the unique Farm 56 *S.* Anatum lineage possessed an IncI1 plasmid and bla_{CMY-2} and was multidrug resistant (MDR) (resistant to amoxicillin-clavulanic acid, ampicillin, cefoxitin, ceftiofur, and ceftriaxone; **Figure 5**). Three of six *S.* Anatum strains comprising the major Farm 56 *S.* Anatum lineage were pan-susceptible. The remaining three isolates were resistant to one of (i) tetracycline, (ii) streptomycin, or (iii) ceftiofur and sulfisoxazole; the streptomycin-resistant isolate additionally exhibited reduced susceptibility to chloramphenicol (**Figure 5**). The tetracycline-resistant isolate additionally possessed both ColpVC and IncI1 plasmids and harbored tetracycline resistance gene *tetC* (**Figure 5**). While these data suggest some *S.* Anatum lineages queried here have recently acquired AMR, the limited number of isolates and the large degree of uncertainty for some phylogeny node ages preclude reliable estimation of AMR acquisition timeframes.

A Closely Related *Salmonella* Cerro Lineage Spans Two New York State Dairy Farms

Thirteen *S.* Cerro strains encompassing two PFGE types (**Supplementary Table 1**) isolated from two dairy farms (12 from Farm 62 and one from Farm 35) were found to share a high degree of genomic similarity; isolates differed by, at most, 12 core SNPs and evolved from a common ancestor that existed circa March 2008 [node age 2008.21, common ancestor (CA) node height 95% HPD interval 2007.6–2008.6; **Figure 6**, **Table 3**, **Supplementary Figure 6**, and **Supplementary Table 5**]. While IncI1 and ColRNAI plasmid replicons were detected in all 13 *S.* Cerro isolates, only one isolate was not pan-susceptible (**Figure 6**). Notably, the isolate from Farm 35 (BOV_CERO_35_10-02-08_R8-2685) was classified as resistant to nine antimicrobials using phenotypic methods (i.e., amoxicillin-clavulanic acid, ampicillin, cefoxitin, ceftiofur, ceftriaxone, chloramphenicol, streptomycin, sulfisoxazole, and tetracycline); based on the most parsimonious explanation for AMR acquisition, this lineage acquired AMR after July 2008 (node age 2008.51, CA node height 95% HPD interval 2008.14–2008.75; **Figure 6** and **Supplementary Figure 6**). However, no genomic determinants known to confer resistance to these antimicrobials were detected in the genome of the MDR isolate (**Figure 6**), and the MDR phenotype was confirmed in a second, independent phenotypic AMR test (**Supplementary Table 4**).

Salmonella Kentucky Strains Isolated Across Five Different New York State Dairy Farms Evolved From a Common Ancestor That Existed Circa 2004

Thirty-six *S.* Kentucky isolates encompassing two PFGE types (**Supplementary Table 1**) isolated across five New York State dairy farms (i.e., five, seven, nine, seven, and eight isolates from each of Farm 14, 16, 17, 19, and 42, respectively) were similar at a genomic level; isolates differed by between 0 and 30 core SNPs and shared a common ancestor that was predicted to have existed circa January/February 2004 (node age 2004.07, CA node height 95% HPD interval 2000.73–2006.8; **Figure 7**, **Table 3**, **Supplementary Figure 7**, and **Supplementary Table 5**). Two farms harbored a total of three *S.* Kentucky isolates, which were not pan-susceptible (two isolates from Farm 16 and one from Farm 17; **Figure 7**). Farm 17 harbored a tetracycline-resistant isolate (ENV_KENT_17_03-11-08_R8-0815), which possessed an IncI1 plasmid and *tetC* (**Figure 7**). The lineage represented by this isolate was predicted to have acquired tetracycline resistance after March 2007 (node height 2007.19, CA node height 95% HPD interval 2006.43–2007.84; **Figure 7** and **Supplementary Figure 7**). The two *S.* Kentucky isolates from Farm 16 additionally showed reduced susceptibility to chloramphenicol, a trait predicted to have been acquired by these lineages after December 2006/January 2007 (for the lineage represented by isolate ENV_KENT_16_12-04-07_R8-0061; node height 2006.98, CA node height 95% HPD interval 2005.95–2007.85) and May 2007 (for the lineage represented by isolate BOV_KENT_16_02-13-08_R8-0838; node height 2007.38, CA node height 95% HPD interval 2006.59–2008.10; **Figure 7** and **Supplementary Figure 7**). No corresponding genes that may encode for reduced chloramphenicol susceptibility were identified in these two isolates.

A Clonal *Salmonella* Meleagridis Lineage Is Distributed Across Two New York State Dairy Farms and Encompasses Isolates Carrying $bla_{CTX-M-1}$

Nineteen *S.* Meleagridis isolates encompassing two PFGE types (**Supplementary Table 1**) were isolated from two dairy farms (13 and six isolates from Farms 01 and 11, respectively) and were highly clonal: isolates differed by fewer than ten core SNPs and evolved from a common ancestor that existed circa May/June 2007 (node age 2007.42, CA node height 95% HPD interval 2006.91–2007.75; **Figure 8**, **Table 3**, **Supplementary Figure 8**, and **Supplementary Table 5**). All but three branches within the *S.* Meleagridis phylogeny had low

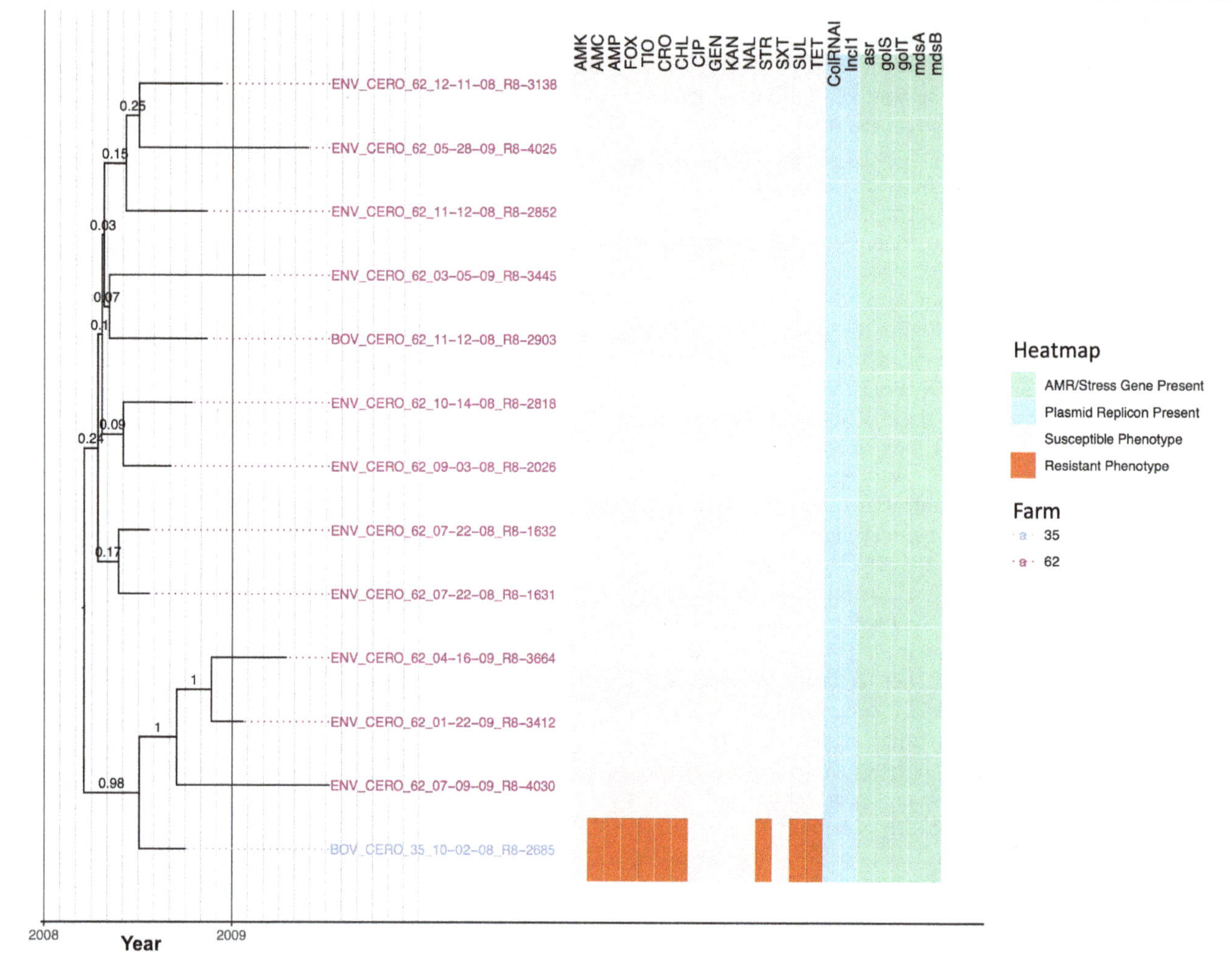

FIGURE 6 | Rooted, time-scaled maximum clade credibility (MCC) phylogeny constructed using core SNPs identified among 13 *Salmonella* Cerro genomes isolated from subclinical bovine sources and the surrounding bovine farm environment. Tip label colors denote the ID of the farm from which each strain was isolated. Branch labels denote posterior probabilities of branch support. Time in years is plotted along the *X*-axis, and branch lengths are reported in years. The heatmap to the right of the phylogeny denotes (i) the susceptible-intermediate-resistant (SIR) classification of each isolate for each of 15 antimicrobials (obtained using phenotypic testing and NARMS breakpoints; orange); (ii) presence of plasmid replicons (detected using ABRicate/PlasmidFinder and minimum nucleotide identity and coverage thresholds of 80 and 60%, respectively; blue); (iii) presence of antimicrobial resistance (AMR) and stress response genes (identified using AMRFinderPlus and default parameters; green). Core SNPs were identified using Snippy. The phylogeny was constructed using the results of ten independent runs using a strict clock model, the Standard_TPM1 nucleotide substitution model, and the Coalescent Bayesian Skyline population model implemented in BEAST version 2.5.1, with 10% burn-in applied to each run. LogCombiner-2 was used to combine BEAST 2 log files, and TreeAnnotator-2 was used to construct the phylogeny using common ancestor node heights. Abbreviations for the 15 antimicrobials are: AMK, amikacin; AMC, amoxicillin-clavulanic acid; AMP, ampicillin; FOX, cefoxitin; TIO, ceftiofur; CRO, ceftriaxone; CHL, chloramphenicol; CIP, ciprofloxacin; GEN, gentamicin; KAN, kanamycin; NAL, nalidixic acid; STR, streptomycin; SXT, sulfamethoxazole-trimethoprim; SUL, sulfisoxazole; TET, tetracycline.

support (PP $\leq$ 0.41; **Figure 8** and **Supplementary Figure 8**), indicating that most nodes were unreliable, likely due to the isolates being highly clonal. All *S.* Meleagridis isolates from Farm 11 were pan-susceptible, possessed no plasmid replicons, and did not possess any acquired AMR genes (**Figure 8**). Among the *S.* Meleagridis isolates from Farm 01, one isolate (ENV_MELA_01_10-02-07_R6-0938) was resistant to ampicillin, ceftiofur, and ceftriaxone, and possessed an IncN plasmid, macrolide resistance gene *mph(A)*, and beta-lactamase $bla_{CTX-M-1}$ (**Figure 8**). Two additional *S.* Meleagridis isolates from Farm 01 each exhibited reduced susceptibility to either (i) cefoxitin, sulfisoxazole, and tetracycline, or (ii) ceftiofur (**Figure 8**).

Kanamycin Resistance Among Each of Three New York State Dairy Farms Harboring a Distinct, Multidrug-Resistant *Salmonella* Newport Lineage Is Farm-Associated

Sixteen *S.* Newport isolates encompassing three PFGE types (**Supplementary Table 1**) were isolated from one

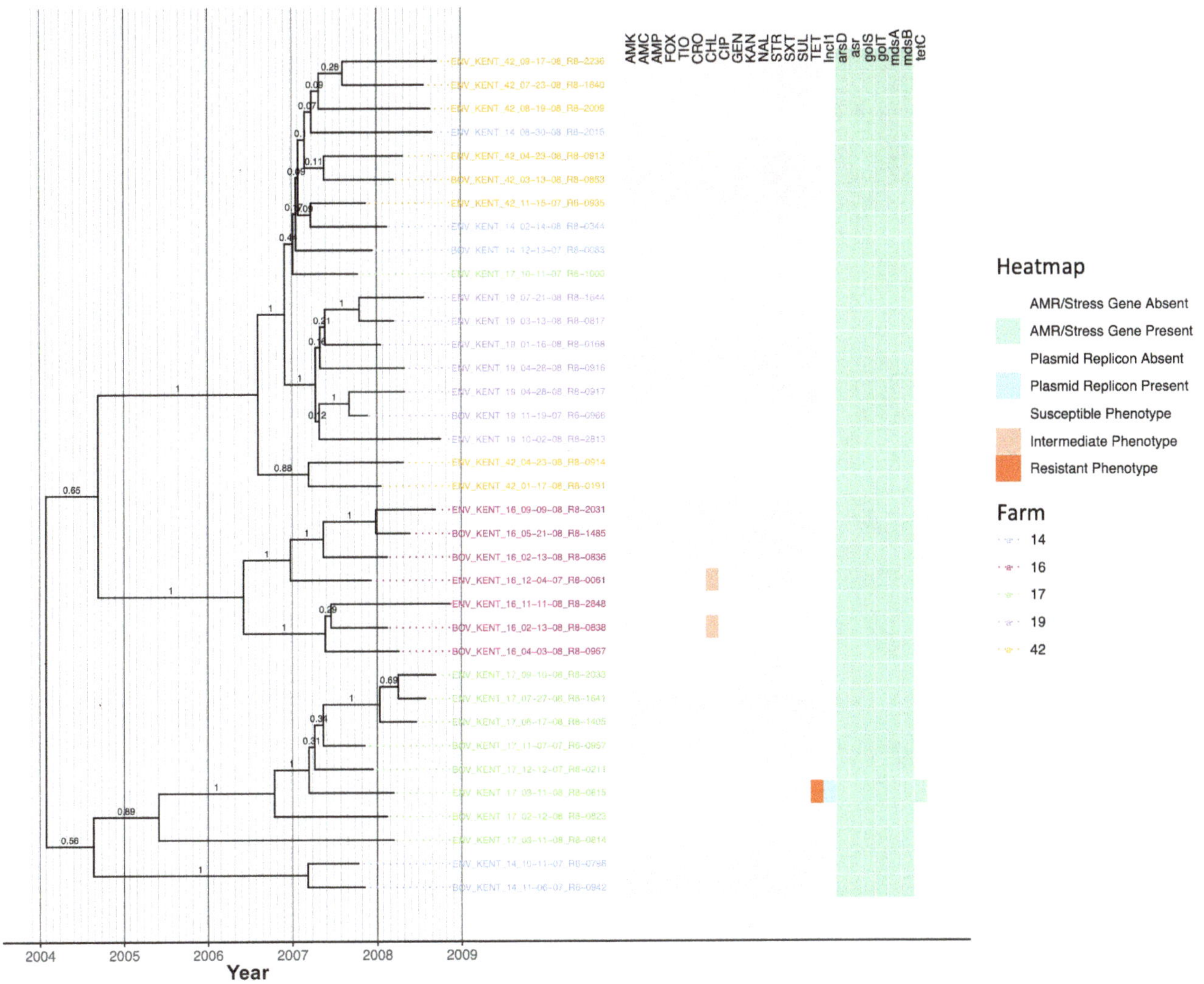

FIGURE 7 | Rooted, time-scaled maximum clade credibility (MCC) phylogeny constructed using core SNPs identified among 36 *Salmonella* Kentucky genomes isolated from subclinical bovine sources and the surrounding bovine farm environment. Tip label colors denote the ID of the farm from which each strain was isolated. Branch labels denote posterior probabilities of branch support. Time in years is plotted along the *X*-axis, and branch lengths are reported in years. The heatmap to the right of the phylogeny denotes (i) the susceptible-intermediate-resistant (SIR) classification of each isolate for each of 15 antimicrobials (obtained using phenotypic testing and NARMS breakpoints; orange); (ii) presence of plasmid replicons (detected using ABRicate/PlasmidFinder and minimum nucleotide identity and coverage thresholds of 80 and 60%, respectively; blue); (iii) presence of antimicrobial resistance (AMR) and stress response genes (identified using AMRFinderPlus and default parameters; green). Core SNPs were identified using Snippy. The phylogeny was constructed using the results of ten independent runs using a relaxed lognormal clock model, the Standard_TVMef nucleotide substitution model, and the Coalescent Bayesian Skyline population model implemented in BEAST version 2.5.1, with 10% burn-in applied to each run. LogCombiner-2 was used to combine BEAST 2 log files, and TreeAnnotator-2 was used to construct the phylogeny using common ancestor node heights. Abbreviations for the 15 antimicrobials are: AMK, amikacin; AMC, amoxicillin-clavulanic acid; AMP, ampicillin; FOX, cefoxitin; TIO, ceftiofur; CRO, ceftriaxone; CHL, chloramphenicol; CIP, ciprofloxacin; GEN, gentamicin; KAN, kanamycin; NAL, nalidixic acid; STR, streptomycin; SXT, sulfamethoxazole-trimethoprim; SUL, sulfisoxazole; TET, tetracycline.

of three farms (four, five, and seven isolates from Farms 17, 35, and 62, respectively); all isolates were resistant to amoxicillin-clavulanic acid, ampicillin, cefoxitin, ceftiofur, ceftriaxone, streptomycin, sulfisoxazole, and tetracycline (**Figure 9**). All *S.* Newport genomes harbored IncA/C2 and ColRNAI plasmids, as well as streptomycin resistance genes *APH(3″)-Ib* and *APH(6)-Id* (i.e., *strAB*), beta-lactamase bla_{CMY-2}, sulfonamide resistance gene *sul2*, and tetracycline resistance gene *tetA* (**Figure 9**). Notably, the *S.* Newport lineage circulating on each farm formed one of three separate clades (PP = 0.99–1.0) that evolved from a common ancestor that existed circa March/April 2004 (node age 2004.23, CA node height 95% HPD interval 2000.42–2007.85; **Figure 9**, **Table 3**, **Supplementary Figure 9**, and **Supplementary Table 5**).

The *S.* Newport lineages present on Farm 17 and Farm 62 were additionally resistant to chloramphenicol and kanamycin and possessed chloramphenicol and kanamycin resistance genes

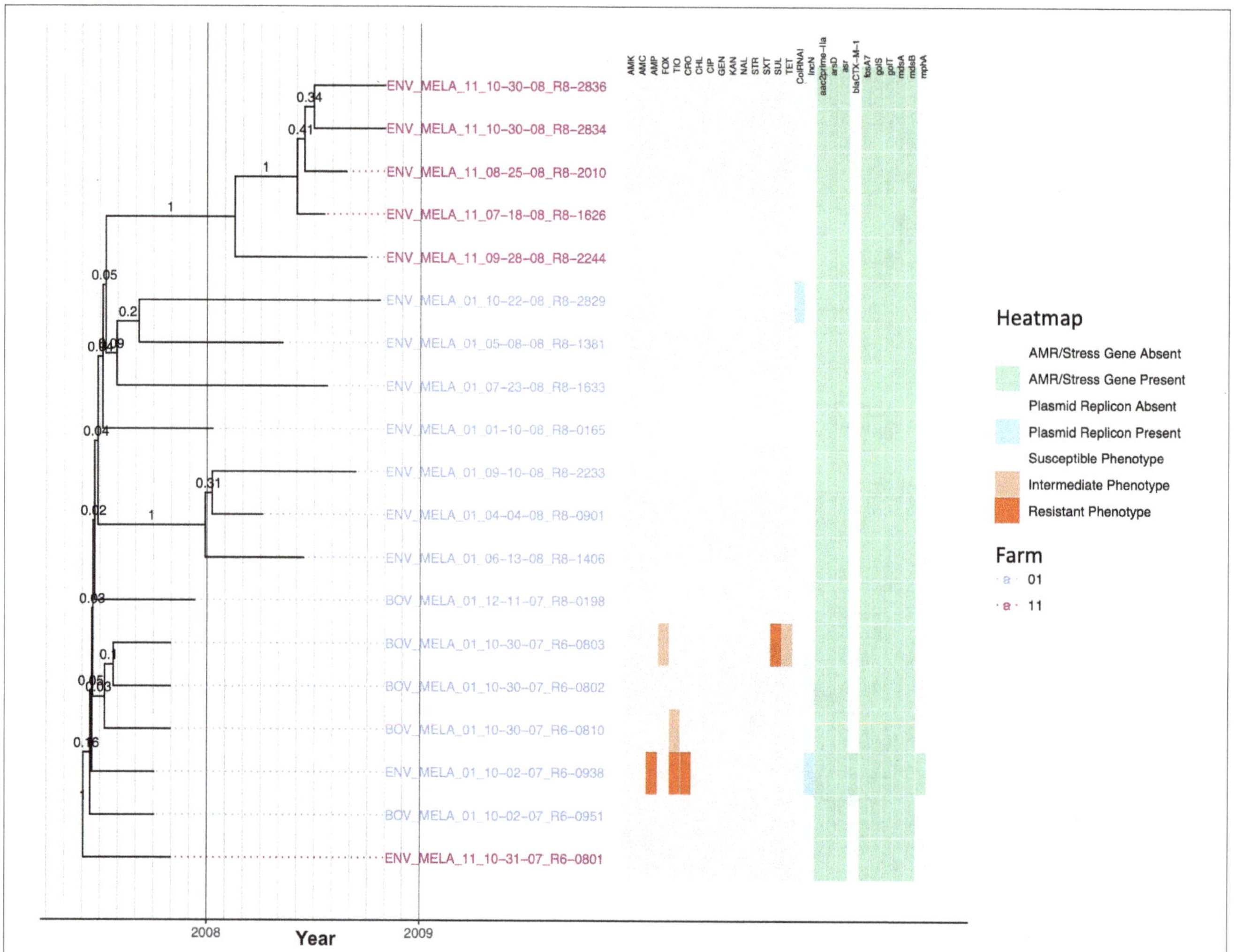

FIGURE 8 | Rooted, time-scaled maximum clade credibility (MCC) phylogeny constructed using core SNPs identified among 19 *Salmonella* Meleagridis genomes isolated from subclinical bovine sources and the surrounding bovine farm environment. Tip label colors denote the ID of the farm from which each strain was isolated. Branch labels denote posterior probabilities of branch support. Time in years is plotted along the *X*-axis, and branch lengths are reported in years. The heatmap to the right of the phylogeny denotes (i) the susceptible-intermediate-resistant (SIR) classification of each isolate for each of 15 antimicrobials (obtained using phenotypic testing and NARMS breakpoints; orange); (ii) presence and absence of plasmid replicons (detected using ABRicate/PlasmidFinder and minimum nucleotide identity and coverage thresholds of 80 and 60%, respectively; blue); (iii) presence and absence of antimicrobial resistance (AMR) and stress response genes (identified using AMRFinderPlus and default parameters; green). Core SNPs were identified using Snippy. The phylogeny was constructed using the results of ten independent runs using a strict clock model, the Standard_TPM2 nucleotide substitution model, and the Coalescent Bayesian Skyline population model implemented in BEAST version 2.5.1, with 10% burn-in applied to each run. LogCombiner-2 was used to combine BEAST 2 log files, and TreeAnnotator-2 was used to construct the phylogeny using common ancestor node heights. Abbreviations for the 15 antimicrobials are: AMK, amikacin; AMC, amoxicillin-clavulanic acid; AMP, ampicillin; FOX, cefoxitin; TIO, ceftiofur; CRO, ceftriaxone; CHL, chloramphenicol; CIP, ciprofloxacin; GEN, gentamicin; KAN, kanamycin; NAL, nalidixic acid; STR, streptomycin; SXT, sulfamethoxazole-trimethoprim; SUL, sulfisoxazole; TET, tetracycline.

floR and *APH(3′)-Ia*, respectively (**Figure 9**). The Farm 17 and Farm 62 lineages evolved from a common ancestor predicted to have existed circa November/December 2005 (node age 2005.91, CA node height 95% HPD interval 2003.77–2007.85; **Figure 9** and **Supplementary Figure 9**). All members of the Farm 17 lineage additionally harbored a ColpVC plasmid and shared a common ancestor dated to circa August/September 2007 (node age 2007.65, CA node height 95% HPD interval 2007.29–2007.85; **Figure 9** and **Supplementary Figure 9**). The Farm 62 lineage, which did not possess the ColpVC plasmid, evolved from a common ancestor circa August/September 2008 (node age 2008.68, CA node height 95% HPD interval 2008.42–2008.78; **Figure 9** and **Supplementary Figure 9**).

Unlike the *S.* Newport lineages present on Farm 17 and Farm 62, the Farm 35 *S.* Newport lineage did not possess kanamycin resistance gene *APH(3′)-Ia* and was kanamycin-susceptible (**Figure 9**). The common ancestor of the Farm 35 *S.* Newport lineage was dated circa May 2008 (node age 2008.38, CA node height 95% HPD interval 2008.06–2008.55). All but one Farm 35 *S.* Newport isolates were additionally resistant to chloramphenicol and possessed *floR*;

TABLE 3 | Summary of within-serotype evolutionary analyses[a].

Serotype	Isolates	Core SNPs (Pairwise Range)[b]	Clock/Population Model[c]	Mean/Median Tree Height in Years (95% HPD Interval)[d]	Mean/Median Evolutionary Rate in Substitutions/Site/Year (95% HPD Interval)[e]
Anatum	15	337 (0–257)	Strict/Skyline	1484.9/1837.0 (549.6–1980.1)	$1.67 \times 10^{-7}/1.48 \times 10^{-7}$ (6.92×10^{-11}–3.86×10^{-7})
Cerro	13	21 (0–12)	Strict/Skyline	2008.2/2008.4 (2007.6–2008.6)	$9.11 \times 10^{-7}/8.94 \times 10^{-7}$ (3.06×10^{-7}–1.57×10^{-6})
Kentucky	36	102 (0–30)	Relaxed/Skyline	2004.1/2005.0 (2000.8–2006.8)	$6.39 \times 10^{-7}/6.34 \times 10^{-7}$ (2.05×10^{-7}–1.07×10^{-6})
Meleagridis	19	27 (0–9)	Strict/Skyline	2007.4/2007.5 (2006.9–2007.7)	$6.88 \times 10^{-7}/6.66 \times 10^{-7}$ (2.90×10^{-7}–1.12×10^{-6})
Newport	16	52 (0–38)	Relaxed/Skyline	2004.2/2004.6 (2000.4–2007.8)	$9.02 \times 10^{-7}/8.22 \times 10^{-7}$ (2.64×10^{-7}–1.65×10^{-6})
Typhimurium (Copenhagen)	27	732 (0–634)	Relaxed/Skyline	1936.0/1943.0 (1864.7–1991.4)	$1.07 \times 10^{-6}/9.66 \times 10^{-7}$ (2.84×10^{-7}–2.05×10^{-6})

[a]*See* ***Supplementary Table 5*** *for an extended version of this table; note that evolutionary rates may be higher than previously reported estimates for Salmonella populations isolated over a longer time frame, due to the small sample sizes and short temporal period characterized here (Moller et al., 2018).*
[b]*Number of core SNPs identified among all genomes within the serotype after removing recombination with Gubbins; the range of pairwise SNP differences between isolates was calculated using the dist.gene function in the ape package in R.*
[c]*The optimal model selected for the data set; can be a combination of a strict or lognormal relaxed molecular clock ("Strict" or "Relaxed," respectively) and a Constant Coalescent or Coalescent Bayesian Skyline population model ("CC" or "Skyline," respectively); see* ***Supplementary Table 5*** *for more details.*
[d]*The tree height parameter and its respective 95% highest posterior density (HPD) interval reported by Tracer.*
[e]*Corresponds to the clock Rate and rate.mean parameters estimated by BEAST2 for models using strict and lognormal relaxed molecular clock models, respectively, as reported by Tracer.*

BOV_NEWP_35_10-02-08_R8-2688 did not possess *floR* and was chloramphenicol-susceptible (**Figure 9**).

Each of Four Major Lineages Composed of *Salmonella* Typhimurium and Its O5-Copenhagen Variant Is Associated With One of Three New York State Dairy Farms

Twenty-seven bovine and farm environmental *S.* Typhimurium and *S.* Typhimurium Copenhagen isolates that encompassed five PFGE types (**Supplementary Table 1**) were isolated from three dairy farms (1, 10, and 16 strains isolated from Farm 17, 22, and 25, respectively). All isolates queried here shared a common ancestor that existed circa 1936 (node age 1935.62, CA node height 95% HPD interval 1864.84–1991.86; **Figure 10**, **Table 3**, **Supplementary Figure 10**, and **Supplementary Table 5**). Notably, the *S.* Typhimurium Copenhagen variant was polyphyletic (**Figure 10**), regardless of whether traditional or *in silico* (i.e., SeqSero2) methods had been used for serotype variant assignment. Additionally, the *S.* Typhimurium/*S.* Typhimurium Copenhagen isolates sequenced here showcased the most diverse AMR phenotypic profiles and AMR gene presence/absence profiles (**Figures 4, 10**).

Isolates from Farm 25 were partitioned into two clades: one containing *S.* Typhimurium isolates, and one containing *S.* Typhimurium Copenhagen isolates (based on SeqSero2's *in silico* serotype assignments; **Figure 10**). Farm 25 isolates assigned to the *S.* Typhimurium Copenhagen variant (i) shared a common ancestor that existed circa December 2007/January 2008 (node age 2007.99, CA node height 95% HPD interval 2007.68–2008.21); (ii) were all resistant to ampicillin, kanamycin, streptomycin, sulfisoxazole, and tetracycline, with reduced susceptibility to additional antimicrobials observed sporadically; (iii) all possessed replicons for IncA/C2, IncFIB(AP001918), and IncFII(s) plasmids; and (iv) all possessed streptomycin resistance genes *aadA12*, *APH(3'')-Ib* and *APH(6)-Id* (i.e., *strAB*), beta-lactamase bla_{TEM-1}, and antiseptic resistance gene *qacE* delta 1, with other AMR/stress response genes present sporadically (**Figure 10** and **Supplementary Figure 10**). Farm 25 isolates assigned to the *S.* Typhimurium clade shared a common ancestor that existed circa July 2007 (node age 2007.55, CA node height 95% HPD interval 2007.18–2007.78; **Figure 10** and **Supplementary Figure 10**). All Farm 25 *S.* Typhimurium isolates were resistant to cefoxitin; resistance to additional antimicrobials, along with presence of IncI1 plasmids and bla_{CMY-2}, was observed sporadically (**Figure 10**).

The isolate from Farm 17 was predicted to belong to the *S.* Typhimurium Copenhagen serotype variant using SeqSero2 and shared a common ancestor with the *S.* Typhimurium isolates from Farm 22, which existed circa 2000 (node age 1999.92, CA node height 95% HPD interval 1991.72–2006.21; **Figure 10** and **Supplementary Figure 10**). Of the ten *S.* Typhimurium strains from Farm 22, seven were pan-susceptible (**Figure 10**). A bovine strain (BOV_TYPH_22_03–14–08_R8–0865) was resistant to ampicillin, ceftiofur, and ceftriaxone and was found to harbor IncI1 and IncI2 plasmids, as well as beta-lactamase $bla_{CTX-M-55}$ (**Figure 10**). The remaining two bovine isolates were intermediately resistant to chloramphenicol and additionally resistant to either (i) amoxicillin-clavulanic acid, ampicillin, and sulfisoxazole, or (ii) tetracycline (**Figure 10**). Overall, isolates from Farm 17 and Farm 22 shared a common ancestor with the Farm 25 *S.* Typhimurium clade that existed circa 1988 (node age 1988.02, CA node height 95%

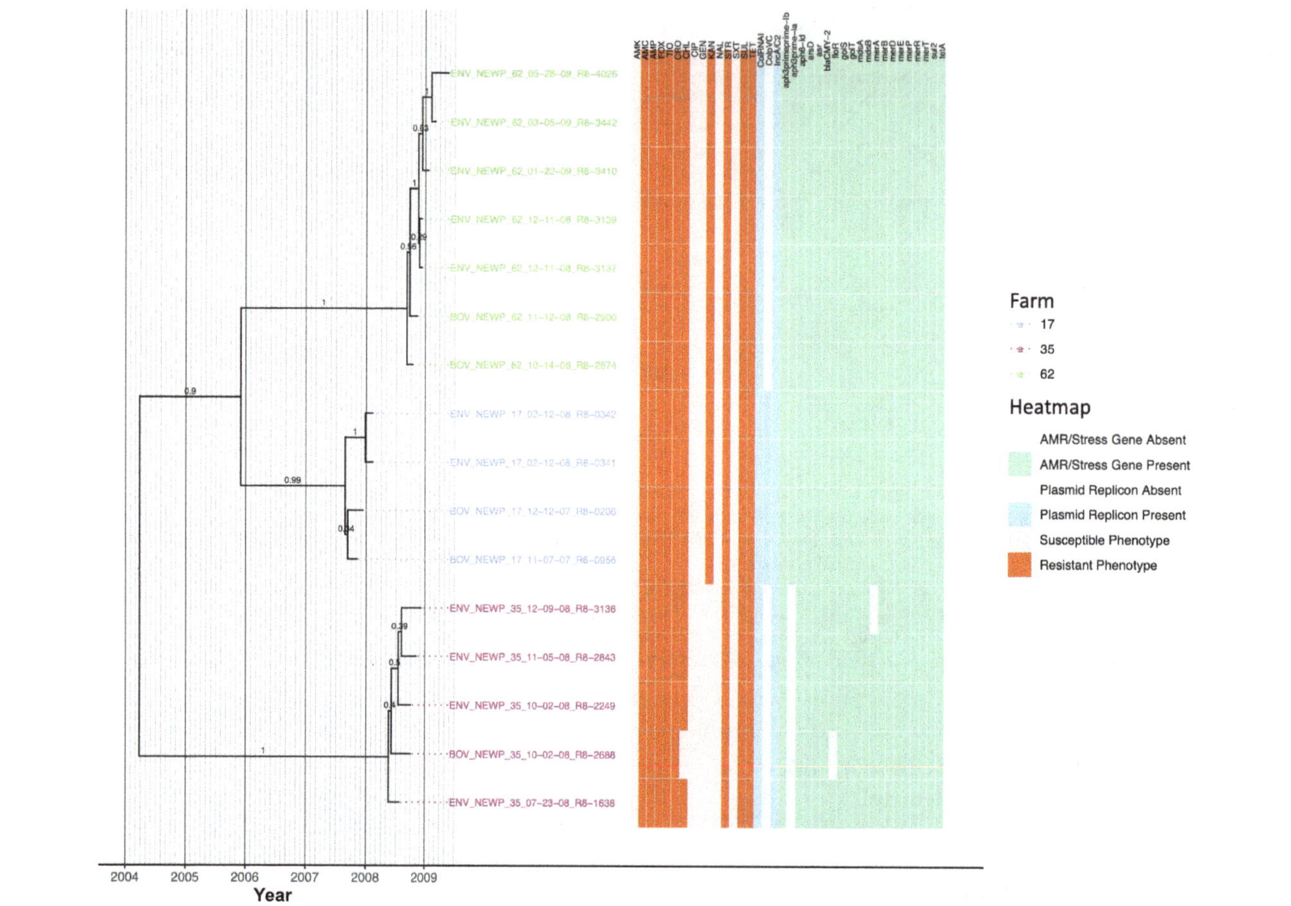

FIGURE 9 | Rooted, time-scaled maximum clade credibility (MCC) phylogeny constructed using core SNPs identified among 16 *Salmonella* Newport genomes isolated from subclinical bovine sources and the surrounding bovine farm environment. Tip label colors denote the ID of the farm from which each strain was isolated. Branch labels denote posterior probabilities of branch support. Time in years is plotted along the *X*-axis, and branch lengths are reported in years. The heatmap to the right of the phylogeny denotes (i) the susceptible-intermediate-resistant (SIR) classification of each isolate for each of 15 antimicrobials (obtained using phenotypic testing and NARMS breakpoints; orange); (ii) presence and absence of plasmid replicons (detected using ABRicate/PlasmidFinder and minimum nucleotide identity and coverage thresholds of 80 and 60%, respectively; blue); (iii) presence and absence of antimicrobial resistance (AMR) and stress response genes (identified using AMRFinderPlus and default parameters; green). Core SNPs were identified using Snippy. The phylogeny was constructed using the results of ten independent runs using a relaxed lognormal clock model, the Standard_TPM1 nucleotide substitution model, and the Coalescent Bayesian Skyline population model implemented in BEAST version 2.5.1, with 10% burn-in applied to each run. LogCombiner-2 was used to combine BEAST 2 log files, and TreeAnnotator-2 was used to construct the phylogeny using common ancestor node heights. Abbreviations for the 15 antimicrobials are: AMK, amikacin; AMC, amoxicillin-clavulanic acid; AMP, ampicillin; FOX, cefoxitin; TIO, ceftiofur; CRO, ceftriaxone; CHL, chloramphenicol; CIP, ciprofloxacin; GEN, gentamicin; KAN, kanamycin; NAL, nalidixic acid; STR, streptomycin; SXT, sulfamethoxazole-trimethoprim; SUL, sulfisoxazole; TET, tetracycline.

HPD interval 1969.24–2002.47; **Figure 10** and **Supplementary Figure 10**).

DISCUSSION

Whole-Genome Sequencing Can Be Used to Monitor Pathogen Microevolution and Temporal Antimicrobial Resistance Dynamics in Animal Reservoirs

Cattle may act as a reservoir for *Salmonella* and may facilitate its transmission to other animals (Mentaberre et al., 2013; Wiethoelter et al., 2015) or humans, either through direct contact or via the food supply chain (Hoelzer et al., 2011; Cummings et al., 2012; Mughini-Gras et al., 2014; An et al., 2017; Gutema et al., 2019). Even outside of a bovine host, *Salmonella* can survive in the farm environment for a prolonged amount of time, making persistent strains a particularly relevant threat to animal and human health (Rodriguez et al., 2006; Cummings et al., 2010b; Gorski et al., 2011; Toth et al., 2011; Tassinari et al., 2019). This threat can be compounded when persistent strains are exposed to antimicrobials, as a number of studies have linked antimicrobial exposure to the emergence of AMR in different foodborne pathogens, including *Salmonella*, *Escherichia coli*, and *Campylobacter* (Boerlin et al., 2001; McDermott et al., 2002; Delsol et al., 2003; Dutil et al., 2010; Hoelzer et al., 2017).

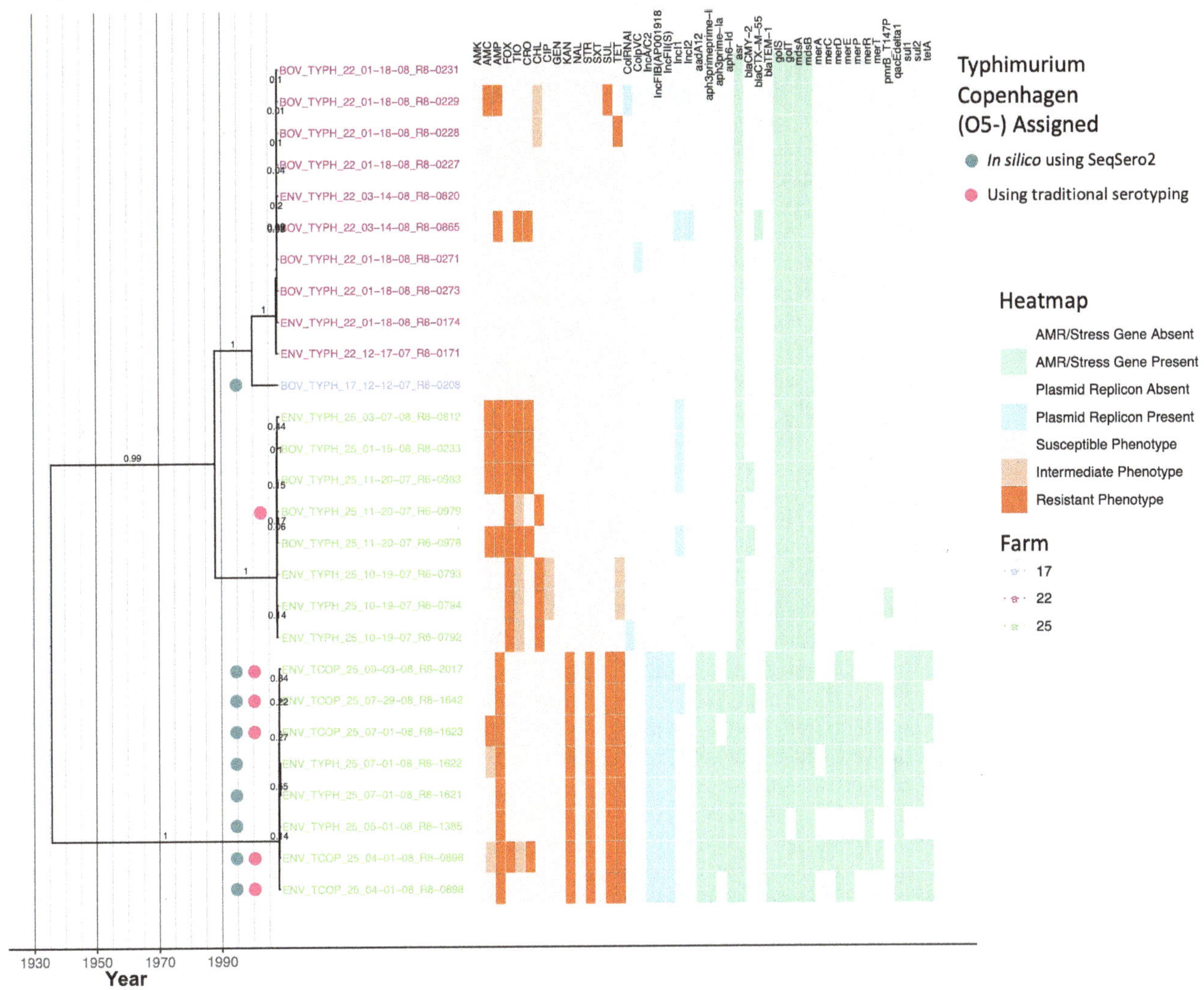

FIGURE 10 | Rooted, time-scaled maximum clade credibility (MCC) phylogeny constructed using core SNPs identified among 27 *Salmonella* Typhimurium and Typhimurium Copenhagen genomes isolated from subclinical bovine sources and the surrounding bovine farm environment. Tip label colors denote the ID of the farm from which each strain was isolated. Circles to the left of tip labels denote isolates that were assigned to the Typhimurium Copenhagen variant of *S.* Typhimurium using SeqSero2 (teal) and/or traditional serotyping (pink). Branch labels denote posterior probabilities of branch support. Time in years is plotted along the *X*-axis, and branch lengths are reported in years. The heatmap to the right of the phylogeny denotes (i) the susceptible-intermediate-resistant (SIR) classification of each isolate for each of 15 antimicrobials (obtained using phenotypic testing and NARMS breakpoints; orange); (ii) presence and absence of plasmid replicons (detected using ABRicate/PlasmidFinder and minimum nucleotide identity and coverage thresholds of 80 and 60%, respectively; blue); (iii) presence and absence of antimicrobial resistance (AMR) and stress response genes (identified using AMRFinderPlus and default parameters; green). Core SNPs were identified using Snippy. The phylogeny was constructed using the results of ten independent runs using a relaxed lognormal clock model, the Standard_TPM1 nucleotide substitution model, and the Coalescent Bayesian Skyline population model implemented in BEAST version 2.5.1, with 10% burn-in applied to each run. LogCombiner-2 was used to combine BEAST 2 log files, and TreeAnnotator-2 was used to construct the phylogeny using common ancestor node heights. Abbreviations for the 15 antimicrobials are: AMK, amikacin; AMC, amoxicillin-clavulanic acid; AMP, ampicillin; FOX, cefoxitin; TIO, ceftiofur; CRO, ceftriaxone; CHL, chloramphenicol; CIP, ciprofloxacin; GEN, gentamicin; KAN, kanamycin; NAL, nalidixic acid; STR, streptomycin; SXT, sulfamethoxazole-trimethoprim; SUL, sulfisoxazole; TET, tetracycline.

However, AMR acquisition among pathogens in livestock environments is far from absolute; in the absence of selective pressures (e.g., antimicrobial exposure), some AMR traits may be associated with a fitness cost for a given organism (Melnyk et al., 2015; Hoelzer et al., 2017; San Millan and MacLean, 2017). Consequently, interventions or changes in farm management practices (e.g., limiting antimicrobial use for all or selected antimicrobials, targeted use of some antimicrobials) may lead to reduced selection of AMR bacteria (Aarestrup, 2015; Tang et al., 2017; Scott et al., 2018). As such, the dynamics of AMR acquisition and loss among livestock-associated bacterial pathogens are complex and influenced by a wide range of factors, including the antimicrobials and treatment regimens used, farm management practices, environmental conditions, and the biology of the pathogens themselves (Aarestrup, 2015;

Hoelzer et al., 2017; Davidson et al., 2018; Pereira et al., 2019; Clarke et al., 2020).

Using a WGS-based approach applied to serially sampled *Salmonella* strains isolated over a short time frame (i.e., less than 2 years), the study detailed here reveals that sporadic acquisition and loss of acquired AMR genes can occur within closely related populations over a short timescale. One particularly notable observation is represented by multiple, independent acquisitions of the beta-lactamase bla_{CMY} among *S.* Typhimurium and *S.* Typhimurium Copenhagen, as all bla_{CMY} acquisition events within this serotype group were confined to the 2000s. bla_{CMY} can confer resistance to cephalosporins, including (i) ceftriaxone, which has been used in human medicine since the early 1980s, and is used to treat invasive salmonellosis cases when fluoroquinolones cannot be used (e.g., for pediatric salmonellosis cases), and (ii) ceftiofur, which has been used in veterinary settings since the late 1980s to treat disease cases among dairy cattle and other animals (Hornish and Kotarski, 2002; Alcaine et al., 2005; Liebana et al., 2013; Yang et al., 2016; Carroll et al., 2017b, 2020a). Because bla_{CMY} often confers resistance to both ceftriaxone and ceftiofur, there has been concern that the use of ceftiofur in livestock can contribute to the dissemination of bla_{CMY} and thus yield bacterial populations that are co-resistant to ceftriaxone (Alcaine et al., 2005; Tragesser et al., 2006; Carroll et al., 2017b, 2020a).

Two independent bla_{CTX-M} acquisition events among *S.* Meleagridis and *S.* Typhimurium were additionally observed. bla_{CTX-M}, which also confers resistance to cephalosporins, was rarely detected in the United States in the 1990s (Lewis et al., 2007; Canton et al., 2012). However, bla_{CTX-M} rapidly increased in prevalence in the United States between 2000 and 2005 (Lewis et al., 2007; Canton et al., 2012), and there is evidence that bacterial populations associated with dairy cattle may have been affected as well. In a study of *E. coli* isolated from dairy cattle in the western United States, the prevalence of bla_{CTX-M} was found to have increased between 2008 and 2012 (Afema et al., 2018). The results of our study are congruent with these findings, as all observed bla_{CTX-M} acquisition events were estimated to have occurred in the 2000s.

Antimicrobial resistance loss events were additionally observed among the bovine-associated, MDR *S.* Newport isolates sequenced here. Prevalence of MDR *S.* Newport among humans increased rapidly in the United States within the late 1990s and early 2000s and was linked to cattle exposure, farm/petting zoo exposure, unpasteurized milk consumption, and ground beef consumption (Spika et al., 1987; Gupta et al., 2003; Karon et al., 2007). While chloramphenicol resistance is often a hallmark characteristic of MDR *S.* Newport, the MDR *S.* Newport lineage represented by an isolate in this study was chloramphenicol-susceptible and was predicted to have lost chloramphenicol resistance gene *floR* after 2008. These results indicate that even well-established MDR pathogens can still be subjected to temporal changes in AMR profile.

Due to the global burden that AMR pathogens impose on the health of humans and animals, numerous agencies have called for improved monitoring of pathogens and their associated AMR determinants along the food supply chain (World Health Organization, 2014, 2017; Centers for Disease Control and Prevention, 2019). The study detailed here showcases how WGS can be used to identify temporal changes in the resistomes of livestock-associated pathogens at the farm level. However, further sequencing efforts querying (i) a larger selection of *Salmonella* strains isolated from livestock on individual farms (ii) over a longer timeframe are needed to determine whether the AMR dynamics observed here are merely sporadic, or rather are indications of larger trends.

Bovine-Associated *Salmonella* Lineages With Heterogeneous Antimicrobial Resistance Profiles May Be Present Across Multiple Farms or Strongly Farm-Associated

Geography has been shown to play an important role in shaping bacterial populations (Achtman, 2008; Strachan et al., 2015), including some *Salmonella* lineages (Carroll et al., 2017b; Palma et al., 2018; Fenske et al., 2019; Liao et al., 2020). However, for some foodborne pathogens, including some *Salmonella* populations, global spread of lineages due to human migration and movement of food and animals can often obfuscate local phylogeographic signals (Wong et al., 2015; Llarena et al., 2016; The et al., 2016; Palma et al., 2018).

In the study detailed here, *Salmonella* lineages isolated from cattle and their associated environments on 13 separate farms in a confined geographic location (i.e., New York State) were found to vary in terms of the farm-specific signal they possessed; some lineages (i.e., *S.* Anatum, *S.* Newport, *S.* Typhimurium, *S.* Typhimurium Copenhagen, some *S.* Kentucky populations) were found to be strongly associated with a particular farm, while other lineages (i.e., *S.* Cerro, *S.* Meleagridis, some *S.* Kentucky populations) were distributed across multiple farms. Multiple scenarios may explain the existence of *Salmonella* lineages distributed across multiple farms, including movement of livestock, humans, pets, and/or wildlife (Skov et al., 2008; Hoelzer et al., 2011; Palma et al., 2018) or introduction via feed; however, additional metadata (e.g., farm geography, proximity to other farms in the study, and management practices) are needed to draw further conclusions. Even with limited metadata available, WGS data can provide important insights into *Salmonella* transmission and introduction on farms, as shown in this study. For example, for one farm (i.e., Farm 25), two *Salmonella* Typhimurium clonal groups were present (i.e., one representing Typhimurium and one representing Typhimurium Copenhagen), each of which shared a common ancestor dated circa 2007. WGS data can be used to identify time frames in which *Salmonella* lineages may have emerged in a given farm or region, which could help pinpoint root causes (e.g., changes in management practices that occurred around the predicted time of emergence).

While the characterization of additional, larger strain sets from more geographically diverse farms is essential, our data suggest that specific *Salmonella* clones may persist on a given farm. This suggests that WGS databases covering isolates from a large number of farms could be used to develop initial hypotheses about farm sources of *Salmonella* strains. While such applications are tempting, it is crucial that these types of data are only used for initial hypothesis generation; rigorous, critical epidemiological investigations are essential before any conclusions regarding strain source are drawn.

In silico Serotyping of Bovine-Associated *Salmonella* Can Outperform Traditional Serotyping

Well into the genomic era, serotyping remains a vital microbiological assay that allows *Salmonella* isolates to be classified into meaningful, evolutionary units. Serotype assignments are used to facilitate outbreak investigations and surveillance efforts, construct salmonellosis risk assessment frameworks, and inform food safety and public health policy and decision-making efforts (Yoshida et al., 2016; Gutema et al., 2019). Importantly, serotyping is used worldwide to monitor salmonellosis cases among humans and animals, including cattle (Gutema et al., 2019; Centers for Disease Control and Prevention, 2020).

In this study, serotypes assigned using traditional phenotypic methods were compared to serotypes assigned using two *in silico* methods (i.e., SISTR and SeqSero2). Notably, both *in silico* serotyping approaches outperformed traditional *Salmonella* serotyping for this data set. Serotypes assigned using SISTR's cgMLST approach and/or SeqSero2 were congruent with the *Salmonella* whole-genome phylogeny and were able to resolve all un-typable, ambiguous, and incorrectly assigned serotypes (**Supplementary Table 1**). It is essential to note that the data set queried here is far too small and, thus, inadequate to formally benchmark these tools. Furthermore, all serotypes studied here were among the ten most frequently reported serotypes of *Salmonella* isolated from subclinical cattle between 2000 and 2017 (Gutema et al., 2019), indicating that they are well-represented in public databases and thus likely do not pose a significant challenge to *in silico* tools. However, the results observed here reflect observations made in several recent studies, which queried greater numbers of isolate genomes and/or a wider array of diverse *Salmonella* serotypes (Yachison et al., 2017; Ibrahim and Morin, 2018; Diep et al., 2019; Banerji et al., 2020; Uelze et al., 2020). In their analysis of 1,624 animal- and food-associated (i.e., non-human) *Salmonella* isolate genomes assigned to 72 serotypes, Uelze et al. (2020) reported that SISTR and SeqSero2 achieved the highest and second-highest accuracy of all tested *in silico Salmonella* serotype assignment tools, correctly serotyping 94 and 87% of isolates, respectively. However, unlike the results observed here, the authors note that neither tool outperformed traditional serotyping conducted by *Salmonella* reference laboratories. Similarly, in a study of 813 *Salmonella* isolates, SISTR outperformed the original version of SeqSero (i.e., SeqSero 1.0) with serotype prediction accuracies of 94.8 and 88.2%, respectively (Yachison et al., 2017).

With WGS data in hand, *in silico* serotyping is rapid, scalable, inexpensive, and reproducible (Uelze et al., 2020). Nevertheless, it is important to be mindful of the strengths and weaknesses of different *in silico* serotyping tools. In their benchmarking study, Uelze et al. (2020) recommended SISTR as the optimal contemporary tool for routine *in silico Salmonella* serotyping based on overall accuracy; however, they additionally report that the raw read mapping approach implemented in SeqSero2 (i.e., "allele mode") outperforms SISTR for prediction of monophasic variants. Banerji et al. (2020) did not assess the performance of SISTR on their data set, as it requires assembled genomes and not raw reads (another potential drawback if a high-quality assembly is not available or obtainable for an isolate of interest); however, they found that both SeqSero and MLST approaches misidentified monophasic variants, particularly among the important monophasic S. Typhimurium lineage. Among the bovine-associated *Salmonella* strains sequenced here, a combination of S. Typhimurium strains that possessed the O5 epitope, and those that did not (i.e., S. Typhimurium Copenhagen) was observed. Importantly, SISTR was unable to differentiate S. Typhimurium from S. Typhimurium Copenhagen, while SeqSero2 could, as reported previously (Ibrahim and Morin, 2018; Zhang et al., 2019). While the differentiation of S. Typhimurium from its O5- counterpart may not be essential for all microbiological applications, it is important to be aware of this limitation; S. Typhimurium Copenhagen has been responsible for outbreaks and illnesses around the world (Luceron et al., 2017; Tack et al., 2020) and can be multidrug-resistant, as demonstrated here and elsewhere (Frech et al., 2003; Tack et al., 2020).

While serotypes assigned *in silico* using SISTR and SeqSero2 are highly accurate and congruent, each tool has strengths and limitations; as such, an approach that utilizes both methods, such as the one employed here, may increase accuracy and minimize potential misclassifications. Results from other studies support this (Yachison et al., 2017; Banerji et al., 2020). For example, in an analysis of 520 primarily human-associated *Salmonella* isolate genomes, Banerji et al. (2020) found that serotypes assigned *in silico* using SeqSero showed 98% concordance with traditional serotyping and outperformed serotype assignment using seven-gene MLST. However, when SeqSero and seven-gene MLST were used in combination, *in silico* serotyping accuracy surpassed 99%, consistent with our results that a combination of SeqSero2 and cgMLST-based serotyping (as implemented in SISTR) improved *in silico* serotyping accuracy. Overall, the results provided here lend further support to the idea that *in silico* serotyping may eventually replace traditional serotyping as WGS becomes more widely used and accessible (Yachison et al., 2017; Banerji et al., 2020; Uelze et al., 2020).

Limitations of the *in silico* Antimicrobial Resistance Method Evaluation Presented Here, and Considerations for Future Antimicrobial Resistance Monitoring Efforts Among Livestock and Beyond

In addition to studying the microevolution and AMR dynamics of bovine *Salmonella* on a genomic scale, the study presented here compared results obtained from numerous *in silico* AMR characterization pipelines that attempt to replicate traditional microbiological assays used to characterize AMR *Salmonella*. More specifically, each of the following tools was applied to the set of 128 bovine-associated *Salmonella* genomes sequenced here: (i) combinations of five *in silico* AMR determinant detection pipelines (i.e., ABRicate, AMRFinderPlus, ARIBA, BTyper, and SRST2) and one to five AMR determinant databases (i.e., ARG-ANNOT, CARD, MEGARes, NCBI, and ResFinder); and (ii) an *in silico* MIC prediction tool (i.e., PATRIC3).

Here, all AMR determinant detection pipelines and AMR determinant databases showed an extremely high degree of concordance; regardless of pipeline or database selection, all tools performed nearly identically on an SIR-prediction task relative to (i) "true" SIR classifications based on NARMS breakpoints and "true" MIC values obtained for a panel of 15 antimicrobials, and (ii) each other. A previous, small-scale (n = 111) WGS-based study of AMR *Salmonella* observed similarly high rates of concordance among several *in silico* AMR determinant detection tools (Cooper et al., 2020). However, in addition to its small sample size, this study also relied on *Salmonella* strains isolated from a single source (broiler chickens) in a single country (Canada) over an extremely short temporal range (December 2012–2013). Similarly, the study detailed here is not a formal benchmarking study, and it is essential that its numerous limitations are pointed out.

First and foremost, the study conducted here relied on WGS data from an extremely small sample of *Salmonella* isolates (n = 128) from a single source (dairy cattle and their surrounding farm environments) in a confined geographic area (New York State, United States) isolated over a short temporal range (fewer than 2 years). While all isolates were "unique" (i.e., each strain was isolated from a separate sampling event of a unique source), many isolates were highly similar at both the genomic and pan-genomic level (e.g., *S.* Cerro, *S.* Meleagridis), indicating that, in some cases, the same lineage was being sampled repeatedly over time. Consequently, this relatively miniscule sample is unrepresentative of AMR pathogens and, more specifically, *Salmonella* as a whole; readers should not infer the general superiority or inferiority of any AMR detection tool or database tested, and the results obtained here should not be extrapolated to external data sets.

Secondly, the data set queried here was heavily biased toward susceptible isolates. More than half of all isolates were pan-susceptible to the 15 antimicrobials included on the panel, and only 21 unique phenotypic SIR profiles were observed. Congruent with this, relatively little diversity was observed in terms of AMR gene profile (e.g., the AMRFinderPlus pipeline produced 20 unique AMR/stress response determinant presence/absence profiles among the 128 isolates sequenced here). This is not particularly surprising; numerous studies have shown that the resistomes of bovine-associated *Salmonella* tend to be less diverse than *Salmonella* isolated from humans (Afema et al., 2015; Carroll et al., 2017b), as well as some other animals (Mellor et al., 2019). Furthermore, the resistomes of *Salmonella* isolated from subclinical cattle, such as the isolates queried in this study, have been shown to be less diverse than the resistomes of *Salmonella* isolated from cattle showing clinical signs of disease (Afema et al., 2015).

The relative homogeneity of the subclinical *Salmonella* bovine resistome and bias toward antimicrobial-susceptible isolates have important implications for the AMR pipeline/database comparison conducted here. For this data set, stringent and conservative approaches are rewarded, as isolates that do not possess AMR determinants are more likely to be predicted to be susceptible. While it is possible that different AMR detection tools may perform better on WGS data from pathogens with more diverse resistomes, very few formal benchmarking studies of *in silico* AMR determinant detection tools currently exist (Hendriksen et al., 2019). The choice of AMR determinant database in combination with the choice of pipeline, on the other hand, can clearly affect AMR determinant identification in a critical way. For example, the ARG-ANNOT database (Gupta et al., 2014), a manually curated AMR determinant database first published in 2014, is not updated as frequently as other AMR databases (e.g., CARD, NCBI, and ResFinder). Since it was last updated in May 2018 (accessed May 25, 2020), at the time of our study, the database does not yet include three novel plasmid-mediated genes (*mcr-8*, *-9*, and *-10*) that can confer resistance to colistin, a last-resort antibiotic used to treat MDR and extensively drug resistant infections (Wang et al., 2018, 2020; Carroll et al., 2019). Similarly, versions of tools that rely on even older versions of this database would not be able to detect all members of the continuously growing repertoire of *mcr* genes. For the low-diversity subclinical bovine *Salmonella* resistomes queried here, the use of a smaller database was inconsequential, as reflected in the high congruency of all methods and databases observed here. For some studies, a manually curated database of AMR genes that is updated conservatively may possibly even be desirable, as such a database may yield less noise and improve interpretability and reproducibility. However, for pathogens with more diverse resistomes (e.g., human clinical isolates, isolates from geographic regions with different antibiotic use practices), the omission of critically important genes could be a disastrous flaw. Similar to our results, a large study (n = 6,242) querying NARMS isolates belonging primarily to the *S. enterica* species (n = 5,425) observed a high degree of concordance between NCBI's AMRFinder tool and ResFinder (this study was used to validate AMRFinder and the NCBI AMR determinant database) (Feldgarden et al., 2019). However, when differences between tools were observed, the vast majority (81%) were attributed to differences in database composition (Feldgarden et al., 2019; Hendriksen et al., 2019).

Thirdly, the small sample size (n = 128) and sparsity of AMR isolates available in this study limited the methods that could be used to formulate the AMR tool/database comparison. The approach used here was similar to the one used to validate the AMRFinder tool (Feldgarden et al., 2019) in that it relied on known AMR-determinant/AMR phenotype associations available in the literature (see Supplementary Table 4 of Feldgarden et al.) (Feldgarden et al., 2019). As such, the approach used here does not account for previously unobserved genotype/phenotype associations. Furthermore, different variants of the same AMR gene may yield different AMR phenotypes; for example, some variants of the OXA beta-lactamases are able to confer resistance to cephalosporins, while others are not (Evans and Amyes, 2014). All AMR determinant detection pipelines tested here produced nearly identical genes calls among the 128 isolates sequenced here, and all detected AMR determinants were manually annotated in a consistent fashion; while the overall accuracy of all pipeline/database combinations tested here could likely be optimized if more accurate, data set-specific AMR genotype/phenotype associations could be derived, congruency among tools/databases would likely remain high.

Classifying bacterial pathogens into discrete SIR groups using AMR determinant detection methods is challenging, as it requires users to have a great degree of prior knowledge regarding the AMR determinants that are detected, the antimicrobials of interest, and the pathogen being studied. PATRIC3's MIC prediction tool (Nguyen et al., 2019) offers a promising departure from this framework, as it allows for the prediction of MIC values directly from WGS data. Interpreting the resulting *in silico* MIC values does not require any prior knowledge on the user end, and results can be harmoniously integrated into the SIR framework using clinical breakpoints. Among the *Salmonella* isolates sequenced here, SIR classification using PATRIC3 resulted in an overall accuracy of 93%. However, all of the limitations of this study described above for AMR determinant detection (e.g., small sample size, AMR sparsity bias, single-source, single geographic region, small temporal range) apply to *in silico* MIC prediction as well; for example, when "intermediate" resistance predictions produced via PATRIC3 are re-classified as "susceptible" (as was done for the AMR determinant detection approaches used here), PATRIC3's accuracy for this data set increases to 96.0% and is on par with all other AMR prediction methods tested here. Readers should thus interpret comparisons among these methods with caution.

Benchmarking and validating AMR detection and prediction tools is notoriously challenging (Feldgarden et al., 2019), and very few researchers have undertaken this task (Hendriksen et al., 2019). While high congruency may be observed among tools (Clausen et al., 2016), identification of a clear "optimal" method for *in silico* AMR characterization has remained elusive, as the few available benchmarking studies differ in terms of the tools tested, the AMR database(s) used, and the data set(s) chosen for benchmarking. Furthermore, the underlying WGS data can affect pipeline performance (Clausen et al., 2016; Feldgarden et al., 2019). For example, assembly quality has been shown to influence AMR determinant detection for methods that rely on assembled genomes (Clausen et al., 2016; Hendriksen et al., 2018, 2019). Thus, whether a read- or assembly-based method performs optimally can depend on a given data set (e.g., sequencing quality, the organism being studied). Another criticism of BLAST-based AMR gene detection methods among assembled genomes has been the choice of thresholds used for considering AMR determinants present or absent (Hendriksen et al., 2019). Here, no significant differences were observed between the accuracy of read-based ARIBA and SRST2 and assembly-based ABRicate, AMRFinderPlus, and BTyper. Additionally, for BLAST-based methods, a relatively wide range of optimal nucleotide identity and coverage values were found to maximize accuracy, with thresholds of 75% identity and 50–60% coverage adequate for most pipeline/database combinations. Overall, when selecting an *in silico* AMR characterization method, researchers should take into account not only practical considerations (e.g., whether reads or assembled genomes are available, the quality of reads and/or assembled genomes), but also the biology of the pathogen being studied (e.g., by querying organism-specific, AMR-conferring point mutations). To assess the robustness of *in silico* AMR predictions, researchers may additionally consider employing multiple *in silico* AMR characterization tools and/or databases in combination, as well as testing various AMR gene detection thresholds.

Finally, it is essential to note that accuracy estimates for *in silico* AMR characterization tools relative to gold-standard phenotypic methods are only as reliable as the phenotypic data they rely on. Previous studies of *Salmonella* that attempted to predict phenotypic AMR using *in silico* methods (McDermott et al., 2016; Cooper et al., 2020) have reported accuracy values between 98 and 100%. For this data set, the highest accuracy achieved was 97.4% (for SRST2/ARG-ANNOT). However, sensitivity (i.e., the ability of an *in silico* pipeline/database combination to correctly classify an isolate as phenotypically resistant to an antimicrobial) was lower for this study (71.8–84.4%) than sensitivity estimates calculated in a study of MDR *Salmonella* that included bovine isolates from New York State (97.2%) (Carroll et al., 2017b). As mentioned above, this could be due to the sparsity of AMR among isolates in this data set (i.e., predicting susceptible, rather than resistant phenotypes, is incentivized here). However, it is important to note that the AMR phenotypes of several isolates were highly incongruent with their respective AMR genotypes, regardless of the tool/database used for *in silico* AMR prediction. For example, one *S.* Cerro isolate (BOV_CERO_35_10-02-08_R8-2685) was reported to be phenotypically resistant to nine antimicrobials but did not possess any acquired AMR determinants known to produce this phenotypic AMR profile. A recent case study in which WGS and phenotypic methods were used to characterize *Salmonella* isolates from raw chicken identified numerous AMR genotype/phenotype discrepancies resulting in both false negative and false positive predictions for *in silico* methods (Zwe et al., 2020). In this case study, the authors attributed these discrepancies to heteroresistant *Salmonella* subpopulations (i.e., a subpopulation of bacteria that exhibits a range of susceptibility to a particular antimicrobial). The possibility that several heteroresistant *Salmonella* populations were characterized here cannot be discounted, as isolates underwent phenotypic AMR characterization and WGS separately (i.e., years apart). Other biological phenomena, such as plasmid loss during storage or culturing, or unknown/undetected resistance genes or mutations, could also contribute to discrepancies (Hendriksen et al., 2018). However, it is also possible that one or more incongruent isolates was mislabeled and/or mishandled during AMR phenotyping, genomic DNA extraction, and/or WGS. While removal of these isolates from the data set would increase overall prediction accuracy, the high congruency among AMR genotyping methods would be unaffected.

AUTHOR CONTRIBUTIONS

LC designed and carried out all computational analyses. AB, AG, JS, KC, and RC collected, analyzed, and/or interpreted all microbiological data. LC and MW conceived the study and co-wrote the manuscript with input from all authors. All authors contributed to the article and approved the submitted version.

FUNDING

This material is based on work supported by the National Science Foundation Graduate Research Fellowship Program under grant No. DGE-1650441. This project was supported in part by the Cornell University Zoonoses Research Units of the Food and Waterborne Diseases Integrated Research Network, funded by the National Institute of Allergy and Infectious Diseases, National Institutes of Health, under contract No. N01- AI-30054.

REFERENCES

Aarestrup, F. M. (2015). The livestock reservoir for antimicrobial resistance: a personal view on changing patterns of risks, effects of interventions and the way forward. *Philos. Trans. R. Soc. Lond. B Biol. Sci.* 370:20140085. doi: 10.1098/rstb.2014.0085

Achtman, M. (2008). Evolution, population structure, and phylogeography of genetically monomorphic bacterial pathogens. *Annu. Rev. Microbiol.* 62, 53–70. doi: 10.1146/annurev.micro.62.081307.162832

Afema, J. A., Ahmed, S., Besser, T. E., Jones, L. P., Sischo, W. M., and Davis, M. A. (2018). Molecular epidemiology of dairy cattle-associated *Escherichia coli* carrying blaCTX-M genes in Washington State. *Appl. Environ. Microbiol.* 84:e02430-17. doi: 10.1128/AEM.02430-17

Afema, J. A., Mather, A. E., and Sischo, W. M. (2015). Antimicrobial resistance profiles and diversity in *Salmonella* from humans and Cattle, 2004-2011. *Zoonoses Public Health* 62, 506–517. doi: 10.1111/zph.12172

Agren, E. C., Wahlstrom, H., Vesterlund-Carlson, C., Lahti, E., Melin, L., and Soderlund, R. (2016). Comparison of whole genome sequencing typing results and epidemiological contact information from outbreaks of *Salmonella* Dublin in Swedish cattle herds. *Infect. Ecol. Epidemiol.* 6:31782. doi: 10.3402/iee.v6.31782

Alcaine, S. D., Sukhnanand, S. S., Warnick, L. D., Su, W. L., Mcgann, P., Mcdonough, P., et al. (2005). Ceftiofur-resistant *Salmonella* strains isolated from dairy farms represent multiple widely distributed subtypes that evolved by independent horizontal gene transfer. *Antimicrob. Agents Chemother.* 49, 4061–4067. doi: 10.1128/AAC.49.10.4061-4067.2005

An, R., Alshalchi, S., Breimhurst, P., Munoz-Aguayo, J., Flores-Figueroa, C., and Vidovic, S. (2017). Strong influence of livestock environments on the emergence and dissemination of distinct multidrug-resistant phenotypes among the population of non-typhoidal *Salmonella*. *PLoS One* 12:e0179005. doi: 10.1371/journal.pone.0179005

Anderson, M. J. (2001). A new method for non-parametric multivariate analysis of variance. *Austral Ecol.* 26, 32–46. doi: 10.1046/j.1442-9993.2001.01070.x

Anderson, M. J. (2006). Distance-Based tests for homogeneity of multivariate dispersions. *Biometrics* 62, 245–253. doi: 10.1111/j.1541-0420.2005.00440.x

Anderson, M. J., and Walsh, D. C. I. (2013). PERMANOVA, ANOSIM, and the Mantel test in the face of heterogeneous dispersions: what null hypothesis are you testing? *Ecol. Monogr.* 83, 557–574. doi: 10.1890/12-2010.1

Andrews, S. (2019). *FastQC: A Quality Control Tool for High Throughput Sequence Data.* 0.11.8 ed.

Banerji, S., Simon, S., Tille, A., Fruth, A., and Flieger, A. (2020). Genome-based *Salmonella* serotyping as the new gold standard. *Sci. Rep.* 10:4333. doi: 10.1038/s41598-020-67917-3

Bankevich, A., Nurk, S., Antipov, D., Gurevich, A. A., Dvorkin, M., Kulikov, A. S., et al. (2012). SPAdes: a new genome assembly algorithm and its applications to single-cell sequencing. *J. Comput. Biol.* 19, 455–477. doi: 10.1089/cmb.2012.0021

Boerlin, P., Wissing, A., Aarestrup, F. M., Frey, J., and Nicolet, J. (2001). Antimicrobial growth promoter ban and resistance to macrolides and vancomycin in enterococci from pigs. *J. Clin. Microbiol.* 39, 4193–4195. doi: 10.1128/JCM.39.11.4193-4195.2001

Bolger, A. M., Lohse, M., and Usadel, B. (2014). Trimmomatic: a flexible trimmer for Illumina sequence data. *Bioinformatics* 30, 2114–2120. doi: 10.1093/bioinformatics/btu170

Boore, A. L., Hoekstra, R. M., Iwamoto, M., Fields, P. I., Bishop, R. D., and Swerdlow, D. L. (2015). *Salmonella enterica* infections in the united states and assessment of coefficients of variation: a novel approach to identify epidemiologic characteristics of individual serotypes, 1996-2011. *PLoS One* 10:e0145416. doi: 10.1371/journal.pone.0145416

Bouckaert, R., Heled, J., Kuhnert, D., Vaughan, T., Wu, C. H., Xie, D., et al. (2014). BEAST 2: a software platform for Bayesian evolutionary analysis. *PLoS Comput. Biol.* 10:e1003537. doi: 10.1371/journal.pcbi.1003537

Bouckaert, R., Vaughan, T. G., Barido-Sottani, J., Duchene, S., Fourment, M., Gavryushkina, A., et al. (2019). BEAST 2.5: an advanced software platform for Bayesian evolutionary analysis. *PLoS Comput. Biol.* 15:e1006650. doi: 10.1371/journal.pcbi.1006650

Camacho, C., Coulouris, G., Avagyan, V., Ma, N., Papadopoulos, J., Bealer, K., et al. (2009). BLAST+: architecture and applications. *BMC Bioinformatics* 10:421. doi: 10.1186/1471-2105-10-421

Canton, R., Gonzalez-Alba, J. M., and Galán, J. C. (2012). CTX-M enzymes: origin and diffusion. *Front. Microbiol.* 3:110. doi: 10.3389/fmicb.2012.00110

Carattoli, A., Zankari, E., Garcia-Fernandez, A., Voldby Larsen, M., Lund, O., Villa, L., et al. (2014). *In silico* detection and typing of plasmids using PlasmidFinder and plasmid multilocus sequence typing. *Antimicrob. Agents Chemother.* 58, 3895–3903. doi: 10.1128/AAC.02412-14

Carroll, L. M., Gaballa, A., Guldimann, C., Sullivan, G., Henderson, L. O., and Wiedmann, M. (2019). Identification of novel mobilized colistin resistance gene mcr-9 in a multidrug-resistant, colistin-susceptible *Salmonella enterica* serotype Typhimurium isolate. *mBio* 10:e00853-19. doi: 10.1128/mBio.00853-19

Carroll, L. M., Huisman, J. S., and Wiedmann, M. (2020a). Twentieth-century emergence of antimicrobial resistant human- and bovine-associated *Salmonella enterica* serotype Typhimurium lineages in New York State. *Sci. Rep.* 10:14428. doi: 10.1038/s41598-020-71344-9

Carroll, L. M., Wiedmann, M., and Kovac, J. (2020b). Proposal of a taxonomic nomenclature for the *Bacillus cereus* group which reconciles genomic definitions of bacterial species with clinical and industrial phenotypes. *mBio* 11:e00034-20. doi: 10.1101/779199

Carroll, L. M., Kovac, J., Miller, R. A., and Wiedmann, M. (2017a). Rapid, high-throughput identification of anthrax-causing and emetic *Bacillus cereus* group genome assemblies via BTyper, a computational tool for virulence-based classification of *Bacillus cereus* group isolates by using nucleotide sequencing data. *Appl. Environ. Microbiol.* 83:e01096-17. doi: 10.1128/AEM.01096-17

Carroll, L. M., Wiedmann, M., Den Bakker, H., Siler, J., Warchocki, S., Kent, D., et al. (2017b). Whole-Genome sequencing of drug-resistant *Salmonella enterica* isolates from dairy cattle and humans in New York and Washington States reveals source and geographic associations. *Appl. Environ. Microbiol.* 83:e00140-17. doi: 10.1128/AEM.00140-17

Centers for Disease Control and Prevention (2019). *Antibiotic Resistance Threats in the United States, 2019.* Atlanta, GA: U.S. Department of Health and Human Services.

Centers for Disease Control and Prevention (2020). *Serotypes and the Importance of Serotyping Salmonella.* CDC. Available online at: https://www.cdc.gov/salmonella/reportspubs/salmonella-atlas/serotyping-importance.html (accessed May 25, 2021).

Centers for Disease Control and Prevention (2021). *Salmonella.* Available online at: https://www.cdc.gov/salmonella/index.html (accessed September 24, 2021).

Chiu, C. H., Su, L. H., and Chu, C. (2004). *Salmonella enterica* serotype Choleraesuis: epidemiology, pathogenesis, clinical disease, and treatment. *Clin. Microbiol. Rev.* 17, 311–322. doi: 10.1128/CMR.17.2.311-322.2004

Clarke, K. R. (1993). Non-parametric multivariate analyses of changes in community structure. *Aust. J. Ecol.* 18, 117–143. doi: 10.1111/j.1442-9993.1993.tb00438.x

Clarke, L., Pelin, A., Phan, M., and Wong, A. (2020). The effect of environmental heterogeneity on the fitness of antibiotic resistance mutations in *Escherichia coli. Evol. Ecol.* 34, 379–390. doi: 10.1007/s10682-019-10027-y

Clausen, P. T., Zankari, E., Aarestrup, F. M., and Lund, O. (2016). Benchmarking of methods for identification of antimicrobial resistance genes in bacterial whole genome data. *J. Antimicrob. Chemother.* 71, 2484–2488. doi: 10.1093/jac/dkw184

Cooper, A. L., Low, A. J., Koziol, A. G., Thomas, M. C., Leclair, D., Tamber, S., et al. (2020). Systematic evaluation of whole genome sequence-based predictions of *Salmonella* serotype and antimicrobial resistance. *Front. Microbiol.* 11:549. doi: 10.3389/fmicb.2020.00549

Croucher, N. J., Page, A. J., Connor, T. R., Delaney, A. J., Keane, J. A., Bentley, S. D., et al. (2015). Rapid phylogenetic analysis of large samples of recombinant bacterial whole genome sequences using Gubbins. *Nucleic Acids Res.* 43:e15. doi: 10.1093/nar/gku1196

Cummings, K. J., Warnick, L. D., Davis, M. A., Eckmann, K., Grohn, Y. T., Hoelzer, K., et al. (2012). Farm animal contact as risk factor for transmission of bovine-associated *Salmonella* subtypes. *Emerg. Infect. Dis.* 18, 1929–1936. doi: 10.3201/eid1812.110831

Cummings, K. J., Warnick, L. D., Elton, M., Grohn, Y. T., Mcdonough, P. L., and Siler, J. D. (2010a). The effect of clinical outbreaks of salmonellosis on the prevalence of fecal *Salmonella* shedding among dairy cattle in New York. *Foodborne Pathog. Dis.* 7, 815–823. doi: 10.1089/fpd.2009.0481

Cummings, K. J., Warnick, L. D., Elton, M., Rodriguez-Rivera, L. D., Siler, J. D., Wright, E. M., et al. (2010b). *Salmonella enterica* serotype Cerro among dairy cattle in New York: an emerging pathogen? *Foodborne Pathog. Dis.* 7, 659–665. doi: 10.1089/fpd.2009.0462

Davidson, K. E., Byrne, B. A., Pires, A. F. A., Magdesian, K. G., and Pereira, R. V. (2018). Antimicrobial resistance trends in fecal *Salmonella* isolates from northern California dairy cattle admitted to a veterinary teaching hospital, 2002-2016. *PLoS One* 13:e0199928. doi: 10.1371/journal.pone.0199928

Delgado-Suarez, E. J., Selem-Mojica, N., Ortiz-Lopez, R., Gebreyes, W. A., Allard, M. W., Barona-Gomez, F., et al. (2018). Whole genome sequencing reveals widespread distribution of typhoidal toxin genes and VirB/D4 plasmids in bovine-associated nontyphoidal *Salmonella. Sci. Rep.* 8:9864. doi: 10.1038/s41598-018-28169-4

Delsol, A. A., Anjum, M., Woodward, M. J., Sunderland, J., and Roe, J. M. (2003). The effect of chlortetracycline treatment and its subsequent withdrawal on multi-resistant *Salmonella enterica* serovar Typhimurium DT104 and commensal *Escherichia coli* in the pig. *J. Appl. Microbiol.* 95, 1226–1234. doi: 10.1046/j.1365-2672.2003.02088.x

Diep, B., Barretto, C., Portmann, A. C., Fournier, C., Karczmarek, A., Voets, G., et al. (2019). *Salmonella* serotyping; comparison of the traditional method to a microarray-based method and an *in silico* platform using whole genome sequencing data. *Front. Microbiol.* 10:2554. doi: 10.3389/fmicb.2019.02554

Dutil, L., Irwin, R., Finley, R., Ng, L. K., Avery, B., Boerlin, P., et al. (2010). Ceftiofur resistance in *Salmonella enterica* serovar Heidelberg from chicken meat and humans, Canada. *Emerg. Infect. Dis.* 16, 48–54. doi: 10.3201/eid1601.090729

Evans, B. A., and Amyes, S. G. B. (2014). OXA β-Lactamases. *Clin. Microbiol. Rev.* 27, 241–263. doi: 10.1128/CMR.00117-13

Ewels, P., Magnusson, M., Lundin, S., and Kaller, M. (2016). MultiQC: summarize analysis results for multiple tools and samples in a single report. *Bioinformatics* 32, 3047–3048. doi: 10.1093/bioinformatics/btw354

Feldgarden, M., Brover, V., Haft, D. H., Prasad, A. B., Slotta, D. J., Tolstoy, I., et al. (2019). Validating the AMRFinder tool and resistance gene database by using antimicrobial resistance genotype-phenotype correlations in a collection of isolates. *Antimicrob. Agents Chemother.* 63:e00483-19. doi: 10.1128/AAC.00483-19

Fenske, G. J., Thachil, A., Mcdonough, P. L., Glaser, A., and Scaria, J. (2019). Geography shapes the population genomics of *Salmonella enterica* dublin. *Genome Biol. Evol.* 11, 2220–2231. doi: 10.1093/gbe/evz158

Frech, G., Kehrenberg, C., and Schwarz, S. (2003). Resistance phenotypes and genotypes of multiresistant *Salmonella enterica* subsp. enterica serovar Typhimurium var. Copenhagen isolates from animal sources. *J. Antimicrob. Chemother.* 51, 180–182. doi: 10.1093/jac/dkg058

Gardner, S. N., and Hall, B. G. (2013). When whole-genome alignments just won't work: kSNP v2 software for alignment-free SNP discovery and phylogenetics of hundreds of microbial genomes. *PLoS One* 8:e81760. doi: 10.1371/journal.pone.0081760

Gardner, S. N., Slezak, T., and Hall, B. G. (2015). kSNP3.0: SNP detection and phylogenetic analysis of genomes without genome alignment or reference genome. *Bioinformatics* 31, 2877–2878. doi: 10.1093/bioinformatics/btv271

Gorski, L., Parker, C. T., Liang, A., Cooley, M. B., Jay-Russell, M. T., Gordus, A. G., et al. (2011). Prevalence, distribution, and diversity of *Salmonella enterica* in a major produce region of California. *Appl. Environ. Microbiol.* 77, 2734–2748. doi: 10.1128/AEM.02321-10

Gupta, A., Fontana, J., Crowe, C., Bolstorff, B., Stout, A., Duyne, S. V., et al. (2003). Emergence of multidrug-resistant *Salmonella enterica* serotype newport infections resistant to expanded-spectrum Cephalosporins in the United States. *J. Infect. Dis.* 188, 1707–1716. doi: 10.1086/379668

Gupta, S. K., Padmanabhan, B. R., Diene, S. M., Lopez-Rojas, R., Kempf, M., Landraud, L., et al. (2014). ARG-ANNOT, a new bioinformatic tool to discover antibiotic resistance genes in bacterial genomes. *Antimicrob. Agents Chemother.* 58, 212–220. doi: 10.1128/AAC.01310-13

Gurevich, A., Saveliev, V., Vyahhi, N., and Tesler, G. (2013). QUAST: quality assessment tool for genome assemblies. *Bioinformatics* 29, 1072–1075. doi: 10.1093/bioinformatics/btt086

Gutema, F. D., Agga, G. E., Abdi, R. D., De Zutter, L., Duchateau, L., and Gabriel, S. (2019). Prevalence and serotype diversity of *Salmonella* in apparently healthy cattle: systematic review and meta-analysis of published studies, 2000-2017. *Front. Vet. Sci.* 6:102. doi: 10.3389/fvets.2019.00184

Harvey, R. R., Friedman, C. R., Crim, S. M., Judd, M., Barrett, K. A., Tolar, B., et al. (2017). Epidemiology of *Salmonella enterica* serotype Dublin infections among humans, United States, 1968-2013. *Emerg. Infect. Dis.* 23, 1493–1501. doi: 10.3201/eid2309.170136

Hendriksen, R. S., Bortolaia, V., Tate, H., Tyson, G. H., Aarestrup, F. M., and Mcdermott, P. F. (2019). Using genomics to track global antimicrobial resistance. *Front. Public Health* 7:242. doi: 10.3389/fpubh.2019.00242

Hendriksen, R. S., Pedersen, S. K., Leekitcharoenphon, P., Malorny, B., Borowiak, M., Battisti, A., et al. (2018). Final report of ENGAGE – establishing next generation sequencing ability for genomic analysis in Europe. *EFSA Support. Publ.* 15:1431E. doi: 10.2903/sp.efsa.2018.EN-1431

Hoang, D. T., Chernomor, O., Von Haeseler, A., Minh, B. Q., and Vinh, L. S. (2018). UFBoot2: improving the ultrafast bootstrap approximation. *Mol. Biol. Evol.* 35, 518–522. doi: 10.1093/molbev/msx281

Hoelzer, K., Moreno Switt, A. I., and Wiedmann, M. (2011). Animal contact as a source of human non-typhoidal salmonellosis. *Vet. Res.* 42:34. doi: 10.1186/1297-9716-42-34

Hoelzer, K., Wong, N., Thomas, J., Talkington, K., Jungman, E., and Coukell, A. (2017). Antimicrobial drug use in food-producing animals and associated human health risks: what, and how strong, is the evidence? *BMC Vet. Res.* 13:211. doi: 10.1186/s12917-017-1131-3

Holschbach, C. L., and Peek, S. F. (2018). *Salmonella* in dairy cattle. *Vet. Clin. North Am. Food Anim. Pract.* 34, 133–154. doi: 10.1016/j.cvfa.2017.10.005

Hornish, R. E., and Kotarski, S. F. (2002). Cephalosporins in veterinary medicine - ceftiofur use in food animals. *Curr. Top. Med. Chem.* 2, 717–731. doi: 10.2174/1568026023393679

Hunt, M., Mather, A. E., Sanchez-Buso, L., Page, A. J., Parkhill, J., Keane, J. A., et al. (2017). ARIBA: rapid antimicrobial resistance genotyping directly from sequencing reads. *Microb. Genom.* 3:e000131. doi: 10.1099/mgen.0.000131

Ibrahim, G. M., and Morin, P. M. (2018). *Salmonella* serotyping using whole genome sequencing. *Front. Microbiol.* 9:2993. doi: 10.3389/fmicb.2018.02993

Inouye, M., Dashnow, H., Raven, L. A., Schultz, M. B., Pope, B. J., Tomita, T., et al. (2014). SRST2: rapid genomic surveillance for public health and hospital microbiology labs. *Genome Med.* 6:90. doi: 10.1186/s13073-014-0090-6

Issenhuth-Jeanjean, S., Roggentin, P., Mikoleit, M., Guibourdenche, M., De Pinna, E., Nair, S., et al. (2014). Supplement 2008-2010 (no. 48) to the White-Kauffmann-Le Minor scheme. *Res. Microbiol.* 165, 526–530. doi: 10.1016/j.resmic.2014.07.004

Jia, B., Raphenya, A. R., Alcock, B., Waglechner, N., Guo, P., Tsang, K. K., et al. (2017). CARD 2017: expansion and model-centric curation of the comprehensive antibiotic resistance database. *Nucleic Acids Res.* 45, D566–D573. doi: 10.1093/nar/gkw1004

Jorgensen, J. H., and Ferraro, M. J. (2009). Antimicrobial susceptibility testing: a review of general principles and contemporary practices. *Clin. Infect. Dis.* 49, 1749–1755. doi: 10.1086/647952

Karon, A. E., Archer, J. R., Sotir, M. J., Monson, T. A., and Kazmierczak, J. J. (2007). Human multidrug-resistant *Salmonella* Newport infections, Wisconsin, 2003-2005. *Emerg. Infect. Dis.* 13, 1777–1780. doi: 10.3201/eid1311.061138

Kodama, Y., Shumway, M., Leinonen, R., and International Nucleotide Sequence Database Collaboration (2012). The sequence read archive: explosive growth of sequencing data. *Nucleic Acids Res.* 40, D54–D56. doi: 10.1093/nar/gkr854

Kruskal, J. B. (1964). Nonmetric multidimensional scaling: a numerical method. *Psychometrika* 29, 115–129. doi: 10.1007/BF02289694

Kuhn, M. (2008). Building predictive models in R using the caret package. *J. Stat. Softw.* 28, 1–26. doi: 10.18637/jss.v028.i05

Lakin, S. M., Dean, C., Noyes, N. R., Dettenwanger, A., Ross, A. S., Doster, E., et al. (2017). MEGARes: an antimicrobial resistance database for high throughput sequencing. *Nucleic Acids Res.* 45, D574–D580. doi: 10.1093/nar/gkw1009

Leinonen, R., Sugawara, H., Shumway, M., and International Nucleotide Sequence Database Collaboration (2011). The sequence read archive. *Nucleic Acids Res.* 39, D19–D21. doi: 10.1093/nar/gkq1019

Lewis, J. S. II, Herrera, M., Wickes, B., Patterson, J. E., and Jorgensen, J. H. (2007). First report of the emergence of CTX-M-type extended-spectrum beta-lactamases (ESBLs) as the predominant ESBL isolated in a U.S. health care system. *Antimicrob. Agents Chemother.* 51, 4015–4021. doi: 10.1128/AAC.00576-07

Liao, J., Orsi, R. H., Carroll, L. M., and Wiedmann, M. (2020). Comparative genomics reveals different population structures associated with host and geographic origin in antimicrobial-resistant *Salmonella enterica*. *Environ. Microbiol.* 22, 2811–2828. doi: 10.1111/1462-2920.15014

Liao, J., Orsi, R. H., Carroll, L. M., Kovac, J., Ou, H., Zhang, H., et al. (2019). Serotype-specific evolutionary patterns of antimicrobial-resistant *Salmonella enterica*. *BMC Evol. Biol.* 19:132. doi: 10.1186/s12862-019-1457-5

Liebana, E., Carattoli, A., Coque, T. M., Hasman, H., Magiorakos, A. P., Mevius, D., et al. (2013). Public health risks of enterobacterial isolates producing extended-spectrum beta-lactamases or AmpC beta-lactamases in food and food-producing animals: an EU perspective of epidemiology, analytical methods, risk factors, and control options. *Clin. Infect. Dis.* 56, 1030–1037. doi: 10.1093/cid/cis1043

Llarena, A. K., Zhang, J., Vehkala, M., Valimaki, N., Hakkinen, M., Hanninen, M. L., et al. (2016). Monomorphic genotypes within a generalist lineage of *Campylobacter jejuni* show signs of global dispersion. *Microb. Genom.* 2:e000088. doi: 10.1099/mgen.0.000088

Luceron, C. O., Meixeira, A. P., Sanz, I. A., Deleyto, V. C., Leon, S. H., and Ruiz, L. G. (2017). Notes from the field: an outbreak of *Salmonella* Typhimurium associated with playground sand in a preschool setting - Madrid, Spain, September-October 2016. *MMWR Morb. Mortal Wkly. Rep.* 66, 256–257. doi: 10.15585/mmwr.mm6609a3

Mather, A. E., Reid, S. W., Maskell, D. J., Parkhill, J., Fookes, M. C., Harris, S. R., et al. (2013). Distinguishable epidemics of multidrug-resistant *Salmonella* Typhimurium DT104 in different hosts. *Science* 341, 1514–1517. doi: 10.1126/science.1240578

McDermott, P. F., Bodeis, S. M., English, L. L., White, D. G., Walker, R. D., Zhao, S., et al. (2002). Ciprofloxacin resistance in *Campylobacter jejuni* evolves rapidly in chickens treated with fluoroquinolones. *J. Infect. Dis.* 185, 837–840. doi: 10.1086/339195

McDermott, P. F., Tyson, G. H., Kabera, C., Chen, Y., Li, C., Folster, J. P., et al. (2016). Whole-genome sequencing for detecting antimicrobial resistance in nontyphoidal *Salmonella*. *Antimicrob. Agents Chemother.* 60, 5515–5520. doi: 10.1128/AAC.01030-16

Mellor, K. C., Petrovska, L., Thomson, N. R., Harris, K., Reid, S. W. J., and Mather, A. E. (2019). Antimicrobial resistance diversity suggestive of distinct *Salmonella* Typhimurium sources or selective pressures in food-production animals. *Front. Microbiol.* 10:708. doi: 10.3389/fmicb.2019.00708

Melnyk, A. H., Wong, A., and Kassen, R. (2015). The fitness costs of antibiotic resistance mutations. *Evol. Appl.* 8, 273–283. doi: 10.1111/eva.12196

Mentaberre, G., Porrero, M. C., Navarro-Gonzalez, N., Serrano, E., Dominguez, L., and Lavin, S. (2013). Cattle drive *Salmonella* infection in the wildlife-livestock interface. *Zoonoses Public Health* 60, 510–518. doi: 10.1111/zph.12028

Minh, B. Q., Nguyen, M. A., and Von Haeseler, A. (2013). Ultrafast approximation for phylogenetic bootstrap. *Mol. Biol. Evol.* 30, 1188–1195. doi: 10.1093/molbev/mst024

Mohammed, M., Le Hello, S., Leekitcharoenphon, P., and Hendriksen, R. (2017). The invasome of *Salmonella* Dublin as revealed by whole genome sequencing. *BMC Infect. Dis.* 17:544. doi: 10.1186/s12879-017-2628-x

Moller, S., Du Plessis, L., and Stadler, T. (2018). Impact of the tree prior on estimating clock rates during epidemic outbreaks. *Proc. Natl. Acad. Sci. U.S.A.* 115, 4200–4205. doi: 10.1073/pnas.1713314115

Mughini-Gras, L., Enserink, R., Friesema, I., Heck, M., Van Duynhoven, Y., and Van Pelt, W. (2014). Risk factors for human salmonellosis originating from pigs, cattle, broiler chickens and egg laying hens: a combined case-control and source attribution analysis. *PLoS One* 9:e87933. doi: 10.1371/journal.pone.0087933

Nguyen, L. T., Schmidt, H. A., Von Haeseler, A., and Minh, B. Q. (2015). IQ-TREE: a fast and effective stochastic algorithm for estimating maximum-likelihood phylogenies. *Mol. Biol. Evol.* 32, 268–274. doi: 10.1093/molbev/msu300

Nguyen, M., Long, S. W., Mcdermott, P. F., Olsen, R. J., Olson, R., Stevens, R. L., et al. (2019). Using machine learning to predict antimicrobial MICs and associated genomic features for nontyphoidal *Salmonella*. *J. Clin. Microbiol.* 57:e01260-18. doi: 10.1128/JCM.01260-18

Oksanen, J., Blanchet, F. G., Friendly, M., Kindt, R., Legendre, P., Mcglinn, D., et al. (2019). *vegan: Community Ecology Package.* R package version 2.5-6. Available online at: https://CRAN.R-project.org/package=vegan (accessed May 22, 2020).

Page, A. J., Cummins, C. A., Hunt, M., Wong, V. K., Reuter, S., Holden, M. T., et al. (2015). Roary: rapid large-scale prokaryote pan genome analysis. *Bioinformatics* 31, 3691–3693. doi: 10.1093/bioinformatics/btv421

Page, A. J., Taylor, B., Delaney, A. J., Soares, J., Seemann, T., Keane, J. A., et al. (2016). SNP-sites: rapid efficient extraction of SNPs from multi-FASTA alignments. *Microb. Genom.* 2:e000056. doi: 10.1099/mgen.0.000056

Palma, F., Manfreda, G., Silva, M., Parisi, A., Barker, D. O. R., Taboada, E. N., et al. (2018). Genome-wide identification of geographical segregated genetic markers in *Salmonella enterica* serovar Typhimurium variant 4,[5],12:i. *Sci. Rep.* 8:15251. doi: 10.1038/s41598-018-33266-5

Parks, D. H., Imelfort, M., Skennerton, C. T., Hugenholtz, P., and Tyson, G. W. (2015). CheckM: assessing the quality of microbial genomes recovered from isolates, single cells, and metagenomes. *Genome Res.* 25, 1043–1055. doi: 10.1101/gr.186072.114

Pereira, R., Williams, D. R., Rossitto, P., Adaska, J., Okello, E., Champagne, J., et al. (2019). Association between herd management practices and antimicrobial resistance in *Salmonella* spp. from cull dairy cattle in Central California. *PeerJ* 7:e6546. doi: 10.7717/peerj.6546

R Core Team (2019). *R: A Language and Environment for Statistical Computing.* 3.6.1 ed. Vienna: R Foundation for Statistical Computing.

Rambaut, A., Lam, T. T., Max Carvalho, L., and Pybus, O. G. (2016). Exploring the temporal structure of heterochronous sequences using TempEst (formerly Path-O-Gen). *Virus Evol.* 2:vew007. doi: 10.1093/ve/vew007

Rodriguez, A., Pangloli, P., Richards, H. A., Mount, J. R., and Draughon, F. A. (2006). Prevalence of *Salmonella* in diverse environmental farm samples. *J. Food Prot.* 69, 2576–2580. doi: 10.4315/0362-028X-69.11.2576

Rodriguez-Rivera, L. D., Wright, E. M., Siler, J. D., Elton, M., Cummings, K. J., Warnick, L. D., et al. (2014). Subtype analysis of *Salmonella* isolated from subclinically infected dairy cattle and dairy farm environments reveals the presence of both human- and bovine-associated subtypes. *Vet. Microbiol.* 170, 307–316. doi: 10.1016/j.vetmic.2014.02.013

San Millan, A., and MacLean, R. C. (2017). Fitness costs of plasmids: a limit to plasmid transmission. *Microbiol. Spectr.* 5, 1–12. doi: 10.1128/microbiolspec. MTBP-0016-2017

Scott, A. M., Beller, E., Glasziou, P., Clark, J., Ranakusuma, R. W., Byambasuren, O., et al. (2018). Is antimicrobial administration to food animals a direct threat to human health? A rapid systematic review. *Int. J. Antimicrob. Agents* 52, 316–323. doi: 10.1016/j.ijantimicag.2018.04.005

Seemann, T. (2014). Prokka: rapid prokaryotic genome annotation. *Bioinformatics* 30, 2068–2069. doi: 10.1093/bioinformatics/btu153

Seemann, T. (2018). *ABRicate: Mass Screening of Contigs for Antimicrobial Resistance or Virulence Genes.*

Seemann, T. (2019). *Snippy: Rapid Haploid Variant Calling and Core Genome Alignment. 4.3.6 ed.*

Skov, M. N., Madsen, J. J., Rahbek, C., Lodal, J., Jespersen, J. B., Jorgensen, J. C., et al. (2008). Transmission of *Salmonella* between wildlife and meat-production animals in Denmark. *J. Appl. Microbiol.* 105, 1558–1568. doi: 10.1111/j.1365-2672.2008.03914.x

Spika, J. S., Waterman, S. H., Hoo, G. W., St Louis, M. E., Pacer, R. E., James, S. M., et al. (1987). Chloramphenicol-resistant *Salmonella* newport traced through hamburger to dairy farms. A major persisting source of human salmonellosis in California. *N. Engl. J. Med.* 316, 565–570. doi: 10.1056/NEJM198703053161001

Strachan, N. J. C., Rotariu, O., Lopes, B., Macrae, M., Fairley, S., Laing, C., et al. (2015). Whole genome sequencing demonstrates that geographic variation of *Escherichia coli* O157 genotypes dominates host association. *Sci. Rep.* 5:14145. doi: 10.1038/srep14145

Tack, B., Phoba, M. F., Barbe, B., Kalonji, L. M., Hardy, L., Van Puyvelde, S., et al. (2020). Non-typhoidal *Salmonella* bloodstream infections in Kisantu, DR Congo: emergence of O5-negative *Salmonella* Typhimurium and extensive drug resistance. *PLoS Negl. Trop. Dis.* 14:e0008121. doi: 10.1371/journal.pntd. 0008121

Tang, K. L., Caffrey, N. P., Nobrega, D. B., Cork, S. C., Ronksley, P. E., Barkema, H. W., et al. (2017). Restricting the use of antibiotics in food-producing animals and its associations with antibiotic resistance in food-producing animals and human beings: a systematic review and meta-analysis. *Lancet Planet Health* 1, e316–e327. doi: 10.1016/S2542-5196(17)30141-9

Tassinari, E., Duffy, G., Bawn, M., Burgess, C. M., Mccabe, E. M., Lawlor, P. G., et al. (2019). Microevolution of antimicrobial resistance and biofilm formation of *Salmonella* Typhimurium during persistence on pig farms. *Sci. Rep.* 9:8832. doi: 10.1038/s41598-019-45216-w

Taylor, D. N., Bied, J. M., Munro, J. S., and Feldman, R. A. (1982). *Salmonella* Dublin infections in the United States, 1979-1980. *J. Infect. Dis.* 146, 322–327. doi: 10.1093/infdis/146.3.322

The, H. C., Thanh, D. P., Holt, K. E., Thomson, N. R., and Baker, S. (2016). The genomic signatures of *Shigella* evolution, adaptation and geographical spread. *Nat. Rev. Microbiol.* 14, 235–250. doi: 10.1038/nrmicro.2016.10

Toth, J. D., Aceto, H. W., Rankin, S. C., and Dou, Z. (2011). Survival characteristics of *Salmonella enterica* serovar Newport in the dairy farm environment. *J. Dairy Sci.* 94, 5238–5246. doi: 10.3168/jds.2011-4493

Tragesser, L. A., Wittum, T. E., Funk, J. A., Winokur, P. L., and Rajala-Schultz, P. J. (2006). Association between ceftiofur use and isolation of *Escherichia coli* with reduced susceptibility to ceftriaxone from fecal samples of dairy cows. *Am. J. Vet. Res.* 67, 1696–1700. doi: 10.2460/ajvr.67.10.1696

Uelze, L., Borowiak, M., Deneke, C., Szabo, I., Fischer, J., Tausch, S. H., et al. (2020). Performance and accuracy of four open-source tools for *in silico* serotyping of *salmonella* spp. based on whole-genome short-read sequencing data. *Appl. Environ. Microbiol.* 86:e02265-19. doi: 10.1128/AEM.02265-19

Uzzau, S., Brown, D. J., Wallis, T., Rubino, S., Leori, G., Bernard, S., et al. (2000). Host adapted serotypes of *Salmonella enterica*. *Epidemiol. Infect.* 125, 229–255. doi: 10.1017/S0950268899004379

Wang, C., Feng, Y., Liu, L., Wei, L., Kang, M., and Zong, Z. (2020). Identification of novel mobile colistin resistance gene mcr-10. *Emerg. Microbes Infect.* 9, 508–516. doi: 10.1080/22221751.2020.1732231

Wang, X., Wang, Y., Zhou, Y., Li, J., Yin, W., Wang, S., et al. (2018). Emergence of a novel mobile colistin resistance gene, mcr-8, in NDM-producing *Klebsiella pneumoniae*. *Emerg. Microbes Infect.* 7:122. doi: 10.1038/s41426-018-0124-z

Wiethoelter, A. K., Beltran-Alcrudo, D., Kock, R., and Mor, S. M. (2015). Global trends in infectious diseases at the wildlife-livestock interface. *Proc. Natl. Acad. Sci. U.S.A.* 112, 9662–9667. doi: 10.1073/pnas.1422741112

Wong, V. K., Baker, S., Pickard, D. J., Parkhill, J., Page, A. J., Feasey, N. A., et al. (2015). Phylogeographical analysis of the dominant multidrug-resistant H58 clade of *Salmonella* Typhi identifies inter- and intracontinental transmission events. *Nat. Genet.* 47, 632–639. doi: 10.1038/ng.3281

World Health Organization (2014). *Antimicrobial Resistance: Global Report on Surveillance.* Geneva: World Health Organization (WHO).

World Health Organization (2017). *Critically Important Antimicrobials for Human Medicine, 5th Revision.* Geneva: World Health Organization.

Worley, J., Meng, J., Allard, M. W., Brown, E. W., and Timme, R. E. (2018). *Salmonella enterica* phylogeny based on whole-genome sequencing reveals two new clades and novel patterns of horizontally acquired genetic elements. *MBio* 9:e02303-18. doi: 10.1128/mBio.02303-18

Yachison, C. A., Yoshida, C., Robertson, J., Nash, J. H. E., Kruczkiewicz, P., Taboada, E. N., et al. (2017). The validation and implications of using whole genome sequencing as a replacement for traditional serotyping for a national *Salmonella* reference laboratory. *Front. Microbiol.* 8:1044. doi: 10.3389/fmicb. 2017.01044

Yang, W.-C., Chan, O.-W., Wu, T.-L., Chen, C.-L., Su, L.-H., and Chiu, C.-H. (2016). Development of ceftriaxone resistance in *Salmonella enterica* serotype Oranienburg during therapy for bacteremia. *J. Microbiol. Immunol. Infect.* 49, 41–45. doi: 10.1016/j.jmii.2014.01.011

Yoshida, C. E., Kruczkiewicz, P., Laing, C. R., Lingohr, E. J., Gannon, V. P., Nash, J. H., et al. (2016). The *Salmonella in silico* typing resource (SISTR): an open web-accessible tool for rapidly typing and subtyping draft *Salmonella* genome assemblies. *PLoS One* 11:e0147101. doi: 10.1371/journal.pone.0147101

Zankari, E., Hasman, H., Cosentino, S., Vestergaard, M., Rasmussen, S., Lund, O., et al. (2012). Identification of acquired antimicrobial resistance genes. *J. Antimicrob. Chemother.* 67, 2640–2644. doi: 10.1093/jac/ dks261

Zhang, S., Den Bakker, H. C., Li, S., Chen, J., Dinsmore, B. A., Lane, C., et al. (2019). SeqSero2: rapid and improved *Salmonella* serotype determination using whole-genome sequencing data. *Appl. Environ. Microbiol.* 85:e01746-19. doi: 10.1128/AEM.01746-19

Zwe, Y. H., Chin, S. F., Kohli, G. S., Aung, K. T., Yang, L., and Yuk, H.-G. (2020). Whole genome sequencing (WGS) fails to detect antimicrobial resistance (AMR) from heteroresistant subpopulation of *Salmonella enterica*. *Food Microbiol.* 91:103530. doi: 10.1016/j.fm.2020.103530

Permissions

All chapters in this book were first published by Frontiers; hereby published with permission under the Creative Commons Attribution License or equivalent. Every chapter published in this book has been scrutinized by our experts. Their significance has been extensively debated. The topics covered herein carry significant findings which will fuel the growth of the discipline. They may even be implemented as practical applications or may be referred to as a beginning point for another development.

The contributors of this book come from diverse backgrounds, making this book a truly international effort. This book will bring forth new frontiers with its revolutionizing research information and detailed analysis of the nascent developments around the world.

We would like to thank all the contributing authors for lending their expertise to make the book truly unique. They have played a crucial role in the development of this book. Without their invaluable contributions this book wouldn't have been possible. They have made vital efforts to compile up to date information on the varied aspects of this subject to make this book a valuable addition to the collection of many professionals and students.

This book was conceptualized with the vision of imparting up-to-date information and advanced data in this field. To ensure the same, a matchless editorial board was set up. Every individual on the board went through rigorous rounds of assessment to prove their worth. After which they invested a large part of their time researching and compiling the most relevant data for our readers.

The editorial board has been involved in producing this book since its inception. They have spent rigorous hours researching and exploring the diverse topics which have resulted in the successful publishing of this book. They have passed on their knowledge of decades through this book. To expedite this challenging task, the publisher supported the team at every step. A small team of assistant editors was also appointed to further simplify the editing procedure and attain best results for the readers.

Apart from the editorial board, the designing team has also invested a significant amount of their time in understanding the subject and creating the most relevant covers. They scrutinized every image to scout for the most suitable representation of the subject and create an appropriate cover for the book.

The publishing team has been an ardent support to the editorial, designing and production team. Their endless efforts to recruit the best for this project, has resulted in the accomplishment of this book. They are a veteran in the field of academics and their pool of knowledge is as vast as their experience in printing. Their expertise and guidance has proved useful at every step. Their uncompromising quality standards have made this book an exceptional effort. Their encouragement from time to time has been an inspiration for everyone.

The publisher and the editorial board hope that this book will prove to be a valuable piece of knowledge for researchers, students, practitioners and scholars across the globe.

List of Contributors

Hui Deng, Shu-Yi Zeng, Jian Sun, Liang-Xing Fang, Run-Shi Yang and Xiao-Ping Liao
National Risk Assessment Laboratory for Antimicrobial Resistance of Animal Original Bacteria, South China Agricultural University, Guangzhou, China
College of Veterinary Medicine, South China Agricultural University, Guangzhou, China

Hong-Bin Si
College of Animal Science and Technology, Guangxi University, Nanning, China

Ya-Hong Liu
National Risk Assessment Laboratory for Antimicrobial Resistance of Animal Original Bacteria, South China Agricultural University, Guangzhou, China
College of Veterinary Medicine, South China Agricultural University, Guangzhou, China
Jiangsu Co-Innovation Centre for Prevention and Control of Important Animal Infectious Diseases and Zoonoses, Yangzhou, China

Daniela Jones-Dias, Inês B. Moura, Vera Manageiro, Eugénia Ferreira and Manuela Caniça
National Reference Laboratory of Antibiotic Resistances and Healthcare Associated Infections, Department of Infectious Diseases, National Institute of Health Doutor Ricardo Jorge, Lisbon, Portugal
Centre for the Studies of Animal Science, Institute of Agrarian and Agri-Food Sciences and Technologies, Oporto University, Oporto, Portugal

Lurdes Clemente and Teresa Albuquerque
Microbiology and Mycology Laboratory, Instituto Nacional de Investigação Agrária e Veterinária, Lisbon, Portugal

Daniel A. Sampaio and Luís Vieira
Innovation and Technology Unit, Human Genetics Department, National Institute of Health Doutor Ricardo Jorge, Lisbon, Portugal

Manuela Caniça
National Reference Laboratory of Antibiotic Resistances and Healthcare Associated Infections, Department of Infectious Diseases, National Institute of Health Doutor Ricardo Jorge, Lisbon, Portugal

Hui Huang, Li Yuan, Yushan Pan, Caihui Ma and Gongzheng Hu
College of Veterinary Medicine, Henan Agricultural University, Zhengzhou, China

Yawei Sun
College of Veterinary Medicine, Henan Agricultural University, Zhengzhou, China
College of Animal Science and Technology, Henan Institute of Science and Technology, Xinxiang, China

Yanlin Gao
Animal Husbandry Bureau of Henan Province, Zhengzhou, China

Haihong Hao and Zonghui Yuan
China MOA Laboratory for Risk Assessment of Quality and Safety of Livestock and Poultry Products, Huazhong Agricultural University, Wuhan, China
National Reference Laboratory of Veterinary Drug Residues (HZAU) and MOA Key Laboratory for the Detection of Veterinary Drug Residues in Foods, Huazhong Agricultural University, Wuhan, China

Pascal Sander
Laboratory of Fougères, French Agency for Food, Environmental and Occupational Safety, Fougères Cedex, France

Zahid Iqbal, Guyue Cheng
China MOA Laboratory for Risk Assessment of Quality and Safety of Livestock and Poultry Products, Huazhong Agricultural University, Wuhan, China

Yulian Wang
National Reference Laboratory of Veterinary Drug Residues (HZAU) and MOA Key Laboratory for the Detection of Veterinary Drug Residues in Foods, Huazhong Agricultural University, Wuhan, China

Ijaz Ahmad
National Reference Laboratory of Veterinary Drug Residues and MAO Key Laboratory for Drug Residues Detection, Huazhong Agriculture University, Wuhan, China

Haihong Hao, Xu Wang, Kuang Xiuhua, Juan Li and Wan Dan
MOA Laboratory for Risk Assessment of Safety and Quality of Livestock and Poultry Products, Huazhong Agriculture University, Wuhan, China

Lingli Huang and Shuyu Xie
MOA Laboratory for Risk Assessment of Safety and Quality of Livestock and Poultry Products, Huazhong Agriculture University, Wuhan, China
Hubei Collaborative Innovation Centre for feed Safety and Animal Nutrition, Huazhong Agricultural University, Wuhan, China

Dongmei Chen and Yanfei Tao
National Reference Laboratory of Veterinary Drug Residues and MAO Key Laboratory for Drug Residues Detection, Huazhong Agriculture University, Wuhan, China
Hubei Collaborative Innovation Centre for feed Safety and Animal Nutrition, Huazhong Agricultural University, Wuhan, China

Pascal Sanders
Laboratory of Fougères, French Agency for Food, Environmental and Occupational Safety, Maisons-Alfort, France

Zonghui Yuan
National Reference Laboratory of Veterinary Drug Residues and MAO Key Laboratory for Drug Residues Detection, Huazhong Agriculture University, Wuhan, China
MOA Laboratory for Risk Assessment of Safety and Quality of Livestock and Poultry Products, Huazhong Agriculture University, Wuhan, China
Hubei Collaborative Innovation Centre for feed Safety and Animal Nutrition, Huazhong Agricultural University, Wuhan, China

Wilbert Sybesma, Ulrich Mehnert and Thomas M. Kessler
Neuro-Urology, Spinal Cord Injury Center and Research, University of Zürich, Balgrist University Hospital, Zürich, Switzerland

Reinhard Zbinden
Institute of Medical Microbiology, University of Zürich, Zürich, Switzerland

Nino Chanishvili and Mzia Kutateladze
The Eliava Institute of Bacteriophage, Microbiology, and Virology, Tbilisi, Georgia

Archil Chkhotua and Aleksandre Ujmajuridze
Tsulukidze National Center of Urology, Tbilisi, Georgia

Ximin Zeng, Barbara Gillespie and Jun Lin
Department of Animal Science, The University of Tennessee, Knoxville, TN, USA

Rafael Graça
National Reference Laboratory of Antibiotic Resistances and Healthcare Associated Infections, Department of Infectious Diseases, National Institute of Health Dr. Ricardo Jorge, Lisbon, Portugal

Teresa Albuquerque, Patrícia Themudo and Lurdes Clemente
Instituto Nacional de Investigação Agrária e Veterinária, Lisboa, Portugal

Christian Penny and Henry-Michel Cauchie
Environmental Research and Innovation Department, Luxembourg Institute of Science and Technology, Esch-sur-Alzette, Luxembourg

Beau Grothendick, Lin Zhang, Connie M. Borror, Duane Barbano and Todd R. Sandrin
School of Mathematical and Natural Sciences, Arizona State University, Phoenix, AZ, USA

Angela J. Cornelius and Brent J. Gilpin
Institute of Environmental Science and Research, Christchurch, New Zealand

Clifton K. Fagerquist and William J. Zaragoza
Agricultural Research Service, United States Department of Agriculture, Albany, CA, USA

Michele T. Jay-Russell
Western Center for Food Safety, University of California at Davis, Davis, CA, USA

Albert J. Lastovica
Department of Biotechnology, University of the Western Cape, Bellville, South Africa

Catherine Ragimbeau
Epidemiological Surveillance of Infectious Diseases, Laboratoire National de Santé, Dudelange, Luxembourg

Puyuan Li, Wenkai Niu, Leijing Guo, Xin Yuan, Huiying Liu and Changqing Bai
Department of Respiratory and Critical Care Diseases, 307th Hospital of Chinese People's Liberation Army, Beijing, China

Huan Li, Wei Liu, Xiangna Zhao, Dayang Zou and Jing Yuan
Institute of Disease Control and Prevention, Academy of Military Medical Sciences, Beijing, China

Hong Lei
Department of Clinical Laboratory 309th Hospital of Chinese People's Liberation Army, Beijing, China

Bingjun Dang
School of Environmental Science and Engineering, Tianjin University, Tianjin, China
Ministry of Education Key Laboratory of Pollution Processes and Environmental Criteria, College of Environmental Science and Engineering, Nankai University, Tianjin, China

Daqing Mao
School of Environmental Science and Engineering, Tianjin University, Tianjin, China

Yi Luo
Ministry of Education Key Laboratory of Pollution Processes and Environmental Criteria, College of Environmental Science and Engineering, Nankai University, Tianjin, China

Maria Bartolomeu, Sónia Rocha, Ângela Cunha and Adelaide Almeida
Departamento de Biologia and Centro de Estudos do Ambiente e do Mar, University of Aveiro, Aveiro, Portugal

M. G. P. M. S. Neves and Maria A. F. Faustino
Departamento de Química and Unidade de Investigação em Química Orgânica, Produtos Naturais e Agroalimentares, University of Aveiro, Aveiro, Portugal

Daniela Jones-Dias and Vera Manageiro
National Reference Laboratory of Antibiotic Resistances and Healthcare Associated Infections, Department of Infectious Diseases, National Health Institute Doutor Ricardo Jorge (INSA), Lisbon, Portugal
Centre for the Studies of Animal Science, Institute of Agrarian and Agri-Food Sciences and Technologies, University of Porto, Porto, Portugal

Conceição Egas and Hugo Froufe
Biocant, Parque Tecnológico de Cantanhede, Cantanhede, Portugal

Daniel A. Sampaio and Luís Vieira
Innovation and Technology Unit, Human Genetics Department, National Health Institute Doutor Ricardo Jorge (INSA), Lisbon, Portugal

Maria Fookes and Nicholas R. Thomson
Wellcome Trust Sanger Institute, Wellcome Trust Genome Campus, Hinxton, UK

Manuela Caniça
National Reference Laboratory of Antibiotic Resistances and Healthcare Associated Infections, Department of Infectious Diseases, National Health Institute Doutor Ricardo Jorge (INSA), Lisbon, Portugal

Yingchao Li
College of Mechanical Engineering and Applied Electronics Technology, Beijing University of Technology, Beijing, China

Hussain H. Al-Mahamedh
Saudi Basic Industries Corporation, Jubail, Saudi Arabia

Dake Xu
Institute of Metal Research, Chinese Academy of Sciences, Shenyang, China

Ru Jia and Tingyue Gu
Department of Chemical and Biomolecular Engineering, Institute for Corrosion and Multiphase Technology, Ohio University, Athens, OH, USA

Venkateswara Reddy Gogulamudi
Department of Parasitology, Postgraduate Institute of Medical Education and Research, Chandigarh, India
Department of Physiology, Tulane University School of Medicine, New Orleans, LA, USA

Mohan Lal Dubey and Rakesh Sehgal
Department of Parasitology, Postgraduate Institute of Medical Education and Research, Chandigarh, India

Deepak Kaul
Department of Experimental Medicine and Biotechnology, Postgraduate Institute of Medical Education and Research, Chandigarh, India

Venkata Subba Rao Atluri
Department of Immunology, Herbert Wertheim College of Medicine, Florida International University, Miami, FL, USA

Alexandra S. Simões and Isabel Couto and Miguel Viveiros
Global Health and Tropical Medicine, Instituto de Higiene e Medicina Tropical, Universidade Nova de Lisboa, Lisbon, Portugal

Cristina Toscano and Elsa Gonçalves
Laboratório de Microbiologia Clínica e Biologia Molecular, Serviço de Patologia Clínica, Hospital de Egas Moniz, Centro Hospitalar de Lisboa Ocidental, Lisbon, Portugal
Centro de Estudos de Doenças Crónicas, NOVA Medical School/Faculdade de Ciências Médicas, Universidade Nova de Lisboa, Lisbon, Portugal

Pedro Póvoa
Centro de Estudos de Doenças Crónicas, NOVA Medical School/Faculdade de Ciências Médicas, Universidade Nova de Lisboa, Lisbon, Portugal
Unidade de Cuidados Intensivos Polivalente, Hospital de São Francisco Xavier, Centro Hospitalar de Lisboa Ocidental, Lisbon, Portugal

Luís V. Lapão
Global Health and Tropical Medicine, Instituto de Higiene e Medicina Tropical, Universidade Nova de Lisboa, Lisbon, Portugal
WHO Collaborating Center for Health Workforce Policy and Planning, Instituto de Higiene e Medicina Tropical, Universidade Nova de Lisboa, Lisbon, Portugal

Amandine Laffite, Naresh Devarajan and Vera I. Slaveykova
Faculty of Science, Earth and Environmental Science Section, F.-A. Forel Institute and Institute of Environmental Sciences, University of Geneva, Geneva, Switzerland

Pitchouna I. Kilunga and Crispin K. Mulaji
Department of Chemistry, Faculty of Science, University of Kinshasa, Kinshasa, Democratic Republic of the Congo

John M. Kayembe
Département de Géographie-Science de l'Environnement, Faculté des Sciences, Université Pédagogique Nationale, Kinshasa, Democratic Republic of the Congo

Gregory Giuliani
Faculty of Science, Earth and Environmental Science Section, F.-A.Forel Institute and Institute of Environmental Sciences, University of Geneva, Geneva, Switzerland
enviroSPACE Lab., Institute for Environmental Sciences, University of Geneva, Geneva, Switzerland
United Nations Environment Programme, Division of Early Warning and Assessment, Global Resource Information Database - Geneva, International Environment House, Geneva, Switzerland

John Poté
Faculty of Science, Earth and Environmental Science Section, F.-A. Forel Institute and Institute of Environmental Sciences, University of Geneva, Geneva, Switzerland
Department of Chemistry, Faculty of Science, University of Kinshasa, Kinshasa, Democratic Republic of the Congo
Département de Géographie-Science de l'Environnement, Faculté des Sciences, Université Pédagogique Nationale, Kinshasa, Democratic Republic of the Congo

Haihong Hao, Yulian Wang and Zonghui Yuan
National Reference Laboratory of Veterinary Drug Residues and MAO Key Laboratory for Detection of Veterinary Drug Residues, Huazhong Agricultural University, Wuhan, China
MOA Laboratory for Risk Assessment of Quality and Safety of Livestock and Poultry Products, Huazhong Agricultural University, Wuhan, China

Shengxi Zhou, Guyue Cheng and Menghong Dai
MOA Laboratory for Risk Assessment of Quality and Safety of Livestock and Poultry Products, Huazhong Agricultural University, Wuhan, China

Xu Wang and Zhenli Liu
National Reference Laboratory of Veterinary Drug Residues and MAO Key Laboratory for Detection of Veterinary Drug Residues, Huazhong Agricultural University, Wuhan, China

Shantelle Claassen-Weitz and Michelle R. Ngwarai
Division of Medical Microbiology, Department of Pathology, Faculty of Health Sciences, University of Cape Town, Cape Town, South Africa

Adebayo O. Shittu
Department of Microbiology, Obafemi Awolowo University, Ile-Ife, Nigeria

Lehana Thabane
Department of Clinical Epidemiology and Biostatistics, McMaster University, Hamilton, ON, Canada

Mark P. Nicol
Division of Medical Microbiology, Department of Pathology, Faculty of Health Sciences, University of Cape Town, Cape Town, South Africa
Institute of Infectious Disease and Molecular Medicine, Faculty of Health Sciences, University of Cape Town, Cape Town, South Africa
National Health Laboratory Service of South, Groote Schuur Hospital, Cape Town, South Africa

Mamadou Kaba
Division of Medical Microbiology, Department of Pathology, Faculty of Health Sciences, University of Cape Town, Cape Town, South Africa
Institute of Infectious Disease and Molecular Medicine, Faculty of Health Sciences, University of Cape Town, Cape Town, South Africa

Xiaotian Dai, Wei Xiong, Guangming Luo, Haijing Wang and Xiangdong Zhou
Department of Pulmonology, Southwest Hospital, Third Military Medical University, Chongqing, China,

Dongsheng Zhou and Jiao Feng
State Key Laboratory of Pathogen and Biosecurity, Beijing Institute of Microbiology and Epidemiology, Beijing, China

Wenbo Luo
State Key Laboratory of Pathogen and Biosecurity, Beijing Institute of Microbiology and Epidemiology, Beijing, China

Department of Pharmacy, Southwest Hospital, Third Military Medical University, Chongqing, China

Fengjun Sun
Department of Pharmacy, Southwest Hospital, Third Military Medical University, Chongqing, China

Laura M. Carroll, Ariel J. Buehler, Ahmed Gaballa, Rachel A. Cheng and Martin Wiedmann
Department of Food Science, Cornell University, Ithaca, NY, United States

Julie D. Siler and Kevin J. Cummings
Department of Population Medicine and Diagnostic Sciences, Cornell University, Ithaca, NY, United States

Index

P

R

S

T

U

V

W

www.ingramcontent.com/pod-product-compliance
Lightning Source LLC
LaVergne TN
LVHW061513220926
848485LV00018B/1028
* 9 7 8 1 6 3 9 2 7 8 8 3 1 *